Psychiatry in Long-Term Care

Psychiatry in Long-Term Care

Second Edition

Edited by
William E. Reichman
Paul R. Katz

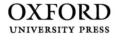

2009

OXFORD
UNIVERSITY PRESS

Oxford University Press, Inc., publishes works that further
Oxford University's objective of excellence
in research, scholarship, and education.

Oxford New York
Auckland Cape Town Dar es Salaam Hong Kong Karachi
Kuala Lumpur Madrid Melbourne Mexico City Nairobi
New Delhi Shanghai Taipei Toronto

With offices in
Argentina Austria Brazil Chile Czech Republic France Greece
Guatemala Hungary Italy Japan Poland Portugal Singapore
South Korea Switzerland Thailand Turkey Ukraine Vietnam

Published by Oxford University Press, Inc.
198 Madison Avenue, New York, New York 10016
www.oup.com

Oxford is a registered trademark of Oxford University Press

Library of Congress Cataloging-in-Publication Data

Psychiatry in long-term care/edited by William E. Reichman,
Paul R. Katz — 2nd ed.
p. ; cm.
Rev. ed. of: Psychiatric care in the nursing home/edited by William E. Reichman,
Paul R. Katz. 1996.
Includes bibliographical references and index.
ISBN 978-0-19-516094-9
1. Nursing home patients—Mental health. 2. Geriatric psychiatry.
I. Reichman, William E. II. Katz, Paul R. (Paul Richard)
III. Psychiatric care in the nursing home.
[DNLM: 1. Mental Disorders. 2. Aged. 3. Assisted Living Facilities.
4. Homes for the Aged. 5. Long-Term Care. 6. Nursing Homes. WT 150 P9673 2009]
RC451.4.N87P78 2009
362.2'3—dc22
2008028747

Originally published as *Psychiatric Care in the Nursing Home*

Printed in the United States of America
on acid-free paper

Preface

Remarkably, it has been 12 years since the publication of *Psychiatric Care in the Nursing Home*, one of the first volumes of its kind. Although the landscape in long-term care has changed over this time, the challenges inherent in the provision of high-quality psychiatric care across what is now a long-term care continuum remain. The literature on this topic has continued to evolve in parallel with new scientific insights, the convening of interdisciplinary professional consensus conferences, and societal demographic trends that put into stark reality the importance of how best to provide physical and mental health care to a rapidly aging population.

The title of this new edition, *Psychiatry in Long-Term Care,* reflects the growing importance of assisted and supportive living environments as alternatives to nursing homes with their own set of unique challenges. Nearly 3 million Americans are cared for in this continuum and as the "baby boomer" population ages, this number is expected to grow dramatically over the next 30 years. Compared with a decade earlier, nursing home residents today are more physically and mentally frail, the majority suffering significant functional disability in the context of multiple medical comorbidities. By all available estimates, the aging baby boom generation expects that the residential health-care system and society as a whole will be able to offer more satisfaction and well-being in their experience of aging than that made available to their grandparents and parents.

The multidisciplinary group of contributors to this second edition have again been chosen based on their hands-on experience and recognized expertise in their respective fields. Our overarching goal for this volume was to provide a practical, evidence-based approach to the most common psychiatric problems encountered in both nursing home and assisted living environments with recommendations based on the most recent review of the academic literature and professional consensus guidelines.

All of the chapters on nursing home care have been extensively updated and where information in the literature exists, references are made to the assisted living setting. As before, we have attempted, whenever appropriate, to structure each chapter to cover a broad range of issues in epidemiology, pathophysiology, differential diagnosis, and contemporary approaches to pharmacological and nonpharmacological treatments. Further, several chapters focus on important "systems issues" in long-term care recognizing that what occurs at the bedside is increasingly affected by regulatory, workforce, and socioeconomic factors.

Admittedly, there is still much about psychiatric practice in the long-term care setting that lacks an adequate evidence base. In these circumstances, treatment approaches are extrapolated from data gathered in other settings and from the authors' clinical experience. While acknowledging the many questions that remain unanswered, we are hopeful that *Psychiatry in Long-Term Care* will provide some much needed building blocks while highlighting the urgent need for more research, education, and policy planning for care delivery in this setting.

We wish to use the publication of this book to acknowledge the commitment of our colleagues across the professional health-care disciplines who dedicate their professional lives to improve the well-being of older persons in the long-term care setting. Those of us in the field know how intellectually and personally rewarding work in this milieu can be. We also wish to thank our many generous collaborators over the years, several of whom have been great mentors to both of us. We are very grateful to our developmental editor, Mark O'Malley, at Oxford University Press for bringing this project to fruition. Last, and most vitally, we dedicate this book to our patients and their families for it is they who have taught us the most about dedication, courage, and strength in the face of great adversity.

William E. Reichman
Toronto, Canada

Paul R. Katz
Rochester, New York

Contents

Part III   Societal Influences

Contributors

Marc E. Agronin, MD
Associate Professor, Department of
  Psychiatry,
University of Miami,
Miller School of Medicine;
Director of Mental Health Services,
Miami Jewish Home & Hospital
  for the Aged,
Miami, FL

Ashok J. Bharucha, MD
Assistant Professor of Psychiatry,
  Psychiatry Department,
University of Pittsburgh School of
  Medicine,
Pittsburgh, PA

Soo Borson, MD
Professor, Department of Psychiatry and
  Behavioral Sciences,
University of Washington;
Director of Geropsychiatry Services,
Psychiatry and Behavioral Sciences,
University of Washington Medical Center,
Seattle, WA

Lisa L. Boyle, MD
Senior Instructor of Psychiatry,
Department of Psychiatry,
University of Rochester Medical
  Center,
Rochester, NY

**Jiska Cohen-Mansfield, PhD,
ABPP**
Professor and Chair,
Health Promotion Department,
Tel-Aviv University,
Tel-Aviv, Israel;
Professor,
Health Care Sciences
  Department,
George Washington University,
Washington, DC
Director, Research Institute
  on Aging, CESLC,
Rockville, MD

David K. Conn, MB, BCh, BAO, FRCPC
Associate Professor, Department of
 Psychiatry,
University of Toronto
Vice President, Medical Services and
 Academic Education,
Baycrest Center for Geriatric Care,
Toronto, Canada

Jeffrey L. Cummings, MD
Augustus Rose Professor of Neurology
 and Director,
Mary S. Easton Center for Alzheimer's
 Disease Research,
David Geffen School of Medicine,
University of California,
Los Angeles, CA

Hannah Day, MS
Doctoral Student,
Department of Epidemiology and
 Preventive Medicine,
University of Maryland,
Baltimore, MD

Jody DelaPena-Murphy, MBA
Community Relations Director,
Stein Institute for Research on Aging,
University of California,
San Diego, CA

Yohannes W. Endeshaw, MD, MPH
Assistant Professor, Diplomate,
American Academy of Sleep Medicine,
Department of Medicine,
Emory University School of Medicine,
Atlanta, GA

Suzanne M. Gillespie, MD
Assistant Professor,
Medicine Division of Geriatrics/Aging,
University of Rochester School of
 Medicine & Dentistry,
Rochester, NY

Ann L. Gruber-Baldini, PhD
Associate Professor,
Department of Epidemiology and
 Preventive Medicine,
University of Maryland,
Baltimore, MD

Solasinee Hemrungrojn, MD
Clinical Instructor,
Department of Psychiatry,
Faculty of Medicine,
Chulalongkorn University;
Professor, Department of Neurology,
David Geffen School of Medicine of
 UCLA,
Los Angeles, CA;
Faculty, Psychiatrist,
Department of Psychiatry,
King Chulallongkorn
 Memorial Hospital,
Bangkok, Thailand

C. Michael Henderson, MD
Associate Professor,
Division of Geriatrics,
Department of Medicine,
University of Rochester School of
 Medicine and Dentistry,
Rochester, NY

Gregory A. Hinrichsen, PhD
Associate Clinical Professor of Psychiatry
 and Behavioral Sciences,
Albert Einstein College of Medicine;
Voluntary Staff,
Department of Psychiatry,
The Zucker Hillside Hospital,
North Shore-Long Island Jewish Health
 System,
New York, NY

Timothy Howell, MD, MA
Associate Professor,
Department of Psychiatry,
University of Wisconsin,
School of Medicine and Public Health;
Director, Geriatric Psychiatry Fellowship
 Program,
University of Wisconsin Hospital and
 Clinics and Madison VA Hospital,
Madison, WI

Steven F. Huege, MD
Assistant Professor of Clinical Psychiatry,
Section of Geriatric Psychiatry,
University of Pennsylvania School of
 Medicine,
Philadelphia, PA

Lee Hyer, PhD, ABPP
Professor of Psychiatry and Health
  Behavior,
Department of Psychiatry and
  Health Behavior,
Mercer School of Medicine,
Georgia Neurological Institute,
Macon, GA

Dilip V. Jeste, MD
Estelle and Edgar Levi Chair in Aging,
Director, Sam and Rose Stein Institute
  for Research on Aging;
Distinguished Professor of Psychiatry
  and Neurosciences,
University of California, San Diego,
VA San Diego Healthcare System,
San Diego, CA

Marshall B. Kapp, JD, MPH
Garwin Distinguished Professor
  of Law and Medicine,
School of Law,
Southern Illinois University,
Carbondale, IL

Jurgis Karuza, PhD
Visiting Professor of Medicine,
Division of Geriatrics/Aging,
University of Rochester School of
  Medicine & Dentistry,
Rochester, NY

Paul R. Katz, MD
Professor of Medicine, Chief,
Division of Geriatrics/Aging,
University of Rochester School
  of Medicine & Dentistry,
Rochester, NY

Daniel S. Kim, MD
Assistant Clinical Professor,
Department of Psychiatry,
University of California,
San Diego, CA

Rene P. Laje, PhD
Research Associate,
Research Institute on Aging,
CESLC,
Rockville, MD

Adrian Leibovici, MD
Clinical Associate Professor of
  Psychiatry,
Department of Psychiatry,
University of Rochester;
Chief of Psychiatry,
Department of Psychiatry,
Highland Hospital University
  of Rochester Medical Center,
Rochester, NY

Jay Magaziner, PhD, MSHyg
Professor and Chair,
Department of Epidemiology
  and Preventive Medicine,
University of Maryland,
Baltimore, MD

Patricia Marino, PhD
Instructor of Psychology,
Department of Psychiatry,
Weill Medical College,
Cornell University,
White Plains, NY

Gary S. Moak, MD
Clinical Associate Professor of
  Psychiatry,
University of Massachusetts
  Medical School,
Worcester, MA;
Director, Moak Center for
  Health Aging,
Westborough, MA

Anton P. Porsteinsson, MD
Associate Professor of
  Psychiatry,
Department of Psychiatry,
University of Rochester
  School of Medicine
  and Dentistry;
Director, Alzheimer's
  Disease Care,
Research and Education
  Program,
University of Rochester
  School of Medicine
  and Dentistry,
Rochester, NY

William E. Reichman, MD
Professor of Psychiatry,
Faculty of Medicine,
University of Toronto;
President and Chief Executive Officer,
Baycrest,
Toronto, Canada

Joy Richards, RN, PhD
Lecturer, Faculty of Nursing,
University of Toronto;
Adjunct Faculty, Health Sciences,
Herber College,
University of New Brunswick;
Adjunct Professor School of Nursing,
York University,
Toronto, Canada

Adam Rosenblatt, MD
Associate Professor,
Department of Psychiatry,
Johns Hopkins School of Medicine;
Director of Neuropsychiatry,
Department of Psychiatry,
Johns Hopkins Hospital,
Baltimore, MD

Amanda Sacks, PhD
Staff Psychologist,
Department of Psychology,
Rusk Institute,
New York University,
New York, NY

Quincy M. Samus, PhD, MS
Instructor, Department of Psychiatry
    and Behavioral Sciences,
The Johns Hopkins University,
Baltimore, MD

Gauri N. Savla, MA, MS
Graduate Student,
Joint Doctoral Program in Clinical
    Psychology,
San Diego State University/University
    of California,
San Diego, CA;
Clinical Psychology Fellow,
Department of Psychiatry,
University of California,
San Francisco,
San Francisco and San Diego, CA

Kenneth Schwartz, MD, FRCP(C)
Assistant Professor,
Department of Psychiatry,
University of Toronto;
Staff Psychiatrist,
Baycrest Geriatric Health Care System,
Toronto, Canada

Daniel D. Sewell, MD
Clinical Professor,
Department of Psychiatry,
University of California,
San Diego, CA

Shailaja Shah, MD
Clinical Assistant Professor,
Department of Geriatric Psychiatry,
UMDNJ-Robert Wood Johnson Medical
    School,
Piscataway, NJ

Joel E. Streim, MD
Professor of Psychiatry,
Geniatric Psychiatry Section,
University of Pennsylvania School of
    Medicine;
Director, Geniatric Psychiatry Program,
Department of Behavioral Health,
Veterans Integrated Services Network 4,
Mental Illness Research, Education,
    and Clinical Center, Philadelphia
    Veterans Affairs Medical Center,
Philadelphia, PA

**Peggy A. Szwabo, PhD, APN, RN,
CC-S, MSW**
Associate Clinical Professor,
Neurology and Psychiatry,
Geriatric Psychiatry Division
    and Internal Medicine,
Division of Geriatric Medicine,
Saint Louis University,
School of Medicine,
St. Louis, MO

Pierre N. Tariot, MD
Research Professor,
Department of Psychiatry,
University of Arizona,
College of Medicine;
Director, Memory Disorders Center,
Banner Alzheimer's Institute,
Phoenix, AZ

Art Walaszek, MD
Assistant Professor,
Department of Psychiatry,
University of Wisconsin School of
  Medicine and Public Health,
Madison, WI

Richard A. Zweig, PhD
Associate Professor of Psychology and
  Director,
Ferkauf Older Adult Program,
Ferkauf Graduate School of Psychology,
Albert Einstein College of Medicine,
Yeshiva University,
New York, NY

PART I

PSYCHIATRIC DISORDERS

1

Epidemiology of Psychiatric Conditions in Nursing Homes

Ann L. Gruber-Baldini, Hannah Day, and *Jay Magaziner*

With the increasing age of the U.S. population, especially among those aged 85 and above, there will be greater numbers of older persons with psychiatric conditions and persons requiring long-term care in the future (American Geriatrics Society & American Association for Geriatric Psychiatry, 2003a, 2003b; Decker, 2005; U.S. Department of Health and Human Services under the direction of the Substance Abuse and Mental Health Services Administration et al., 2001). It is estimated that 4% to 5% of persons 65 years and older reside in a nursing home (Sirrocco, 1994; U.S. Bureau of the Census, 1993a) and that as many as 50% of older adults will enter a nursing home at some point in their lives (Cohen et al., 1986; Murtaugh et al., 1990). Also, the increasing prevalence of Alzheimer's Disease and Related Dementia (ADRD) with older age (Gallo & Lebowitz, 1999; Graham et al., 1997) will lead to more persons with ADRD and related behavioral symptoms in both community and long-term-care settings. In general, the prevalence of ADRD, depression, and other psychiatric conditions are higher in nursing home residents than in community-dwelling elderly; this may be due to the increased need for care among persons with psychiatric conditions, especially ADRD (Hybels & Blazer, 2003). Concomitant medical illnesses are also frequent among those requiring nursing home care, and these comorbid illnesses are associated with higher rates of psychiatric conditions (Evans et al., 2005). For example, high rates of depression are common among patients hospitalized

3

with hip fracture (Lyons et al., 1989; Mossey et al., 1990; Nightingale et al., 2001; Zimmerman et al., 1999), stroke (Aben et al., 2003; Ostir et al., 2002), or myocardial infarction (Aben et al., 2003), all of which are frequent causes of nursing home admission (Wells et al., 2003). Prevalence of depression is also higher among persons with ADRD (Evans et al., 2005), which is another typical reason for nursing home admission (Welch et al., 1992).

OVERVIEW OF CHANGES IN NURSING HOMES SINCE 1995

In the decade since the previous edition of this book, nursing homes have changed dramatically. From 1977 to 1999, data from the National Nursing Home Study (Decker, 2005) report that the number of residents in nursing homes increased by 27%. Residents are being cared for in larger nursing homes (the number of beds per facility has increased by 32% and the number of facilities with less than 50 beds has decreased by almost 75%); the average age of residents in nursing homes has also increased, as has the amount of functional limitations and disability among residents (Sahyoun et al., 2001).

Accompanying these changes in nursing home structure and resident composition, large policy and other industry changes have occurred and have probably affected changes in the number and characteristics of nursing home residents in the past 10 years. Medicare instituted the nursing home prospective payment system (NH PPS) in 1999, as part of the Balanced Budget Refinement Acts of 1997 and 1999 (Centers for Medicare and Medicaid Services). This shift to prospective payment has resulted in nursing homes becoming sites that provide services that emphasize greater rehabilitation and treatment for those with more medical illnesses since the reimbursement rates for these resource utilization groups are higher (Centers for Medicare and Medicaid Services). Prior to the implementation of NH PPS, the Omnibus Budget Reconciliation Act of 1987 (OBRA-87) instituted the Minimum Data Set (MDS) assessment (done at admission and at least quarterly during nursing home stay) as part of a standard data collection form to support care planning activities (Hawes et al., 1997). The MDS is now used as part of the NH PPS and provides a standard assessment of the prevalence of some mental health conditions. Preadmission screening for appropriate placement of psychiatric patients and the Olmstead decision in 1999 mandating community care alternatives for the severely mentally ill have also impacted the case-mix of psychiatric cases in the nursing home setting (Bartels et al., 2003; Borson et al., 1997).

The rapid growth of assisted living as an alternate care setting for persons requiring help with activities of daily living (ADL) has also affected the case-mix of nursing homes. It is believed that the availability of these alternate care settings may have removed many of the persons with mild-to-moderate dementia without complicating medical illnesses, who might have previously been treated in the nursing home. The emergence of assisted living facilities may be one of the reasons that the percent of nursing home residents requiring assistance with ADL, such as dressing and bathing, has increased in the nursing home setting from 1977 to 1999 (Decker, 2005; Sahyoun et al., 2001). There are also indications of an increase in cognitive and mental disorders (excluding schizophrenia) in nursing homes during this same time period (Mechanic & McAlpine, 2000; Sahyoun et al., 2001). It is important to point out that many residents initially admitted to assisted living are eventually admitted to a nursing home (Phillips et al., 2003; Rosenberg et al., 2006; Zimmerman et al., 2005), again suggesting that the most severely impaired physically and mentally will wind up living the remainder of their lives in nursing homes.

Finally, there have been changes in the treatment of psychiatric conditions in nursing home settings. The implementation of OBRA-87 was following by a decrease in the use of typical antipsychotics to treat behavioral symptoms in the nursing home setting (Borson & Doane, 1997; Cohen-Mansfield et al., 1996) and also required better documentation for the prescribing of these medications. In addition, the availability of atypical antipsychotics has increased (Jeste et al., 2005; Schneider et al., 2006), treatments for depression have expanded to include selective serotonin reuptake inhibitors (SSRIs) (Brown et al., 2002; Lapane & Hughes, 2004), and there was the emergence of cholinesterase inhibitors and memantine to help slow the progression of ADRD (Forchetti, 2005; Tariot et al., 2004). In addition, there is now a growing awareness of the potential of environmental modifications and behavioral approaches to treatment of psychiatric conditions (Cohen-Mansfield & Mintzer, 2005; Landreville et al., 2006; Lantz et al., 1996). OBRA-87 was also responsible for regulating the use of physical restraints (Castle, 2006). Many of these changes and approaches will be discussed in subsequent chapters, but it is important to keep them in mind when considering all of the psychiatric conditions seen in the nursing home setting.

MEASUREMENT ISSUES

In addition to changes in the nursing home setting, there are important measurement issues to consider when assessing the prevalence and incidence of psychiatric conditions in nursing homes. In the late 1980s and early 1990s, a fairly substantial amount of research summarized the high prevalence of dementia, depression, and other psychiatric conditions in the nursing home (as summarized in the previous edition (Kim & Rovner, 1996) and other reviews (Kim & Rovner, 1995; Streim et al., 1997). Many of these studies identified methodological issues that arise from relying on documented chart diagnoses. In general, the research showed that more detailed assessment by psychiatrists results in a larger prevalence than relying on chart diagnosis (Rovner et al., 1990). Alternate approaches, such as the use of screening tools and panel adjudication of data, result in prevalence rates that typically fall between chart diagnoses and detailed clinical workups (Magaziner et al., 2000). In addition, the use of current nursing home residents versus assessment of residents at admission results in very different estimates of prevalence, depending on how likely it is for residents with conditions to have longer stays (especially the case for ADRD; Garrard et al., 1993; Magaziner et al., 2000) and whether new conditions develop or resolve over the course of stay (e.g., adjustment stress; German et al., 1992; Keister, 2006). There has been little data across all of these conditions on the incidence of new psychiatric conditions in nursing homes.

Since the implementation of the MDS system, many prevalence reports have relied on either the recorded diagnoses or the associated scales derived from the MDS to identify and characterize residents with psychiatric conditions and as screening tools to identify residents for treatment. A large body of literature on the validity of the MDS has appeared since 1994. In general, diagnoses on the MDS appear to be similar to those captured in the chart (Gruber-Baldini et al., 1999). The validity of psychiatric-related scales has ranged from good for the cognitive items to fair or poor for the depression scales, with behavioral symptoms measures falling in between (Gruber-Baldini et al., 2000; Horgas & Margrett, 2001; Lawton et al., 1998). However, not all of these findings have been consistent, especially those regarding the validity of the MDS to assess depression (see some positive depression scale reviews such as Schnelle et al., 2001; Simmons et al., 2004). Since the MDS is a mandated instrument collected on all residents, the advantages of these large available samples need to be weighed against the potential misclassification (typically undercounting) from data provided.

NATIONAL ESTIMATES OF PSYCHIATRIC CONDITIONS FROM MDS DATA

MDS data from December 2005 suggest that 46.5% of nursing home residents have dementia, 46.8% have depression, 30.0% display behavioral symptoms, 2.8% have mental retardation, and 20.1% have another psychiatric diagnosis (such as schizophrenia or anxiety disorder; American Health Care Association, 2005). Overall, the prevalence of dementia and depression reported by the MDS has increased in recent years (Mechanic & McAlpine, 2000; Sahyoun et al., 2001) and is higher than the chart reports cited in the previous edition of this book (Kim & Rovner, 1996). This increase might be due to either the changes in case-mix and nursing home structures discussed previously or better recognition and documentation of these conditions in the nursing home chart. In any case, as detailed below, these numbers still remain underestimates of the true burden of psychiatric conditions in nursing homes.

ALZHEIMER'S DISEASE AND RELATED DEMENTIAS, COGNITIVE IMPAIRMENT, AND DELIRIUM

In the previous edition of this book, Kim and Rovner (1996) reported a prevalence of ADRD at admission of 67%, with Alzheimer's disease in over half of these cases (38% of the entire sample) and multi-infarct dementia in 17.8% of the overall sample. These data relied on extensive psychiatric assessment of 454 new admissions to eight nursing homes in the Baltimore area. Since that study was completed, a larger study of 2285 new admissions to 59 Maryland nursing homes utilized an expert panel of geriatric psychiatrists, neurologists, and a geriatrician to determine the prevalence of dementia on admission and found a rate of 48.2% of entering residents with ADRD at admission, which was higher than the 35% diagnosed with dementia by either chart or recorded on the MDS (Magaziner et al., 2000). These two studies represent the most intensive adjudication of dementia in nursing homes at admission, and their prevalence estimates (48%–67%) are higher than reported in other studies that relied on medical chart diagnoses, which found that 25% to 40% of new admission had ADRD (Engle & Graney, 1993; Garrard et al., 1993). All of these studies included cohorts enrolled prior to 1995. Few studies have examined the prevalence of dementia of all current residents with such detail, and most were done prior to 1990, with the exception of two smaller studies from the early 1990s that found prevalences of 46% to 68% (Class et al., 1996; Tariot et al., 1993). The most recent (and largest) study of current nursing home residents with ADRD was reported as part of the Canadian Study of Health and Aging; that study reported an overall ADRD prevalence of 57% (37% Alzheimer's and 12% vascular dementia) in a clinical examination of 1255 nursing home residents (Canadian Study of Health and Aging Working Group, 1994; Graham et al., 1997). Since the most recent MDS of 2005 identified 46.5% as having dementia, and it is well known that the MDS and charts underestimate the prevalence of dementia, it is therefore reasonable to postulate that well over half of all current nursing home residents have some form of ADRD.

In addition to frank dementia, there is a growing interest in broader definitions of cognitive impairment, and in the predementia state of "mild cognitive impairment." One study of cognitive impairment without dementia that included nursing home residents reported that around 19.3% of the sample had cognitive impairment and 69.2% had dementia, such that only 11.5% of the sample of 104 nursing home residents could be considered cognitively "normal" (Unverzagt et al., 2001). Studies using the MDS cognition scales have found that between 56% and 64% of residents have some cognitive impairment and 21% to 38% have severe impairment at nursing home admission (Gruber-Baldini et al., 2000). Overall, studies in cross-sectional samples report that 71% to 75% have some cognitive impairment and that 40% to 57% are severely cognitive impaired (Hartmaier et al., 1994; Mor et al., 1997). These percentages included residents with dementia, but again, the data substantiate that the nursing home is a setting in which cognitive impairment affects the majority of the residents.

Finally, there has been increasing attention given to the prevalence and outcomes related to delirium in the nursing home setting. Streim et al. (1997) summarized the literature in the early 1990s and reported a point prevalence of 6% to 7%, although they acknowledged that this was an underestimate. More recent work by Kiely et al. (2003) examined large samples of residents on admission to nursing homes for postacute care and found a prevalence of delirium of 16%, with an additional 13% of admissions having two or more delirium symptoms (subclinical delirium). This group also found that subjects with delirium and high delirium symptoms were less likely to recover functional ability (Marcantonio et al., 2005).

DEPRESSION

Similar to ADRD, the prevalence of depression in nursing homes varies quite widely, depending on the method of ascertainment and time frame of study. Estimates of the prevalence of clinical depression among elderly nursing home residents range from 9% to 30% (Gruber-Baldini et al., 2005; Parmelee et al., 1989; Payne et al., 2002; Rovner, 1993), with rates of high depressive symptomatology ranging from 25% to up to 66% (Gruber-Baldini et al., 2005; McCurren et al., 1999; Ryden et al., 1999). Reports from the 1996 Medical Expenditure Panel Survey–Nursing Home Component (MEPS-NHC) used diagnoses derived from the MDS and found an overall prevalence of 20.3% (Jones et al., 2003), which is much less than the 46.8% with depression reported using national MDS data in 2005 (American Health Care Association, 2005), but higher than the 11% identified by the MDS in the early 1990s (Brown et al., 2002). Studies using more intense depression assessments in the early 1990s found prevalences of 5% to 31% for major depression and 35% to 42% for depressive symptoms (Teresi et al., 2001). However, it is widely acknowledged that these estimates were low. Teresi et al. (2001) found prevalence rates of 14.4% for major depression, 16.8% for minor depression, and 44.2% for significant depressive symptomatology (including minor and major depression) when psychiatrists assessed residents directly. This same study found that staff recognition of depression was low, such that only 37% to 45% of cases diagnosed by psychiatrists were recognized as depressed by staff.

One of the few studies that investigated the incidence of depression in nursing homes was limited to 201 residents of a single Maryland nursing home, which is targeted for those with memory and dementia impairments (Payne et al., 2002). At admission, they found 19.9% of the residents had depression, with only 15% remaining depressed through 6 months and 7.5% at 12 months. Incidence of new depression was low, with 1.8% at 6 months and 6.4% at 12 months, resulting in a cumulative prevalence of depression of 26.4% over the year. These results mirror some of the earlier reports on transition stress that appeared in the nursing home literature in the 1980s (German et al., 1992; Keister, 2006). Thus, while the prevalence of ADRD increases with nursing home length of stay, rates of depression may actually decrease over time, due to either spontaneous recovery, attrition, or the effect of treatment.

Many studies have determined that depression is underdetected (Bagley, 2000; Gruber-Baldini et al., 2005; Rovner et al., 1991; Ryden et al., 1999) and undertreated in nursing homes (Brown et al., 2002; Webber et al., 2005), especially among residents with dementia (Brown et al., 2002). Depression has been the target of a number of initiatives for improvement in the nursing home setting, and these initiatives could eventually affect the rates of recognition and treatment in nursing homes. Michigan's Quality Improvement Organization reported on a quality-improvement project in 14 nursing homes and found that 26% of newly admitted nursing home residents had symptoms of depression at admission, with an additional 12% recognized within 2 weeks of admission (Boyle et al., 2004). Treatment rates were high, with 79% to 81% of those identified receiving treatment in the initial 2 weeks of their stay (Boyle et al., 2004).

ANXIETY

Despite the substantial prevalence of anxiety disorders among the elderly as a whole, it has been given very little attention in the nursing home literature (Hybels & Blazer, 2003). Rates of anxiety in community-dwelling elderly have been estimated at 11.4% (Gallo & Lebowitz, 1999; U.S. Department of Health and Human Services under the direction of the Substance Abuse and Mental Health Services Administration et al., 2001). We could find articles from only two groups that studied anxiety in nursing homes, and these studied a limited number of nursing homes in the Netherlands (Smalbrugge et al., 2005) and in Australia (Cheok et al., 1996). These studies found a prevalence of 5.7% to 11.0% for generalized anxiety, 4.2% for subthreshold anxiety disorders, and 29.7% for anxiety symptoms. Anxiety was associated with depression and also with medical conditions, such as stroke.

SCHIZOPHRENIA AND OTHER MENTAL PROBLEMS

MDS data from 2005 suggest a relatively low prevalence of other mental disorders in the nursing home setting (20.1% in aggregate, but low for specific disorders; American Health Care Association, 2005). The prevalence of schizophrenia in nursing homes was observed to decline over time. In the 1985 National Nursing Home Survey, 9.8% had schizophrenia and in the 1987 Medical Expenditure

Survey, 9.2% had schizophrenia; these percentages decreased to 7.1% in 1995 and 5.9% in 1996 (respective studies; Mechanic & McAlpine, 2000). Rates declined most in those under age 65, perhaps because of the attention given from the preadmission screening mandated under OBRA-87.

BEHAVIORAL SYMPTOMS

In addition to categorized psychiatric conditions, behavioral symptoms associated with dementia and other conditions are a frequent mental health concern in nursing homes. Behavioral symptoms have become recognized as not only "problems" for nursing home staff but also potential manifestations of other conditions or states within the resident, such as pain, infection, depression, medication side effects, environmental stressors, and issues related to caregiving (American Geriatrics Society & American Association for Geriatric Psychiatry, 2003a, 2003b). Studies of behavioral symptoms among elderly people in nursing homes have typically categorized them into three types: aggressive (e.g., cursing, grabbing, kicking, and pushing), physically nonaggressive (e.g., pacing, wandering, and general restlessness), and verbal (constant request for attention, verbal bossiness, and complaining; Cohen-Mansfield & Billig, 1986; Cohen-Mansfield et al., 1989). Behavioral symptoms are a common stressor in nursing homes, leading to staff burnout and turnover (Maslach & Jackson, 1981).

The prevalence of behavioral symptoms can be estimated by three general methods: staff or family caregiver ratings, chart review, or direct observation. Prevalence estimates vary based on the method of detection and on the definition. Larger estimates are reported for the presence of any behavioral symptom, while smaller estimates are generated when examining a single behavior or a combination of several behaviors or when frequency or severity criteria are applied. The most recent reports from the 1995 MEPS suggest that 30% of nursing home residents exhibited some form of behavioral symptoms (wandering, disruptive, or physically aggressive) within the prior 2 weeks (Krauss & Altman, 1998; Rhoades & Krauss, 1999). Other nursing home studies from the 1980s, which vary in ascertainment of behavioral symptoms, reported cross-sectional prevalences of behavioral symptoms ranging from 24% to 93% (Cohen-Mansfield et al., 1989; Jackson et al., 1997; Rovner et al., 1990; U.S. Department of Health and Human Services, 1989; Zimmer et al., 1984). These percentages are highest among residents with dementia, with reports of around 66% in dementia subsamples in the nursing home (Boustani et al., 2005). The prevalence of behavioral symptoms, the high burden that they present to nursing home staff and the potential for misuse of physical and chemical restraints to treat them, has resulted in them perhaps being given the most attention for treatment and regulation within the nursing home setting.

CONCLUSIONS

Given the high rates of ADRD, depression, behavioral problems, and other psychiatric conditions, many have argued that nursing homes are de facto psychiatric hospitals (Kim & Rovner, 1996). While that point can be debated, the nursing home certainly remains a site of care for a large number of people with psychiatric needs. It is important to consider that in addition to being a care environment, for many residents it is also their final living environment (residence). There is clearly a need for psychiatrists and allied mental health professionals to improve the quality of psychiatric care in this environment. In the past 10 years, the prevalence of dementia, behavioral problems, and perhaps depressive symptoms has increased in the nursing home setting; these increases have been accompanied by changes in the structure of the nursing home, resident case-mix, and policy changes. However, the growth of treatments (both pharmaceutical and behavioral) for psychiatric conditions and nursing home care initiatives might allow for better care provision in the future. The importance of this issue was highlighted in a 2003 consensus statement from the American Geriatrics Society and the American Association for Geriatric Psychiatry, which presented recommendations for management of depression and behavioral symptoms in nursing homes, as well as recommendations for related policies (American Geriatrics Society & American Association for Geriatric Psychiatry, 2003a, 2003b). Given the changes in nursing home case-mix reviewed earlier, it is likely that not only will a greater proportion of residents in nursing homes have psychiatric conditions but also the residents being treated in these facilities will be more medically complex.

Acknowledgments   The authors would like to thank Yvonne Aro for her help with formatting this chapter. Some of the research reported in this chapter was supported by grants from the National Institute on Aging (R01 AG8211; R29 AG11407).

REFERENCES

Aben, I., Verhey, F., Strik, J., et al. (2003). A comparative study into the one year cumulative incidence of depression after stroke and myocardial infarction. *Journal of Neurology, Neurosurgery, and Psychiatry, 74*, 581–585.

American Geriatrics Society & American Association for Geriatric Psychiatry. (2003a). The American Geriatrics Society and American Association for Geriatric Psychiatry recommendations for policies in support of quality mental health care in U.S. nursing homes. *Journal of the American Geriatrics Society, 51*(9), 1299–1304.

American Geriatrics Society & American Association for Geriatric Psychiatry. (2003b). Consensus statement on improving the quality of mental health care in U.S.

nursing homes: Management of depression and behavioral symptoms associated with dementia. *Journal of the American Geriatrics Society, 51,* 1287–1298.

American Health Care Association. (2005, December). *Medical condition—mental status—CMS OSCAR data current surveys.* Retrieved October 18, 2006, from http://ahca.org/research/oscar/rpt_MC_mental_status_200512.pdf

Bagley, H., Cordingley, L., Burns, A., et al. (2000). Recognition of depression in staff in nursing and residential homes. *Journal of Clinical Nursing, 9*(3), 445–450.

Bartels, S. J., Miles, K. M., Dums, A. R., & Levine, K. J. (2003). Are nursing homes appropriate for older adults with severe mental illness? Conflicting consumer and clinician views and implications for the Olmstead decision. *Journal of the American Geriatrics Society, 51*(11), 1571–1579.

Borson, S., & Doane, K. (1997). The impact of OBRA-87 on psychotropic drug prescribing in skilled nursing facilities. *Psychopharmacology Series, 48*(10), 1289–1296.

Borson, S., Loebel, J. P., Kitchell, M., et al. (1997). Psychiatric assessments of nursing home residents under OBRA-87: Should PASARR be reformed? *Journal of the American Geriatrics Society, 45*(10), 1173–1181.

Boustani, M., Zimmerman, S., Williams, C. S., et al. (2005). Characteristics associated with behavioral symptoms related to dementia in long-term care residents. *Gerontologist, 45*(1), 56–61.

Boyle, V. L., Roychoudhury, C., Beniak, R., et al. (2004). Recognition and management of depression in skilled-nursing and long-term care settings: Evolving targets for quality improvement. *American Journal of Geriatric Psychiatry, 12*(3), 288–295.

Brown, M. N., Lapane, K. L., & Luisi, A. F. (2002). The management of depression in older nursing home residents. *Journal of the American Geriatrics Society, 50*(1), 69–76.

Canadian Study of Health and Aging Working Group. (1994). Canadian Study of Health and Aging: Study methods and prevalence of dementia. *Canadian Medical Association Journal, 150*(6), 899–913.

Castle, N. G. (2006). Mental health outcomes and physical restraint use in nursing homes. *Administration and Policy in Mental Health, 33*(6), 686–704.

Centers for Medicare and Medicaid Services. Retrieved May 15, 2006, from http://www.cms.hhs.gov/SNFPPS/09_RUGRefinement.asp

Cheok, A., Snowdon, J., Miller, R., & Vaughan, R. (1996). The prevalence of anxiety disorders in nursing homes. *International Journal of Geriatric Psychiatry, 11,* 405–410.

Class, C. A., Unverzagt, F. W., Gao, S., et al. (1996). Psychiatric disorders in African American nursing home residents. *American Journal of Psychiatry, 153*(5), 677–681.

Cohen, M. A., Tell, E. J., & Wallack, S. S. (1986). The lifetime risks and costs of nursing home use among the elderly. *Medical Care, 24*(12), 1161–1172.

Cohen-Mansfield, J., & Billig, N. (1986). Agitated behaviors in the elderly: A conceptual review. *Journal of the American Geriatrics Society, 34*(10), 711–721.

Cohen-Mansfield, J., Lipson, S., Gruber-Baldini, A. L., et al. (1996). Longitudinal prescribing patterns of psychotropic drugs in nursing home residents. *Experimental and Clinical Psychopharmacology, 4*(2), 224–233.

Cohen-Mansfield, J., Marx, M. S., & Rosenthal, A. S. (1989). A description of agitation in a nursing home. *Journal of Gerontology, 44*(3), M77–M84.

Cohen-Mansfield, J., & Mintzer, J. E. (2005). Time for change: The role of nonpharmacological interventions in treating behavior problems in nursing home residents with dementia. *Alzheimer Disease and Associated Disorders, 19*(1), 37–40.

Decker, F. H. (2005). *Nursing homes (1977–1999): What has changed, what has not?* Hyattsville, MD: National Center for Health Statistics.

Engle, V. F., & Graney, M. J. (1993). Stability and improvement of health after nursing home admission. *Journal of Gerontology: Social Sciences, 48*(1), S17–S23.

Evans, D. L., Charney, D. S., Lewis, L., et al. (2005). Mood disorders in the medically ill: Scientific review and recommendations. *Biological Psychiatry, 58*(3), 175–189.

Forchetti, C. M. (2005). Treating patients with moderate to severe Alzheimer's disease: Implications of recent pharmacologic studies. *Primary Care Companion to the Journal of Clinical Psychiatry, 7*(4), 155–161.

Gallo, J. J., & Lebowitz, B. D. (1999) The epidemiology of common late-life mental disorders in the community: Themes for the new century. *Psychiatry Service, 50*(9), 1158–1166.

Garrard, J., Buchanan, J. L., Ratner, E. R., et al. (1993). Differences between nursing home admissions and residents. *Journal of Gerontology: Social Sciences, 48*(6), S301–S309.

German, P. S., Rovner, B. W., Burton, L., et al. (1992). The role of mental morbidity in the nursing home experience. *The Gerontologist, 32*(2), 152–158.

Graham, J. E., Rockwood, K., Beattie, B. L., et al. (1997). Prevalence and severity of cognitive impairment with and without dementia in an elderly population. *Lancet, 349*(9068), 1793–1796.

Gruber-Baldini, A. L., Magaziner, J., Zimmerman, S. I., et al. (1999). MDS assessment of dementia compared to an expert panel [abstract]. *The Gerontologist, 39* (special issue 1), 88.

Gruber-Baldini, A. L., Zimmerman, S., Boustani, M., et al. (2005). Characteristics associated with depression in long-term care residents with dementia. *The Gerontologist, 45*(1), 50–55.

Gruber-Baldini, A. L., Zimmerman, S. I., Mortimore, E., & Magaziner, J. (2000). The validity of the Minimum Data Set in measuring the cognitive impairment of persons admitted to nursing homes. *Journal of the American Geriatrics Society, 48*(12), 1601–1606.

Hartmaier, S., Sloane, P. D., Guess, H., & Koch, G. (1994). The MDS Cognition Scale: A valid instrument for identifying and staging nursing home residents with dementia using the Minimum Data Set. *Journal of the American Geriatrics Society, 42*, 1173–1179.

Hawes, C., Mor, V., Phillips, C. D., et al. (1997). The OBRA-87 nursing home regulations and implementation of the Resident Assessment Instrument: Effects on process quality. *Journal of the American Geriatrics Society, 45*(8), 977–985.

Horgas, A. L., & Margrett, J. A. (2001). Measuring behavioral and mood disruptions in nursing home residents using the Minimum Data Set. *Outcomes Management for Nursing Practice, 5*(1), 28–35.

Hybels, C. F., & Blazer, D. G. (2003). Epidemiology of late-life mental disorders. *Clinics in Geriatric Medicine, 19*(4), 663–696.

Jackson, M. E., Spector, W. D., & Rabins, P. V. (1997). Risk of behavior problems among nursing home residents in the United States. *Journal of Aging and Health, 9*(4), 451–472.

Jeste, D. V., Dolder, C. R., Nayak, G. V., & Salzman, C. (2005). Atypical antipsychotics in elderly patients with dementia or schizophrenia: Review of recent literature. *Harvard Review of Psychiatry, 13*(6), 340–351.

Jones, R. N., Marcantonio, E. R., & Rabinowitz, T. (2003). Prevalence and correlates of recognized depression in U.S. Nursing Homes. *Journal of the American Geriatrics Society, 51*(10), 1404–1409.

Keister, K. J. (2006). Predictors of self-assessed health, anxiety, and depressive symptoms in nursing home residents at week 1 postrelocation. *Journal of Aging and Health, 18*(5), 722–742.

Kiely, D. K., Bergmann, M. A., Murphy, K. M., et al. (2003). Delirium among newly admitted postacute facility patients: Prevalence, symptoms, and severity. *Journals of Gerontology Series A: Biological Sciences and Medical Sciences, 58*(5), M441–M445.

Kim, E., & Rovner, B. (1995). Epidemiology of psychiatric disturbances in nursing homes. *Psychiatric Annals, 25*(7), 409–412.

Kim, E., & Rovner, B. W. (1996). *The nursing home as a psychiatric hospital. Psychiatric care in the nursing home.* New York: Oxford University Press, 1996.

Krauss, N. A., & Altman, B. M. (1998). *Characteristics of nursing home residents— 1996.* Rockville, MD: Agency for Health Care Policy and Research.

Landreville, P., Bedard, A., Verreault, R., et al. (2006). Non-pharmacological interventions for aggressive behavior in older adults living in long-term care facilities. *International Psychogeriatrics, 18*(1), 47–73.

Lantz, M. S., Giambanco, V., & Buchalter, E. N. (1996). A ten-year review of the effect of OBRA-87 on psychotropic prescribing practices in an academic nursing home. *Psychiatric Services, 47*(9), 951–955.

Lapane, K. L., & Hughes, C. M. (2004). An evaluation of the impact of the prospective payment system on antidepressant use in nursing home residents. *Medical Care, 42*(1), 48–58.

Lawton, M. P., Casten, R., Parmelee, P. A., et al. (1998). Psychometric characteristics of the minimum data set II: Validity. *Journal of the American Geriatrics Society, 46*(6), 736–744.

Lyons, J. S., Strain, J. J., Hammer, J. S., et al. (1989). Reliability, validity and temporal stability of the Geriatric Depression Scale in hospitalized elderly. *International Journal of Psychiatry in Medicine, 19*(2), 203–209.

Magaziner, J., German, P., Zimmerman, S. I., et al. (2000). The prevalence of dementia in a statewide sample of new nursing home admissions aged 65 and older: Diagnosis by expert panel. *Gerontologist, 40*(6), 663–672.

Marcantonio, E. R., Kiely, D. K., Simon, S. E., et al. (2005). Outcomes of older people admitted to postacute facilities with delirium. *Journal of the American Geriatrics Society, 53*(6), 963–969.

Maslach, C., & Jackson, S. E. (1981). The measurement of experienced burnout. *Journal of Occupational Behavior* 2(3), 99–113.

McCurren, C., Dowe, D., Rattle, D., & Looney, S. (1999). Depression among nursing home elders: Testing an intervention strategy. *Applied Nursing Research, 12*(4), 185–195.

Mechanic, D., & McAlpine, D. D. (2000). Use of nursing homes in the care of persons with severe mental illness: 1985 to 1995. *Psychiatric Services, 51*(3), 354–458.

Mor, V., Intrator, O., Fries, B. E., et al. (1997). Changes in hospitalization associated with introducing the Resident Assessment Instrument. *Journal of the American Geriatrics Society, 45*(8):1002–1010.

Mossey, J. M., Knott, K., & Craik, R. (1990). The effects of persistent depressive symptoms on hip fracture recovery. *Journal of Gerontology, 45*(5), M163–M168.

Murtaugh, C., Kemper, P., & Spillman, B. (1990). The risk of nursing home use in later life. *Medical Care, 28*(10), 952–962.

Nightingale, S., Holmes, J., Mason, J., & House, A. (2001). Psychiatric illness and mortality after hip fracture. *Lancet, 357*, 1264–1265.

Ostir, G. V., Goodwin, J. S., Markides, K. S., et al. (2002). Differential effects of premorbid physical and emotional health on recovery from acute events. *Journal of the American Geriatrics Society, 50*, 713–718.

Parmelee, P. A., Katz, I. R., & Lawton, M. P. (1989). Depression among institutionalized aged: Assessment and prevalence estimation. *Journal of Gerontology, 44*(1), M22–M29.

Payne, J. L., Sheppard, J. M., Steinberg, M., et al. (2002). Incidence, prevalence, and outcomes of depression in residents of a long-term care facility with dementia. *International Journal of Geriatric Psychiatry, 17*(3), 247–253.

Phillips, C. D., Munoz, Y., Sherman, M., et al. (2003). Effects of facility characteristics on departures from assisted living: Results from a national study. *Gerontologist, 43*(5), 690–696.

Rhoades, J., & Krauss, N. (1999). *Nursing home trends, 1987 and 1996*. Rockville, MD: Agency for Health Care Policy and Research.

Rosenberg, P. B., Mielke, M. M., Samus, Q. M., et al. (2006). Transition to nursing home from assisted living is not associated with dementia or dementia-related problem behaviors. *Journal of the American Medical Directors Association, 7*(2), 73–78.

Rovner, B. W. (1993). Depression and increased risk of mortality in the nursing home patient. *American Journal of Medicine, 94*(5A), 19S–22S.

Rovner, B. W., German, P. S., Brant, L. J., et al. (1991). Depression and mortality in nursing homes. *JAMA, 265*(8), 993–996.

Rovner, B. W., German, P. S., Broadhead, J., et al. (1990). The prevalence and management of dementia and other psychiatric disorders in nursing homes. *International Psychogeriatrics, 2*(1), 13–24.

Ryden, M. B., Pearson, V., Kaas, M. J., et al. (1999). Nursing interventions for depression in newly admitted nursing home residents. *Journal of Gerontological Nursing, 25*(3), 20–29.

Sahyoun, N. R., Pratt, L. A., Lentzner, H., et al. (2001). *The changing profile of nursing home residents: 1985–1997. Aging trends; No. 4*. Hyattsville, MD: National Center for Health Statistics.

Schneider, L. S., Tariot, P. N., Dagerman, K. S., et al. (2006). Effectiveness of atypical antipsychotic drugs in patients with Alzheimer's disease. *New England Journal of Medicine, 355*(15), 1525–1538.

Schnelle, J. F., Wood, S., Schnelle, E. R., & Simmons, S. F. (2001). Measurement sensitivity and the Minimum Data Set depression quality indicator. *The Gerontologist, 41*(3), 401–405.

Simmons, S. F., Cadogan, M. P., Cabrera, G. R., et al. (2004). The minimum data set depression quality indicator: Does it reflect differences in care processes? *The Gerontologist, 44*(4), 554–564.

Sirrocco, A. (1994). *Nursing homes and board and care homes. Advance data from Vital and Health Statistics*. Hyattsville, MD: National Center for Health Statistics.

Smalbrugge, M., Pot, A. M., Jongenelis, K., et al. (2005). Prevalence and correlates of anxiety among nursing home patients. *Journal of Affective Disorders, 88*(2), 145–153.

Streim, J. E., Oslin, D., Katz, I. R., & Parmelee, P. A. (1997). Lessons from geriatric psychiatry in the long-term care setting. *Psychiatric Quarterly, 68*(3), 281–307.

Tariot, P. N., Farlwo, M. R., Grossberg, G. T., et al. (2004). Memantine treatment in patients with moderate to severe Alzheimer disease already receiving donepezil: A randomized controlled trial. *JAMA, 291*(3), 317–324.

Tariot, P. N., Podgorski, C. A., Blazina, L., & Leibovici, A. (1993). Mental disorders in the nursing home: Another perspective. *American Journal of Psychiatry, 150*(7), 1063–1069.

Teresi, J., Abrams, R., Holmes, D., et al. (2001). Prevalence of depression and depression recognition in nursing homes. *Social Psychiatry and Psychiatric Epidemiology, 36*(12), 613–620.

Unverzagt, F. W., Gao, S., Baiyewu, O., et al. (2001). Prevalence of cognitive impairment: Data from the Indianapolis study of health and aging. *Neurology, 57*(9), 1655–1662.

U.S. Bureau of the Census. (1993a). *Nursing home population: 1990.* Washington, DC: U.S. Government Printing Office.

U.S. Department of Health and Human Services. (1989). *Nursing home utilization by current residents: United States, 1985.* Hyattsville, MD: National Center for Health Statistics.

U.S. Department of Health and Human Services under the direction of the Substance Abuse and Mental Health Services Administration, Center for Mental Health Services, in partnership with the National Institute of Mental Health, and National Institutes of Health. (2001). *Mental health: A report of the surgeon general.* Chapter 5: Older adults and mental health. Retrieved from www.surgeongeneral.gov/library/mentalhealth/chapter5/sec1.html

Webber, A. P., Martin, J. L., Harker, J. O., et al. (2005). Depression in older patients admitted for postacute nursing home rehabilitation. *Journal of the American Geriatrics Society, 53*(6), 1017–1022.

Welch, H. G., Walsh, J. S., & Larson, E. B. (1992). The cost of institutional care in Alzheimer's disease: Nursing home and hospital use in a prospective cohort. *Journal of the American Geriatrics Society, 40,* 221–224.

Wells, J. L., Seabrook, J. A., Stolee, P., et al. (2003). State of the art in geriatric rehabilitation. Part I: Review of frailty and comprehensive geriatric assessment. *Archives of Physical Medicine and Rehabilitation, 84*(6), 890–897.

Zimmer, J. G., Watson, M., & Treat, A. (1984). Behavioral problems among patients in skilled nursing facilities. *American Journal of Public Health, 74,* 1118–1121.

Zimmerman, S., Sloane, P. D., Eckert, J. K., et al. (2005). How good is assisted living? Findings and implications from an outcome study. *Journal of Gerontology: Social Sciences, 60*(B), S195–S204.

Zimmerman, S. I., Smith, H. D., Gruber-Baldini, A., et al. (1999, September). Short-term persistent depression following hip fracture: A risk factor and target to increase resilience in elderly people. *Social Work Research, 23*(3), 187–196.

2

Dementia in Nursing Home Patients: Assessment and Management

Solasinee Hemrungrojn and *Jeffrey L. Cummings*

Currently 4 million Americans suffer from dementia. Without effective treatment, the number of patients with dementia, primarily Alzheimer's disease (AD), is estimated to reach 13.2 million by 2050 (Hebert et al., 2003). Most patients with dementia are eventually admitted to nursing homes, and patients with dementia comprise a large segment of the nursing home population. Dementia afflicts 50% of the residents in nursing homes in the United States (Delacourte et al., 1999). In a Swedish study, Fratiglioni and colleagues found that 77% of patients with moderate to severe dementia were inpatient residents in nursing homes. Similarly, many survey studies report that the number of severely demented patients is high in institutions of long-term care (Fratiglioni, 1996). Mayeux (1994) and colleagues noted that the proportion of severely demented patients living in nursing homes in the state of New York was 65%. It is estimated that in the year 2020 there will be more than 3 million severely demented patients requiring long-term care (Teresi et al., 1994). The cost for dementia care in nursing homes is a major national health care expenditure. The estimated annual nursing cost for dementia in 1986 was $22,458.00 per patient per year, rising to $42,230.00 in 1997 (O'Brien & Caro, 2001).

Disclosure: Dr. Cummings has provided consultation to the following pharmaceutical companies: AstraZeneca, Avanir, Bristol-Myers Squibb, Eisai, Forest, Janssen, Lilly, Memory, Neurochem, Novartis, Ono, Pfizer, Sanofi-Aventis, and Wyeth.

In this chapter, we consider the prevalence, characteristics, and management of dementia in long-term care settings.

PREVALENCE OF DEMENTIA IN THE NURSING HOME

A nursing home survey conducted by the National Center for Health Statistics identified 19,180 Nursing Homes in the United States with 1,491,400 residents. Data collected from the residents' medical records found that 47% of all residents had "senile dementia" or "chronic organic brain syndrome." Rovner et al. (1990) studied the prevalence of psychiatric disorders in nursing homes and found that 80.2% had a psychiatric disorder and 67.4% manifested a dementia syndrome. Forty percent of demented patients had additional psychiatric syndromes such as delusions or depression. A population-based study done by Matthews et al. (2002) in the United Kingdom found that most elderly were living in their own homes and only 4.4% were living in residential care or nursing homes. Nevertheless, they observed that dementia prevalence in the nursing home was as high as 62% and was slightly higher in women than in men (Matthews & Dening, 2002). Dementia in nursing homes is underdiagnosed, leading to the underestimation of the magnitude of the residential dementia population. One-third of patients with dementia in nursing homes are not formally diagnosed according to nursing home medical records (Nygaard & Ruths, 2003). Dementia also is very common in institutions that are not registered to care for dementia patients (MacDonald et al., 2002).

BEHAVIORAL PROBLEMS ASSOCIATED WITH DEMENTIA IN NURSING HOMES

Behavioral symptoms of dementia, which include restlessness, agitation, aggression, psychosis, wandering, and resistiveness, are so disturbing to family caregivers that many are forced to relinquish care and institutionalize their loved one. These symptoms are much more common in nursing homes than in the community and often necessitate the use of physical restraint and psychotropic medications.

Pacing. Inappropriate pacing has been found in 23% to 40% of severely demented patients. Pacing is linked to cognitive and functional deterioration.

Agitation and aggression. Studies report prevalence rates of agitation in nursing home patients with dementia of 30% to 75% depending on the patient population and definition of agitation. Physical and verbal aggression is frequently related to severe dementia, particularly in patients with impaired verbal skills and difficulty expressing themselves. Agitation may lead to injury to both patients and caregivers, require use mechanical or drug treatment, and contribute to increased stress of staff.

Hallucinations and delusions. The reported prevalence of hallucinations among nursing home residents with dementia varies from 12% to 53%. Related factors are increasing severity of cognitive disorder and decreasing visual acuity. Most common are visual hallucinations followed by auditory hallucinations. The frequency of delusions has been found to be between 38% and 73%; most are of the paranoid type. In advanced dementia, the problem of diminished verbal expression interferes with the diagnosis of both hallucinations and delusions. Theft of property is a common paranoid delusion; other common delusions involve infidelity of the spouse or the delusion that the spouse is not the spouse.

Screaming episodes. These occur with a frequency of 17% to 25% in severe dementia patients. Patients with screaming tend to be dependent in activities of daily living, to have multiple medical problems, to be restrained, and to be receiving psychotropic drugs.

Self-destructive behavior. Self-destructive behaviors in nursing home residents are common. Indirect behaviors such as refusal to eat, take medication or cooperate with staff occur in about 60% of patients at least weekly. Direct behaviors such as cutting, hitting, and ingesting foreign objects occur at least weekly in 15%.

Depression. Depression may be underdiagnosed in dementia patients. The prevalence of depression in nursing homes is higher than in community settings, varying from 17% to 35%. It is more difficult to estimate or diagnose depression in patients with dementia because of disturbances in the patient's ability to identify or communicate depressive symptoms such as feeling of sadness, hopelessness, worthlessness, or anhedonia. Depression among dementia patients may not meet research criteria for major depression. Tearfulness, feelings of guilt, long-lasting depressed mood, and anhedonia are good indicators of depression in dementia patients. Depression may present with atypical symptoms such as inversion of the day–night cycle, aggressiveness or agitation, severe anxiety, social withdrawal, refusal of activities, and staying in bed.

MEDICAL COMORBIDITY

Most nursing home residents have extensive medical comorbidity, and medical illness may contribute to psychiatric symptoms in the elderly. Rapid identification of these potential causes of behavioral change will help physicians reduce these symptoms without psychotropic medications (Sutor et al., 2001). A study in patients with AD found that 60% had three or more comorbid medical illnesses; medical comorbidity increased with dementia severity.

INCONTINENCE

Incontinence (urinary and fecal) occurs in 53% to 90% of severely demented patients. It is estimated that the expense of caring for urinary incontinence in nursing homes will exceed $25 billion annually in the United States by the year 2025. Loss of sphincter control may be related to lesions at the posterior part of the superior frontal and anterior cingulate gyri and intervening white matter. Medical causes of incontinence include infection, prostate problems, and side effects of medications. Difficulty in finding or seeing the toilet, impaired mobility, difficulty undressing, and reduced ability to express toileting needs exacerbate this problem.

RECOGNITION OF DEMENTIA IN NURSING HOMES

Dementia is typically the product of a progressive neurodegenerative disorder manifested by cognitive and memory deterioration and progressive impairment of activities of daily living. These impairments are severe enough to disturb the ability to function independently and represent a decline from a previously higher level of function. People living in nursing home settings have few cognitively demanding tasks in everyday life and their dementia may be overlooked. One study found that only half of nursing home residents with Mini-Mental State Examination (MMSE) scores less than 15 were recognized as demented by nursing staff. Dementia may predispose to confusion from medications, delirium, falls, and fractures.

ALZHEIMER'S DISEASE

Recent demographic data suggest that AD could affect up to 14 million men and women in the United States by the year 2050. It is the fourth leading cause of death in the United States with annual treatment costs of nearly $100 billion.

Diagnosis

Alzheimer's disease is the most common form of dementia in the elderly. The commonly recognized criteria are those of the *Diagnostic and Statistical Manual of Mental Disorders*, 4th edition (American Psychiatric Association, APA, 2000), and those of the National Institute of Neurologic and Communicative Disorders and Stroke-Alzheimer's Disease and Related Disorders Association (Doraiswamy et al., 2002) (Table 2.1). The latter defines three levels of diagnosis: *Definite*— clinical diagnosis and histologic confirmation; *probable*—typical clinical syndrome without histologic confirmation; *possible*—typical clinical syndrome

TABLE 2.1. Clinical Diagnostic Criteria for Alzheimer's Disease

DSM-IV DEMENTIA OF THE ALZHEIMER'S TYPE (McKHANN ET AL., 1984)	NINCDS-ADRDA PROBABLE ALZHEIMER'S DISEASE (DORAISWAMY ET AL., 2002)

A. The development of multiple cognitive deficits manifest both by
  1. Memory impairment (amnesia) and
  2. At least one of the following cognitive disturbances:
    a) Aphasia
    b) Apraxia
    c) Agnosia
    d) Disturbed executive functioning (planning, organizing sequencing, abstracting).
B. Cognitive deficits cause significant impairment in social-occupational functioning and represent a significant decline from previous level of functioning
C. The course is characterized by gradual onset and continuing cognitive decline
D. The cognitive deficits are not due to other brain-induced, systemic, or substance-induced condition
E. The deficits do not occur exclusively during the course of delirium
F. The disturbance is not accounted for by another Axis I diagnosis (e.g., major depressive disorder, schizophrenia)
	Dementia established by clinical examination (mental status testing) and documented by mental status scales (confirmed by neuropsychological testing)
	• Deficits in two or more cognitive areas
	• Progressive worsening of memory and other cognitive functions
	• No disturbance in consciousness
	• Onset between 40 and 90 years of age
	• Absence of systemic disorders or other brain diseases that could account for the progressive deficits in memory and cognition
	Diagnosis supported by
	• Progressive deficits in language (aphasia), motor skills (apraxia), and perception (agnosia)
	• Impaired activities of daily living and altered patterns of behavior
	• Family history of similar disorders
	• Consistent laboratory or radiologic results (e.g., cerebral atrophy on computed tomography)

without histologic confirmation or atypical clinical features with no alternative diagnosis apparent and no histologic confirmation (Doraiswamy et al., 2002).

Cognition

Memory. The early stage of AD is characterized by deficits in episodic memory; as dementia progresses amnesia becomes more prominent and deficits of remote memory become more severe (Sagar et al., 1988).

Language. In the early stage of impairment, the patients may suffer from word finding difficulty or mild aphasia. There may be an inability to retrieve words with circumlocution and poor word list generation for words in a given semantic category (e.g., number of animals named in 1 min). The disease progresses to include poor naming. Eventually, comprehension of speech and conversation may be affected. In the final stages, there may be echolalia (the tendency to repeat the words of others), palilalia (the tendency to repeat their own words), logoclonia (repetition of the final syllable of a word), and nonverbal vocalization (unrecognizable as language) or even mutism (Mendez et al., 2003).

Visuospatial function. Patients evidence a progressive inability to orient themselves in their surroundings although basic visual functions are spared. AD patients in the early stages may have impairment of visual attention, visual search, and global pattern recognition. Neuropsychological tests may reveal an inability to copy elementary figures or three-dimensional representations and impairment in accurately drawing a clock. With progression, patients may get lost in unfamiliar surroundings, lose their way while driving, and eventually become disorientated in their own homes or the nursing home (Suzuki et al., 2003).

Executive function. Impairments of executive function occur in the early stages of AD. The first manifestations are decreased awareness of their deficits and impaired performance on executive tests such as Trail Making B. Frontal executive disturbances include impairments in insight, planning, goal-directed behavior, abstraction, judgment, and reasoning.

Motor function. Motor disturbances are not common in AD patients until the late stages when there is limb rigidity and progressive loss of the ability to walk.

Primitive reflexes. In AD, the frequency of primitive reflexes is 20% to 50%, the snout, grasp, and palmomental reflexes being the most frequent. These changes are common late in the disease.

Apraxia. Apraxia is a failure to produce a learned movement in the absence of weakness, sensory loss, incoordination, incomprehension, or inattention to commands. The common types of apraxia associated with AD are ideomotor and ideational apraxia. They occur in 70% to 80% of patients in middle and late stages of the disease. First, patients manifest ideomotor apraxia with spatial and temporal errors in the execution of a motor act or the use of a body part as a substitute for an object. Thereafter, patients have ideational apraxia with difficulty in sequencing events of a complex motor plan.

Behavioral Changes in Alzheimer's Disease Patients in Nursing Homes

Neuropsychiatric symptoms become more frequent in populations of AD patients as the underlying disease worsens; patients with more severe cognitive abnormalities are more likely to exhibit behavioral changes (Cummings, 2003). Behavior changes are nearly universally present in AD patients residing in nursing homes.

Apathy. Apathy, a syndrome composed of decreased initiation, diminished social engagement, emotional indifference, and reduced motivation is the most common neuropsychiatric symptom reported in AD patients. Apathy often occurs early in the course and increases in severity as the illness progresses, affecting approximately 70% of patients in the mild—moderate stages and over 90% of patients in the later stages (Boyle & Malloy, 2004).

Depression and apathy commonly co-occur, but apathy can occur in the absence of depression and is not necessarily a manifestation of depression. In addition, apathy may coexist with both aberrant motor behavior such as pacing, wandering, and rummaging, as well as agitation because patients with apathy are not necessarily continuously hypokinetic. Apathy has been associated with impaired executive function including impaired set shifting and reduced verbal fluency (Cummings, 2003). Apathy is significantly associated with impairment of both instrumental activities of daily living (IADL) and basic activities of daily living (BADL; Boyle et al., 2003).

Agitation. Agitation was one of the most common behavioral disturbances in AD. It is strongly correlated with degree of cognitive impairment. Most definitions include aggressive, destructive, and resistive behaviors such as threats, pushing, hitting, shouting, and cursing, and it may also comprise less severe behaviors such as repeatedly asking questions, pacing, and repetitive stereotyped motor behaviors (Cummings 2003). The most common agitated behavior is verbal aggressiveness, reported in 75% of patients; the least is physical aggressiveness, reported in 50% of patients. A trigger initiating the symptoms of agitation is present in 60% of cases; the most frequently reported factors are psychosocial stresses including death of a spouse, absence of a family member, or being asked to do something they did not want to do (i.e., take a shower). Factors such as side effects from medications, recent surgical interventions, and pain may be significant causes of agitation (Leger et al., 2002).

AD patients with agitation tend to have executive dysfunction indicative of frontal lobe involvement. They exhibit a dysregulation syndrome with a loss of ability to modulate behavioral responses to environmental provocations or emotional disturbances arising from comorbid neuropsychiatric disorders such as psychosis or depression (Cummings, 2003).

Depression. Depressive symptoms are common at the onset of AD, and they remain common with disease progression. Prevalence rates of major depression among AD patients attending clinics is 1.5% to 25%, minor depression occurs at a frequency of 10% to 30%; incidence of depression in dementia over one year is at least 6% and may be higher. Clinically, dysphoric symptoms (sadness, feelings of guilt, self-criticism, helplessness, and hopelessness) can help distinguish depression from apathy (Lee & Lyketsos, 2003; Table 2.2). Nearly a third of AD patients experience delusions or hallucinations during their major depressive episodes (Zubenko et al., 2003).

Psychosis. Psychosis in AD is defined by the occurrence of delusions or hallucinations that have their onset after the appearance of the dementia syndrome; have been present at least intermittently for 1 month or longer; and are severe enough to disrupt the patient's function (Cummings, 2003; Table 2.3).

Prevalence rates of psychosis in patients with AD range from 10% to 73% in clinic populations, and from 7% to 20% in community and clinical trial populations (Schneider & Dagerman, 2004). The combined prevalence of delusions

TABLE 2.2. Provisional Diagnostic Criteria for Depression of Alzheimer's Disease (Olin et al., 2002)

A. Three (or more) of the following symptoms have been present during the same 2-week period and represent a change from previous functioning:

At least one of the symptoms is either (1) depressed mood or (2) decreased positive affect or pleasure

Note: Do not include symptoms that, in your judgment, are clearly due to a medical condition other than Alzheimer's disease, or are a direct result of non-mood-related dementia symptoms (e.g., loss of weight due to difficulties with food intake).

Clinically significant depressed mood (e.g., depressed, sad, hopeless, discouraged, tearful)

Decreased positive affect or pleasure in response to social contacts and usual activities

Social isolation or withdrawal

Disruption in appetite

Disruption in sleep

Psychomotor changes (e.g., agitation or retardation)

Irritability

Fatigue or loss of energy

Feelings of worthlessness, hopelessness, or excessive or inappropriate guilt

B. Recurrent thoughts of death, suicidal ideation, plan or attempt. All criteria are met for dementia of the Alzheimer's type (*DSM-IV-TR*)

C. The symptoms cause clinically significant distress or disruption in functioning

D. The symptoms do not occur exclusively during the course of a delirium

E. The symptoms are not due to the direct physiological effects of a substance (e.g., a drug of abuse or a medication)

The symptoms are not better accounted for by other conditions such as major depressive disorder, bipolar disorder, bereavement, schizophrenia, schizoaffective disorder, psychosis of Alzheimer's disease, anxiety disorders, or substance-related disorder

Specify if	*Specify*
Co-occurring onset: if onset antedates or co-occurs with the AD symptoms	With psychosis of Alzheimer's disease
Post-AD onset: if onset occurs AD symptoms	With other significant behavioral signs or symptoms
	With past history of mood disorders

---

and hallucinations in cross-sectional studies is 40% to 65% (Cummings, 2003). Among a clinical sample of 329 AD patients, the incidence of delusions and hallucinations in people with probable AD who did not have psychosis at initial evaluation was 20% at 1 year, 36% at 2 years, and 50% at 3 years (Cook et al., 2003). Delusions have a higher frequency among nursing home patients (Schneider & Dagerman, 2004) than among outpatients.

The delusions that occur in AD are typically paranoid type, nonbizarre, and simple. Misidentification delusions (e.g., Capgras syndrome) are common in AD

TABLE 2.3. Diagnostic Criteria for Psychosis of Alzheimer's Disease

Characteristic symptoms

Presence of one (or more) of the following symptoms:
 Visual or auditory hallucinations
 Delusions
Primary diagnosis: All the criteria for dementia of the Alzheimer type are met

Chronology of the onset of symptoms of psychosis vs. onset of symptoms of dementia

There is evidence from the history that the symptoms in Criterion A have not been
 present continuously since prior to the onset of the symptoms of dementia

Duration and severity

The symptom(s) in Criterion A have been present, at least intermittently, for 1 month
 or longer. Symptoms are severe enough to cause some disruption in patients' and/or
 others' functioning

Exclusion of schizophrenia and related psychotic disorders

Criteria for schizophrenia, schizoaffective disorder, delusional disorder, or mood
 disorder with psychotic features have never been met

Relationship to delirium

The disturbance does not occur exclusively during the course of a delirium

Exclusion of other causes of psychotic symptoms

The disturbance is not better accounted for by another general-medical condition or
 direct physiological effects of a substance (e.g., a drug of abuse, a medication)

Associated features (*specify* if associated)

With agitation: When there is evidence, from history or examination, of prominent
 agitation with or without physical or verbal aggression
With negative symptoms: When prominent negative symptoms, such as apathy, affective
 flattening avolition, or motor retardation, are present
With depression: When prominent depressive symptoms, such as depressed mood,
 insomnia or hypersomnia, feelings of worthlessness or excessive or inappropriate
 guilt, or recurrent thoughts of death, are present

Source: Jeste and Finkel (2000).

patients. Typical delusions include the belief that people are stealing things from
them, they are in danger and others are planning to harm them, their spouse or
other caregiver is an imposter, their house is not their home, their spouse is having
an affair, or their family members are planning to abandon them (Schneider &
Dagerman, 2004).

   Sundowning. Sundowning is defined by Rindlisbacher and Hopkins (1992) as
"an exacerbation of symptoms indicating increased arousal or impairment in late

afternoon, evening, or at night among elderly demented individuals." The estimated rate of sundowning prevalence in AD ranges from 12% to 25% (Bliwise, 2004). Sleep disturbances were more frequent in patients with sundowning than those without. Bright light has been reported to improve sundowning and nocturnal agitation in AD. Restlessness, as observed in sundowning, also responds to bright light (Lebert et al., 1996). The sundowning syndrome increases the burden on caregivers as it occurs when the institutional caregiving staff is at the lowest levels.

Sleep disturbances. Nocturnally disturbed sleep may affect as many as 25% of AD patients during some stage of their illness. Patients often have excessive daytime napping and sleepiness, thus contributing to a cycle of excessive sleepiness during the day- and nighttime wakefulness. Sleep architecture studies show that wakefulness after sleep onset increases with the severity of dementia, just as nocturnal total sleep time, sleep efficiency (e.g., proportion of time in bed asleep), and rapid eye movement (REM) sleep decrease. The latency to the first REM episode of the night is increased (Cummings, 2003).

Kluver–Bucy syndrome. Some AD patients may have a Kluver–Bucy syndrome, characterized by change in dietary habits with bulimia, emotional placidity (marked change in emotional behavior), psychic blindness (sensory agnosia), hypermetamorphosis (compulsive exploration of objects in the environment), and hypersexuality and hyperorality (Cummings & Mega, 2003).

Weight loss and loss of appetite. Weight loss is common in AD. This can contribute to loss of muscle mass and increased risk of decubitus ulcers. Weight loss frequently occurs in the first stages of the disease, even though the patients have adequate food intake. Weight loss is more common with progression of AD. It is important to consider the balance of low-energy intake and high expenditure with pacing, agitation, and repetitive behaviors. An imbalance of only a few hundred calories per day can lead to substantial weight loss over weeks or months. Swallowing abnormalities in patients with advanced dementia may increase weight loss (Gillette-Guyonnet et al., 2000; White et al., 2004).

Treatment of Alzheimer's Disease

Donepezil hydrochloride. Several placebo-controlled trials demonstrated significant improvement of cognition and global function in patients with mild to moderate AD treated with donepezil. The agent also improved behavioral symptoms and activities of daily living in patients with more advanced AD. Feldman et al. (2003) reported that donepezil improved cognition, behavior, and function compared with placebo in patients with moderate to severe AD. There was significant improvement in anxiety, apathy/indifference, and irritability/lability. This was associated with reduced requirement for caregiving time and lower levels of caregiver stress (Feldman et al., 2003; Gauthier et al., 2002). Similarly,

Winblad and colleagues (2006) showed that nursing home residents with severe dementia derive cognitive and functional benefit from donepezil.

Donepezil is safe and well tolerated with a low incidence of adverse effects. Nausea, insomnia, diarrhea, or vivid dreams and nightmares may occur with the agent. Administration in the morning or slowing titration is recommended to ameliorate these problems. Some studies show that maintenance of cognition and function continue for at least one year, but the total duration of benefit is not known (Smith Doody, 2003; Tariot et al., 2001). Donepezil is initiated at a dose of 5 mg once daily and increased to 10 mg once daily after a month of therapy. Donepezil is approved for treatment of mild, moderate, and severe AD.

Galantamine. Galantamine has two mechanisms for increasing cholinergic activity: the first is inhibition of acetylcholinesterase, and the second is allosteric modulation of the presynaptic nicotinic receptor, which increases acetylcholine release. Short-term trials of galantamine indicate cognitive benefit during 6 months of treatment (Cummings et al., 2004). AD patients with mild to moderate dementia treated with galantamine had better total Neuropsychiatric Inventory scores and showed less aberrant motor behavior, agitation, anxiety, apathy, and disinhibition than patients receiving placebo. Galantamine also decreased behavior-related caregiver distress (Cummings et al., 2004). The recommended dose of galantamine is 4 mg twice daily at initiation. After 1 month, it is increased to a dose of 8 mg twice daily; 12 mg twice daily is the target dose (Cummings, 2003). Galantamine sustained-release form is administered once daily. Galantamine is approved for treatment of mild to moderate AD.

Rivastigmine. This inhibitor of acetylcholinesterase and butyrylcholinesterase is approved for the treatment of mild to moderate AD. Several double-blind placebo-controlled studies have reported that rivastigmine improves activities of daily living, behavior, cognition, and global functioning in mild to moderate AD compared with placebo. Some patients may have adverse effects such as nausea, vomiting, diarrhea, and weight loss. Slower titration may reduce the prevalence of these symptoms (Farlow, 2003).

Effective therapy requires titration from an initial dosage of 3 to 6 mg/d with additional increases to 9 or 12 mg/d. Dosage increments occur at 1-month intervals. Twice per day dosing is suggested. Rivastigmine is indicated for mild–moderate AD.

Memantine. Memantine is a low to moderate affinity, uncompetitive *N*-methyl-D-aspartate (NMDA) receptor antagonist. This mechanism is thought to reduce overstimulation of the NMDA receptor antagonist. This mechanism may be neuroprotective by preventing cellular calcium entry and neuronal death (Wilcock, 2003). Recent studies in moderate-to-severe AD patients (MMSE 3–14) found that there are benefits of memantine treatment on global, cognitive, and functional measures (Reisberg, 2003). Beneficial effects of memantine were found on the Severe Impairment Battery, the Functional Assessment Staging scale, and the Resource Utilization in Dementia instrument (Wilcock, 2003). In a study of moderate-to-severe AD patients who received stable doses of done- pezil and were randomized to memantine or placebo significantly better out- comes on measures of cognition (Severe Impairment Battery), activities of daily living, global assessment, and behavior measures resulted (Tariot et al., 2004). Memantine is well tolerated in clinical trials; however, side effects have been reported, including agitation, urinary incontinence, insomnia, diarrhea, diz- ziness, headache, falls, and hallucinations. These have typically been of mild to moderate severity (Wilcock, 2003). Memantine is begun at a dose of 5 mg daily and titrated in 5 mg increments weekly to doses of 10 mg twice daily. Memantine is indicated for moderate–severe AD (See Table 2.4).

VASCULAR DEMENTIA

Vascular dementia (VaD) is the second or third most common dementing dis- ease in most series of cases (Heidebrink, 2002). The prevalence of VaD rises with increasing age in all countries and is generally more common in men, rang- ing from 3.2% to 4.8% in men and 2.2% to 2.9% in women between 70 and 79 years and from 3.5% to 16.3% in men and 2.8% to 9.2% in women between 80 and 89 years (Qizilbash et al., 2002). However, VaD is the most common cause of dementia in residents aged 65 years and above in Japan, where it accounts in some studies for more than 50% of all cases. VaD is becoming more frequent in China and Russia (Qizilbash et al., 2002). The annual incidence (per 100,000) of VaD varies from 20 to 40 in 60 to 69 year-olds and from 200 to 700 in those over 80 years of age. The incidence rate has declined over the past 2 decades, probably as a consequence of effective antihypertensive and stroke prevention programs (Leys et al., 1998). The following factors increase the risk of dementia after stroke: Old age, lower education level and income, smoking, lower blood pressure, orthostatic hypotension, and larger and recurrent strokes.

The most widely used criteria for VaD are the *Diagnostic and Statistical Manual of Mental Disorders* (*DSM-IV*), the International Classification of Diseases (ICD-10), and the National Institute of Neurological Disorders and Stroke—Association Internationale pour la Recherche et l'Enseignement en Neuroscience (NINDS-AIREN; Table 2.5). The NINDS-AIREN research crite- ria for VaD defined cerebrovascular disease by the presence of focal neurological signs and detailed imaging evidence of ischemic changes in the brain. A rela- tionship between dementia and cerebrovascular disorder is based on the onset of dementia within 3 months following a recognized stroke, abrupt deterioration in cognitive function or fluctuating, stepwise progression of cognitive deficits. The

TABLE 2.4. Clinical Pharmacology of Agents Useful for Improving Cognition in Alzheimer's Disease

CHARACTERISTIC	DONEPEZIL	RIVASTIGMINE	GALANTAMINE	MEMANTINE
Time to maximal serum concentration (h)	3–5	0.5–2	0.5–1	3–7
Absorption affected by food	No	Yes	Yes	No
Serum half-life (h)	70–80	2*	5–7	60–80
Protein binding (%)	96	40	0–20	45
Metabolism (hepatic)	CYP2D6, CYP3A4	Nonhepatic	CYP2D6, CYP3A4	Nonhepatic
Dose (initial/maximal)	5 mg daily/10 mg daily	1.5 mg twice daily/6 mg twice daily	4 mg twice daily/12 mg twice daily	5 mg daily/10 mg twice daily
Mechanism of action	Cholinesterase inhibitor	Cholinesterase inhibitor	Cholinesterase inhibitor	NMDA–receptor antagonist

Source: Cummings (2004).

Note: CYP2D6, cytochrome P-450 enzyme 2D6; CYP3A4, cytochrome P-450 enzyme 3A4; and NMDA, *N*-methyl-D-aspartate.

* Rivastigmine is a pseudo-irreversible acetylcholinesterase inhibitor that has an 8-h half-life for the inhibition of acetylcholinesterase in the brain.

TABLE 2.5. Clinical Diagnostic Criteria for Vascular Dementia

Probable vascular dementia

Dementia (decline from previous higher level of cognitive function, impairment
  of two or more cognitive domains deficits severe enough to interfere with
  activities of daily living and not due to physical effects of stroke alone,
  absence of delirium/psychosis/aphasia/sensorimotor impairment that precludes
  neuropsychologic testing and absence of any other disorder capable of producing
  a dementia syndrome)
Cerebrovascular disease, neurologic signs, and evidence of relevant cerebrovascular
  disease by imaging
A relationship between dementia and cerebrovascular disease
    Onset of dementia within 3 months of a recognized stroke
    Abrupt onset and stepwise fluctuating course of dementia

Features supporting a diagnosis of vascular dementia

Subtle onset and variable course of cognitive deficits
Early gait disturbances
Unsteadiness or frequent unprovoked falls
Early urinary frequency, urgency, and other urinary symptoms not explained by
  urologic disease
Pseudobulbar palsy
Personality change, abulia, depression, emotional incontinence, pseudobulbar affect,
  psychomotor retardation

Features against a diagnosis of vascular dementia

Early prominent amnesia, aphasia, apraxia, or agnosia without focal imaging
  correlates
Absence of focal signs
Absence of cerebrovascular lesions on brain computed tomography or magnetic
  resonance imaging scans

Definite vascular dementia

Presence of clinical criteria for probable vascular dementia
Histopathologic evidence of cerebrovascular disease from biopsy or autopsy study
Absence of neurofibrillary tangles and neuritic plaques exceeding that expected
  for age
Absence of other clinical or pathologic disorder capable of producing dementia

Source: Roman et al. (1993).

inter-rater reliability of the NINDS-AIREN criteria has been shown to be moderate to substantial (kappa 0.46–0.72; Lopez et al., 1994). In a neuropathological
series, the sensitivity of the NINDS-AIREN criteria was 58%, and specificity
was 80%. Compared with other criteria, the NINDS-AIREN were more specific,
while the most sensitive criteria for VaD are those of the State of California
Alzheimer's Disease Diagnostic and Treatment Centers (Gold et al., 1997).

Subtypes of VaD

VaD is a group of heterogeneous syndromes and takes several clinical forms depending on the region of brain affected. Subtypes of VaD included in current classifications are cortical VaD or multi-infarct dementia, subcortical ischemic VaD (e.g., lacunar state; white matter disease) or small vessel dementia and strategic infarct dementia (Erkinjuntti, 2002; Table 2.6).

Multi-infarct dementia

Thromboembolic occlusion of multiple cerebral vessels produced by cardiac embolic events is the major cause of multi-infarct dementia. Clinical features may vary with the location of the strokes. Lateralized sensorimotor changes are common (Mendez & Cummings, 2003; Suzuki et al., 2003).

Strategic infarct dementia

Multiple cognitive impairments may be caused by small focal ischemic lesions involving sites critical for higher cortical function and behavior. These areas include the angular gyrus and thalamus.

Lacunar state

The vessels commonly associated with lacunes are the lenticulostriate branches of the middle cerebral artery or the thalamogeniculate, choroidal, and thalamoperforator branches of the posterior communicating and posterior cerebral arteries. The most commonly affected site for lacunar infarction is the frontal lobe white matter. Patients typically have a frontal-subcortical cognitive deficit. Patients may have lacunar syndromes such as pure motor hemiplegia, pure sensory stroke, dysarthria-clumsy hand syndrome, homolateral ataxia, pseudobulbar pulsy, small-stepped gait, and urinary incontinence.

White matter injury and Binswanger's disease

Ischemia causes periventricular leukoencephalopathy that typically spares the arcuate subcortical U-fibers. Binswanger's disease (dementia associated with white matter ischemic injury) has its onset in the 6th or 7th decade and is associated with significant hypertension. Clinical features in the early phase are episodes of mild motor signs (weakness, reflex asymmetry, incoordination), gait disorder (lower half parkinsonism with diminished stride length and diminished step height), imbalance, urinary frequency and incontinence, and extrapyramidal signs. Dementia has features of frontal-subcortical dysfunction with mood changes (Suzuki et al., 2003).

Mixed Alzheimer's disease and cerebrovascular disease

Many patients diagnosed with VaD clinically have coexistent pathologic changes of AD at autopsy. For AD with cerebrovascular disorder or mixed

TABLE 2.6. Signs and Symptoms by Subtype of Vascular Dementia (Cummings, 2003; Mendez & Cummings, 2003)

SUBTYPE	LESION	SIGNS AND SYMPTOMS
Multi-infarct dementia	Lt. Middle cerebral artery	Aphasia, apraxia, depression
	Rt. Middle cerebral artery	Visuospatial deficit: left hemispatial neglect, dressing disturbances, aprosody, impaired visuomotor performance
		Balint's syndrome, Man-in-the-barrel syndrome
Strategic infarct dementia	Bilateral watershed infarctions	Memory impairment, psychomotor slowing, decreased attention and mental control, apathy, decreased spontaneity, reduced verbal fluency, poor abstracting ability
	– Bilateral paramedian thalamic infarctions	Verbal memory impairment, aphasic disturbance with spare repetition, executive dysfunction
	– Isolated left-sided thalamic infarctions	Hemispatial neglect, visuospatial processing deficits
	– Isolated right-sided thalamic infarctions	Apathy, hypokinesia
	– Dorsolateral part of caudate nucleus	Disinhibition, impulsiveness
	– Ventromedial part of caudate nucleus	Fluent aphasia, alexia with agraphia, Gerstman syndrome
	– Left angular gyrus	Attention deficit with fluctuating alertness
	– Anterior cingulate gyrus	Apathy, akinetic mutism, abulia, memory loss
	– Basal forebrain/the genu of internal capsule	– Emotional bluntness
		– Decline in performance IQ
		– Laconic speech with simplified syntax
		– Decreased spontaneity
		– Depression/agitation/irritability/impulsivity
		– Apathy/abulia
		– Psychosis with persecutory delusion

Lacunar infarction	Frontal lobe white matter; basal ganglia; thalamus	Frontal—subcortical cognitive impairment – Impairment in psychomotor speed – Impairment in sustained and divided attention – Impairment in set shifting – Impairment in verbal fluency, working memory and response inhibition
Binswanger's disease	White matter of hemisphere	Frontal executive deficit – Decline in functional abilities – Lack of insight, apathy, listlessness Reduced speed of information processing – Deficit of sustained and divided attention – Frontal—executive dysfunctions – Memory retrieval impairment

Source: Cummings (2003); Mendez and Cummings (2003).

dementia, patients may have a clinical history and signs of cerebrovascular disorder, clinically resembling VaD. This group of patients has reliable biological markers of clinical AD such as early and significant medial temporal lobe atrophy on magnetic resonance imaging (MRI), bilateral parietal hypoperfusion on single photon emission computed tomography (SPECT), change in cerebrospinal fluid (CSF) beta amyloid and tau-protein, and increased frequency of the apolipoprotein (APOE) 4 allele.

Cognition

Early cognitive changes of subcortical VaD include a dysexecutive syndrome with slowed information processing and impairment in goal formulation, initiation, planning, organizing, sequencing, executing, and abstracting ability. The memory deficit of VaD is characterized by impaired recall, relatively intact recognition, less severe forgetting, and greater benefits from cues. Behavior and psychological symptoms of VaD include depression, personality change, emotional lability, inertia, emotional bluntness, and psychomotor retardation (Erkinjuntti, 2002).

Behavioral Changes in Vascular Dementia

Depression. The prevalence rate of major depression in VaD is higher than in AD. The prevalence rate of major depression is 4% to 10% for AD and 20% to 25% (varying from 6% to 45%) for VaD (Newman, 1999). Persistent depression was significantly associated with older age.

Anxiety disorders. Anxiety disorders are common in those who suffer from VaD, with prevalence rates of 17% to 38% (Moroney et al., 1997).

Psychosis. Nearly 50% of VaD patients have psychotic symptoms. These include visual hallucinations, delusions, delusional misidentification, and auditory hallucinations. The most common symptoms are persecutory delusions and phantom boarder delusions. Visual hallucinations are significantly associated with more severe cognitive impairment (Moroney et al., 1997).

Treatment of VaD

The therapeutic goals in treating VaD include treating both the underlying disease and the cognitive deterioration.

Primary prevention. Reduction of the progression of VaD depends on eliminating the main risk factors related to cerebrovascular disease, such as arterial hypertension, atrial fibrillation, myocardial infarction, coronary heart disease, diabetes, artherosclerosis, lipid abnormalities, and smoking. Inappropriate decreases of nocturnal blood pressure may lead to lacunar infarction and require management.

Secondary prevention. The goals of secondary prevention are to limit the extent of ischemic brain injury and prevent recurrence of stroke. Selective treatment according to the etiology of the cerebrovascular disorder including small vessel disease, hypodynamic problems, and hypoxic ischemia may have a role. Platelet antiaggregants, such as aspirin, are commonly used. Systolic blood pressure should be maintained within the range of 135 to 150 mmHg in patients who have VaD and stroke because mild systolic blood pressure elevation may be necessary to normalize cerebral perfusion.

Tertiary treatment. The specific strategy for treatment of the cognitive changes of VaD is use of cholinesterase inhibitors and possibly memantine.

Donepezil. There are large-scale, 24-week, randomized, double-blind, parallel-group controlled trials, of mild-to-moderate probable or possible VaD, using donepezil 5 or 10 mg daily compared with placebo. The donepezil group showed significantly better performance than the placebo group on the cognitive, functional, and global measures. Most side effects were transient including nausea, diarrhea, anorexia, and cramps (Malouf et al., 2004).

Rivastigmine. A small open label study of patients, with subcortical VaD, reported that rivastigmine can improve cognitive function and behavior. Patients also showed a slight improvement in executive functions (Moretti et al., 2003).

Galantamine. Patients with probable VaD treated with galantamine showed significant improvement in cognition, compared with the baseline at 6 months. They showed significant benefits in activities of daily living, behavior, and global function compared with patients receiving placebo. Some patients experience nausea and vomiting; using a slower dose escalation may improve tolerability. The effective dose is 16 to 24 mg/d (Erkinjuntti et al., 2002).

Memantine. In a 28-week randomized placebo-controlled trial study in patients with mild to moderate VaD, memantine 20 mg/d improved cognition, MMSE, and the Gottfries-Brane-Steen Scale intellectual function subscale. These were no effect on a global measure. Adverse effects included agitation, confusion, and dizziness with no significant difference from adverse events experienced by the placebo group (Orgogozo et al., 2002).

PARKINSON'S DISEASE

Parkinson's disease (PD) is a slowly progressive neurodegenerative disorder. The characteristics of the disorder include bradykinesia, resting tremor, rigidity, flexed posture, loss of postural reflexes, and the freezing phenomenon (Table 2.7; Cummings, 2003). Patients with PD respond to treatment with dopaminergic agents.

PD can develop at any age; however, it most commonly begins around age 60 years. The risk increases with age, with lifetime risk at 2% to 4%. There are

TABLE 2.7. Clinical Diagnostic Criteria for Idiopathic Parkinson's Disease

Clinically possible: one of

1. Asymmetric resting tremor
2. Asymmetric rigidity
3. Asymmetric bradykinesia

Clinically probable: any two of

1. Asymmetric resting tremor
2. Asymmetric rigidity
3. Asymmetric bradykinesia

Clinically definite

1. Criteria for clinically probable
2. Definitive response to anti-Parkinson drugs

Exclusion criteria

1. Exposure to drugs that can cause parkinsonism such as neuroleptics, some antiemetic drugs, tetrabenazine, reserpine, flunarizine, and cinnarizine
2. Cerebellar signs
3. Corticospinal tract signs
4. Eye movement abnormalities other than slight limitation of upward gaze
5. Severe dysautonomia
6. Early moderate to severe gait disturbance or dementia
7. History of encephalitis, recurrent head injury (such as seen in boxers), or family history of Parkinson's disease in two or more family members
8. Evidence of severe subcortical white-matter disease, hydrocephalus, or other structural lesions on MRI that may account for parkinsonism

Source: Calne et al. (1992); Samii et al. (2004).

850,000 PD patients in the United States. Males have greater prevalence and incidence rates than females. While there is no specific diagnostic laboratory test for PD, using ligands for the dopamine transporter with positron emission tomography (PET) or SPECT have shown decreased dopaminergic nerve terminals in the striatum in PD.

Most patients begin with an asymmetric resting tremor, intermittent at first and insidiously progressive. Bradykinesia is an early feature with slowness, slower and smaller handwriting, and decreased amplitude of voice. As PD worsens, flexed posture, the freezing phenomena, and loss of postural reflexes occur. These correlate with disability and loss of independence. In addition, PD patients may suffer from nonmotor symptoms such as autonomic instability, hypotension, constipation, sexual dysfunction, bladder problems, sensory abnormalities (numbness, burning sensation, pain in limbs), and sleep disturbances (excessive daytime sleepiness, REM sleep behavior disorder, sleep fragmentation).

Parkinson's Disease in the Nursing Home

Studies from population-based databases found a prevalence of PD in nursing homes of 5.2% to 6.8% with peak prevalence between ages 75 and 84 years. Seventy to eighty percent of PD patients had moderate-to-severe cognitive impairment and moderate-to-severe functional disability with a greater rate of functional decline than nursing home residents without PD. Communication and swallowing problems, bowel and bladder incontinence, and the use of restraints also were common in the PD group. PD patients had more severe neuropsychiatric symptoms than residents without PD: 10% had anxiety and 34% had depressive symptoms. A study of mortality in nursing home residents demonstrated that advancing age, severe functional and cognitive disability, male gender, and the occurrence of pneumonia or congestive heart failure were the strongest predictors of death (Fernandez & Lapane, 2002; Lapane et al., 1999; Mitchell et al., 1996).

Cognition and Dementia in Parkinson's Disease

Early in the course of PD, there may be subtle cognitive dysfunction, mainly executive abnormalities. Minor deficits in set-shifting and attention, mild disturbance of retrieving learned material, reduced verbal fluency, and visuospatial impairment are common. Neuropsychological profiles of PD patients with dementia have shown a progressive dysexecutive syndrome. Those with PD and dementia have better recognition and a slower rate of forgetting than AD (Bosboom et al., 2004; McKeith, 2004).

Risk factors for developing dementia in PD include older age at onset, older current age, longer duration of motor symptoms, greater severity of motor impairment, akinetic rigid syndrome, early hallucinations, prior history of depression, and poor response to levodopa (McKeith, 2000). The risk for developing dementia in PD is up to six times greater compared with age-matched control subjects (Emre, 2003). Recent studies have shown that 60% to 80% of people with PD will develop dementia, typically after 10 to 15 years of motor disability. Annual incidence rates range from 30 to 120 cases per 1000 (Aarsland et al., 2003). Dementia in PD is thought to be the result of a combination of subcortical and cortical pathological changes. Mechanisms include dopaminergic deficiency, cortical cholinergic deficiency, and cortical Lewy bodies (Bosboom et al., 2004).

Depression

Depression is common in PD. A recent population-based study of 97 patients found that 36.1% reported mild depressive symptoms, 10.3% reported moderate symptoms, and 9.3% reported severe depression (Anderson & Weiner, 2002).

Advancing disease, a history of recent decline in function, falls, patient's perception of their perceived disability rather than actual disability, and cognitive impairment are associated with depressed mood. Characteristics of depression complicating PD are lowered arousal, apathy, diminished self-initiated planning, psychomotor retardation, marked decrease in concentration, dysphoria, pessimism, irritability, sadness, and suicidal thinking. Suicidal behavior is not common (Cummings, 1992; Slaughter et al., 2001). There is significantly greater cognitive impairment in PD with major depression than without depression.

Many physicians prefer to use selective serotonin reuptake inhibitors (SSRIs) in treating depression in PD. These agents have few side effects and no anticholinergic properties. Tricyclic antidepressants (TCAs) may be used as antidepressant therapy; however, their anticholinergic effects may include unwanted effects such as delirium, greater memory impairment, orthostatic hypotension, urinary retention, and constipation (Richard et al., 1997).

Psychotic Symptoms

Psychotic symptoms are common in PD with dementia, where their prevalence rate is 25% to 44%. They correlate with older age, advanced stage of PD, history of depression, and coexistent sleep disorder (altered dream phenomenon, sleep fragmentation). Common features are visual hallucinations with nonthreatening vivid, colorful visions of people or animals. Most patients retain insight into hallucinations, but when cognition becomes more impaired and disease progresses, delusional interpretation and deterioration of reality testing occur (Anderson & Weiner, 2002).

Treatment of psychosis should begin by evaluating for underlying infection or other medical illness. Reducing the antiparkinsonian treatment may be warranted. If the symptoms disturb the patient's function, atypical antipsychotics are the treatment of choice because they have fewer effects of motor symptoms than conventional neuroleptics. Clozapine is the most widely studied medication and produces significant improvement in psychotic symptoms. However, the risk of leukopenia requires regularly monitoring of white blood cells. Other agents such as olanzapine and risperidone also have shown efficacy in treating psychotic symptoms, but they may worsen motor symptoms. An atypical agent that may be less prone to exacerbate parkinsonism is quetiapine. Open label studies demonstrate efficacy without worsening motor symptoms. The initial dose is 12.5 mg/d and a target dose is 100 to 200 mg/d (Anderson & Weiner, 2002).

Recent Food and Drug Administration (FDA) warnings of the risk of stroke and death with antipsychotic use in the elderly mandate caution in the use of these agents.

Anxiety and Panic

Compared with other neurologic and medical illnesses, PD patients have higher rates of anxiety disorders. Simple phobia is seen in 35%, agoraphobia in 15%, obsessive disorder in 15%, panic disorder in 10%, and social phobia in 5% (Anderson & Weiner, 2002).

Symptomatic Treatment of Parkinson's Disease

Symptomatic treatment is initiated when symptoms disturb function or compromise independence. In the elderly, levodopa is the preferred drug because dopamine agonists may enhance adverse effects such as nausea, hypotension, leg edema, vivid dreams, hallucinations (particularly in dementia patients), and somnolence. Levodopa remains the most potent antiparkinson drug and provides the majority of treatment throughout the entire course. Side effects are nausea, hypotension, and vivid dreams. Long-term complications of levodopa treatment are motor fluctuation and the on-off phenomenon (unpredictable sudden switches between mobility and immobility). These occur in 25% to 50% of patients on lovodopa for 5 years or longer (Calne et al., 1992).

Dopamine agonists are highly effective in the management of both advanced PD as an adjuvant with levodopa and in early stage as monotherapy. Catechol-*O*-methyl transferase (COMT) inhibitors may be used to potentiate levodopa therapy.

Treatment Specific for the Dementia of Parkinson's Disease

Cholinesterase inhibitors are effective in PD with dementia. In a 24-week randomized multicenter double-blind placebo-controlled parallel group study, assessing the efficacy, tolerability, and safety of 3 to 12 mg of rivastigmine, it was found that there were benefits in cognition, function, behavioral symptoms, and global performance (Emre, 2003). Other open label studies with rivastigmine have shown similar outcomes. There was no worsening of motor function although 10% of patients experienced an increase in tremor (Giladi et al., 2003). Donepezil improved cognition (MMSE score) and was well tolerated in a study of PD with dementia. In open label studies with galantamine, cognition and hallucinations improved without significant worsening of extrapyramidal features (Samii et al., 2004). Rivastigmine is approved by the U.S. FDA for the treatment of PD dementia.

DEMENTIA WITH LEWY BODIES DISEASE

Dementia with Lewy bodies (DLB) is the second most common cause of neuro-degenerative dementia in older people, accounting for 10% to 15% of cases at autopsy (McKeith et al., 2004; Table 2.8).

TABLE 2.8. Consensus Guidelines for the Clinical Diagnosis of Probable and Possible Dementia with Lewy Bodies

---

Central features

Progressive cognitive decline of sufficient magnitude to interfere with normal social and occupational function; prominent or persistent memory impairment does not necessary occur in the early stages but is evident with progression in most cases; deficits on tests of attention and of frontal-subcortical skills and visuospatial ability can be especially prominent

Core features (two core features essential for a diagnosis of probable, one for possible, DLB)

1. Fluctuating cognition with pronounced variations in attention and alertness
2. Recurrent visual hallucinations that are typically well formed and detailed
3. Spontaneous motor features of parkinsonism

Supportive features

Repeated falls, syncope, transient loss of consciousness, neuroleptic sensitivity, systematized delusions, hallucinations in other modalities, REM sleep behavior disorder, depression

Features less likely to be present

1. History of stroke, evident as focal neurological signs or on brain imaging
2. Evidence on physical examination and investigation of any other physical illness or brain disorder sufficient to interfere with cognitive performance

---

Source: McKeith (2002); McKeith et al. (2004).

Clinical Features of DLB

Core clinical features of DLB are fluctuating cognitive impairment, recurrent visual hallucinations, and parkinsonism. Syncopal attacks with loss of consciousness and muscle tone may occur. Fluctuation of attention and cognition including transient episodes of unresponsiveness, occurs in 15% of DLB cases at presentation, and in 46% during the course of the illness. Extrapyramidal signs are reported in 25% to 50% of patients with DLB, at diagnosis, and most develop some signs during the course.

Sleep. DLB patients may have REM sleep behavior disorder (parasomnia manifested by vivid and frightening dreams, associated with simple or complex motor behavior during REM sleep), daytime hypersomnolence, hallucinations, and cataplexy. Sleep disorders also contribute to the fluctuations of DLB (McKeith et al., 2004).

Cognitive dysfunction in DLB. Cognitive impairment is the presenting feature of DLB, evidenced as recurrent episodes of confusion on a background of progressive intellectual deterioration (McKeith, 2002; Noe et al., 2004).

Prominent memory impairment is not common early in the course but develops in most patients as the disease progresses. It is predominantly a retrieval deficit syndrome. DLB patients without AD pathology do not have the poor retention and propensity to produce intrusion errors on cued recall characteristic of AD. Disproportionate visuospatial impairment and visuoconstructional dysfunction as manifested by poor performance on block design and clock drawing is evident. Executive impairment is prominent.

Attention may vary over minutes, hours, or days. This fluctuation occurs 50% to 75% at the time of presentation. Excessive daytime drowsiness with transient confusion on waking can occur and may last from a few seconds to several hours.

Behavioral and psychiatric symptoms of DLB. Psychiatric manifestations are common in DLB. Visual hallucinations, delusions, apathy, and anxiety are commonly present early and tend to persist over the course of the disease. Visual hallucinations are well-formed, detailed animate figures. Auditory hallucinations occur in 19% of cases. Olfactory and tactile hallucinations can occur in some cases. Delusions also are common in DLB, occurring in 50% of cases. Delusions may have a fixed, complex, bizarre content.

Treatment of DLB

The dementia of DLB may respond to treatment with cholinesterase inhibitors. Psychotic phenomenon may be ameliorated by quetiapine or other atypical antipsychotics. There is a high risk of worsening parkinsonism in DLB with antipsychotic agents and they must be used only with caution (McKeith et al., 1996).

MANAGEMENT OF ADVANCED DEMENTIA

The management strategies for individuals with severe dementia include

1. General medical care
2. Nonpharmacological management of behavioral symptoms
3. Pharmacological management of behavioral symptoms.

General Medical Care

Infections. Geriatric patients are more susceptible to infections than younger individuals. Infection is a nearly inevitable complication of the dementia process because of loss of ambulation, incontinence, malnutrition, and aspiration. These cause recurrent infections, especially pneumonia. Another common site of infection is the skin. Neglect of skin care in the elderly may lead not only to the infection but also to poor quality of life. The most common skin problems found in elderly nursing home residents are scabies, cellulitis, herpes zoster, pressure ulcers, and lichen simplex chronicus (Norman, 2003).

Nursing home patients with restricted mobility, poor nutrition, and incontinence are at risk for decubitus ulcer formation. Bed-ridden patients should be turned from side to side at 30° angles at least every 2 h. Special mattresses, splints, cradle boots, barrier ointments, and absorptive products may help to reduce the likelihood of developing ulcerations. Scheduled toileting for incontinence may prevent dampness, and good nutritional status is essential.

Hydration/nutrition. The main cause of malnutrition in dementia is that nursing home residents have eating difficulties and weight loss. Other causes of eating abnormalities such as depression should be sought. Treatment with antidepressants can enhance food intake even in advanced stages of dementia.

In those with advanced dementia, there are simple maneuvers such as modifying the consistency of the food or treating dental problems that may facilitate eating. Patients with problems opening the mouth or swallowing spontaneously may benefit from verbal cues when feeding, gentle massaging of the cheeks to prevent pouching of food, or using straws to promote drinking of liquid nutrition supplements. Thick liquids may induce less choking than thin liquids.

Dronabinol is associated with increased food intake when used as an antiemetic in cancer patients; it also enhances appetite and sense of well-being, as well as weight gain in acquired immunodeficiency syndrome patients. In a placebo-controlled crossover design study in 15 AD patients with food refusal, body weight of patients increased more with dronabinol treatment than placebo. Euphoria, somnolence, and tiredness were observed more commonly during the dronabinol treatment period (Volicer et al., 1997).

Feeding tubes may be considered in patients unresponsive to these strategies. Approximately 10% of advanced dementia patients living in United States nursing homes have feeding tubes. The goal of insertion of a feeding tube is to provide adequate nutrients and sufficient calories to facilitate weight gain and increase serum albumin. However, no randomized controlled studies have examined the effectiveness of feeding tubes in prolonging life, and retrospective studies suggest that there is no survival benefit (Gillick, 2001). Similarly, there is no evidence that feeding tubes prevent aspiration. On the contrary, aspiration pneumonia is a leading cause of death in nursing home patients with feeding tubes. Nursing home patients with feeding tubes are often restrained to prevent self-extubation leading to agitation and infringement of personal dignity.

Urinary incontinence. Urinary incontinence (UI) is highly prevalent in nursing homes, affecting 50% to 70% of institutionalized dementia patients. UI may cause increased moisture in the perineal area, irritation, pressure ulcers, delayed wound healing, and urinary tract infections. Detailed urodynamic studies indicate that detrusor overactivity is the predominant cause. The first management step is to evaluate medical causes and medication side effects. Modifying the environment, placing signs or pictures on bathroom doors, and ensuring adequate lighting may reduce incontinence. Behavioral modification is reported to be helpful. Toileting every 2 h while awake, restricting bedtime liquids, and providing physiotherapy to improve gait speed may reduce incontinence episodes (Holroyd, 2004; Sutor et al., 2001; Volicer, 2001).

Management of Behavioral Symptoms of Dementia: Nonpharmacological Approaches

Patients with dementia have an impaired ability to learn or reason. Caregivers who spend time trying to reorient, "teach" new information, or provide full explanations will often be frustrated. Caregivers who learn what to expect as the disease progresses can anticipate cognitive and functional limitations as well as behavioral changes (Sutor et al., 2001). Despite advancing cognitive loss, older adults with dementia retain basic human needs, including the need to belong, to be loved, to be touched, and to feel useful. Unfortunately, meaningful relationships and appropriate social groups are often unavailable or insufficiently matched to the functional level of such patients.

Staff education. Staff may benefit from education in the use of structured guidelines for the management of behavioral symptoms including appropriate use of psychotropic drugs for behavioral management and alternative management strategies. Teaching coping skills and stress reduction techniques or providing new information about the disease and its treatment lead to better management of behaviorally disturbed nursing home patients.

Environmental modification. Behavioral symptoms are closely related to a patient's caregiver, social environment, and physical environment. Different environmental modifications work best for patients in each stage of impairment.

The physical and psychological environment should be familiar to help patients remain oriented and increase the person's sense of identity by stimulating memory (Alzheimer's Association Australia, 2000). In addition, the environment should encourage patients to participate in tasks and activities. Activities should be adjusted to balance security and safety with patient independence.

To limit wandering, doors leading to the outside should be locked, alarmed, or controlled (Teresi et al., 2000). Hearing aids and glasses and appropriate use of lighting may reduce confusion. In addition, glare from windows or noise from televisions may annoy the patient and lead to restlessness. Falls may be prevented by removing hazardous furniture that is difficult to see and replacing extension cords and telephone lines that may trip. Installation of grab bars by the toilet and in the shower may reduce falls.

Behavioral interventions. The American Academy of Neurology Practice Guidelines for dementia supported use of several evidence-based nonpharmacological behavioral interventions. Interventions such as short-term educational programs or support group programs may increase caregivers' disease knowledge and satisfaction and increase confidence and the ability to cope. An intensive long-term education and support program for caregivers delayed time to nursing home placements by 12 to 24 months. In addition, specialized training of staff in nursing homes can significantly diminish the use of antipsychotic medication in AD patients without increasing disruptive behaviors (Doody et al., 2001). Behavioral modification is another effective strategy for management in dementia patients. Graded assistance with positive reinforcement can improve performance in daily activities. Scheduled toileting and prompted voiding are strongly recommended for urinary incontinence. Occupational rehabilitation such as memory training, creative activities, improving sensorimotor functions, and self-management therapy can improve cognitive performance, psychosocial functioning, emotional balance, and subjective well-being.

Music can reduce agitation, aggression, and mood disturbances particularly while eating or bathing. One-on-one social interaction or videotapes of family members may reduce verbally disruptive behaviors. Walking and light exercise are helpful for demented individuals, reducing wandering, aggression, and agitation (Doody et al., 2001).

Pharmacologic Management

Antipsychotic agents: More than 40% of patients with dementia living in residential or nursing home care facilities are prescribed antipsychotic drugs (Furniss et al., 1998). In a survey study of antipsychotic prescriptions in 909 elderly residents to nursing homes in Glasgow, without history of schizophrenia or other major psychoses, it was found that 17% were given a prescription for an antipsychotic drug within 100 days and 24% within 1 year of their index date (Bronskill et al., 2004). In another survey, 24% of residents were taking antipsychotic drugs regularly, but only 12% of this use was appropriate according to treatment guidelines (McGrath et al., 1996). No antipsychotics are specifically approved for treatment of patients with dementia, and their usage must be balanced between perceived benefits and risks. Table 2.9 lists the antipsychotic agents commonly used to treat nursing home residents.

Risperidone has been used to treat agitation in older patients with dementia. The 1988 Expert Consensus Guideline for the treatment of agitation of older people with dementia recommended starting doses of 0.25 to 0.5 mg/d with an average target dose of 0.5 to 1.5 mg/d (Kasckow et al., 2004). Extrapyramidal symptoms may be precipitated and require careful monitoring.

Olanzapine also has been studied for the ability to reduce psychosis and agitation in nursing home residents with AD. Olanzapine doses of 5 and 10 mg produced significant reduction in these symptoms. Adverse effects included somnolence and abnormal gait (Street et al., 2000). In addition, olanzapine can produce of orthostasis and weight gain (Kasckow et al., 2004).

TABLE 2.9. Comparative Side Effects of Atypical Antipsychotic Drugs and Haloperidol

	HALOPERIDOL	RISPERIDONE	OLANZAPINE	QUETIAPINE
EPS	+++	0 to ++	0 to +	0
Metabolic syndrome	+	+ to ++	+++	+ to ++
TD	+++	0 to +	0 to +	0 to +
Prolactin elevation	+++	+++	0 to +	0
Hypotension	+	+ to ++	+	+ to ++
QTc prolongation	0	0	0	0
Weight gain	+	++	++ to +++	++
Sedation	+	+	+ to ++	+ to ++
Anticholinergic effect	0 to +	0 to +	+ to ++	0 to +
Seizures		0 to +	0 to +	0 to +

Source: Adapted from Tandon and Jibson (2003); Tandon et al. (1999).
Note: 0, absent; +, minimal; ++, moderate; +++, severe; EPS, extrapyramidal side effects; TD, tardive dyskinesia.

Quentiapine may reduce agitation and psychosis in dementia without precipitating parkinsonism. The optimal dose is 200 mg/d; sedation is the most common side effect.

Atypical antipsychotics have been associated with an increased risk of all-cause mortality in the elderly. They must be used with caution and sparingly in this population.

Antiepileptic drugs. Antiepileptics have been reported to reduce agitation, aggression, irritability, and impulsivity across a wide range of illnesses including dementia. A randomized, multisite, parallel-group study of 51 nursing home patients with dementia and agitation showed greater reduction of agitation after 6 weeks in the carbamazapine-treated patients than in the placebo group. There was a decrease in agitation and aggression without change in cognition. Side effects included drowsiness, disorientation, ataxia, and postural instability (Tariot et al., 1998). Treatment is initiated with a dose of 100 mg/d, advancing in 50 mg or 100 mg increments every 3 to 7 days until clinical benefits or toxicity are seen. The usual daily dose ranges from 300 to 500 mg (Qizilbash et al., 2002).

The anticonvulsant valproate also has been reported to be effective in the management of behavioral disturbances in dementia and tends to have fewer drug–drug interactions compared with carbamazapine. A randomized placebo-controlled study of divalproex sodium conducted in 56 demented nursing home patients with agitation found significantly reduced agitation in those treated with the active agent (Porsteinsson et al., 2001). Negative studies also have been reported (Tariot et al., 2005). Valproate can cause symptoms of nausea, sedation, gastrointestinal distress, and diarrhea. In addition, dose-dependent liver enzyme elevation may occur and, rarely, hepatotoxicity. Other effects such as mild thrombocytopenia, weight gain, and hair loss may occur. Available evidence suggests initiating treatment at a dose of 125 mg/b.i.d., increasing in 125 mg increments every 3 to 5 days until benefit is seen or toxicity occurs. The usual daily dose ranges from 750 to 1250 mg (Qizilbash et al., 2002).

Antidepressants. With the superior side effects of profiles of SSRIs compared with TCAs, recent studies have addressed the use of these agents in managing depression in patients with dementia. Citalopram and sertraline have been demonstrated to reduce mood symptoms in this setting (Lebert et al., 1994; Martinon-Torres et al., 2004; Nyth et al., 1992; Peskind, 2003; Roose et al., 2003). Side effects included orthostasis, falls, and somnolence.

Anxiolytics. Benzodiazepines previously were commonly used to treat agitated behavior in demented patients. Oxazepam was commonly prescribed and one double-blind placebo-controlled study showed superior effects of oxazepam compared with chlordiazepoxide in reducing the anxiety symptoms (Qizilbash et al., 2002). Side effects such as increasing confusion, oversedation, dizziness, ataxia, paradoxical agitation, tolerance, and withdrawal limit use of these compounds in the elderly.

Buspirone, a serotonergic 5-HT1A agonist with anxiolytic effects, has also been used to treat aggression in dementia patients in doses ranging from 15 to 60 mg/d. Agitation, oppositional behavior, sexual disinhibition, verbal and physical aggression, screaming, and catastrophic reactions improved. Buspirone is as a well-tolerated drug without sedation, drowsiness, or confusional effects (Erkinjuntti, 2002).

Hypnotics. No hypnotics have been approved specifically for use in dementia. Zolpidem is a nonbenzodiazepine hypnotic agent that acts via γ-aminobutyrate (GABA)-A receptors to induce sleep with no significant suppression of REM sleep and unchanged slow-wave sleep. Zolpidem in average doses of 10 to 15 mg before bed time can increase sleep from 2–3 to 7–8 h each night (Shelton & Hocking, 1997). Zolpidem has few reported adverse effects, a low rate of dependence and is well tolerated for elderly: There are infrequent reports of confusion, anterograde amnesia, and somnambulism occurring within 30 to 60 min of ingestion. Rare patients have headaches, drowsiness, and nightmares (Wortelboer et al., 2002). Other nonbenzodiazepine hypnotics and melatonin receptor agonists may benefit sleep in patients with dementia. Evidence with regard to the utility of melatonin in improving sleep is mixed. Some studies report a beneficial effect (Brusco et al., 1999), whereas others found no sleep enhancement (Serfaty et al., 2002; Singer et al., 2003).

NURSING HOME STAFF

Annual turnover of staff in nursing homes ranges from 40% to 96% in the United States (Cohen-Mansfield, 1997). This high turnover reflects work stress and poor job satisfaction. Staff stress is associated with working with cognitive impaired patients, resident aggression, and difficult and unpredictable resident behavior

(Brodaty et al., 2003; Rodney, 2000). When stress levels become overwhelming, role conflict, goal ambiguity, poor self-esteem, and burnout may occur (Mobily et al., 1992). Over 30% of the staff report that there were not enough opportunities at work to discuss the psychological stress of the job and over 55% felt that they knew too little about the residents' disease and treatments. Caregiver education, providing support, and developing coping skills may help reduce turnover rate and stress (Brodaty et al., 2003).

FAMILY CAREGIVERS OF NURSING HOME PATIENTS

The cognitive deterioration and behavioral manifestations of dementia regularly cause great emotional stress in the lives of family caregivers and eventually may lead to patient institutionalization. Although relocation may relieve caregivers from complete responsibility, they must develop a different role in caring for their institutionalized relatives. Stress may increase from loss of a positive relationship and from their guilt about placing the patient in a nursing home. There may be feelings of confinement imposed by the obligations to provide care and from conflict with staff caregivers who may see family as intruders. Institutionalization may offer the opportunity for the family caregiver to devote more time to support, enhancing the patient's quality of life, improving their relationship, introducing behavior modification, or participating in specific supportive care for their relative. Nevertheless, most family caregivers lack knowledge of how to adapt to their new role in caring. Families should be oriented to nursing home facilities. They require education about involvement in care: they will need to develop a partnership with the care giving staff. This intervention may improve the experience of family members with patients in nursing homes and can positively improve nursing home staff attitudes toward family members (Maas et al., 2004). Spouses are the caregivers who remain the most actively involved with patients after nursing home placement. Almost half of spouses who visit the nursing home daily have high levels of depression and anxiety both before and after placement. They lack adequate support from others, may require intervention as part of the placement process, and may need pharmacologic treatment for anxiety and depression as well as the support of family and friends (Schulz et al., 2004).

CONCLUSION

Dementia is common in nursing home residents and is complicated by behavioral disturbances, progressive loss of functions, and increasing medical comorbidity. Preventive treatments and therapy of active problems can reduce symptoms and improve quality of life.

Acknowledgments   The author is supported by a National Institute on Aging Alzheimer's Disease Research Center Grant (P50AG16570) and Alzheimer's Disease Research Center of California Grant, the Sidell-Kagan Foundation, and the Deane F. Johnson Alzheimer's Research Foundation.

REFERENCES

Aarsland, D., Andersen, K., Larsen, J. P., Lolk, A., & Kragh-Sorensen, P. (2003). Prevalence and characteristics of dementia in Parkinson disease: An 8-year prospective study. *Archives of Neurology, 60*, 387–392.

American Psychiatric Association. (2000). *Diagnostic and statistical manual of mental disorders* (4th ed., text revision). Washington, DC: Author.

Anderson, K. E., & Weiner, W. J. (2002). Psychiatric symptoms in Parkinson's disease. *Current Neurology and Neuroscience Reports, 2*, 303–309.

Australia Alzheimer's Association. (2000). *At home with dementia: The environment and dementia.* Author. http://www.add.nsw.gov.au

Bliwise, D. L. (2004). Sleep disorders in Alzheimer's disease and other dementias. *Clinical Cornerstone, 6*(Suppl 1A), 16–28.

Bosboom, J. L., Stoffers, D., & Wolters, E. (2004). Cognitive dysfunction and dementia in Parkinson's disease. *Journal of Neural Transmission, 111*, 1303–1315.

Boyle, P. A., & Malloy, P. F. (2004). Treating apathy in Alzheimer's disease. *Dementia and Geriatric Cognitive Disorders, 17*, 91–99.

Boyle, P. A., Malloy, P. F., Salloway, S., Cahn-Weiner, D. A., Cohen, R., & Cummings, J. L. (2003). Executive dysfunction and apathy predict functional impairment in Alzheimer disease. *American Journal of Geriatric Psychiatry, 11*, 214–221.

Brodaty, H., Draper, B., Low, L. F. (2003). Nursing home staff attitudes towards residents with dementia: strain and satisfaction with work. *Journal of Advanced Nursing, 44*, 583–590.

Bronskill, S. E., Anderson, G. M., Sykora, K., et al. (2004). Neuroleptic drug therapy in older adults newly admitted to nursing homes: Incidence, dose, and specialist contact. *Journal of the American Geriatric Society, 52*, 749–755.

Brusco, L. I., Fainstein, I., Marquez, M., & Cardinali, D. P. (1999). Effect of melatonin in selected populations of sleep-disturbed patients. *Biological Signals and Receptors, 8*, 126–131.

Calne, D. B., Snow, B. J., & Lee, C. (1992). Criteria for diagnosing Parkinson's disease. *Annals of Neurology, 32*(Suppl), 125–127.

Cohen-Mansfield, J. (1997). Turnover among nursing home staff. A review. *Nursing Management, 28*, 59–62, 64.

Cook, S. E., Miyahara, S., Bacanu, S. A., et al. (2003). Psychotic symptoms in Alzheimer disease: Evidence for subtypes. *American Journal of Geriatric Psychiatry, 11*, 406–413.

Cummings, J. (2003). *The neuropsychiatry of Alzheimer's disease and related dementias.* London, England: Martin Dunitz.

Cummings, J. L. (1992). Depression and Parkinson's disease: A review. *American Journal of Psychiatry, 149*, 443–454.

Cummings, J. L. (2004). Drug therapy: Alzheimer's disease. *New England Journal of Medicine, 351*, 56–67.

Cummings, J. L., & Mega, M. S. (2003). *Neuropsychiatry and behavioral neuroscience.* New York: Oxford University Press.

Cummings, J. L., Schneider, L., Tariot, P. N., Kershaw, P. R., & Yuan, W. (2004). Reduction of behavioral disturbances and caregiver distress by galantamine in patients with Alzheimer's disease. *American Journal of Psychiatry, 161,* 532–538.

Delacourte, A., David, J. P., Sergeant, N., et al. (1999). The biochemical pathway of neurofibrillary degeneration in aging and Alzheimer's disease. *Neurology, 52,* 1158–1165.

Doody, R. S., Stevens, J. C., Beck, C., et al. (2001). Practice parameter: Management of dementia (an evidence-based review). Report of the Quality Standards Subcommittee of the American Academy of Neurology. *Neurology, 56,* 1154–1166.

Doraiswamy, P. M., Leon, J., Cummings, J. L., Marin, D., & Neuman, P. (2002). Prevalence and impact of medical comorbidity in Alzheimer's disease. *Journal of Gerontology Series A: Biological Sciences and Medical Sciences, 57,* 173–177.

Emre, M. (2003). Dementia associated with Parkinson's disease. *Lancet Neurology, 2,* 229–237.

Erkinjuntti, T. (2002). Diagnosis and management of vascular cognitive impairment and dementia. *Journal of Neural Transmission Supplement, 63*(Suppl), 91–109.

Erkinjuntti, T., Kurz, A., Gauthier, S., et al. (2002). Efficacy of galantamine in probable vascular dementia and Alzheimer's disease combined with cerebrovascular disease: A randomised trial. *Lancet, 359,* 1283–1290.

Farlow, M. R. (2003). Update on rivastigmine. *The Neurologist, 9,* 230–234.

Feldman, H., Gauthier, S., Hecker, J., et al. (2003). Efficacy of donepezil on maintenance of activities of daily living in patients with moderate to severe Alzheimer's disease and the effect on caregiver burden. *Journal of the American Geriatric Society, 51,* 737–744.

Fernandez, H. H., & Lapane, K. L. (2002). Predictors of mortality among nursing home residents with a diagnosis of Parkinson's disease. *Medical Science Monitor, 8,* 241–246.

Fratiglioni, L. (1996). Epidemiology of Alzheimer's disease and current possibilities for prevention. *Acta Neurologica Scandinavica Supplementum, 165,* 33–40.

Furniss, L., Craig, S. K., & Burns, A. (1998). Medication use in nursing homes for elderly people. *International Journal of Geriatric Psychiatry, 13,* 433–439.

Gauthier, S., Feldman, H., Hecker, J., et al. (2002). Efficacy of donepezil on behavioral symptoms in patients with moderate to severe Alzheimer's disease. *International Psychogeriatrics, 14,* 389–404.

Giladi, N., Shabtai, H., Gurevich, T., Benbunan, B., Anca, M., & Korczyn, A. D. (2003). Rivastigmine (Exelon) for dementia in patients with Parkinson's disease. *Acta Neurologica Scandinavica, 108,* 368–373.

Gillette-Guyonnet, S., Nourhashemi, F., Andrieu, S., et al. (2000). Weight loss in Alzheimer's disease. *American Journal of Clinical Nutrition, 71,* 637S–642S.

Gillick, M. (2001). When the nursing home resident with advanced dementia stops eating: What is the medical director to do? *Journal of American Medical Directors Association, 2,* 259–263.

Gold, G., Giannakopoulos, P., Montes-Paixao, C., et al. (1997). Sensitivity and specificity of newly proposed clinical criteria for possible vascular dementia. *Neurology, 49,* 690–694.

Hebert, L. E., Scherr, P. A., Bienias, J. L., Bennett, D. A., & Evans, D. A. (2003). Alzheimer disease in the US population: Prevalence estimates using the 2000 census. *Archives of Neurology, 60,* 1119–1122.

Heidebrink, J. L. (2002). Is dementia with Lewy bodies the second most common cause of dementia? *Journal of Geriatric Psychiatry and Neurology, 15,* 182–187.

Holroyd, S. (2004). Managing dementia in long-term care settings. *Clinics in Geriatric Medicine, 20*, 83–92.

Jeste, D. V., & Finkel, S. I. (2000). Psychosis of Alzheimer's disease and related dementias. *American Journal of Geriatric Psychiatry, 8*, 29–34.

Kasckow, J. W., Mulchahey, J. J., & Mohamed, S. (2004). The use of novel antipsychotics in the older patient with neurodegenerative disorders in the long-term care setting. *Journal of the American Medical Directors Association, 5*, 242–248.

Lapane, K. L., Fernandez, H. H., & Friedman, J. H. (1999). Prevalence, clinical characteristics, and pharmacologic treatment of Parkinson's disease in residents in long-term care facilities. SAGE Study Group. *Pharmacotherapy, 19*, 1321–1327.

Lebert, F., Pasquier, F., & Petit, H. (1994). Behavioral effects of trazodone in Alzheimer's disease. *Journal of Clinical Psychiatry, 55*, 536–538.

Lebert, F., Pasquier, F., & Petit, H. (1996). Sundowning syndrome in demented patients without neuroleptic therapy. *Archives of Gerontology and Geriatrics, 22*, 49–54.

Lee, H. B., & Lyketsos, C. G. (2003). Depression in Alzheimer's disease: Heterogeneity and related issues. *Biological Psychiatry, 54*, 353–362.

Leger, J. M., Moulias, R., Robert, P., et al. (2002). Agitation and aggressiveness among the elderly population living in nursing or retirement homes in France. *International Psychogeriatric Association, 14*, 405–416.

Leys, D., Pasquier, F., & Parnetti, L. (1998). Epidemiology of vascular dementia. *Haemostasis, 28*, 134–150.

Lopez, O. L., Larumbe, M. R., Becker, J. T., et al. (1994). Reliability of NINDS-AIREN clinical criteria for the diagnosis of vascular dementia. *Neurology, 44*, 1240–1245.

Maas, M. L., Reed, D., Park, M., et al. (2004). Outcomes of family involvement in care intervention for caregivers of individuals with dementia. *Nursing Research, 53*, 76–86.

Macdonald, A. J., Carpenter, G. I., Box, O., Roberts, A., & Sahu, S. (2002). Dementia and use of psychotropic medication in non-"Elderly Mentally Infirm" nursing homes in South East England. *Age and Ageing, 31*, 58–64.

Malouf, R., & Birks, J. (2004). Donepezil for vascular cognitive impairment. *Cochrane Database Systemic Review*, CD004395.

Martinon-Torres, G., Fioravanti, M., & Grimley, E. J. (2004). Trazodone for agitation in dementia. *Cochrane Database Systemic Review*, CD004990.

Matthews, F. E., & Dening, T. (2002). Prevalence of dementia in institutional care. *Lancet, 360*, 225–226.

Mayeux, R. (1994). Diagnostic problems in nursing home patients with dementia: Why we should and how we can improve accuracy. *Alzheimer Disease and Associated Disorders, 8*(1), S184–S187.

McGrath, A. M., & Jackson, G. A. (1996). Survey of neuroleptic prescribing in residents of nursing homes in Glasgow. *BMJ, 312*, 611–612.

McKeith, I. (2004). Dementia in Parkinson's disease: Common and treatable. *Lancet Neurology, 3*, 456.

McKeith, I., Mintzer, J., Aarsland, D., et al. (2004). Dementia with Lewy bodies. *Lancet Neurology, 3*, 19–28.

McKeith, I. G. (2000). Spectrum of Parkinson's disease, Parkinson's dementia, and Lewy body dementia. *Neurology Clinic, 18*(4), 865–902.

McKeith, I. G. (2002). Dementia with Lewy bodies. *British Journal of Psychiatry, 180*, 144–147.

McKeith, I. G., Galasko, D., Kosaka, K., et al. (1996). Consensus guidelines for the clinical and pathologic diagnosis of dementia with Lewy bodies (DLB): Report of the consortium on DLB international workshop. *Neurology, 47*, 1113–1124.

McKhann, G., Drachman, D., Folstein, M., Katzman, R., Price, D., & Stadlan, E. M. (1984). Clinical diagnosis of Alzheimer's disease: Report of the NINCDS-ADRDA Work Group under the auspices of Department of Health and Human Services Task Force on Alzheimer's Disease. *Neurology, 34,* 939–944.

Mendez, M. F., & Cummings, J. L. (2003). *Dementia: A clinical approach* (3rd ed.). Philadelphia, PA: Butterworth Heinemann,.

Mitchell, S. L., Kiely, D. K., Kiel, D. P., & Lipsitz, L. A. (1996). The epidemiology, clinical characteristics, and natural history of older nursing home residents with a diagnosis of Parkinson's disease. *Journal of the American Geriatric Society, 44,* 394–399.

Mobily, P. R., Maas, M. L., Buckwalter, K. C., & Kelley, L. S. (1992). Staff stress on an Alzheimer's unit. *Journal of Psychosocial Nursing and Mental Health Services, 30,* 25–31.

Moretti, R., Torre, P., Antonello, R. M., Cazzato, G., & Bava, A. (2003). Rivastigmine in subcortical vascular dementia: A randomized, controlled, open 12-month study in 208 patients. *American Journal of Alzheimer's Disease and Other Dementias, 18,* 265–272.

Moroney, J. T., Bagiella, E., Desmond, D. W., et al. (1997). Meta-analysis of the Hachinski Ischemic Score in pathologically verified dementias. *Neurology, 49,* 1096–1105.

Newman, S. C. (1999). The prevalence of depression in Alzheimer's disease and vascular dementia in a population sample. *Journal of Affective Disorders, 52,* 169–176.

Noe, E., Marder, K., Bell, K. L., Jacobs, D. M., Manly, J. J., & Stern, Y. (2004). Comparison of dementia with Lewy bodies to Alzheimer's disease and Parkinson's disease with dementia. *Movement Disorders, 19,* 60–67.

Norman, R. A. (2003). Long-term care dermatology. *Dermatologic Therapy, 16,* 186–194.

Nygaard, H. A., & Ruths, S. (2003). Missing the diagnosis: Senile dementia in patients admitted to nursing homes. *Scandinavian Journal of Primary Health Care, 21,* 148–152.

Nyth, A., Gottfries, C., Lyby, K., et al. (1992). A controlled multicenter clinical study of citalopram and placebo in elderly depressed patients with and without concomitant dementia. *Acta Psychiatrica Scandinavica, 86,* 138–145.

O'Brien, J. A., & Caro, J. J. (2001). Alzheimer's disease and other dementia in nursing homes: Levels of management and cost. *International Psychogeriatrics, 13,* 347–358.

Olin, J. T., Schneider, L. S., Katz, I. R., et al. (2002). Provisional diagnostic criteria for depression of Alzheimer disease. *American Journal of Geriatric Psychiatry, 10,* 125–128.

Orgogozo, J. M., Rigaud, A. S., Stoffler, A., Mobius, H. J., & Forette, F. (2002). Efficacy and safety of memantine in patients with mild to moderate vascular dementia: A randomized, placebo-controlled trial (MMM 300). *Stroke, 33,* 1834–1839.

Peskind, E. R. (2003). Management of depression in long-term care of patients with Alzheimer's disease. *Journal of American Medical Directors Association, 4,* S141–S145.

Porsteinsson, A. P., Tariot, P. N., Erb, R., et al. (2001). Placebo-controlled study of divalproex sodium for agitation in dementia. *American Journal of Geriatric Psychiatry, 9,* 58–66.

Qizilbash, N., Broadaty, H., Chiu, H., & Kaye, J. (2002). *Evidence-based dementia practice.* Cambridge, MA: Blackwell.

Reisberg, B., Doody, R., Stoffler, A., Schmitt, F., Ferris, S., & Mobius, H. J. (2003). Memantine in moderate-to-severe Alzheimer's disease. *New England Journal of Medicine, 348,* 1333–1341.

Richard, I. H., Kurlan, R., & Group, P. S. (1997). A survey of antidepressant drug use in Parkinson's disease. *Neurology, 49,* 1168–1170.

Rindlisbacher, P., & Hopkins, R. W. (1992). An investigation of the sundowning syndrome. *International Journal of Geriatric Psychiatry, 7,* 15–23.

Rodney, V. (2000). Nurse stress associated with aggression in people with dementia: Its relationship to hardiness, cognitive appraisal and coping. *Journal of Advances in Nursing, 31,* 172–180.

Roman, G. C., Tatemichi, T. K., Erkinjuntti, T., et al. (1993). Vascular dementia: Diagnostic criteria for research studies: Report of the NINDS-AIREN international workshop. *Neurology, 43,* 250–260.

Roose, S. P., Nelson, J. C., Salzman, C., Hollander, S. B., & Rodrigues, H. (2003). Open-label study of mirtazapine orally disintegrating tablets in depressed patients in the nursing home. *Current Medical Research and Opinion, 19,* 737–746.

Rovner, B. W., German, P. S., Broadhead, J., et al. (1990). The prevalence and management of dementia and other psychiatric disorders in nursing home. *International Psychogeriatrics, 2,* 13–24.

Sagar, H. J., Cohen, N. J., Sullivan, E. V., Corkin, S., & Growdon, J. H. (1988). Remote memory function in Alzheimer's disease and Parkinson's disease. *Brain, 111*(Pt 1), 185–206.

Samii, A., Nutt, J. G., & Ransom, B. R. (2004). Parkinson's disease. *Lancet, 363,* 1783–1793.

Schneider, L. S., & Dagerman, K. S. (2004). Psychosis of Alzheimer's disease: Clinical characteristics and history. *Journal of Psychiatric Research, 38,* 105–111.

Schulz, R., Belle, S. H., Czaja, S. J., McGinnis, K. A., Stevens, A., & Zhang, S. (2004). Long-term care placement of dementia patients and caregiver health and well-being. *JAMA, 292,* 961–967.

Serfaty, M., Kennell-Webb, S., Warner, J., Blizard, R., & Raven, P. (2002). Double-blind randomised placebo controlled trial of low dose melatonin for sleep disorders in dementia. *International Journal of Geriatric Psychiatry, 17,* 1120–1127.

Shelton, P. S., & Hocking, L. B. (1997). Zolpidem for dementia-related insomnia and nighttime wandering. *Annals of Pharmacotherapy, 31,* 319–322.

Singer, C., Tractenberg, R. E., Kaye, J., et al. (2003). A multicenter, placebo-controlled trial of melatonin for sleep disturbance in Alzheimer's disease. *Sleep Medicine Review, 26,* 893–901.

Slaughter, J. R., Slaughter, K. A., Nichols, D., Holmes, S. E., & Martens, M. P. (2001). Prevalence, clinical manifestations, etiology, and treatment of depression in Parkinson's disease. *Journal of Neuropsychiatry and Clinical Neurosciences, 13,* 187–196.

Smith Doody, R. (2003). Update on Alzheimer drugs (donepezil). *Neurologist, 9,* 225–229.

Street, J., Clark W. S., Gannon, K. S., et al. (2000). Olanzapine treatment of psychotic and behavioral symptoms in patients with Alzheimer's disease in nursing care facilities. A double-blind, randomized, placebo-controlled trial. *Archives of General Psychiatry, 57,* 968–976.

Sutor, B., Rummans, T. A., & Smith, G. E. (2001). Assessment and management of behavioral disturbances in nursing home patients with dementia. *Mayo Clinic Proceedings, 76,* 540–550.

Suzuki, K., Otsuka, Y., Endo, K., et al. (2003). Visuospatial deficits due to impaired visual attention: Investigation of two cases of slowly progressive visuospatial impairment. *Cortex, 39,* 327–341.

Tandon, R., & Jibson, M. D. (2003). Safety and tolerability: How do second-generation atypical antipsychotics compare? Current Science, 1, 15–21.

Tandon, R., Milner, K., & Jibson, M. D. (1999) Antipsychotics from theory to practice: Integrating clinical and basic data. Journal of Clinical Psychiatry, 60(Suppl 8), 21–28.

Tariot, P. N., Cummings, J. L., Katz, I. R., et al. (2001). A randomized, double-blind, placebo-controlled study of the efficacy and safety of donepezil in patients with Alzheimer's disease in the nursing home setting. Journal of the American Geriatric Society, 49, 1590–1599.

Tariot, P. N., Erb, R., Podgorski, C., et al. (1998). Efficacy and tolerability of cabamazepine for agitation and aggression in dementia. American Journal of Psychiatry, 155, 54–61.

Tariot, P. N., Farlow, M. R., Grossberg, G. T., Graham, S. M., McDonald, S., & Gergel, I. (2004). Memantine treatment in patients with moderate to severe Alzheimer disease already receiving donepezil: A randomized controlled trial. JAMA, 291, 317–324.

Tariot, P. N., Raman, R., Jakimovich, L., et al. (2005). Divalproex sodium in nursing home residents with possible or probable Alzheimer Disease complicated by agitation: A randomized, controlled trial. American Journal of Geriatric Psychiatry, 13, 942–949.

Teresi, J., Lawton, M. P., Ory, M., & Holmes, D. (1994). Measurement issues in chronic care populations: Dementia special care. Alzheimer Disease and Associated Disorders, 8(Suppl 1), 144–183.

Teresi, J. A., Holmes, D., & Ory, M. G. (2000). The therapeutic design of environments for people with dementia: Further reflections and recent findings from the National Institute on Aging Collaborative studies of Dementia special care units. The Gerontologist, 40, 417–421.

Volicer, L. (2001). Management of severe Alzheimer's disease and end-of-life issues. Clinics in Geriatric Medicine, 17, 377–391.

Volicer, L., Stelly, M., Morris, J., McLaughlin, J., & Volicer, B. J. (1997). Effects of dronabinol on anorexia and disturbed behavior in patients with Alzheimer's disease. International Journal of Geriatric Psychiatry, 12, 913–919.

White, H. K., McConnell, E. S., Bales, C. W., & Kuchibhatla, M. (2004). A 6-month observational study of the relationship between weight loss and behavioral symptoms in institutionalized Alzheimer's disease subjects. Journal of the American Medical Directors Association, 5, 89–97.

Wilcock, G. K. (2003). Memantine for the treatment of dementia. Lancet Neurology, 2, 503–505.

Winblad, B., Kilander, L., Eriksson, S., et al. (2006). Donepezil in patients with severe Alzheimer's disease: Double-blind, parallel-group, placebo-controlled study. Lancet, 367, 1057–1065.

Wortelboer, U., Cohrs, S., Rodenbeck, A., & Ruther, E. (2002). Tolerability of hypno-sedatives in older patients. Drugs Aging, 19, 529–539.

Zubenko, G. S., Zubenko, W. N., McPherson, S., et al. (2003). A collaborative study of the emergence and clinical features of the major depressive syndrome of Alzheimer's disease. American Journal of Psychiatry, 160, 857–866.

3

Delirium in the Nursing Home Setting

Steven F. Huege and *Joel E. Streim*

Although extensively studied in the acute care setting, the syndrome of delirium—also referred to as acute confusion—has been a subject of relatively few studies in the long-term care (LTC) setting. Delirium represents a significant source of morbidity and mortality for patients in nursing homes. Studies indicate that the incidence of acute confusion in residents of LTC facilities ranges from 14% to 40% (Culp et al., 1997; Mentes et al., 1999). Although cognitive impairment is common in the nursing home setting, in some instances it may be reversible. Sabin et al. (1982) found that 25% of LTC facility residents with impaired cognition had a potentially reversible condition, and 6% to 12% of nursing home residents with dementia showed improvement in cognitive performance over the course of 1 year (Katz, 1991). However, it is not known what proportion of the patients in these studies actually met criteria for a diagnosis of delirium.

Nursing home residents may require transfer to a hospital because of the acute onset of confusion due to an undiagnosed medical illness; or they may be admitted for an acute medical illness with unrecognized confusion or change in mental status. Levkoff et al. (1991) found that 52% of hospitalized older adults admitted from institutional settings suffered from delirium. Conversely, elderly patients are often discharged to LTC facilities with unresolved delirium after initial inpatient treatment of an acute illness. Among these are patients without a previous need for nursing home placement. With the introduction of diagnosis-related groups

(DRGs) and other prospective payment systems (PPS), acute care facilities face increasing pressure to reduce lengths of stay in the hospital. As a result, many elderly patients are discharged early from inpatient hospital beds and are admitted to subacute care beds located in nursing homes if additional time is required for rehabilitation or convalescence before returning home. These patients commonly have residual symptoms of delirium, including cognitive impairment, as they recover from their underlying acute medical illness. The presence of delirium may be a reason for admission to a nursing home and might also serve as an impediment to successful care and rehabilitation while the patient is recovering in the nursing home.

Because of the prevalence and possible adverse consequences of delirium in nursing homes, including revolving door transfers between hospitals and nursing homes, it is critical that health-care professionals working in the LTC setting are competent in the recognition, diagnosis, and management of acute confusion in LTC residents.

DIAGNOSIS

The syndrome of delirium consists of a variety of psychiatric symptoms that are manifestations of one or more underlying medical conditions or medication effects (including substance intoxication and substance withdrawal). The *Diagnostic and Statistical Manual of Mental Disorders* (4th ed., text revision, *DSM-IV-TR,* American Psychiatric Association, APA, 2000) delineates four diagnostic criteria that must be met to make the diagnosis of delirium:

Criterion A is the presence of a disturbance of consciousness, with a reduced ability to focus, sustain, or shift attention.

Criterion B is a change in cognition (such as memory deficit, disorientation, language disturbance) or the development of a perceptual disturbance that is not better accounted for by a preexisting, established, or evolving dementia.

Criterion C is that the disturbance develops over a short period of time (usually hours or days) and tends to fluctuate during the course of the day.

Criterion D is that there is evidence from the history, physical examination, or laboratory findings that the disturbance is caused by the direct physiological consequences of a general medical condition. (APA, 2000)

The core clinical features of acute confusion include disturbances in consciousness, attention, perception, and cognition (APA, *Practice Guidelines*, 1999). Altered level of consciousness (Criterion A), however, is the hallmark feature of acute confusion that distinguishes it from the syndrome of dementia (in which memory impairment is paramount). Delirium typically develops over the course of hours to days, and the symptoms fluctuate, sometimes dramatically and within a short time frame (often within the same day), as the illness progresses (Burns et al., 2004).

Patients with alteration in level of consciousness demonstrate a reduced awareness of their environment, which does not approach the level of stupor or coma.
Manifestations of impaired level of consciousness include difficulty focusing,
sustaining, or shifting attention and being easily distracted (APA, 1999, 2000).
Delirium often causes disruptions in the sleep–wake cycle leading to daytime
sleepiness, nighttime agitation (sometimes referred to as "sundowning"), and
insomnia. Delirious patients can experience fragmentation of sleep continuity
and even complete reversal of night–day sleep–wake cycles.

Both hypoactive and hyperactive subtypes of delirium have been described in
the literature (Burns et al., 2004; Lipowski, 1983). Patients with the hyperactive
variant usually present with vivid hallucinations, delusions, agitation, nighttime
wakefulness, and irritability. These patients may refuse care and become physically
combative with caregivers. Whereas these hyperactive patients often come to the
attention of LTC staff quickly, patients with a hypoactive picture may be noticed
less than their hyperactive counterparts. Their symptoms—which include lethargy,
increased daytime sleepiness/drowsiness, lowered cognitive ability, diminished
interaction with caregivers, and inability to perform previously performable ADLs
do not cause the disruptions in staff activities and peer interactions that result from
hyperactive symptoms. Like the hyperactive delirium patient, those with hypoactive delirium can have serious underlying illnesses (Burns et al., 2004). There is
conflicting literature on whether or not the presence of one type of delirium or
another correlates with the acuity of the patient's medical condition (de Rooij,
2005). Hypoactive delirium, however, carries a poorer prognosis and accounted for
28% of cases of acute confusion in one study examining delirium in LTC residents
(Cacchione, Culp, Laing, & Tripp-Reimer, 2003; Potter & George, 2006). As the
clinical course of delirium typically fluctuates, some individuals may alternately
exhibit hypoactive and hyperactive symptoms during a single episode of delirium.

Cognitive impairment can present as disorientation to time and place (though
rarely to self) and problems with recent/short-term memory. Language and
speech disturbances such as dysarthria, dysnomia, and even aphasia can occur
in patients with acute confusion.

Delirium can lead to disturbances in perception: misinterpretations, hallucinations, and illusions. For example, an LTC resident with delirium may misinterpret a staff member's removal of the resident's laundry as the theft of his
possessions. Items on a food tray may appear as animate objects, such as insects
(illusion). While visual hallucinations are common, auditory, tactile, gustatory,
and olfactory hallucinations can also occur with delirium.

ETIOLOGY AND RISK FACTORS

A disruption in the normal functioning of any organ system can lead to delirium, especially in a vulnerable patient. Known causes of delirium cited in the

literature from the acute care setting include infections, adverse effects of medications (particularly those with anticholingeric properties), metabolic/electrolyte abnormalities, hypoxemia, urinary and fecal retention, pain, and neurological injuries (Nayeem, 2003). A study of LTC residents by Cacchione, Culp, Laing, and Tripp-Reimer (2003) found that the most common causes of acute confusion in order of occurrence were infections (pneumonia, urinary tract infection, and other), dehydration, anticholinergic medications, intracranial problems, and electrolyte disturbances (Table 3.1).

Not all patients who experience a precipitating medical illness develop acute confusion. Delirium requires the presence of two necessary conditions: a vulnerable patient and precipitating factors (Inouye, 1994; Inouye & Charpentier, 1996). A vulnerable patient can have any or all of the following triad of patient vulnerabilities to delirium: decreased cognitive reserves (advanced age, preexisting cognitive impairment), decreased physiological reserves (multiple illnesses/frailty), and decreased biochemical reserves (multiple medications, alcohol use, major organ failure) (Mentes et al., 1999). Many of the "vulnerability factors" found in Table 3.2 occur in residents of nursing homes. Rovner (1990) found that 67.8% of new nursing home admissions have dementia. Other risk factors for developing acute confusion found in LTC residents include dehydration, polypharmacy, and infection (Culp et al., 1997). A study by Cacchione, Culp, Laing, and Tripp-Reimer (2003) found the following risk factors associated with developing delirium in nursing home residents: pulmonary disorder, an abnormal serum sodium or potassium level, and hearing deficit. In this same study, antidepressant therapy approached statistical significance as a possible risk factor for developing delirium. Visually impaired seniors in nursing homes and those with dual sensory impairment (vision and hearing) are also at greater risk of developing delirium (Cacchione, Culp, Dyck, & Laing, 2003). Culp et al. (2004) demonstrated that an increased BUN/Cr ratio of greater than 21:1 was found to increase the risk of acute confusion. This elevated ratio, usually interpreted as an indicator of prerenal azotemia, is often associated with dehydration or intravascular volume depletion. It can also be elevated in patients with gastrointestinal bleeding.

EVALUATION AND ASSESSMENT

The diagnosis of delirium in nursing home residents requires vigilance for changes in behavior and level of functioning. Although laboratory and radiological tests can aid in determining the underlying medical conditions causing or contributing to acute confusion, the diagnosis of delirium is based mainly on clinical observation and examination of the patient. Three general types of delirium assessment methods exist for nursing home staff (APA, 1999): instruments for screening, diagnosis, and severity ratings.

TABLE 3.1. Common Precipitating Causes of Delirium

Medications/drugs	• Alcohol or sedative hypnotic withdrawal • Anticholinergics • Gastrointestinal: histamine (H2) antagonists, metaclopramide, cisapride • Cardiac: digoxin, antiarrythymics, calcium channel blockers • Anti-inflammatories: steroids, NSAIDs • Opioids: morphine, Darvocet, merperidine • Psychotropics: benzodiazepines, antidepressants • Neurological: antiparkinson agents (dopamine agonists), anticonvulsants • Over-the-counter agents: antihistamines, anticholinergics, hypnotics, pseudoephedrine, caffeine
Neurological illness	• Stroke, TIA • Seizures • Subdural hematoma
Infections	• Urinary tract infection • Pneumonia • Cellulitis • Sepsis
Metabolic disturbances	• Hypoglycemia • Hyponatremia, hypernatremia • Hypokalemia • Hypercalcemia • Hypomagnesemia • Hepatic failure: hyperammonemia • Renal failure: azotemia, uremia
Hypoperfusion and hypoxemia	• Cardiac failure • Left ventricular dysfunction • Arrhythmia • Hypotension, cardiovascular shock • Dehydration, intravascular volume depletion • Pulmonary insufficiency or respiratory failure • Pulmonary embolism
Urinary and fecal retention Pain Use of physical restraint Bladder catheter use	

Source: Adapted from Nayeem (2003) and CMS Resident Assessment Protocol (1990).

TABLE 3.2. Vulnerability Factors for the Development of Acute Confusion

DECREASED COGNITIVE RESERVES	DECREASED PHYSIOLOGICAL RESERVES	DECREASED BIOCHEMICAL RESERVES
Advanced age	Multiple illness/comorbidity	Multiple medications
Pre-existing cognitive impairment, such as dementia	Frailty	Previous alcoholism Major organ exhaustion

Source: Adapted from Mentes et al. (1999).

Screening tools can help staff identify those LTC residents with symptoms that might indicate the presence of delirium. Many of these were designed to be administered by nurses. The NEECHAM was developed by Neelon and colleagues (1996) and assesses for acute confusion. It is divided into three categories: (1) level of responsiveness, (2) level of behavior, and (3) level of integrative and physiological control. The Mini Mental State Examination (MMSE) developed by Folstein et al. (1975) can help detect cognitive impairment. These instruments are designed for screening and aid in the detection and recognition of possible cases of delirium, but they do not establish or confirm the diagnosis.

Several diagnostic instruments have been developed to assist in making a formal diagnosis of delirium. The Confusion Assessment Method (CAM) was developed by Inouye et al. (1990). It uses four characteristic items to evaluate for acute confusion: acute change in mental status, inattention, altered level of consciousness, and disorganized thinking (Table 3.3).

Using the CAM, a diagnosis of delirium requires the presence of features 1 and 2 and either 3 or 4. The other five features (5–9) were not included in the diagnostic algorithm of the CAM (features 1–4) because they did not increase sensitivity or specificity (Inouye et al., 1990).

Staff can also measure the severity of delirium by using symptom severity scales. Instruments such as the Delirium Rating Scale (DRS) and the Memorial Delirium Assessment Scale (MDAS) can help staff to monitor the progress of a resident's delirium over time and can provide a measure of effectiveness of treatments and interventions.

Delirium screening and evaluation is also supported by elements of the Resident Assessment Instrument, including the Minimum Data Set (MDS) and Resident Assessment Protocols (RAPs) that were developed and implemented in response to the federal mandate for comprehensive, standardized, periodic assessment of nursing home residents in the United States (HCFA, 1992). Every Medicare/Medicaid certified nursing home is required to administer the MDS on admission and at least quarterly (Morris et al., 1990). If a rating on the MDS indicates a potential change or deterioration in a resident's clinical status, this may "trigger"

TABLE 3.3. Items from the Confusion Assessment
Method Instrument Used to Detect Delirium

NUMBER	FEATURES
1	Acute onset
2	Inattention
3	Disorganized thinking
4	Altered level of consciousness
5	Disorientation
6	Memory impairment
7	Perceptual disturbances
8	Psychomotor agitation
9	Altered sleep–wake cycle

Source: Adapted from Inouye et al. (1990).

a RAP for evaluation of possible delirium. Items on the MDS 2.0 that can trigger
the delirium RAP include the following: being easily distracted, periods of altered
perception or awareness, episodes of disorganized speech, periods of restlessness,
periods of lethargy, variation in mental functioning over the course of the day,
decline in cognitive status, decline in mood, or behavioral symptoms (CMS RAI
Version 2.0). If any of these are recorded on a resident's MDS, then staff are
required to complete a RAP. RAPs are designed to help nursing home staff (1)
recognize signs of clinically significant problems, (2) evaluate potential causal
and contributing factors, and (3) determine if treatment plans need to be altered
to address the underlying problem (Streim & Katz, 2007).

RAPs for delirium include advice for helping nurses detect signs and symptoms of delirium. They also identify and direct nursing staff to search for the
most common causes of delirium with the goal of changing treatment or patient
care to minimize or eliminate the causative agent. The delirium RAP addresses
important psychosocial and environmental stressors that may occur with or even
be contributing to the acute confusion.

Using MDS risk variables, Mentes et al. (1999) found that inadequate fluid
intake, dementia, sensory deficits, and experiencing a fall within the past 30
days were associated with acute confusion.

By utilizing the MDS and other assessment tools, nursing home staff can
diagnose delirium at an early stage and implement treatment in a timely manner
so as to minimize adverse consequences and improve patient outcomes.

CMS is currently developing MDS version 3.0, which is designed to improve
the detection of cognitive impairment. CMS has also proposed the development
and implementation of electronic RAPs with the hope that this will improve
evaluation and care of nursing home patients with common conditions such as
delirium.

TREATMENT

The cornerstone of delirium treatment is prompt diagnosis and management of the underlying medical condition causing the acute confusion. Nursing care is essential and should focus on assuring the safety of the patient in the nursing home setting, especially of those whose confusion is associated with hyperactivity. Monitoring for impulsive or agitated behaviors that represent a danger to self or others can help avert serious injuries. Nurses should be available to provide necessary supervision or assistance for patients whose combination of confusion, agitation, and lack of safety awareness makes it dangerous for them to transfer or ambulate independently or whose combination of confusion, impulsivity, and poor judgment puts them at risk for aspiration during unsupervised self-feeding.

Specific treatment of delirium usually involves symptomatic relief of behavioral disturbances and problems with sleep–wake cycle abnormalities.

Antipsychotics remain the agents of choice in treating delirium symptoms. Haloperidol is the most established treatment and has demonstrated efficacy in treating acute confusion. It may be administered intramuscularly (IM), orally (PO), or intravenously (IV). Although IV administration is not FDA approved, it is commonly used in practice in acute care settings (APA, 1999). IV administration may be associated with a lower risk of extrapyramidal side effects, but an increased risk of hypotension compared with other routes of administration. In nursing home settings, where IV administration is often not available or not practical, IM administration may be the only available parenteral route. Given concerns about side effects of haloperidol such as extrapyramidal symptoms and sedation, there has been interest in studying the use of atypical antipsychotics for the treatment of acute confusion. Limited studies have shown newer agents, such as risperidone and olanzapine, to be effective in treating delirium and perhaps better tolerated (Sipahimalani & Masand, 1998). Case reports have also demonstrated efficacy of aripiprazole in treating delirium (Alao et al., 2005).

Although atypicals appear to provide some benefit in symptom relief in patients with acute confusion, they are not FDA approved for treatment of delirium. It is worth noting that the recent CATIE-AD study concluded that adverse effects of atypical antipsychotics outweighed benefits of treatment for agitation and psychosis of Alzheimer's disease (Schneider, 2006), though the study was not designed to examine patients with a diagnosis of dementia with delirium. Pooled safety data from other studies revealed that elderly dementia patients treated with atypicals have a 1.6 to 1.7 times greater risk of death than those treated with placebo (FDA, 2005). While the risks of atypical use in dementia patients is known, the safety of using atypicals in the treatment of acute confusion has not been systematically examined (Boettger & Breitbart, 2005). Until such studies have been done in elderly patients with delirium, clinicians should carefully weigh the benefits and uncertain risks when using atypical antipsychotics in the management of delirium.

The use of benzodiazepines alone in treating acute confusion should be limited to delirium caused by acute sedative/hypnotic or alcohol withdrawal (delirium tremens). Benzodiazepines, especially when used as the sole agent of treatment, have not shown efficacy in the treatment of most cases of delirium. They may provide benefit when used in conjunction with antipsychotics (APA, 1999). Although the use of benzodiazepines in delirium has mostly been studied in the acute care setting, lorazepam use has been shown to be an independent risk factor for transition to delirium in ICU patients (Pandharipande, 2004). Given the known and unknown risks and benefits of medications in treatment of acute confusion, any pharmacological intervention must be done cautiously and with careful monitoring for efficacy and side effects.

Nonpharmacological interventions include frequent orienting of patients with clocks and calendars, having people and objects (photographs, etc.) familiar to the patient within the patient's field of vision or reach, ensuring proper lighting or darkening of rooms at appropriate times during the day/night, and minimizing overstimulation by noise or peers (APA, 1999).

OUTCOMES

With prompt diagnosis and appropriate management of the underlying medical illness, delirium can resolve. For cases of delirium caused by reversible medical conditions, the patient may not incur any permanent injury and disability can often be averted. In nonnursing home settings, with treatment of the underlying medical condition, some cases of delirium have been observed to resolve within a few hours or days, while other cases have persisted for weeks or even months. The typical duration of acute confusion is 10 to 12 days, with up to 15% of patients having their delirium persist for 30 days or beyond (APA, 1999). A small minority of patients can have symptoms lasting 6 months or greater (Burns et al. 2004).

Furthermore, patients with delirium can have residual cognitive impairment that lingers after the acute confusion resolves, which may be due to a previously undiagnosed, underlying dementia. In this scenario, an older adult in the early stages of a dementing illness that has not yet been recognized or diagnosed may be at increased risk for developing delirium; it is sometimes after an episode of acute delirium, superimposed on a "subclinical" dementia, that residual cognitive impairment first brings the underlying dementia to attention.

Acute confusion constitutes a medical emergency, however, and should be evaluated and managed aggressively. Urgent treatment is especially important in nursing home residents, given their underlying susceptibilities and generally frail condition. When delirium is associated with medical illness that is refractory to treatment, mortality rates are high. The danger of delirium in nursing home residents was demonstrated by Cacchione, Culp, Dyck, and Laing (2003) who found that 34% of residents with acute confusion in an LTC facility died within 3 months of their assessment. Hyperactive delirium symptoms can lead to falls and injuries, whereas hypoactive symptoms may place nursing home residents at risk for pressure sores, urinary incontinence, and infections that can prolong or exacerbate an episode of acute confusion (Nayeem, 2003). Hypoactive delirium may also be associated with poor oral intake, resulting in dehydration and nutritional compromise in nursing home residents.

Although patients with delirium often have cognitive impairment that limits their ability to understand what is happening to them, they may still be able to benefit from simple explanations and reassurances during the course of the illness; they should be debriefed when possible after the delirium resolves. Staff should educate families and LTC residents about the causes, consequences, and prevention of delirium. It should be conveyed that a diagnosis of delirium does not equate with a diagnosis of an underlying psychiatric illness, such as schizophrenia, bipolar disorder, or dementia and that confusion, cognitive impairment, and other symptoms like agitation and hallucinations will likely resolve as the delirium clears.

PREVENTION

Given the high mortality rate and significant morbidity of delirium in nursing home residents, staff should seek to prevent and minimize the risks for developing acute confusion before it occurs. Nursing and other staff with direct and daily resident contact represent the front line of delirium prevention and early detection in LTC residents. Nurses and physicians can reduce or even eliminate certain risk factors for acute confusion in nursing home residents. Streamlining medication usage and stopping medications no longer needed, especially those that are likely to cause delirium, such as medications with anticholinergic side effects, may limit LTC residents' chances of becoming delirious.

Residents with impaired mobility or ability to feed themselves risk dehydration and electrolyte abnormalities that can lead to delirium. Culp et al. (1997) found in a pilot study that LTC residents who drank four or more 8-ounce glasses of water daily had a lowered chance of developing acute confusion.

Sensory impairment occurs commonly in seniors in nursing homes and sometimes is the reason they were admitted to the LTC facility in the first place. Nursing home staff must familiarize themselves with residents' sensory limitations and ensure that residents have access to assistive devices and equipment, such as hearing aids and eye glasses, that can help reduce levels of visual and auditory impairment. Optimal lighting, and regulation of lighting levels to correspond to time of day or night, may also be helpful in reducing the risk of acute confusion in these residents.

Helping nursing home residents, especially those with cognitive decline who may feel unfamiliar with their environment, maintain a sense of orientation to time and place can reduce confusion. Simple interventions, such as the use of calendars, clocks, and objects recognizable to the patient, may reduce resident disorientation. Working to normalize sleep patterns, reducing daytime sleeping, developing good sleep hygiene, and reducing environmental stimulation at night help reduce sleep deprivation and fatigue and may reduce chances of developing acute confusion. A trial of a multicomponent intervention demonstrated a reduction in the incidence acute confusion and the duration of delirium in hospitalized older patients. The interventions targeted the following delirium risk factors: cognitive impairment, sleep deprivation, immobility, visual/hearing impairment, and dehydration. The protocol included interventions such as use of cognitively stimulating activities, boards with orienting information such as staff names and schedules, noise reduction strategies, ear wax disimpaction, easy-to-read books, early recognition of dehydration, and minimizing use of immobilizing equipment (Inouye et al., 1999). Although this work focused on hospitalized patients, many of these interventions could be applied to LTC residents as well.

Educating nursing home staff about the symptoms of delirium and how they differ from those of chronic, long-term cognitive decline—as seen in dementia—can increase the likelihood of early detection and prompt treatment of the acute illness/condition causing the delirium. Integrating tools such as MDS and CAM into patient care and treatment planning can identify those nursing home residents most at risk for delirium, as well as those who have already developed acute confusion.

CONCLUSION

Delirium is a commonly occurring syndrome that threatens the health and well-being of nursing home residents. By virtue of the illnesses and conditions that have resulted in their need for nursing home care, LTC residents face a substantial risk of delirium. Impaired ability to perform ADLs, cognitive decline, multiple medical illnesses and pharmacological treatments, and sensory impairments represent just a few of the potential contributors to the development of delirium in nursing home residents. Like any serious medical illness, acute confusion must be approached with a rigorous program of prevention, early detection, prompt treatment of the underlying etiology, and rapid, effective management of the cognitive and behavioral symptoms. Nursing homes and their staff are in a unique position to reduce the risk of delirium and, when it does occur, to ensure improved clinical outcomes.

REFERENCES

Alao, A., Soderberg, M., Pohl, E., & Koss, M. (2005). Aripiprazole in the treatment of delirium. *International Journal of Psychiatry in Medicine, 35*(4), 429–433.

American Psychiatric Association. (1999). *Practice guidelines for the treatment of patients with delirium.* Washington, DC: Author.

American Psychiatric Association. (2000). *Diagnostic and statistical manual of mental disorders* (4th ed., text revision). Washington, DC: Author.

Boettger, S. & Breitbart, W. (2005, September). Atypical antipsychotics in the management of delirium: A review of the empirical literature. *Palliative & Supportive Care, 3*(3): 227–237.

Burns, A., Gallagley, A., & Byrne, J. (2004). Review: Delirium. *Journal of Neurology, Neurosurgery, and Psychiatry, 75,* 362–367.

Cacchione, P. Z., Culp, K., Laing, J., & Tripp-Reimer, T. (2003). Clinical profile of acute confusion in the long-term care setting. *Clinical Nursing Research, 12*(2), 145–158.

Cacchione, P. Z., Culp, K., Dyck, M. J., & Laing, J. (2003). Risk for acute confusion in sensory-impaired, rural, long-term care elders. *Clinical Nursing Research, 12*(4), 340–355.

RAI Version 2.0. Centers for Medicare and Medicaid Services. Revised December 2002, Appendix C.

Culp, K. R., Tripp-Reimer, T., Wadle, K., et al. (1997). Screening for acute confusion in elderly long-term care residents. *Journal of Neuroscience Nursing, 29*(2), 86–88, 95–100.

Culp, K. R., Wakefield, B., Dyck, M. J., Cacchione, P. Z., DeCrane, S., & Decker, S. (2004). Bioelectrical impedance analysis and other hydration parameters as risk factors for delirium in rural nursing home residents. *Journal of Gerontology: Medical Sciences, 59A*(8), 813–817.

De Rooij, S. E., Schuurmans, M. J., van der Mast, R. C., & Levi, M. (2005). Clinical subtypes of delirium and their relevance for daily clinical practice: A systematic review. *International Journal of Geriatric Psychiatry, 20,* 609–615.

FDA. (2005, April). Public Health Advisory: Deaths with antipsychotics in elderly patients with behavioral disturbances. Washington, DC: US Food and Drug Administration/ Center for Drug Evaluation and Research. Retrieved from http://www.fda.gov/cder/ drug/advisory/antipsychotics.htm

Folstein, M., Folstein, S., & McHugh, P. (1975). Mini-mental state: A practical method for grading the cognitive state of patients for the clinician. *Journal of Psychiatric Research, 12*(3), 189–198.

Health Care Financing Administration. (1992). Medicare and Medicaid: Resident assessment in long-term care facilities. *Federal Register, 57,* 61614–61733.

Inouye, S. K., van Dyck, C. H., Alessi, C. A., Balkin, S., Sigal, A. P., & Horowitz, R. I. (1990). Clarifying confusion: The confusion assessment method. A new method for detection of delirium. *Annals of Internal Medicine, 113,* 941–948.

Inouye, S. (1994). The dilemma of delirium: Clinical and research controversies regarding diagnosis and evaluation of delirium in hospitalized elderly medical patients. *American Journal of Medicine, 97,* 278–288.

Inouye, S., & Charpentier, P. (1996). Precipitating factors for delirium in hospitalized elderly persons. Predictive model and interrelationship with baseline vulnerability. *JAMA, 275,* 852–857.

Inouye, S. K., Bogardus, S. T., Charpentier, P. A., et al. (1999). A multicomponent inter-vention to prevent delirium in hospitalized older patients. *New England Journal of Medicine, 340*(9), 669–676.

Katz, I. R., Parmelee, P. A., & Brubaker, K. (1991). Toxic and metabolic encephalopa-thies in long-term care patients. *International Psychogeriatrics, 3*, 337–347.

Levkoff, S., Cleary, P., Liptzin, B., & Evans, D. A. (1991). Epidemiology of delirium: An overview of research issues and findings. *International Psychogeriatrics, 3*, 149–167.

Lipowski, Z. J. (1983). Transient cognitive disorders (delirium, acute confusional states) in the elderly. *American Journal of Psychiatry, 140*(11), 1426–1436.

Mentes, J., Culp, K., Maas, M., & Rantz, M. (1999). Acute confusion indicators: Risk fac-tors and relevance using MDS data. *Research in Nursing and Health, 22*, 95–105.

Morris, J. N., Hawes, C., Fries, B. E., et al. (1990) Designing the national resident assess-ment instrument for nursing homes. *The Gerontologist, 30*, 293–307.

Nayeem, K., & O'Keeffe, S. T. (2003). Delirium. *Clinical Medicine, 3*(5), 412–415.

Neelon, V., Champagne, M., Carlson, J., & Funk, S. (1996). The NEECHAM Confusion Scale: Construction, validation, and clinical testing. *Nursing Research, 45*, 324–330.

Pandharipande, P., Shintani, A., Peterson, J., & Ely, E. W. (2004). Sedative and anal-gesic medications are independent risk factors in ICU patients for transitioning into delirium. *Critical Care Medicine, 32*, A19.

Potter, J., & George, J. (2006) The prevention, diagnosis and management of delirium in older people: Concise guidelines. *Clinical Medicine, 6*, 303–308.

Rovner, B. W., German, P. S., Braodhead, J., et al. (1990). The prevalence and manage-ment of dementia and other psychiatric disorders in nursing homes. *International Psychogeriatrics, 2*(1), 13–24.

Sabin, T. D., Vitug, A. J., & Mark, V. H. (1982). Are nursing home diagnosis and treat-ment inadequate? *JAMA, 248*, 321–322.

Schneider, L.S., Tariot, P. N., Dagerman, K. S., et al. (2006). Effectiveness of atypical antipsychotic drugs in patients with Alzheimer's disease. *New England Journal of Medicine, 355*, 1525–1538.

Streim, J., & Katz, I. (2006). Clinical psychiatry in the nursing home. In D. G. Blazer, E. W. Burse, D. C. Steffens (Eds.), *Essentials of Geriatric Psychiatry* (pp. 375–403). Washington, DC: American Psychiatric Publishing.

Sipahimalani, A. & Masand, P. (1998). Olanzapine in the treatment of delirium. *Psychosomatics, 39*, 422–430.

4

Mood Disorders

Ashok J. Bharucha and *Soo Borson*

Mood disorders are psychiatric syndromes defined by prominent changes in emotional tone. To recognize disordered mood states and to separate them from normal and expected responses to life events, sustained changes in social behavior—interest, attitudes, energy, thinking, judgment, and patterns of eating and sleeping—must accompany the change in mood. The identification of mood disorders is a clinical task based on familiarity with standards of diagnosis and skilled observation and interaction with patients. Certified nurses' aides (CNAs) in long-term care settings, who provide the vast majority of direct care to residents, can be trained in the observational skills needed to report concerns about possible mood disorders in patients, but a full diagnostic assessment requires specialized interviewing skills and knowledge of the patient's history and medical status. Uncomplicated mood disorders can be evaluated by general psychiatrists, primary care physicians, psychologists, nurses, and social workers experienced in differential diagnosis of psychiatric disorders in the elderly; more complex presentations are in the domain of the geriatric psychiatrist. In this chapter, we review the clinical features, diagnosis, prevalence, etiology, and management of manic and depressed elderly residents encountered in long-term care settings, encompassing the broad range of residential/assisted living facilities and nursing homes.

MANIC AND MANIC-LIKE STATES

Epidemiology

The relative plethora of information on depression contrasts sharply with a minimal literature on mania or bipolar disorder. In this section, we briefly summarize the presentation and treatment of mania in the elderly, based predominantly on studies of elderly psychiatric inpatients and outpatients. A comprehensive critical review of bipolar disorder in older adults notes that the illness becomes less common with age, accounts for 8% to 10% of late-life psychiatric admissions, is associated more commonly with neurological factors in the late-onset groups, and evolves clinically along multiple possible trajectories (Depp & Jeste, 2004). Moreover, manic-like states in older adults represent a heterogeneous group of syndromes with an extensive differential diagnosis. This includes not only strictly defined bipolar disorder but also secondary ("symptomatic") mood disorders, delusional disorders, paranoid schizophrenia, schizoaffective disorder, and, in some cases, delirium and dementia (Mirchandani & Young, 1993). These diagnostic distinctions are important as they often determine the focus of treatment: for example, an excited delirious patient might occasionally appear manic and a bipolar patient in a prolonged manic state can appear delirious. The frequency of mania in nursing home residents is unknown. Weissman et al. (1991) cited a 1-year incidence of 9.7% bipolar affective episodes (mania or depression) among residents of nursing homes included in the Epidemiological Catchment Area (ECA) study. In addition, Tariot et al. (1993) reported a 3% prevalence rate of bipolar disorder in a randomly selected sample of 80 residents in one public facility. Current rates could be lower consequent to the enactment of the Omnibus Budget Reconciliation Act (OBRA 87; Public Law 100–203) in 1987, mandating prescreening of patients for mental illness requiring active treatment and permitting the exclusion of chronically mentally ill persons from nonpsychiatric facilities.

Clinical Features

Clinical diagnostic criteria for mania are presented in Table 4.1. When the elderly patient presents with affective signs and symptoms of a pressured, driven, or accelerated nature, the possibility of mania, hypomania, bipolar disorder, and other diagnoses as noted above must be considered. A prudent first step lies in careful assessment of the patient for an organic mood disorder or "secondary mania." Krauthammer and Klerman (1978) defined this as a manic episode involving an elated and/or irritable mood and classic manic symptoms causally linked to a medical or pharmacological condition. Importantly, elderly patients are more likely than younger adults to have mania as a symptom of another

TABLE 4.1. Diagnostic Criteria for Mania and Related States

Manic episode

A. A distinct period of abnormally and persistently elevated, expansive, or irritable mood, lasting at least 1 week (or any duration if hospitalization is necessary)
B. During the period of mood disturbance, three (or more) of the following symptoms have persisted (four if the mood is only irritable) and have been present to a significant degree:
   (1) inflated self-esteem or grandiosity
   (2) decreased need for sleep (e.g., feels rested after only 3 h of sleep)
   (3) more talkative than usual or pressure to keep talking
   (4) flight of ideas or subjective experience that thoughts are racing
   (5) distractibility (i.e., attention too easily drawn to unimportant or irrelevant external stimuli)
   (6) increase in goal-directed activity (either socially, at work or school, or sexually) or psychomotor agitation
   (7) excessive involvement in pleasurable activities that have a high potential for painful consequences (e.g., engaging in unrestrained buying sprees, sexual indiscretions, or foolish business investments)
C. The symptoms do not meet criteria for a Mixed Episode
D. The mood disturbance is sufficiently severe to cause marked impairment in occupational functioning or in usual social activities or relationships with others, or to necessitate hospitalization to prevent harm to self or others, or there are psychotic features
E. The symptoms are not due to the direct physiological effects of a substance (e.g., a drug of abuse, a medication, or other treatment) or a general medical condition (e.g., hyperthyroidism)

Note: Manic-like episodes that are clearly caused by somatic antidepressant treatment (e.g., medication, electroconvulsive therapy, light therapy) should not count toward a diagnosis of Bipolar I Disorder

Hypomanic episode

A. Similar to manic episode except mood duration is at least 4 days
B. Similar to manic episode
C. The episode is associated with an unequivocal change in functioning that is uncharacteristic of the person when not symptomatic
D. The disturbance in mood and the change in functioning are observable by others.
E. The episode is not severe enough to cause marked impairment in social or occupational functioning, or to necessitate hospitalization, and there are no psychotic features
F. Similar to E for manic episode

Note: Hypomanic-like episodes that are clearly caused by somatic antidepressant treatment (e.g., medication, electroconvulsive therapy, light therapy) should not count toward a diagnosis of Bipolar II Disorder

Continued

TABLE 4.1. Continued

Mixed manic—depressive episode

Meets criteria for both manic episode (above) and major depressive episode
  (Table 4.2) for at least 1 week, with symptoms present at least nearly every day

Secondary manic episode

Similar to manic episode except that evidence of a specific causal factor is present:
  substance abuse, medication or other treatment effect, or a medical condition
  known to be a potential direct cause (e.g., stroke, hyperthyroidism)

Source: Adapted from the *DSM-IV-TR* (APA, 2000).

disorder rather than of primary bipolar disorder. Secondary manic episodes are
more likely to begin later in life than primary bipolar disorder, and family history is less often positive for mood disorders (Krauthammer & Klerman, 1978;
Rubin, 1988). Many cerebral organic pathologies have been implicated as causes
of secondary mania in the elderly. Among the most important are cerebral infarction (stroke, particularly right-sided), infection (e.g., viral encephalitis, neuro-
syphilis), tumors, and substance abuse, including alcohol (Goyal et al., 2006;
Gupta & Basu 1997). Medications may also cause a manic syndrome, including
agents such as L-dopa, corticosteroids, anticholinergics, psychostimulants, and
antidepressants (Mendez, 2000; Mirchandani & Young, 1993). Occasionally, a
manic episode occurs as a complication of an acute nonneurological disease
such as myocardial infarction.

The clinical picture of mania may be muted in elderly patients. For example,
Secondary and primary manic episodes cannot be reliably distinguished on
the basis of symptoms as manic syndromes due to medical disorders or drugs
frequently meet all diagnostic criteria defining a primary manic episode except
etiology (i.e., the patient has no history of primary bipolar mood disorder; Rubin,
1988). A history of prior episodes beginning in early or middle adulthood usually
identifies elderly patients with primary bipolar disorder, and thorough medical
assessment (including medications) usually reveals potential causes in secondary manic states.

The clinical picture of mania may be muted in elderly patients. For example,
Post in 1965 noted that flight of ideas is often replaced in elderly manics by
"senile anecdotal and circumstantial garrulity" (shallow overtalkativeness).
Slater and Roth (1977) observed that euphoria in elderly manics often is not
"infectious"; speech and thought are "threadbare and repetitious," lacking the
typical "sparkle and versatility" of younger patients; and that while overall
severity of illness may be "relatively mild," "hostility and resentment" are often
marked.

Several clinical presentations of mania in the elderly patient are noteworthy.
Confusion may be marked, giving rise to the clinically useful concept of "manic

delirium" or "delirious mania." These terms highlight the potential for manic states to impair intellectual function in elderly patients and the difficulty of distinguishing between psychiatric and neurological causes of cognitive dysfunction in actively manic patients. Moreover, preliminary evidence supports the clinical observation that many older bipolar patients continue to exhibit significant neuropsychological deficits even during euthymic mood states (Gildengers et al., 2004).

Inconsistent evidence suggests that *mixed bipolar episodes* are more frequently encountered in elderly than in young patients with bipolar disorder (Depp & Jeste, 2004). Mixed episodes share features of both mania and depression admixed or alternating in rapid succession. *Mania with psychotic features* may be difficult to distinguish clinically from other psychotic states of the elderly. *Chronic hypomanic states* occasionally occur in elderly patients but have not been well characterized. A history of long-standing primary bipolar disorder is the usual backdrop for these presentations, and narcissistic, self-centered, and demanding personality features are common.

Clinicians who treat the elderly will encounter both patients with late-onset mania and those with recurrent primary bipolar disorder beginning earlier in life. In late-onset mania, comorbid neurological disorders are much more common than in elderly patients with early-onset and multiple prior episodes of mania, though clinical phenomenology is largely indistinguishable except for the possibility of focal neurological findings in late-onset mania with neurological involvement (Depp & Jeste, 2004). In addition, mania can cause a dementia syndrome (Charron et al., 1991). In three demented manic patients, successful lithium therapy led to complete clearing of cognitive dysfunction and abandonment of the dementia diagnosis. On the other hand, some patients with neurodegenerative or other dementias, most often frontotemporal dementia (but also some post-stroke and posttraumatic dementias and occasionally Alzheimer's disease), develop manic features. In frontotemporal dementia, psychiatric disorder may be the first detected sign of the evolving neurodegenerative process, particularly in patients with relatively early onset (e.g., the 50s and 60s). In these cases, a careful search for earlier features of cognitive inefficiency, apathy, and other commonly associated features of early frontotemporal dementia can help but are often confused with a depressive episode that keeps the underlying etiology masked for months or a year or two. In the other dementias that occasionally present with manic-like states, the clinical history and examination usually indicate the presence of predisposing brain disease or injury.

In both secondary and primary manic episodes, lithium remains the treatment of choice when not contraindicated by other medical illness, primarily some renal and cardiac diseases. Although physicians in recent years have been preferentially prescribing divalproex over lithium, direct comparisons of these agents in this population do not unequivocally support this choice, and lithium can be considered a first-line agent unless medically contraindicated (Shulman et al., 2003). Risks associated with lithium toxicity in older adults must be monitored closely. These risks include interactions with some diuretics, rapid development of dehydration with lithium-induced nephrogenic diabetes insipidus or any cause of vomiting or diarrhea, and the long-term risk of renal insufficiency. Treatment with all antimanic agents must be followed regularly, due to the potential for toxicity caused by problems with adherence and inadequate supervision by others. These risks are more likely to be a problem for patients living at home than in long-term care settings where close monitoring can be more readily achieved. Other mood-stabilizing agents, such as carbamazepine, divalproex, or lamotrigine, may be utilized in lieu of lithium when medically necessary or after an adequate trial of lithium has proven unsuccessful or too difficult to regulate. In addition to mood stabilizers, antipsychotic (preferably atypical) or benzodiazepine anxiolytic drugs may be needed in the short-term treatment of acute mania in the elderly for control of psychotic symptoms, excessive overactivity, and sleep disturbance. These agents are increasingly used for their mood stabilizing effects in maintenance therapy but have not been systematically compared with classical mood stabilizers in clinical trials in older adults. Adequate randomized controlled trials of antimanic agents focused specifically on older patients are not available. Young et al. (2004) discuss management of bipolar disorder in the elderly in depth, with attention to alternative treatments as well. Many acutely manic patients are likely to require inpatient psychiatric treatment for stabilization; a few may be managed successfully with stepped-up psychiatric and nursing care in the long-term care setting.

Example. A 72-year-old man with a long history of primary bipolar disorder and binge drinking while manic was observed to be leaving his nursing home at frequent intervals to visit a local tavern. When psychiatric consultation was requested, his behavior had deteriorated to the point of chronic confusion, hyperactivity, hostility, and crawling about the floor barking like a dog, and he was sleeping less than 3 h/day. His lithium level was 0.5 mEq/L. Antipsychotic treatment was initiated with risperidone and titrated to a final dose of 2 mg qhs over a week. Lithium dose was also increased to achieve a level of 1.0 mEq/L. He was denied access to local bars with the aid of constant staff supervision. Over the course of a week, his manic episode was brought under control and no signs or symptoms of alcohol withdrawal were observed. Within three weeks, antipsychotic treatment was successfully discontinued and his lithium level was maintained at 0.8 mEq/L without recurrence of mania or alcohol abuse for the next several years.

DEPRESSION

Depressions newly arising or recurring in nursing home residents are often the outcome of multiple interacting causal factors. These include individual psychological and neurobiological vulnerabilities, ill health and disability, specific losses and stresses, and qualities of the physical and social environment that set the stage for development of depression or contribute to its chronicity. Depressions are a major cause of personal suffering among nursing home residents, impair participation in activity and social life, and impose particular burdens on families and staff caring for these residents.

Depressions are the most common remediable psychiatric disorders in the elderly. All depressive subtypes commonly recognized in younger and medically healthy persons, and some that are specific to the elderly, are represented in this population. These include the currently recognized *Diagnostic and Statistical Manual of Mental Disorders* (4th ed., text Revision, *DSM-IV-TR*, American Psychiatric Association, APA, 2000) syndromes of major depression (with and without agitation or psychosis), minor ("subsyndromal" or "subthreshold") depression, dysthymia, depression due to a general medical condition or substance abuse, as well as the proposed syndromes of "depression without sadness" (withdrawal, apathy, and lack of vitality; Gallo et al., 1997), "vascular depression" (depressive symptoms with prominent executive dysfunction; Alexopoulos et al., 1997), and the more recently conceptualized "depression of Alzheimer's disease" (Olin et al., 2002). Diagnostic criteria for all of the depressive subtypes currently recognized in the *DSM-IV*, and those for "depression of Alzheimer's disease," are shown in Table 4.2.

TABLE 4.2. Diagnostic Criteria for Depressions

Major depressive episode

A. Five (or more) of the following *symptoms* have been present during the same 2-week period and represent a change from previous functioning; at least one of the symptoms is either (1) *depressed mood* or (2) loss of interest or pleasure
Note: Do not include symptoms that are clearly due to a general medical condition, or *mood-incongruent delusions* or *hallucinations*
   (1) depressed mood most of the day, nearly every day, as indicated by either subjective report (e.g., feels sad or empty) or observation made by others (e.g., appears tearful)
   (2) markedly diminished interest or pleasure in all, or almost all, activities most of the day, nearly every day (as indicated by either subjective account or observation made by others)

Continued

TABLE 4.2. Continued

    (3) significant weight loss when not dieting or weight gain (e.g., a change of more than 5% of body weight in a month), or decrease or increase in appetite nearly every day

    (4) insomnia or hypersomnia nearly every day

    (5) psychomotor agitation or retardation nearly every day (observable by others, not merely subjective feelings of restlessness or being slowed down)

    (6) fatigue or loss of energy nearly every day

    (7) feelings of worthlessness or excessive or inappropriate guilt (which may be delusional) nearly every day (not merely self-reproach or guilt about being sick)

    (8) diminished ability to think or concentrate, or indecisiveness, nearly every day (either by subjective account or as observed by others)

    (9) recurrent thoughts of death (not just fear of dying), recurrent suicidal ideation without a specific plan, or a suicide attempt or a specific plan for committing suicide

B. The symptoms do not meet criteria for a mixed episode

C. The symptoms cause clinically significant distress or impairment in social, occupational, or other important areas of functioning

D. The symptoms are not due to the direct physiological effects of a substance (e.g., a drug of abuse, a medication) or a general medical condition (e.g., hypothyroidism)

E. The symptoms are not better accounted for by bereavement, i.e., after the loss of a loved one, the symptoms persist for longer than 2 months or are characterized by marked functional impairment, morbid preoccupation with worthlessness, suicidal ideation, psychotic symptoms, or psychomotor retardation

Dysthymic disorder

A. Depressed mood for most of the day, for more days than not, as indicated either by subjective account or observation by others, for at least 2 years

B. Presence, while depressed, of two (or more) of the following:

    (1) poor appetite or overeating

    (2) insomnia or hypersomnia

    (3) low energy or fatigue

    (4) low self-esteem

    (5) poor concentration or difficulty making decisions

    (6) feelings of hopelessness

C. During the 2-year period (1 year for children or adolescents) of the disturbance, the person has never been without the symptoms in Criteria A and B for more than 2 months at a time

D. No major depressive episode has been present during the first 2 years of the disturbance (1 year for children and adolescents); i.e., the disturbance is not better accounted for by chronic major depressive disorder, or major depressive disorder in partial remission

Note: There may have been a previous Major Depressive Episode, provided there was a full remission (no significant signs or symptoms for 2 months) before development of the Dysthymic Disorder. In addition, after the initial 2 years (1 year in children or adolescents) of Dysthymic Disorder, there may be superimposed episodes of Major Depressive Disorder, in which case both diagnoses may be given when the criteria are met for a Major Depressive Episode

Continued

TABLE 4.2. Continued

E. There has never been a manic episode, a mixed episode, or a hypomanic episode, and criteria have never been met for cyclothymic disorder
F. The disturbance does not occur exclusively during the course of a chronic psychotic disorder, such as schizophrenia or delusional disorder
G. The symptoms are not due to the direct physiological effects of a substance (e.g., a drug of abuse, a medication) or a general medical condition (e.g., hypothyroidism)
H. The symptoms cause clinically significant distress or impairment in social, occupational, or other important areas of functioning

Mood disorder due to general medical condition

A. A prominent and persistent disturbance in mood predominates in the clinical picture and is characterized by either (or both) of the following:
  (1) depressed mood or markedly diminished interest or pleasure in all, or almost all, activities
  (2) elevated, expansive, or irritable mood
B. There is evidence from the history, physical examination, or laboratory findings that the disturbance is the direct physiological consequence of a general medical condition
C. The disturbance is not better accounted for by another mental disorder (e.g., adjustment disorder with depressed mood in response to the stress of having a general medical condition)
D. The disturbance does not occur exclusively during the course of a delirium.
E. The symptoms cause clinically significant distress or impairment in social, occupational, or other important areas of functioning

Substance-induced mood disorder

A. A prominent and persistent disturbance in mood predominates in the clinical picture and is characterized by either (or both) of the following:
  (1) depressed mood or markedly diminished interest or pleasure in all, or almost all, activities
  (2) elevated, expansive, or irritable mood
B. There is evidence from the history, physical examination, or laboratory findings of either (1) or (2):
  (1) the symptoms in Criterion A developed during, or within 1 month of, substance intoxication or withdrawal
  (2) medication use is etiologically related to the disturbance
C. The disturbance is not better accounted for by a mood disorder that is not substance induced. Evidence that the symptoms are better accounted for by a mood disorder that is not substance induced might include the following: the symptoms precede the onset of the substance use (or medication use); the symptoms persist for a substantial period of time (e.g., about a month) after the cessation of acute withdrawal or severe intoxication or are substantially in excess of what would be expected given the type or amount of the substance used or the duration of use; or there is other evidence that suggests the existence of an independent non-substance-induced mood disorder (e.g., a history of recurrent major depressive episodes)

Continued

TABLE 4.2. Continued

D. The disturbance does not occur exclusively during the course of a delirium.

E. The symptoms cause clinically significant distress or impairment in social, occupational, or other important areas of functioning

Note: This diagnosis should be made instead of a diagnosis of substance intoxication or substance withdrawal only when the mood symptoms are in excess of those usually associated with the intoxication or withdrawal syndrome and when the symptoms are sufficiently severe to warrant independent clinical attention.

Depression not otherwise specified (NOS)

DSM-IV-TR recognizes several depressive patterns under this category: subsyndromal depressions common in nursing home patients are classified here.

Minor depressive disorder: Episodes of 2 weeks or more of depressive symptoms, but with fewer than the 5 items required for major depressive disorder

Recurrent brief depressive disorder: Meets all criteria for major depression except duration. Episodes last from 2 days to 2 weeks and occur intermittently, but at least monthly for a year

Source: Adapted from the *DSM-IV-TR* (APA, 2000).

Provisional diagnostic criteria for depression of Alzheimer's disease

A. Three (or more) of the following symptoms have been present during the same 2-week period and represent a change from previous functioning: at least one of the symptoms is either depressed mood or decreased positive affect or pleasure
   1. clinically significant depressed mood (e.g., depressed, sad, hopeless, discouraged, tearful)
   2. decreased positive affect or pleasure in response to social contact and usual activities
   3. social isolation or withdrawal
   4. disruption in appetite
   5. disruption in sleep
   6. psychomotor changes (e.g., agitation or retardation)
   7. irritability
   8. fatigue or loss of energy
   9. feelings of worthlessness, hopelessness, or excessive or inappropriate guilt
   10. recurrent thoughts of death, suicidal ideation, plan or attempt

B. All criteria are met for dementia of the Alzheimer's type (*DSM-IV-TR*)

C. The symptoms cause clinically significant distress or disruption in functioning

D. The symptoms do not occur exclusively during the course of a delirium

E. The symptoms are not due to the direct physiological effects of a substance (e.g., a drug of abuse or a medication)

F. The symptoms are not better accounted for by other conditions such as Major Depressive Disorder, Bipolar Disorder, Bereavement, Schizophrenia, Schizoaffective Disorder, Psychosis of Alzheimer's disease, Anxiety disorders, or Substance-related disorder

Source: Adapted from Olin et al. (2002).

Apathy, a state of contented lack of initiative associated with executive dysfunction (but a concept still lacking a universally agreed upon clinical definition), is important in the context of such complex depressive and depression-like states particular to older adults. Operationalized for research by a rating scale, apathy has been identified as a prodromal stage or risk factor for depression following hip fracture (Lenze et al., 2007), but should be considered distinct from depression unless negative mood states are specifically identified. In a study of the temporal stability of symptoms of major and minor depression and apathy in AD over an average of 17 months, Starkstein et al. (2005) noted significant declines in depressive symptoms in half the study sample, but no change in apathy, further confirming the distinctness of the two behavioral domains.

Epidemiology

Results of numerous studies of the prevalence of depressive disorders in nursing homes published since the late 1970s have been summarized in several reports and reviews (Abrams et al., 1992; Ames, 1991; Gerety et al., 1994; German et al., 1992; Koenig & Blazer, 1992; Parmelee et al., 1989). The prevalence of major depression varies across studies from 5% to 43%, while that of less severe and pervasive (subsyndromal or "minor") depressions appears much higher, at 16% to over 60%. When diagnosis is based on criteria from earlier iterations of the *DSM,* the prevalence of major depressive syndromes approximates 15% to 20%, of minor depressions 25% to 40%, and of significant unhappiness and emotional suffering nearly 50% (Foster et al., 1991; Katz et al., 1989; Katz & Parmelee, 1994). Moreover, a growing evidence base reports similar prevalence rates of all depressive disorders (and other psychopathology) in assisted living facilities (Rosenblatt et al., 2004).

Using a psychiatric diagnostic evaluation for case identification, Teresi et al. (2001) estimated the prevalence of depression among nursing home residents and its recognition by nursing home staff. In a simple random sample of 319 nursing home residents from six downstate New York nursing homes, the prevalence of probable and/or definite major depressive disorder among testable subjects was 14.4%; 15.4% could not be assessed due to refusal or physical or cognitive limitations. The prevalence of minor depression and clinically significant depressive symptoms were 16.8% and 44.2%, respectively. Alarmingly, only 37% to 45% of cases diagnosed by psychiatrists were recognized as depressed by nurses, nurses' aides, and social workers.

Longitudinal studies indicate that depressive symptoms may fluctuate over time, with some patient improving, others worsening, and some remaining chronically depressed (Berger et al., 1998; Foster et al., 1991; Katz et al., 1989; Parmelee et al., 1992b; Rovner et al., 1991; Samuels & Katz, 1995). These and other data (Blazer, 2003; Katz & Parmelee, 1994) support the notion that the various depressive subtypes occupy the same spectrum of disorder and emphasize that patients with all forms of depression deserve detailed evaluation and serious treatment consideration.

Among institutionalized patients with dementia, the prevalence of depressive disorders is less clear. This question is of more than academic importance: dementias are the chief cause of psychiatric morbidity in nursing homes (Burns et al., 1988; Goldfarb, 1962; Teeter et al., 1976; Rovner et al., 1986) and can alter the presentation and treatment of concurrent depression. Investigations of the prevalence of all types of depression among individuals with dementia report a range of 14% to 39% (Cohen et al., 1995; Cohen et al., 1998). In a demented long-term care sample, Payne et al. (2002) noted a 20% prevalence of depression upon admission to the nursing home, most often in persons with a prior depressive history. By 6 months, only 40% of the originally depressed cohort was still depressed, whereas at 12 months only 7.5% remained depressed. Including these and residents not depressed at admission, the cumulative likelihood of depression over 1 year in this demented sample was 26%.

The reported prevalence of depression in AD varies depending on the diagnostic criteria used, and agreement among different diagnostic schemes is low (Vilalta-Franch et al., 2006). In a cross-sectional observational study of 491 AD patients, the prevalence of depression was estimated as 4.9% according to the *International Classification of Diseases*, 10th revision (ICD-10) criteria, 9.8% according to the Cambridge Examination for Mental Disorders of the Elderly (CAMDEX), 13.4% according to *DSM-IV*, 27.4% according to the Provisional Diagnostic Criteria for depression in AD (PDC-dAD), and 43.7% when using questions from the Neuropsychiatric Inventory (NPI) depression subscale (Vilalta-Franch et al., 2006). In addition, some controversy remains as to whether the overall prevalence of depression is lower in studies that include both demented and nondemented nursing home subjects (German et al., 1992; Parmelee et al., 1989), but others do not provide convincing evidence that moderately demented patients are protected from depression (Kafonek et al., 1989; Rovner et al., 1986; Snowden, 1986).

Why does the prevalence of depression vary so widely in different studies? Clearly, agreement on how to diagnose depression is a major factor, but patient case-mix and heterogeneity across facilities in styles of care that influence residents' mood, and varying rates and types of treatment, probably account for most of the difference. Nevertheless, reports from international studies in Singapore, South Africa, Australia, Italy, the United Kingdom, Scotland, and Japan, using a variety of approaches, all support the finding that depressive morbidity is high (Abrams et al., 1992; Ames, 1993; Koenig & Blazer, 1992; Rovner & Katz, 1993).

Complications of Depression: Medical Morbidity and Mortality

Research over the past decade more clearly establishes that depression can contribute to deteriorating health and death among older persons. Its impact is exerted through direct effects on food and fluid intake, resulting in weight loss, undernutrition, dehydration, and impaired resistance to infection (Schleifer et al., 1989). Increased mortality from preexisting cardiac disease (Whooley, 2006) is postulated to be mediated through excessive sympathetic nervous system arousal (Gold & Chrousos, 2002). In a 6-year longitudinal study, depression increased the risk for activities of daily living (ADL) disability and mobility disability by 67% and 73%, respectively (Penninx et al., 1999). Even after adjusting for baseline characteristics and chronic medical conditions, the risks for ADL and mobility disability remained 39% and 45% higher, respectively, than the nondepressed control group. More recently, Jiang et al. (2004) reported 120% higher risk for basic ADL impairment and 329% higher risk for decline in instrumental ADL in depressed elderly even after controlling for confounding factors in an 8-year longitudinal study conducted in Beijing. Similar findings are available from a 5-year longitudinal epidemiological study from Finland as well (Kivela & Pahkala, 2001). Moreover, depression has been shown to increase the risk for onset of coronary artery disease and stroke (Larson et al., 2001; Wulsin & Singal, 2003) and is an independent risk factor for the development of type II diabetes mellitus (Kawakami et al., 1999). Many pathophysiological mechanisms have been implicated in depression's adverse interactions with medical outcomes, including platelet activation (especially in the presence of the serotonin transporter promoter region 5-HTTLPR polymorphism), poorer T-cell immune response, increased systemic inflammatory activity, increased bone resorption, and neuroendocrine dysregulation (McEwan, 2003; Michelson et al., 1996; Thomas et al., 2005; Whyte et al., 2001). Attitudinal, motivational, and cognitive states associated with depression likely also contribute to morbidity and mortality by undermining health promoting behaviors (e.g., compliance with medications, exercise, and smoking cessation) (Ciechanowski et al., 2000).

The effect of depression on mortality has been confirmed in long-term care studies, with relative risks of 1.5 to 3 (Ashby et al., 1991; Katz et al., 1989; Parmelee et al., 1992a, 1992b; Rovner et al., 1991), but the effect is less obvious when rigorous methods are used to control for the effects of medical illness, functional disability, and cognitive status (Parmelee et al., 1992a, 1992b). In contrast, in mixed-age depressed populations, there appears to be a 3- to 4-fold increased risk of death 5 years (and beyond) after an acute myocardial infarction or a stroke (Lesperance et al., 2002; Morris et al., 1993). Further study is needed to resolve the question of whether depression plays a direct causal role in hastening death and whether treatment of depression alters mortality.

Clinical Features of Depression in Nursing Home Patients

Classic major depression and other dysphoric states

The work of Ames (1991), Katz et al. (1989), and Rovner and Katz (1993) demonstrates that standard diagnostic criteria for depression are effective in long-term care residents. Diagnostic ambiguity, while frequent, is no different in principle from that encountered in other groups of older patients with serious medical illness and functional disabilities, just "more so." However, factors related specifically to long-term care settings require that psychiatrists, other mental health professionals, and nursing home staff recognize presentations of mood pathology that are not straightforward. The institutional environment itself may impede recognition of depression by submerging residents' individual symptoms in the press of care or attributing them to personality characteristics. Long-term care patients rarely request treatment for depression, and the diagnostic process must often rely heavily on collateral information from staff whose knowledge of their patients' histories or inner life may be scanty. A detailed understanding of depression in individual patients may require more time and skill than staff can commit. Finally, untreated long-lasting depressions often lose their mood signatures, leaving only a residue of functional impairment and apathy that obscures their original character.

Masked depressions in nursing home patients: Special considerations

Masked depression was eloquently conceptualized early in the history of geriatric psychiatry in the original work of Lesse (1964). This classic of descriptive psychopathology is recommended reading for all who supervise the care of elderly persons in institutional settings. In a modern data-based study, Loebel et al. (1991) compared reasons for referral with subsequent psychiatric diagnosis in 197 patients residing in six Seattle nursing homes. Among the 38 (19%) patients with a depression or anxiety disorder, mood symptoms were identified by staff as the chief presenting problem in only 61%. Behavior problems were predominant in 34%, and "staff concern" with no specific problem stated was noted in 24%. Psychotic features were primary in 13%, somatic symptoms or signs in 11%, impaired function in 3%, and a mixed group of symptoms (including suicidal ideas or acts, cognitive impairment, and nursing home adjustment failure) in 13%. Further evidence for the "masking" phenomenon comes from Fenton et al. (2004) who reported a psychiatric consultation rate of only 20% in a nursing home cohort of 2285 residents, of whom those with a quiet or retarded depression were most likely to be overlooked. Not surprisingly, residents who were agitated or psychomotorically activated were the most likely to be referred for psychiatric consultation. These data emphasize that "masking" of depressive syndromes in the nursing home setting is common and takes many forms.

Extreme social withdrawal, accompanied by voluntary efforts to reduce human contact and sensory stimulation, descriptively termed "cocooning" by Baker and Miller (1991), is strongly associated with depressive disorder and its improvement with antidepressant treatment.

Anxiety, agitation, uncooperativeness, and aggressive or abusive behavior can mask depression. Anxiety in its many forms (including panic disorder, other anxiety disorder diagnoses, and psychological and somatic symptoms of anxiety) is strongly associated with depression in elderly nursing home patients. Three-quarters of anxious patients are depressed, and the majority of patients with major depression are anxious (Parmelee et al., 1993a). Depressed affect and clinical depression, and several of their correlates—such as sleep disturbance, pain, recent life-threatening experience, and poor quality of relationships—are predictors of a variety of agitated behaviors or uncooperativeness (Cohen-Mansfield et al., 1990; Cohen-Mansfield et al., 1992; Menon et al., 2001; Rovner et al., 1992; Talerico et al., 2002). In patients with advanced dementia, agitated behaviors such as screaming, verbal and physical aggression, and dysphoric motor overactivity can represent behavioral expression of a depressive syndrome that cannot be verbally articulated. Regardless of cognitive status, anxious or agitated patients should be carefully examined for clinical features of a depressive syndrome. Even when the clinical picture is not typical, antidepressant pharmacotherapy may improve behavioral symptoms (Friedman et al., 1992; Schneider & Sobin, 1992; Rojas-Fernandez et al., 2001). Important and useful psychodynamic and psychotherapeutic perspectives are provided in the edited volume of Brink (1987) and recently summarized in a state-of-the-evidence review of "talk therapies" in long-term care settings (Bharucha et al., 2006).

Pain is an important mask for depression among nursing home residents. Chronic pain, common in geriatric care settings, is undetected by physicians and certified nurses' aides in at least two-thirds of affected patients who can describe it clearly (Horgas & Dunn, 2001; Winn & Dentino, 2004). With cognitively impaired patients who may express their pain only through behavioral symptoms, failure rates are even higher (Leonard et al., 2006; Sengstaken & King, 1993). Several new scales validly and reliably assess pain in those who are in the advanced stages of dementia and/or are noncommunicative (Cohen-Mansfield, 2006; Snow et al., 2004; Warden et al., 2003), representing major advances over previously available techniques.

Chronic pain should be treated as a potential marker for depression (Gruber-Baldini et al., 2005). Parmelee et al. (1991) reported that, after controlling for medical causes, patients with major depression have both more intense pain and a greater number of pain complaints than do those with subsyndromal or no depression. This finding has been replicated using caregiver reports (Cohen-Mansfield & Marx, 1993), where special attention was given to assessing demented patients, whose self-reported pain complaints are often discounted and ignored (Parmelee et al., 1993b).

Other somatic symptoms and signs may obscure the presence of depression in patients with significant medical illnesses. Depression amplifies symptoms of chronic medical disorders (Arnow et al., 2006; Borson et al., 1986; Katon, 1984; Shahpeshandy, 2005). In medically ill elderly, effective treatment of depression can reduce physical symptoms and disability usually attributed to the underlying medical disorder (Borson et al., 1992). Despite advances in the recognition and treatment of depression over the past 20 years, treatable depression is still underrecognized in the chronically ill (Schnittker, 2005). It is clear that chronic illness is a risk factor for comorbid depression (Borson et al., 1986; Koenig & Blazer, 1992; Kukull et al., 1986), and dysphoria or other depressive indicators accompanying disabling medical illness should prompt psychiatric diagnostic evaluation, as depressed mood is among the strongest predictors of declining health in a nursing home population (Parmelee, et al., 1998).

Eating disorders may be the primary presenting symptom of depression and, when severe, may lead to extreme weight loss (Hsu & Zimmer, 1988; Miller et al., 1991; Price et al., 1985). Weight loss and protein-calorie malnutrition are common in elderly persons residing in long-term care facilities (Crogan & Pasvogel, 2003; Silver et al., 1988); significant undernutrition has been reported in as many as 85% of nursing home residents and carries the potential for serious impairment of resistance to disease and even death in this population (Asplund et al., 1981; Kersteller et al., 1992; Ridman & Feller, 1989). Depression and food intake interact in a complex fashion. Undereating can cause mild depression, and depression can cause reduced food intake by a variety of mechanisms. Some depressed patients stop eating as a form of passive suicide, and others refuse to eat as a way of influencing caregivers ("hunger strike"). Perhaps most commonly, depressed people eat less due to direct effects of depression on appetite: these patients may require special attention at meals and provision of favorite foods in addition to antidepressant treatment. The Centers for Medicare and Medicaid Services' (CMS) final rule permitting a long-term care facility to use paid feeding assistants to supplement the services of certified nurse aides is an important service and can be applied to residents who are experiencing unplanned weight loss or dehydration, even those who are relatively cognitively intact (CMS, 2003).

Alcohol abuse and overuse of sedatives is common, may reflect an underlying depression, and adversely impact depression treatment in long-term care residents (McCullough, 1991; Oslin et al., 2003; Weverer et al., 1999). The widespread prescription of sedatives in nursing homes has raised questions as to the proper indications for their use and prompted experimental efforts to reduce overuse. Two important studies have examined the effects on patients of facility wide reductions in sedative prescribing. Avorn et al. (1992) found that depressive symptoms increased, but Salzman et al. (1992) found that cognitive function improved. These results suggest that many depressed patients are treated for only the associated anxiety and accept oversedation, at the expense of their cognitive capacity, to reduce their suffering.

Example. A 73-year-old woman demented after an episode of herpes encephalitis, presented with dysphoria, agitation, confusion, crying spells, and addiction to alprazolam. A gradual dose taper resulted in marked improvement of cognitive function and emergence of profound and disabling agitated depression.

Cognitive impairment (depressive "pseudodementia") was first described in withdrawn nursing home patients assumed to be demented but found, upon clinical examination, to be suffering from severe depression (Kiloh, 1961). The severe cognitive impairments seen years ago in nondemented depressed patients have fortunately become rare, owing to improvements in nursing home care and the universal availability of antidepressant pharmacotherapy, but cognitive complaints remain common in depressed patients. Cognitive deficits caused by severe depression can usually be distinguished from those due to primary dementing disorders (Poon, 1992), but as new data have emerged on the overlap between dementia and depression in patients with brain diseases of later life, a more inclusive "both and" approach has tended to replace this earlier "either-or" conceptualization. The use of simple bedside cognitive screening tests is appropriate in the evaluation of depressed *long-term care* residents. The familiar Mini-Mental State Exam or the newer, briefer Mini-Cog (Borson et al., 2000; Scanlan & Borson, 2001) are useful as screens for general cognitive impairment; more specific executive screens such as the *exit* interview are considerably longer and require specialized administration techniques but more definitively identify executive dysfunction (Royall et al., 1992). Depressive cognitive dysfunction preferentially affects attention, motivation, and energy to engage in activities requiring mental effort; access to and use of stored information is impaired as a result. Similar deficits are often seen in patients with damage to frontal-subcortical systems even in the absence of clinical mood disorder (Aizenstein et al., 2002). New learning can be impeded by distractability in patients with anxious depressions, due to marked forgetfulness, short attention span, and spells of apparent confusion, about which they may complain bitterly, convinced that "their minds are gone." Patients with severe depressive retardation may appear quite dull and apathetic, have great difficulty recalling information they knew just a short time before the development of their mood disorder, or be unable to participate effectively in diagnostic interviews. These cognitive deficits, due to the psychobiology of depression itself, typically develop in tandem with the onset or worsening of the mood disorder and are reversible with effective treatment in up to 50% of patients (Dobie, 2002). In contrast, patients with cognitive deficits due only to dementing illness can usually pay attention, try their best to perform (often becoming frustrated with the effort), and minimize their mental difficulties. Their cognitive problems develop and persist regardless of the presence of mood disorder, often appearing after a known brain insult or displaying a pattern characteristic of a specific dementia diagnosis.

In actual geriatric practice, varying degrees and types of dementia and depression often coexist, and most research data support the view of experienced geropsychiatrists that patients who present with prominent signs of both dementia and depression probably have both disorders. In patients with a primary dementia, the development of depression amplifies the impact of brain dysfunction on day-to-day life, and antidepressant drugs or other treatments may improve function. In addition, a typical treatment-responsive depressive episode may be the first presenting problem seen in patients who are developing a dementing illness. It is not usually necessary (nor is it always possible) to determine in advance whether depression accounts for all of the cognitive deficits observed in a given patient; far more important is the clinician's recognition of the depression and appropriate therapeutic response to it. The issue will usually be clarified in time by the response of the cognitive impairment to effective treatment. In spite of effective treatment, approximately 50% of patients with pseudodementia will develop a true Alzheimer's type dementia over the next 5 years (Alexopoulos et al., 1993; Nebes et al., 2003). The standard of care in long-term care facilities must include provisions of sufficiently competent psychiatric services to ensure that both dementia and depression are accurately diagnosed and adequately managed.

Cognitive, neurological, and behavioral disturbances of brain disease can influence the way depression manifests itself. In patients with diffuse or multifocal brain disease, damage to the integrity of the central nervous system may prevent the development of the most easily recognized features of syndromal depressions, obscuring them beneath cognitive, motor, or other behavioral deficits more readily observed by caregivers. Both verbal and nonverbal expression of affect may be impaired in patients with brain disease (Blonder et al., 2005); as a result, observable behavioral indicators of depression assume special salience in brain-damaged patients.

Newly refined clinical and imaging techniques and evolving conceptual frameworks now identify a relationship between frontostriatal dysfunction and depression in late life that in some cases appears to be mediated by damage to the linking white matter tracts (Alexopoulos et al., 2005; Ballmaier et al., 2004; Firbank et al., 2004). Functional neuroimaging studies further implicate frontal-subcortical and neo-vs archicortical metabolic changes in depressive states (Alexopoulos, 2002; Drevets, 2003). Hippocampal abnormalities, both in terms of volume and function, have also been associated with late-life depression (Sheline, 2003). Finally, a recent postmortem study of late-life depression lends support to the vascular etiopathology and the importance of the dorsolateral prefrontal cortex as a target site in the pathogenesis of late-life depression (Thomas et al., 2003).

Neurological damage itself can be a direct cause of depressive syndromes when it affects brain pathways important in mood and psychomotor neurovegetative function. Frontotemporal degenerative dementia can cause depressive and anxious symptoms, especially when right frontal and anterior temporal disease predominates (Mendez et al., 2006). Parkinson's disease and "Parkinson-Plus" syndromes such as Shy-Drager syndrome and Progressive Supranuclear Palsy, stroke (frontal, deep lacunar, and brainstem infarction, especially), Huntington's disease, and other disorders are commonly associated with various depressive disorders as a result of neural damage. Other nondepressive disorders of affect regulation, such as lability of mood and emotional expression, also occur in neurological diseases and may be responsive to antidepressant pharmacotherapy (van Wattum & Chiles, 2001). Any sustained period of emotional distress should be viewed as potentially reflecting a treatable depression or related state. It is important to note that a neurological cause for depression does not imply unresponsiveness to antidepressant pharmacotherapy or some other somatic or psychosocial treatments. Contrariwise, a history of major depression might accelerate the neuropathogenesis of an underlying dementing disease (Rapp et al., 2006), though such a mechanism is not firmly established.

Excess disability and motivational failure are core components of depressions in long-term care patients and may be their chief presenting symptom. For individual patients, determining how much disability is "excessive" and how much motivation should be expected (and to what end) can be difficult in the presence of disabling medical conditions and in the setting of under- or overstimulating environments frequently prevailing in *long-term care* facilities. Detailed assessments and sophisticated clinical skills are usually required to identify the presence of and reasons for excess disability and rehabilitation failures; the intimate familiarity with patients and the clinical psychiatric assessment needed for this task are often beyond the reach of direct-care staff. It is important that such problems not escape the attention of those at higher levels.

Example. A 79-year-old married African American woman was admitted to an inner-city nursing home after amputation of a leg because of severe burns caused when she rushed to remove a pan of flaming motor oil from the stove. Discharge home was planned once she had learned to walk with a prosthesis. When 3 months passed with little progress in rehabilitation, she was referred for psychiatric consultation to improve her motivation. She was found to be experiencing a major depressive episode, precipitated by the loss of her leg. Her motivational failure was due to desire to avoid returning home to her demented husband, who had put the oil in the stove to warm it. The discovery of this previously hidden problem led to placement of her husband in a nursing home, rapid progress in her rehabilitation, resolution of her depression without other treatment, and successful return to her life in the community.

Risk factors for depression in long-term care patients

Medical illness and disability are primary risk factors for the development of both major and minor depressive syndromes. Rates of depression in long-term care settings generally exceed those reported in samples of elderly persons residing in the community, including those with chronic diseases (reviewed by Koenig & Blazer, 1992) and increase with functional dependency and level of care (Gurland et al., 1983; Katz & Parmelee, 1994; Parmelee et al., 1989). A recent cross-sectional study of 333 nursing home residents in the Netherlands found pain, functional limitations, visual impairment, stroke, loneliness, lack of social support, negative life events, and perceived inadequacy of care to be strong predictors of risk for depression (Jongenelis et al., 2004). For subclinical depression, the same risk indicators applied, with the exception of lack of social support. A *prior history of depression, dysphoric response to change, or high level of need for personal intimacy* probably elevates risk following institutionalization, but this has not been studied. A fruitful area for future investigation is the relative power of individual versus institutional variables in predicting onset and persistence of depression.

Placement in a long-term care facility is a major life event rarely undertaken happily. Indeed, patients awaiting nursing home admission appear to have rates of depression comparable with those in patients actually admitted (Zenmore & Eames, 1979), and anticipation of nursing home placement appears to be a risk factor for completed suicide (Loebel et al., 1991). Admission to a nursing home usually results from important prior losses and brings new ones: the decision for nursing home care is the result of loss of capacity for independent function and lack of available, adequate in-home care, and placement adds losses of personal control, privacy, and proximity to remaining family and friends (Osgood, 1992). This suggests that it is not the transition to institutional life itself that confers added risk for depression but the nature and personal significance of the disability that make placement necessary. Prospective studies that capture the adjustment process to long-term care placement are much needed before it can be translated into clinical practice (Castle, 2001).

Moving into long-term care could, in principle, ameliorate or prevent mood disorders in frail older persons by simplifying burdensome daily chores and providing easy access to support and assistance, medical care, and opportunities for friendship, social interaction, and activities appropriate to functional ability. There is conflicting evidence about whether a supportive nursing home environment can in fact achieve this goal. Snowden and Donnelly (1986) found lower severity of depressive symptoms in long-term than recently admitted residents.

Parmelee et al. (1992b) found, in a facility providing clinical care for depression, that about half of patients with major depression at the time of admission were improved a year later, but most continued to experience some degree of depressive symptomatology; in this study, long-stay residents fared no better than newly admitted patients. Ames (1991) reported low recovery rates (<30%) after 1 year, despite the availability of psychiatric consultation and management. This suggests that the combination of a supportive care environment and psychiatric treatment is not sufficient to improve the outlook for depression in long-term care settings. It is possible that programmatic changes could help nursing homes realize their potential as therapeutic environments.

What *environmental factors* might make a difference? Clinical and theoretical considerations suggest that institutional factors are important in depression, but no studies have been designed to test this idea. For suicide, however, Osgood (1992) identified several institutional factors associated with risk: larger facility size, less privacy for residents, higher staff turnover, lower charges for care (possibly reflecting fewer available services and a less enriched environment), and religious affiliation. More recently, Gruber-Baldini et al. (2005) have also identified for-profit facility status as a risk factor for depression in demented nursing home residents. Because suicide is most commonly associated with depression, particularly among the elderly (Conwell, 1994), it is likely that environmental factors figure prominently in suicide through their effects both on psychosocial risks for development of depression and on its recognition and treatment (Brant & Osgood, 1990).

We propose that an institutional factor important in initiating or maintaining depression in residents of long-term care facilities is *contagion of dysphoria and dysfunction* among patients and staff. Especially important are residents' relationships with nurses' aides, which are among the most intimate and sustaining that patients in long-term care settings have. Some 80% to 100% of personal care is provided by relatively untrained and unskilled workers who come from sociocultural, linguistic, and economic backgrounds often far different from those of their patients; patient contact with a nurse averages only 12 min/day, and lower direct-care times with a nurse are strongly correlated with a variety of poor medical outcomes (Dorr et al., 2005; Institute of Medicine, 1986). The high aide turnover rates common in many facilities, estimated at 45% to 119% per year (Castle, 2006) add recurring emotional losses to those experienced by patients as a result of long-term care placement, poor health, and attrition of family and friends. Moreover, the turnover is not limited to nurses' aides; the 1-year turnover rate for licensed practical nurses (89%), registered nurses (87%), administrators (57%), and directors of nursing (48%) are alarmingly high (Castle, 2006).

Not unexpectedly, research has shown a correlation between residents' emotional well-being and satisfaction with care and the level of job satisfaction among nurses' aides. Aides' length of employment, wages, level of benefits, and perceptions of the fairness and competence of the charge nurse all correlate with patient satisfaction (Kruzich et al., 1992). Even when job assignments are stable, aides' many responsibilities often limit the more time-consuming emotional aspects of personal care (Bowers & Becker, 1992). It is interesting that vulnerability to the disruptive effects of high staff turnover is highest among the most functionally impaired residents, who are also most vulnerable to depression.

Sources of poor morale and job dissatisfaction among aides are several. As a group, aides are often multiply burdened by adversity at home and at work in ways that create a cycle of distress and indignity in their own lives (V. Tellis-Nayak & M. Tellis-Nayak, 1989). On the job, high workload, inadequate skills—especially in the care of cognitively impaired patients with disruptive behavior—and the physical and emotional demands built into the care of disabled elderly persons contribute to feelings of pressure, burden, and burnout and set the stage for a cycle of abuse that reverberates throughout staff and patients. These factors have been explored in depth in the ground-breaking studies of Foner (1994), using anthropological fieldwork methods.

Abusive behavior of aides toward residents is disturbingly prevalent in nursing homes and probably contributes to depression as well as general misery among residents. In an important series of studies, nursing assistants disclosed high rates of abusive behavior toward their patients—40% acknowledged at least one act of physical abuse (Pillemer & Bachman, 1991; Pillemer & Moore, 1989, 1990). Missing from these studies is the fact that abuse is rarely habitual; most abusive acts appear in a flash of anger reflecting aides' exhaustion and repeated mistreatment by patients whose social restraint has been lost due to mental impairments (Foner, 1994). Episodes of purposeful taunting and humiliation of residents by angry aides also occur and are likely to cluster around patients whose reputation for insulting, threatening, and otherwise ugly and aggressive behavior has spread throughout the facility and affected many caregivers. Regular scapegoating of the most vulnerable residents by aides may signify a response to habitual mistreatment by their superiors, inadequate or insensitive supervisory practices, or frank psychopathology.

Several models of intervention to reduce patient abuse have been developed. Pillemer and Hudson (1993) described a brief curriculum for abuse prevention, based on increasing staff awareness of the dynamics of abuse, ability to recognize abuse-prone situations, and capacity for conflict avoidance and resolution. A study conducted in 10 very diverse nursing homes in the greater Philadelphia area confirmed high rates of self-reported abusive behavior by staff. In the month preceding training, yelling in anger at a resident was reported by 51% and insulting or swearing at a resident by 23%. Threats of physical harm and actual physical abuse (including excessive restraint; pushing, shoving, grabbing, or slapping; throwing something at a resident; kicking; and hitting with the fist) were also reported, but at substantially lower rates. Following abuse prevention training, positive effects were noted on aides' attitudes toward patients and caregiving, levels of conflict experienced, resident aggression toward aides, and number of abuse events. Although patient satisfaction with care and mood were not examined in this study, reduction in abusive interactions with caregivers can be expected to improve both—at least in relation to day-to-day care. Institutional changes to reduce workload and explicit skills training reduce aide burnout (Chappell & Novak, 1992), a major causal factor in patient abuse. Other forms of aide training focused on interactional dynamics have been known, for nearly 30 years, to improve aides' job satisfaction (Goldman & Woog, 1975; Moses, 1982).

Patient welfare on a day-to-day basis is clearly dependent on the well-being of aides. Therefore, the function and fate of these primary caregivers may be fundamental to the psychogenesis of despondency, disengagement, and clinical depression in residents; to the failure of staff to recognize and intervene in them; and to the failure of psychiatric care of patients to solve the epidemiological problem. Much more attention should be given to developing mechanisms for improving aides' satisfaction and safety from emotional and physical abuse by patients who are no longer in control of their own behavior. Among these mechanisms may be such diverse activities as unionization of aides with the anticipated result of improved working conditions, wages and benefits (Foner, 1994), interpersonal training, open recognition by nurses and administrators of the effects on aides of the personally stressful nature of work, and institutional efforts to provide regular, constructive ways of discharging accumulated job tensions before they are played out in abusive behavior toward patients. Conversely, habitual abuse of aides by a patient should be made an explicit and valid reason for psychiatric consultation and management and not merely couched in vague terms such as "agitation."

Many facilities are participating in quality improvement initiatives that may well have positive effects in terms of preventing abuse or neglect (Hawes, 2002). The Wellspring Initiative, started in Wisconsin with spread to Texas and Illinois, is one example. It involves both empowerment of nurses' aides and enhanced clinical training for all staff from a Geriatric Nurse Practitioner as well as peer facilities. An early evaluation, presented by Hawes (2000) to the U.S. Senate Finance Committee, found reduced staff turnover and audit deficiencies among the participating facilities. Other facilities, such as the Pioneers, those participating in the Eden Alternative, and innovators, such as Kendall-Crossland in Pennsylvania and Benedictine in Oregon, may also shed light on how to prevent abuse and neglect. Recognition of the needs of both aides and patients for a humane, supportive, and safe environment is an important step toward its realization.

Detection of Depression and Utilization
of Mental Health Services

Heston et al. (1992) examined medical records of nearly 6000 nursing home patients admitted to 60 Minnesota nursing homes during the 1970s and 1980s and reported that primary care physicians had made a diagnosis of depression or affective psychosis in about 15% of these, a rate of about half that reported from epidemiological surveys for all depressions combined. Of the depressed patients, only 10% were receiving an antidepressant drug and over half received no psychotropic medication. Recognition of depression by nurses and awareness of treatment options are likely to be critical to improvements in patient care; however, Rovner et al. (1992) found that nurses' ratings of patients' depressive symptoms were neither sensitive to nor specific for clinically diagnosed depression. Rovner et al. (1991), studying a cohort of patients admitted in the late 1980s, reported prior recognition of depression in only 14% of patients diagnosed as depressed by psychiatrists and active treatment in only one-quarter of patients so diagnosed. Even when primary care internists identify depressive symptoms in their elderly patients and formulate appropriate treatment plans, they often do not implement them (Barsa et al., 1986).

In contrast to the discouraging findings pertaining to the recognition and treatment of depression prior to the implementation of OBRA-87 (Public Law 100–203), more recent reports from the CMS indicate that, from 1992 to 2000, the percentage of nursing home residents prescribed an antidepressant nearly tripled from 12.6% to 35.5% (Crutchfield, 2001). While the recognition of depression in such facilities has improved over the past decade, many nursing home residents continue to receive inadequate doses of antidepressants for inadequate periods of time (Brown et al., 2002; Weintraub et al., 2003). Moreover, as Weintraub et al. (2002) point out, best next-step practices for partial and nonresponders need to be developed, in addition to optimally maintaining the acute response over the continuation and maintenance phases of antidepressant treatment. Notwithstanding this encouraging progress, a recent review of the provision of mental health services reports persistent, severe inadequacies in the availability of skilled geropsychiatrists (Moak & Borson, 2000). Moreover, the same report expresses the view of directors of nursing that there is a tremendous need for and lack of expertise in nonpharmacological approaches to behavioral and emotional problems.

In the first large-scale systematic study of mental health services utilization by nursing home patients, Burns et al. (1993) reported that only 6% of all patients with a mood disorder diagnosed received any mental health treatment and only 3.5% had contact with a specialty-trained mental health provider. Geographic factors and age influenced mental health treatment. Patients residing in the northeastern part of the United States and younger geriatric patients were most likely to be treated by specialists. Unfortunately, the oldest patients—who are most likely to be severely functionally impaired, who present complex clinical problems, and who are in greatest need of evaluation and management by geropsychiatrists—appear least likely to get it. What will remedy this state of affairs? Effective methods for identifying depressed persons are a priority for health services research and application. Provisions of OBRA-87 recognizing that mental health diagnosis and treatment are integral to high-quality nursing home care are a significant step, as demonstrated by the increased prescription rates for antidepressants over the past decade (Crutchfield, 2001). However, the utility of the mandated Minimum Data Set (MDS) and Resident Assessment Protocols (RAPs) as screens for depressive disorders has not been established and at best can be only as good as the skills of the staff who complete them.

In a cross-sectional study of 1492 nursing homes, only 11% were identified as depressed on the MDS (Brown et al., 2002). These low rates of depression detection have placed into question the utility of the MDS Mood Disturbance items as a screen for depression. The validity of the MDS has been compared with other routinely used research instruments, as well as with modified versions of the original MDS (Burrows et al., 2000; Datto et al., 2002; Frederiksen et al., 1996; Hawes et al., 1995; Lawton et al., 1998; McCurren et al., 1999). These studies report limited criterion validity for MDS as routinely collected by the nursing home staff (correlation coefficients .15 to .44). In response to this poor performance, experts recommend concurrent use of a self-report scale, such as the Geriatric Depression Scale (GDS), for those with minimal cognitive impairment, and an interviewer-rated scale such as the Cornell Scale for Depression in Dementia (CSDD) for those with significant cognitive impairment. Alternatively, the MDS Mood Disturbance items may be reliably and validly administered via self-report to persons scoring at least 12 on the Mini-Mental State Exam (Ruckdeschel et al., 2004). The latter approach obviates the disadvantage of training nursing home staff in the use of research assessment instruments such as the GDS and CSDD since the MDS is a federal requirement.

Inclusion of psychiatric nurse clinicians as members of nursing home staff can have an important impact, and nurse gerontologists are a valuable and underutilized resource for assessment and treatment (Kolcaba & Miller, 1989; Santmyer & Roca, 1991). Several alternative models for providing comprehensive psychiatric service to nursing home patients have been described but not yet tested for their contribution to quality of care. Libow and Starer (1989) have emphasized that the best nursing homes nationwide are characterized by the ready availability of expert geropsychiatric consultation; meeting these manpower needs within current mandates for cost containment remains a significant and growing challenge (Borson et al., 2001).

Caring for Depressed Patients in Long-Term Care

Clinical assessment and treatment planning

Depressed patients usually look sad, worried, or withdrawn when observed unobtrusively. Many try hard to conceal their distress. Some respond to staff interest by seeming brighter, only to withdraw again when left alone. Many patients make frequent calls for help or complain loudly about lack of assistance. Staff often respond by insisting that these patients can do more for themselves than they do. Patients may pick at their food, refuse to go to meals, or disparage the quality of food served. They may wake frequently at night, ask for sleeping pills, seem too tired to function during the day, or complain loudly about physical symptoms for which medical treatment has already been optimized. When asked about what interests them, they may be unable to think of anything.

Diagnostic criteria for the various subtypes of depression are provided in Table 4.2. It is important to note that many medical illnesses and disabilities as well as the interactive effects of polypharmacy can give rise to some of the symptoms of depression but not all of its features. Most nondepressed patients adapt to their physical limitations by developing new sources of stimulation, enjoyment, and meaning in their lives.

The elements of comprehensive diagnostic assessment are shown in Table 4.3. A clinical judgment must be made as to the possible contribution of medical factors to the depressive syndrome. Early undiagnosed pneumonia, poorly controlled congestive heart failure or excessive diuresis, overtreatment of hypertension, inappropriate polypharmacy (either medical or psychotropic drugs), inability to eat because of swallowing problems, specific neurological disorders, respiratory insufficiency requiring adjustment of medications, electrolyte imbalance, or sensory deficits such as hearing and visual loss can all contribute to some of the signs and symptoms of depression. These should be considered and appropriately treated. In general, drug regimens should be simplified whenever this is consistent with good medical practice.

Psychosocial, environmental, and psychological factors with the potential to affect mood should be assessed with the help of the attending physician, nursing and aide staff, family when available, social worker, and recreational therapist. Practical interventions can be developed from this information; they include help in resolving conflictual relations between patient and roommate or aide, prescription of an activity program, or planning a regular program of visitation by family members or volunteers. Environmental modifications may be pertinent, especially for patients with sensory, motor, or cognitive deficits and those who have become severely withdrawn from others. Staff and visitors should be educated about ways to improve communication with hearing—or vision-impaired patients (e.g., audibly identifying all visitors to a blind patient's room, speaking to the "good ear" of a hearing-impaired patient). Frequent, brief, but personal contacts are helpful with confused or fearful patients, and providing adequate light can partly compensate for some visual impairments. Predictable assignment of compatible aides furnishes great comfort to depressed patients.

Medical treatments for depression are required when depression is severe enough to interfere with day-to-day activities, cause intense personal suffering,

TABLE 4.3. Psychiatric Evaluation and Treatment Planning for the Depressed Patient

---

Identify patient with possible mood disorder
Consolidate history and observations made by staff: symptoms, behavior changes,
    duration, effects on others
Examine patient
    Define depressive symptoms and signs
    Assess cognitive and behavioral problems
    Determine medical, neurological, and functional status
    Inquire about prior psychiatric history
    Identify specific relationship problems
    Evaluate attitudes toward care, awareness of problem, emotional understanding
Review medical record
    Diagnoses present and omitted
    Psychiatric, psychosocial history
    Recent physical examination
    Physicians' orders and medication sheets
    Physicians' and nurses' notes: sleep, eating, mood, behavior
    Social work, physical and activity therapy notes
    Minimum Data Set and Preadmission Screening and Annual Review evaluations
Synthesize and record data
    Are further tests needed?
    Assign best-estimate psychiatric diagnosis
    Formulate reasonable pathogenetic hypotheses
    Identify risks relevant to treatment planning: medical, pharmacological factors;
        suicide
Develop and record treatment plan
    Is hospitalization needed?
    Psychosocial, environmental, and sensory approaches
    Antidepressant drug therapy
    Electroconvulsive therapy
Specify how results will be evaluated
    Responsibility for treatment components—who?
    Monitors for treatment response and adverse effects—what, how often?
    Plan for follow-up

Source: Reprinted with permission from the first edition of this textbook.

or is beyond the reach of psychological or psychosocial interventions. This is almost always the case when mood disturbance takes the form of a major depression, is associated with sustained changes in physical function (sleep, appetite, energy, psychomotor agitation or retardation), or is accompanied by anxiety, fearfulness, or psychotic features. Milder chronic depressions frequently require medical therapy as well. Many such illnesses cause protracted but relatively invisible suffering and represent the residue of untreated prior major depressive episodes. Medical treatments for depression include prescription of antidepressant drugs and electroconvulsive therapy.

Antidepressant pharmacotherapy

In the first published randomized controlled trial of an antidepressant specifically in a nursing home setting, Katz et al. (1990) reported the superiority of active treatment with nortriptyline over placebo in patients with major depression. With a conventional dosing paradigm, about half of patients who tolerated the drug experienced useful benefit (mean nortriptyline plasma level at study completion = 75.6 ± 48.4 ng/mL), while placebo response was negligible. However, 7 of 30 experienced adverse events necessitating discontinuation. Since then, 10 double blind or open trials of antidepressant therapy involving nursing home residents exclusively have been published in English peer-reviewed journals (Table 4.4). Sertraline has been the most frequently examined agent (six reports), followed by nortriptyline (two reports), fluoxetine (two reports), paroxetine (two reports), venlafaxine (one report), and mirtazapine (one report). A total of 469 subjects have participated in these trials with 89 (19%) dropouts. The study design, key entry criteria, and primary outcomes of each of these trials are detailed in Table 4.4.

All classes of antidepressant drugs have been used safely in clinical treatment of individual patients, including selective serotonin reuptake inhibitors (SSRIs), serotonin norepinephrine reuptake inhibitors (SNRIs), tricyclics, heterocylics, monoamine oxidase inhibitors, and psychostimulants such as methylphenidate or dextroamphetamine (please refer to the psychopharmacology chapter of this textbook for the pharmacological properties of specific agents). The choice of drug should be made on the basis of risks and side-effect profiles and the patient's prior response to a particular agent (if any). Some antidepressant drugs may be hazardous for patients with specific medical vulnerabilities. Examples include tricyclic antidepressants, which are inadvisable for patients with cardiac conduction defects, and monoamine oxidase inhibitors, which are contraindicated in patients taking meperidine for pain. The compatibility of specific antidepressants with medically essential drugs must be considered before initiating treatment. Once a drug is chosen, treatment is initiated with the lowest appropriate dose. A conservative program of incremental dosing, based on contingencies of response and anticipated or observed side effects, can be scheduled in advance. Specific nursing staff should be assigned to supervise and monitor treatment. Concrete guidelines for monitoring should be spelled out and must include side-effect detection strategies (e.g., serial blood pressure and electrocardiograms in patients at risk, constipation, and behavioral and cognitive assessments). Details of the overall treatment plan and requisite monitors should be spelled out clearly in the patient's chart. When psychiatrists provide only intermittent consultation, telephone monitoring via nursing staff is necessary and usually sufficient, provided the next visit is scheduled no longer than one month away.

TABLE 4.4. Published English Language Trials of Antidepressant Pharmacotherapy for Depression in Long-Term Care Residents

STUDY	SAMPLE; AGE (MEAN, SD, AND/OR RANGE, IF REPORTED); SC	DESIGN	KEY ENTRY CRITERIA	OUTCOME MEASURES	RESULTS
Tricyclic antidepressants (nortriptyline)					
Katz et al. (1990)	$N = 30$ Age = 84.1 SC = 23/30	7-week randomized double-blind placebo-controlled trial of nortriptyline titrated to plasma levels of 80–120 ng/mL; completer analysis	*DSM-III* diagnosis of MDD; 21-item HAM-D ≥ 18; "mild to moderate cognitive impairment" included in the sample	HAM-D, CGI, GDS	Significant drug-placebo differences apparent in CGI and HAM-D but not GDS; mean ± SD nortriptyline plasma level at termination 75.6 ± 48.4 ng/mL
Streim et al. (2000)	$N = 69$ Age = 79.5 (76.9–82) SC = 25/47 in regular-dose arm; 16/22 in low-dose arm	10-week randomized regular dose (60–80 mg/day) vs. low fixed doses (1/6 the regular doses at each time point) of nortriptyline; endpoint sample analyses; plasma level-response relationships considered for those who completed ≥ 28 days of treatment	*DSM-IV* diagnosis of major or minor depression or dysthymia; GDS ≥ 10 and/or > 2 on item 1 of HAM-D; score > 12 on 17-item HAM-D; duration of depressive symptoms > 1 month; BIMCT score ≤ 18	21-item HAM-D; CGI, GDS; response defined as a decrease of at least 33% on the HAM-D or GDS and by a rating of "much" or "very much improved" on the CGI	Nortriptyline dose correlated with clinical improvement and quadratic plasma level—response relationship; clinical improvement noted at lower plasma levels in cognitively impaired patients

Continued

TABLE 4.4. Continued

STUDY	SAMPLE; AGE (MEAN, SD, AND/OR RANGE, IF REPORTED); SC	DESIGN	KEY ENTRY CRITERIA	OUTCOME MEASURES	RESULTS
Selective serotonin reuptake inhibitors					
Oslin et al. (2000); sertraline	N = 28 Age = 83.1 (80–86) SC = 15/28	10-week open label treatment with sertraline, up to 100 mg/day, compared with the regular vs. low dose nortriptyline study by Streim et al.; ITT and completer analyses	Same as Streim et al. study except these subjects had contraindications to treatment with nortriptyline or were early dropouts from the Streim et al. study	21-item HAM-D; response defined as per the Streim et al. study	Sertraline was less effective than optimal dose of nortriptyline (regular dose for the cognitively intact subjects and low dose for the cognitively impaired), irrespective of cognitive status and with no significant improvement in tolerability
Weintraub et al. (2003); sertraline	N = 23 Age = 81.6 (SD 9.7) SC = 16/23	8-week extension phase of sertraline dose increased up to 200 mg/day for subjects with 17-item HAM-D scores ≥ 12 after 10 weeks of treatment with sertraline 100 mg/day	Completion of the 10-week acute phase with the final dose of sertraline of 100 mg/day and 17-item HAM-D score ≥ 12; acute phase criteria same as Streim et al. (2000)	21-item HAM-D; response defined as per Streim et al. study	52% of subjects in the extension phase of treatment were responders compared with 37% for the acute phase; of the acute phase nonresponders, 39% responded during the extension phase

Study; drug	Sample	Design	Criteria	Measures	Results
Rosen et al. (2000); sertraline	$N = 12$ Age = 83.2 (SD 7.8) SC = 12/12	6-week open label trial of sertraline 50–100 mg/day	*DSM-IV* minor depression; baseline MMSE 20 (range 11–29)	HAM-D; GAS; response defined as decrease of HAM-D score by ≥ 50% of HAM-D score < 10 for those with baseline HAM-D score > 10	67% subjects met criteria for full remission
Magai et al. (2000); sertraline	$N = 31$ (all female) Age = 89.2 (SD 6.3) SC = 27/31 analyses	8-week double-blind trial of sertraline (25–100 mg/day) vs. placebo; ITT and completer analyses	NINCDS-ADRDA criteria for probable or possible AD; CSDD ≥ 3 or GS ≥ 1; *DSM-IV* criteria for major or minor depression; GDS stage 6 or 7	CSDD, GS	No differences between the sertraline and placebo groups in the proportion showing ≥ 50% improvement
Burrows et al. (2002); paroxetine	$N = 24$ Age = 87.9 (80–97) SC = 20/24	8-week randomized double-blind placebo-controlled trial of paroxetine (10–30 mg/day) vs. placebo; ITT and completer analyses	*DSM-IV* nonmajor depression; MMSE score < 10	CGI-C (primary); HAM-D; CSDD; 15-item GDS; primary outcome defined as ≥ 25% improvement on CGI-C	No difference in improvement between the paroxetine and placebo groups; 2 subjects on paroxetine experienced delirium and, as a group, were more likely to experience decrease in MMSE score; no difference in serum anticholinergicity between the groups; 45% placebo response rate

Continued

TABLE 4.4. Continued

STUDY	SAMPLE; AGE (MEAN, SD, AND/OR RANGE, IF REPORTED); SC	DESIGN	KEY ENTRY CRITERIA	OUTCOME MEASURES	RESULTS
Trappler & Cohen (1996); fluoxetine	*N* = 29 Age = 89 (75–101) SC = 26/29	12-week open label treatment with fluoxetine 10–30 mg/ day; completer analysis	*DSM-IV* diagnosis of MDD, AD with MDD, VD with MDD, MDD caused by stroke; mean MMSE score of 22 (range 10–29)	21-item HAM-D; 20-item Zung Self-Rating Depression Scale; response defined as ≥ 50% improvement on HAM-D or psychiatric examination no longer indicating fulfillment of *DSM-IV* depression criteria	81% did not meet *DSM-IV* criteria for MDD at 12-week follow-up; 50% met the operational definition of response using the HAM-D; all nonresponders had coexisting dementia or stroke
Trappler & Cohen (1998); fluoxetine, sertraline, paroxetine	*N* = 52 Age = 89 (80–98) SC = 50/52	12-week prospective, open-label fluoxetine (10–30 mg/day) vs. sertraline (50–150 mg/day) vs. paroxetine (10–30 mg/day); completer analysis	*DSM-IV* major depression; AD with MDD; VD with MDD; MDD due to a medical condition; mean MMSE score for "non-CNS-associated depression" was 25, and 17 for "CNS-related depression"	21-item HAM-D; response defined as ≥ 50% drop in Ham-D score at 12-week follow-up	42% of entire sample responded; no difference in response by SSRI; 93% of those without dementia and 20% of those with dementia responded

Serotonin norepinephrine reuptake inhibitors

Study	Sample	Design	Inclusion criteria	Measures	Outcome
Roose et al. (2003); mirtazapine	N = 119; Age = 82.9 (SD 6.58); SC = 110 of total 124 in all-subjects-treated (AS) group	12-week open label trial of mirtazapine (15–45 mg/day) at 30 nursing homes across USA; ITT analysis	Age ≥ 70 years; physician diagnosis of depression; MMSE score ≥ 10	16-item HAM-D; CSDD; CGI; response defined as ≥50% decrease in HAM-D score and percentage of patients "very much" or "much improved" on CGI	At endpoint, 54% "very much" or "much improved" on CGI; 47% responders per HAM-D
Oslin et al. (2003); sertraline, venlafaxine	N = 52; Age = 82.5 (61–99); SC = 40/52	10-week randomized double-blind trial of venlafaxine (up to 150 mg/day) vs. sertraline (up to 100 mg/day); ITT and completer analyses	GDS score ≥ 10 and/or a rating of > 2 on item 1 of 17-item HAM-D; score > 12 on HAM-D; DSM-IV diagnosis of major or minor depression, dementia with depression or dysthymia; BIMCT score < 21	21-item HAM-D; CSDD; GDS; CGI	Tolerability estimated by time to termination was lower for venlafaxine than sertraline without evidence for an increase in efficacy

Note: AD, Alzheimer's disease; BIMCT, Blessed Information Memory Concentration Test; CGI, Clinical Global Impression scale; CNS, central nervous system; CSDD, Cornell Scale for Depression in Dementia; *DSM-III* and *IV, Diagnostic and Statistical Manual,* 3rd and 4th editions; GAS, Global Assessment Scale; GDS, Geriatric Depression Scale; GS, Gestalt Scale; HAM-D, Hamilton Depression Rating Scale; ITT, intent-to-treat analysis; MDD, major depressive disorder; MMSE, Mini Mental State Exam; NINCDS-ADRDA, National Institute of Neurological and Communicable Diseases and Stroke–Alzheimer's Disease and Related Disorders Association; SC, study completers; SD, standard deviation; SSRI, selective serotonin reuptake inhibitor; VD, vascular dementia.

Electroconvulsive therapy

Electroconvulsive therapy (ECT) is indicated and underutilized for treatment of severe depression or mania in nursing home patients for whom pharmaco-therapy is unsafe or ineffective. In fact, outcomes with ECT are often better in older than younger depressed patients (O'Connor et al., 2001; Sackheim, 1993). The increasing availability of outpatient continuation/maintenance ECT in urban medical centers has made ECT a more attractive treatment option when medically indicated. Nursing home staff, however, may be unaware of the indications for, or the safety and efficacy of ECT, and thus be unable to sup-port reluctant patients or family members in considering a recommendation for its use.

Example. A 75-year-old woman with a history of early-onset recurrent major depression, and one major suicide attempt in which she jumped out of a fourth story window, had failed multiple trials of antidepressant monotherapy and aug-mentation strategies involving antidepressants of other chemical classes, mood stabilizers, and atypical antipsychotics over several decades. When ECT became available through her local community mental health center's contract with a local hospital, she received 12 inpatient ECT treatments followed by biweekly outpatient ECT. Though still requiring close clinical monitoring, she became nonpsychotic, complied with treatment, and began to dine with other residents in her nursing home, an activity she had refused during her depressive relapses.

Psychosocial treatments

Few psychological or psychosocial treatments for depression have been tested rigorously in long-term care populations. However, a systematic review found some promising group and individual "talk therapies" (see Table 4.5; Bharucha et al., 2006). Studies included in this review were (a) randomized controlled tri-als published in English, (b) having the primary aim of improving depression or psychological well-being, (c) using at least one specific outcome measure of depression or psychological well-being, and (e) involving individual or group psychotherapy in at least one arm of the intervention. Studies involving subjects with cognitive impairment were also included so long as the therapeutic inter-vention was individual or group psychotherapy. Exclusion criteria included (a) anecdotal clinical reports, case studies, and dissertations, (b) publications in a language other than English, (c) studies in which the formal or informal caregiver was the actual focus of the intervention rather than the subject him-/herself, and (d) psychosocial interventions directed primarily at curbing disruptive behaviors associated with dementia or an intervention other than "talk therapy" since these have been reviewed in detail elsewhere (Cohen-Mansfield, 2001). A total of 1074 subjects have participated in these trials, with one study accounting for 256 of

TABLE 4.5. Published Controlled English Language Trials of Psychotherapy for Long-Term Care Residents

AUTHORS; THERAPEUTIC MODALITY	STUDY DESIGN AND SAMPLE	AGE (MEAN, SD, AND/OR RANGE, IF REPORTED)	STUDY COMPLETERS (n)	KEY ENTRY CRITERIA	ASSESSMENT POINTS	OUTCOME MEASURES	RESULTS
Control relevant interventions							
Langer & Rodin (1976)	Random assignment by floor *Experimental condition:* communication stressing personal responsibility and choice (N = 24) *Control:* communication stressing staff responsibility for subjects (N = 28)	65–90	Not reported; total subjects = 91 but data reported on only 52	Only exclusion criteria reported: bedridden or nonverbal subjects	1 week before and 3 weeks after the communication	*Self-report:* questionnaire rating happiness, activity, perceived control *Interviewer:* nurses ratings of time spent visiting residents and others, talking to staff, watching staff, alertness	Significantly improved alertness, active participation and a general sense of well-being in the experimental group; nurses rated 93% of subjects in experimental condition vs. 21% of control subjects as being improved; at 18-month follow-up, decline in the above measures significantly smaller for the responsibility-induced group (N = 20) than comparison group (N = 14), and 15% of subjects in the experimental group deceased compared with 30% in control group

Continued

TABLE 4.5. Continued

AUTHORS; THERAPEUTIC MODALITY	STUDY DESIGN AND SAMPLE	AGE (MEAN, SD, AND/OR RANGE, IF REPORTED)	STUDY COMPLETERS (n)	KEY ENTRY CRITERIA	ASSESSMENT POINTS	OUTCOME MEASURES	RESULTS
Schulz (1976)	Random assignment *Experimental conditions:* subjects offered controllability (N = 10) over frequency and duration of visits by a college student; subjects offered predictability (N = 10) about visits but not over other details; random visits (N = 10) *Control:* no visits	81.5 (67–96)	40/40	Nursing home residents who could walk and talk	Pre- and post 2-month intervention	4 questionnaires entitled "Activities," "My Usual Day," "Future Diary," and Wohlford Hope Scale; number of medications taken per day	Predictability and controllability groups performed significantly better on indicators of physical and psychological health and activity levels; significantly lesser increase in the number of medications used by the predictability and control groups; no differences evident between the controllability and predictability groups

Study	Conditions	Age	N	Inclusion criteria	Assessment timing	Measures	Results
Rosen et al. (1997)	Random assignment for first 22 patients *Experimental condition:* activities planned with a recreational therapist, 1–2 h twice a day, 5 days a week for 8 weeks (N = 11 + 9 added later without randomization) *Control:* waiting list (N = 11)	78.7 (50–96)	31/31	MMSE > 18, resident of facility for >3 months, diagnosis of minor (*DSM-IV*) or major depression (*DSM-III-R*, mild to moderate severity)	Preintervention, postintervention (8 weeks), 8 weeks after study discontinuation	Responder defined as "significantly improved" functioning by an RN and LPN; GDS, HAM-D, PCS, SCES, AES, EXIT, CIRS-G, Keitel and Barthel Index	0/11 subjects on waiting list were responders; 4/11 subjects randomized to intervention were responders; total 14/31 subjects participating in the intervention were responders (45%); HAM-D and GDS scores improved significantly for the responders but not the nonresponders

Reminiscence or life review

Study	Conditions	Age	N	Inclusion criteria	Assessment timing	Measures	Results
Goldwasser et al. (1987)	Random assignment; group therapy—30 min 2x/week for 5 weeks *Experimental conditions:* REM (N = 9); support group (N = 9) *Control:* no treatment (N = 9)	82.6 (70–97)	27/27	Clinical diagnosis of dementia, presence of symptoms associated with dementia, ability to communicate, ability to function within a group	1 week before intervention, 1 week after intervention, and 5 weeks after termination	MMSE, BDI, Katz ADL	REM reduced depression scores; no change in cognition or ADL measures

Continued

TABLE 4-5. Continued

AUTHORS; THERAPEUTIC MODALITY	STUDY DESIGN AND SAMPLE	AGE (MEAN, SD, AND/OR RANGE, IF REPORTED)	STUDY COMPLETERS (n)	KEY ENTRY CRITERIA	ASSESSMENT POINTS	OUTCOME MEASURES	RESULTS
Rattenbury & Stones (1989)	Random assignment; group therapy—2x/ week for 30 min during weeks 3–6 *Experimental conditions*: REM and current topics group *Control*: no treatment Total *N* = 24	83–87	Not reported	Volunteers with adequate hearing and vision, no overt cognitive impairment	Pre- and posttest, 8 week trial	MUNSH, MUNAI, SGRS, MUMS	Significantly improved psychological well-being for both experimental groups relative to control; greater participation associated with greater improvement
Orten et al. (1989)	Random assignment; group therapy—45 min sessions weekly for 16 weeks *Experimental condition*: REM *Control*: regular milieu therapy Total *N* = 56	82.6 (58–101)	54/56	"Moderately confused but without other diagnosable psychiatric conditions or physical illnesses that might cause such states."	Baseline, weeks 8 and 16	ESBS	No significant improvement in social behavior between or within groups

Study	Design	Age	N	Inclusion criteria	Timing	Instruments	Results
Cook (1991)	Random assignment; group therapy —1 h a week for 16 weeks *Experimental condition:* REM (N = 18) *Controls:* current events group (N = 18) and no treatment group (N = 18)	81.3 (65–96)	41/54	>65 years age, institutionalized >1 month, able to participate orally, able to complete instruments, free of mental illness, and free of organic brain impairment	Pre- and posttest, 16 week trial	LSI-A, GDS, RSES	REM did not increase life satisfaction or self-esteem and did not decrease depression; positive socializing effect for those who participated in REM or current events group
McMurdo & Rennie (1993)	Random assignment by nursing home; group therapy *Experimental condition:* 45 min exercise sessions 2×/week (N = 20) *Control:* 45 min REM 2×/week (N = 24)	81 (63–91)	41/44	Only residents with severe communication difficulties excluded	Baseline and 28 weeks	Postural sway, grip strength, knee flexion/ extension, spinal flexion, Barthel Index, GDS, LSI, MMSE	Motor performance improved in exercise group while declining in REM group; depression decreased in both groups, exercise > REM

Continued

TABLE 4.5. Continued

AUTHORS; THERAPEUTIC MODALITY	STUDY DESIGN AND SAMPLE	AGE (MEAN, SD, AND/OR RANGE, IF REPORTED)	STUDY COMPLETERS (*n*)	KEY ENTRY CRITERIA	ASSESSMENT POINTS	OUTCOME MEASURES	RESULTS
Haight et al. (1998)	Random assignment; Solomon Four Experimental Design (2 groups with premeasurement, and 2 without premeasurement); group therapy *Experimental condition*: life review 1 h × 6 weeks *Control*: friendly visit 1 h × 6 weeks Total *N* = 256	79.6 (60–104)	201 at 8 weeks; 122 at 1 year (of total 256)	>60 years age, within 6 weeks of relocation to nursing home, free of clinical depression as per DIS, oriented to time, place, and person	Pretest, 8 and 52 weeks	ABS, LSI-A, RSES, BDI, HS, SI	Life review was effective in decreasing hopelessness and depression; this change was apparent at 52 weeks but not at 8 weeks; annual follow-up of remaining 52 subjects indicated significant improvements on measures of depression, life satisfaction, and self-esteem for those receiving the intervention. The depression scores in the control group declined significantly.

		Age	N	Sample	Timing	Measures	Results
Jones (2003)	Random assignment; pre- and posttest quasi experimental design. *Experimental condition:* NIC REM (a structured form of REM) 45 min sessions 2 ×/week for 3 weeks (N = 15). *Control:* standard REM 45 min sessions 2 ×/week for 3 weeks (N = 15)	81.7 (61–97)	30/30	Women aged >60 years residing in assisted living facilities for >3 months, ability to give consent, MMSE >15	Pre- and post 3 weeks of REM	GDS	Significantly greater reduction in GDS in the experimental group compared with control group

Problem-solving, cognitive or cognitive behavior therapy

		Age	N	Sample	Timing	Measures	Results
Hussian & Lawrence (1981); social reinforcement; problem-solving therapy	Random assignment; Group therapy—five 30 min sessions over 2 weeks. *Experimental conditions:* social reinforcement (N = 12); problem-solving (N = 12). *Control:* waiting list (N = 12)	73.6 (69–75)	22/36	>60 years age; not deaf or blind; not on an antidepressant; top 36 scorers on the BDI	Baseline, weeks 1, 2, and 12 for BDI, HAS; self-rating of depression 3 ×/week	BDI, HAS	Problem-solving therapy produced greatest decline in depression scores early in treatment but effects not maintained at 12-week follow-up

Continued

TABLE 4.5 Continued

AUTHORS; THERAPEUTIC MODALITY	STUDY DESIGN AND SAMPLE	AGE (MEAN, SD, AND/OR RANGE, IF REPORTED)	STUDY COMPLETERS (*n*)	KEY ENTRY CRITERIA	ASSESSMENT POINTS	OUTCOME MEASURES	RESULTS
Zerhusen et al. (1991)	Random assignment; group therapy for 10 weeks *Experimental condition:* cognitive therapy (*N* = 20) *Controls:* music therapy (*N* = 20) and usual care (*N* = 20)	77 (70–82)	59/60	Moderately to severely depressed per BDI, free from organic brain syndrome	Pre- and posttest, 10-week trial	BDI	Significant decline in depression in CT group compared with music therapy and usual care
Abraham et al. (1992, 1997) (reanalysis of cognitive data)	Random assignment by nursing home; group therapy *Experimental conditions:* CBT (*N* = 30); focused visual imagery group (*N* = 29)	84.3 (71–97)	42/76	> 11 on GDS, adequate hearing and vision, and verbal and comprehension skills, absence of major cognitive	4 weeks before intervention, 8 and 20 weeks after intervention initiation, 4 weeks after intervention termination	3MS, GDS, HS, LSI-Z	Neither CBT nor focused visual imagery reduced depressive symptomatology; however, both experimental conditions improved cognitive

Control: education-discussion group (N = 17)			impairment, free of antidepressants. no history of endogenous depression			performance with focused visual imagery >CBT; improved ability to recognize and associate objects, improved ability to concentrate and execute, and improvements in abstraction, conceptual thinking, linguistic manipulation, and execution of auditorily presented language skills
Miscellaneous approaches						
Moran & Gatz (1987); task- and insight-oriented groups	76.3	59/59	Not listed	Pre- and posttest, 12 week trial	IELCS, ITS, BAPC, SDS, LSI-A	Both experimental conditions superior to control condition. Significant increase in life satisfaction in the task group; significant increase in internal locus of control for both experimental groups; significant increase in trust for insight group
Random assignment; group therapy—once a week for twelve 75-min sessions *Experimental conditions*: task-oriented group (N = 20); insight-oriented group (N = 21) *Control*: waiting list (N=18)						

Continued

TABLE 4-5. Continued

AUTHORS; THERAPEUTIC MODALITY	STUDY DESIGN AND SAMPLE	AGE (MEAN, SD, AND/OR RANGE, IF REPORTED)	STUDY COMPLETERS (n)	KEY ENTRY CRITERIA	ASSESSMENT POINTS	OUTCOME MEASURES	RESULTS
Frey et al. (1992); self-esteem protocol	Random assignment; group therapy —weekly for 12 weeks *Experimental condition*: Frey and Carlock's protocol to improve self-esteem (N = 9) *Control*: current events group (N = 12)	72.5	21/21	Male residents of a Veterans Administration Medical Center for >1 year, age >60 years, competent for informed consent process, >20 on MMSE	Baseline, 6 and 12 weeks	MMSE, CFSEI, RSES	Significantly improved self-esteem at posttreatment, however, the pattern of change was nonlinear over the study period (worse self-esteem at 6 weeks but improved at 12 weeks), controlling for the fact that the experimental group was more cognitively impaired at baseline

Study	Design	Age	N	Inclusion	Assessment times	Measures	Results
Toseland et al. (1997); validation therapy	Random assignment; group therapy 4 times a week, 30 min each, for 52 weeks *Experimental condition:* validation therapy (*N* = 31) *Controls:* social contact (*N* = 29) or usual care (*N* = 28)	88 (SD = 6.5)	66/88	Mild to moderate dementia (<8 errors on SPMSQ) with behavioral disturbances	2 weeks prior to intervention, 3 and 12 months	SPMSQ; VSI; SCES; MOSES; CMAI; GIPB	No change in depression scores in VT group but significant increase in social contact group; VT reduced problem behaviors but social contact and usual care did not
McCurren et al. (1999); volunteer program	Random assignment *Experimental condition:* initial and weekly evaluation by a master's prepared geropsychiatric nurse augmented with trained volunteers delivering supportive therapy *Control:* usual care of depression	84 (SD = 6.5)	61/85	Age > 65, GDS > 10, MMSE > 19	Baseline, 12 and 24 weeks	GDS, MMSE, LSES	Depressive symptomatology significantly reduced in experimental group but not in controls. The decline in GDS scores was not related to antidepressant use

Continued

TABLE 4-5 Continued

AUTHORS; THERAPEUTIC MODALITY	STUDY DESIGN AND SAMPLE	AGE (MEAN, SD, AND/OR RANGE, IF REPORTED)	STUDY COMPLETERS (n)	KEY ENTRY CRITERIA	ASSESSMENT POINTS	OUTCOME MEASURES	RESULTS
Spector et al. (2001); reality orientation	Random assignment; group therapy 15, 45-min, twice weekly sessions *Experimental condition:* reality orientation *Control:* usual care of depression	85.7 (SD = 6.7)	27/35	*DSM-IV* diagnosis of dementia; no severe visual, hearing, or communication difficulties; no serious health problems, no disruptive behaviors	Week prior to 1st group session and week after last group session	MMSE, ADAS-Cog, HCS, CDR, CSDD, RAID, BRS, GHQ-12, RS	Depression scores declined significantly in RO group but not controls; trend toward improvement in cognition and anxiety also noted with RO

Note: 3MS, Modified Mini-Mental Status Examination: ABS. Psychological Well-Being; ADAS-Cog. Alzheimer's Disease Assessment Scale—Cognition; AES, Apathy Evaluation Scale; BAPC, Behavioral Attributes of Psychosocial Competence Scale; BDI, Beck Depression Inventory; BRS, Behavior Rating Scale; CBT, Cognitive Behavior Therapy; CDR, Clinical Dementia Rating; CFSEI, Culture-Free Self-Esteem Inventory; CIRS-G, Cumulative Illness Rating Scale for Geriatrics; CMAI, Cohen-Mansfield Agitation Inventory; CSDD, Cornell Scale for Depression in Dementia; CT, Cognitive Therapy; *DSM-III-R* and *IV, Diagnostic and Statistical Manual*. 3rd edition, revised and 4th edition, APA; ESBS, Evaluation of Social Behavior Scale; EXIT, Executive Interview; GDS, Geriatric Depression Scale; GHQ-12, General Health Questionnaire; GIPB, Geriatric Indices of Positive Behavior; HAM-D, Hamilton Rating Scale for Depression; HAS, Hospital Adjustment Scale; HCS, Holden Communication Scale; HS, Hopelessness Scale; IELCS, Internal-External Locus of Control Scale; ITS, Interpersonal Trust Scale; Katz ADL, Activities of Daily Living; LPN, Licensed Practical Nurse; LSES, Salamon-Conte Life Satisfaction in the Elderly Scale; LSI-A, Life Satisfaction Index-A; LSI-Z, Life Satisfaction Index—short version; MMSE, Mini Mental Status Examination; MOSES, Multidimensional Observation Scale for Elderly Subjects; MUMS, Memorial University Mood Scale; MUNAI, Memorial University of Newfoundland Activities Inventory; MUNSH, Memorial University of Newfoundland Scale of Happiness; NIC, Nursing Intervention Classification; PCS, Perceived Competence Scale; RAID, Rating Anxiety in Dementia; REM, reminiscence therapy; RN, Registered Nurse; RO, Reality Orientation; RS, Relative's Stress Scale; RSES, Rosenberg Self-Esteem Scale; SCES, Sheltered Care Environment Scale; SD, standard deviation; SDS, Social Desirability Scale; SGRS, Stockton Geriatric Rating Scale; SI, Beck Suicide Ideation Scale; SPMSQ, Short Portable Mental Status Questionnaire; SR, Social Reinforcement; VSI, Validation Screening Instrument.

the total (Haight et al., 1998). The mean age of the subjects was 80.9 years (range of 50–104 years), with 71% of the participants being female. The average sample size for all studies was 60 (SD = 53), with a median of 48 subjects. Approximately 78% of the subjects completed their respective intervention trial. The percentage of sessions missed by subjects was usually not systematically reported. The most frequently reported therapeutic modalities were as follows: structured or unstructured reminiscence (seven reports), control-relevant interventions (three reports), cognitive, cognitive behavioral, or problem-solving therapy (three reports), and a host of miscellaneous approaches (five reports).

In total, approximately half of the reviewed studies reported short-term (8–12 week trials) improvements in one or more dimensions of psychological well-being (depression, hopelessness, self-esteem, trust, locus of control). Moreover, some of these reports noted longer term (12–18 months) benefits, such as increased socialization, which were not among the hypothesis-driven primary outcomes of the study (Cook, 1991; Haight et al., 2000). The mildly encouraging results of published reports appear to argue for continued and expanded work in this area. Future studies must include a well-defined therapeutic focus and study entry criteria, clearly articulated intervention protocol with a measure(s) of fidelity of implementation, longer trial duration, replication in diverse settings, and outcome measures that are sensitive and specific to the enhanced capacity for coping and adaptation to the long-term care environment that may be achieved through psychotherapy. In addition, future studies must move beyond group psychotherapy, which has been the only area of emphasis to date; to our knowledge, not a single controlled trial of conventionally applied individual psychotherapy, such as cognitive behavioral, interpersonal, or problem-solving therapy, has been reported in a peer-reviewed journal. However, a notable book chapter describes the process and outcomes of individual psychotherapy in small pilot studies conducted at the Philadelphia Geriatric Center (Frazer, 1997). Finally, the process and outcomes of both individual psychotherapy and combined or sequential psychotherapy/pharmacotherapy and caregiver intervention approaches also await investigation.

In addition, studies of primary prevention of depression in long-term care settings are sorely lacking. In the sea of change that characterizes both the intrapersonal and extrapersonal experience of residents, there are predictable nodal points, such as the time of admission, impending, or actual loss of a spouse, and so forth, when vulnerable persons may benefit from proactive interventions that marshal social and emotional resources and enhance the capacity for adaptive coping. Blazer has recently reviewed such approaches to enhance self-efficacy, and these merit further conceptual and operational attention from long-term care researchers (Blazer, 2002).

A major obstacle that must be addressed in future trials of psychotherapy is how best to take into account the impact of comorbid cognitive impairment, physical and functional decline, premorbid personality traits, comorbid psychiatric disorders, environmental impoverishment and polypharmacy on the incidence and persistence of depression and psychological distress, and their response to psychotherapy. To what extent are depression, hopelessness, and psychological distress realistic reactions to progressively deteriorating physical and cognitive abilities, suboptimal person-environment fit, and diminished opportunities for "meaning making"? At what point, measured either as severity or duration of these responses, should clinical intervention be considered essential? What are appropriate, expectable outcomes of psychotherapy in this population, and how should they be measured? It is likely that new measures are needed to assess the unique features of learning to cope with lasting, undesirable conditions of life while finding meaning and satisfaction. Given the often advanced stage of medical conditions and attendant cognitive, emotional and functional sequelae in many residents of long-term care facilities, symptom measurement scales by themselves are unlikely to capture the full range of benefits that may be derived from psychotherapy, such as enhanced self-esteem, vitality, engagement within the larger social milieu, improved sense of security in the new environment, and other dynamic adaptive responses. Ethnographic studies have identified the loss of autonomy, wounded self-esteem, and purposelessness as seminal existential issues for long-term care residents, lending credence to the need for measures of adaptive coping and self-efficacy as appropriate outcome foci (Fiveash, 1998; Kahn, 1999). On the other hand, inclusion of currently existing psychopathology rating instruments in future investigations will remain important as a reference point and conceptual bridge to the existing literature.

Cognitive impairment, in particular, has generally been viewed by third party payors, at least in the United States, as precluding meaningful short— and longer-term gains from psychotherapy. While the need for preserved cognitive functioning clearly has face validity for the potential effectiveness of psychotherapies that rely on self-directed change, the specific cognitive abilities required for benefit from psychotherapeutic care require further conceptual and empirical exploration. The capacity for emotional attachment and relationship may be much more important than cognitive abilities in determining which patients can benefit. Moreover, appropriate expectations for style and duration of care for specific patients, and what outcomes and predictors should be measured, deserve attention in designing trials for long-term care patients. In the absence of a scientific database that sheds light on the constellation of functions necessary for benefit from psychotherapy, third party payors will likely continue to deny psychotherapy services to many who otherwise could experience important gains. Recent work indicates that bringing caregivers into a modified interpersonal psychotherapy (IPT) approach can extend the applicability of IPT to outpatients with mild or even moderate levels of dementia (Miller & Reynolds, 2007).

PROGRAMMATIC CHANGES IN NURSING HOME CARE

Depressions in their protean forms can be viewed as the product of multiple causal factors that include individual psychodynamics and psychobiology, systemic and neuropsychiatric illness, functional disability (including sensory impairments), concurrent drug treatments, and social and institutional factors affecting the giving and receiving of daily care. Viewed from the perspective of the nursing home as a health-care institution, the high depressive morbidity found there demands focused programmatic change to improve its detection, accurate differential diagnosis, and treatment. Individual nursing homes, like individual patients, may need different approaches based upon resident profiles, staffing patterns, existing services, and commitment to improvement in the quality of care. Preceding sections allude to several such approaches, such as systematic attention to the needs of aides. Others may include periodic facility-wide professional review of the use of psychotropic medications, changes in administrative structure, regular staff retreats, mandatory continuing education of physicians and nurses in the art and science of recognizing and treating depression, and regular interactive staff meetings to review the nursing home mission.

Several recent reviews have focused attention on the inadequate manpower and geropsychiatric skill needs and provided state-of-the-evidence reviews of mental health care in long-term care facilities (American Geriatrics Society & American Association for Geriatric Psychiatry, 2003; Bartels et al., 2002; Borson et al., 2001; Moak & Borson, 2000; Snowden et al., 2003; Streim et al., 2002; Wagenaar et al., 2003). Although there is overwhelming appreciation for the fact that depression in the long-term care setting responds effectively to treatment and management, there is considerable skepticism as to the feasibility of implementing standardized protocols (Wagenaar et al., 2003). Indeed, given the cost constraints of the managed care environment, psychiatric consultants (when available) tend to limit their work to assessment and diagnosis and confine treatment principally to pharmacotherapy of major psychiatric syndromes (delirium, psychosis, dementia, major depression, etc.). As nursing home mental health support is increasingly provided by psychiatric nurse practitioners, supervising psychiatrists may have minimal face-to-face contact with the patient. In this regard, the training and implementation of a masters-level mental health-care specialist ("Long-term care Mental Health Manager"), similar to the depression care specialist employed successfully in the Prevention of Suicide in Primary Care Collaborative Trial (PROSPECT) and Improving Mood-Promoting Access to Collaborate Treatment (IMPACT), may prove to be valuable and cost-effective (Bruce et al., 2004; Unutzer et al., 2002). The same clinician would be ideally situated to provide ongoing staff training in the management of difficult patients and situations, coordinate group therapies with a recreational therapist, and provide liaison with family members.

CONCLUSIONS

Mood disorders are prevalent, persistent, disabling, and deadly conditions in elderly long-term care residents; however, they can be effectively and proactively diagnosed with currently available clinical assessment tools for both those with and without cognitive impairment. Evaluation of mania and depression in patients with severe dementias, mixed behavioral syndromes or atypical presentations, or multiple major medical comorbidities is more difficult and is a task for specialty-trained geropsychiatrists and continuing geropsychiatric research. Medical, neurobiological, psychological, social, environmental, and administrative dimensions form a causal matrix for depression, interacting to create affective illness in ways that are unique for each patient. Effective interventions may be derived from consideration of each of these causal domains, and combinations of several approaches are generally most effective. Although psychiatrists must participate actively and often take the lead in developing effective institutional programs and providing treatment for patients, no single clinical discipline can be entrusted with the full responsibility for this fundamentally collaborative task. Notwithstanding the progress that has been made over the past decade, substantial improvements are needed in recognition of the spectrum of depressive morbidity, timely and adequate (therapeutic) well-targeted treatment and follow up, and application of programmatic innovations that can reduce the burden of depressive morbidity noted worldwide in the setting of long-term care. Mental health services models that improve outcomes of depression in the outpatient primary care of older adults offer a starting point for a new generation of long-term care research.

REFERENCES

Abraham, I. L., Neundorfer, M. M., & Currie, L. J. (1992). Effects of group interventions on cognition and depression in nursing home residents. *Nursing Research, 41*, 196.

Abraham, I. L., Onega, L. L., & Reel, S. J. (1997). Effects of cognitive group interventions on depressed frail nursing home residents. In R. L. Rubinstein & M. P. Lawton (Eds.), *Depression in long term and residential care: Advances in research and treatment.* New York: Springer, 1997.

Abrams, R. C., Teresi, J. A., & Butin, D. N. (1992). Depression in nursing home residents. *Clinics in Geriatric Medicine, 8*, 309.

Aizenstein, H. J., Nebes, R. D., Meltzer, C. C., et al. (2002). The relation of white matter hyperintensities to implicit learning in healthy older adults. *International Journal of Geriatric Psychiatry, 17*, 664.

Alexopoulos, G. S. (2002). Frontostriatal and limbic dysfunction in late-life depression. *American Journal of Geriatric Psychiatry, 10*, 687.

Alexopoulos, G. S., Meyers, B. S., Young, R. C., et al. (1993). The course of geriatric depression with "reversible dementia": A controlled study. *American Journal of Psychiatry, 150*, 1693.

Alexopoulos, G. S., Meyers, B. S., Young, R. C., et al. (1997). "Vascular depression" hypothesis. *Archives of General Psychiatry, 54*, 915.

Alexopoulos, G. S., Schultz, S. K., & Lebowitz, B. D. (2005). Late-life depression: A model for medical classification. *Biological Psychiatry, 58*, 283.

American Geriatrics Society & American Association for Geriatric Psychiatry. (2003). The American Geriatrics Society and American Association for Geriatric Psychiatry recommendations for policies in support of quality mental health care in U.S. nursing homes. *Journal of the American Geriatrics Society, 51*, 1299.

American Psychiatric Association. (2000). *Diagnostic and statistical manual of mental disorders* (4th ed., text revision). Washington, DC: Author.

Ames, D. (1990). Depression among elderly residents of local-authority residential homes: Its nature and efficacy of intervention. *British Journal of Psychiatry, 156*, 667–675.

Ames, D. (1991). Epidemiological studies of depression among the elderly in residential and nursing homes. *International Journal of Geriatric Psychiatry, 6*, 347.

Ames, D. (1993). Depressive disorders among elderly people in long-term institutional care. *Australian and New Zealand Journal of Psychiatry, 27*, 379.

Arnow, B. A., Hunkeler, E. M., Blasey, C. M., et al. (2006). Comorbid depression, chronic pain, and disability in primary care. *Psychosomatic Medicine, 68*, 262.

Ashby, D., Ames, D., West, C., et al. (1991). Psychiatric morbidity as a predictor of mortality for residents of local authority homes for the elderly. *International Journal of Geriatric Psychiatry, 6*, 567.

Asplund, K., Normark, M., & Petterson, V. (1981). Nutritional assessment of psychogeriatric patients. *Age and Ageing, 10*, 87.

Avorn, J., Soumerai, S. B., Everitt, D. E., et al. (1992). A randomized trial of a program to reduce the use of psychoactive drugs in nursing homes. *New England Journal of Medicine, 327*, 1683.

Baker, F. M., & Miller, C. L. (1991). "Cocooning": A clinical sign of depression in geriatric patients. *Hospital and Community Psychiatry, 42*, 845.

Ballmaier, M., Toga, A. W., Blanton, R. E., et al. (2004). Anterior cingulate, gyrus rectus, and orbitofrontal abnormalities in elderly depressed patients: An MRI-based parcellation of the prefrontal cortex. *American Journal of Psychiatry, 161*, 99.

Barsa, J., Toner, J., Gurland, B., et al. (1986). Ability of internists to recognize and manage depression in the elderly. *International Journal of Geriatric Psychiatry, 1*, 57.

Bartels, S. J., Moak, G. S., & Dums, A. R. (2002). Models of mental health services in nursing homes: A review of the literature. *Psychiatric Services, 53*, 1390.

Berger, A. K., Small, B. J., Forsell, Y., et al. (1998). Preclinical symptoms of major depression in very old age: A prospective longitudinal study. *American Journal of Psychiatry, 155*, 1039.

Bharucha, A. J., Dew, M. A., Miller, M. D., et al. (2006). Psychotherapy in long-term care: A review. *Journal of the American Medical Directors Association, 7*, 568.

Blazer, D. G. (2002). Self-efficacy and depression in late-life: A primary prevention proposal. *Aging and Mental Health, 6*, 315.

Blazer, D. G. (2003). Depression in late life: Review and commentary. *Journal of Gerontology Series B: Biological Sciences and Medical Sciences, 58*, 249.

Blonder, X. L., Heilman, K. M., Ketterson, T., et al. (2005). Affective facial and lexical expression in aprosodic versus aphasic stroke patients. *Journal of the International Neuropsychological Society, 11*, 677.

Borson, S., Barnes, R. A., Kukull, W. A., et al. (1986). Symptomatic depression in elderly medical outpatients. *Journal of the American Geriatrics Society, 34*, 341.

Borson, S., Bartels, S. J., Colenda, C. C., et al. (2001, Summer). Geriatric mental health services research: Strategic plan for an aging population: Report of the Health Services Work Group of the American Association for Geriatric Psychiatry. *American Journal of Geriatric Psychiatry, 9,* 191.

Borson, S., McDonald, G. J., Gayle, T., et al. (1992). Improvement in mood, physical symptoms, and function with nortriptyline for depression in patients with chronic obstructive pulmonary disease. *Psychosomatics, 33,* 190.

Borson, S., Scanlan, J., Brush, M., Vitaliano, P., & Dokmak, A. (2000). The Mini-Cog: A cognitive "vital signs" measure for dementia screening in multiethnic elderly. *International Journal of Geriatric Psychiatry, 15,* 1021.

Bowers, B., & Becker, M. (1992). Nurses' aides in nursing homes: The relationship between organization and quality. *The Gerontologist, 32,* 360.

Brant, B. A., & Osgood, N. (1990). The suicidal patient in long-term care institutions. *Journal of Gerontological Nursing, 16,* 15.

Brink, T. L. (1987). *The elderly uncooperative patient.* New York: Haworth Press.

Brown, M. N., Lapane, K. L., & Luisi, A. F. (2002). The management of depression in older nursing home residents. *Journal of the American Geriatrics Society, 50,* 69.

Bruce, M. L., Ten Have, T. R., Reynolds, C. F., 3rd, et al. (2004). Reducing suicidal ideation and depressive symptoms in depressed older primary care patients: A randomized controlled trial. *JAMA, 291,* 1081.

Burns, B. J., Larson, I. D., Goldstrom, W. E., et al. (1988). Mental disorder among nursing home patients: Preliminary findings from the national nursing home pretest. *International Journal of Geriatric Psychiatry, 3,* 27.

Burns, B. J., Wagner, H. R., Taube, J. E., et al. (1993). Mental health service use by the elderly in nursing homes. *American Journal of Public Health, 83,* 331.

Burrows, A. B., Morris, J. N., Simon, S. E., et al. (2000). Development of a Minimum Data Set-based depression rating scale for use in nursing homes. *Age and Ageing, 29,* 165.

Burrows, A. B., Salzman, C., Satlin, A., et al. (2002). A randomized, placebo-controlled trial of paroxetine in nursing home residents with non-major depression. *Depression and Anxiety, 15,* 102.

Castle, N. G. (2001) Relocation of the elderly. *Medical Care Research and Review, 58,* 291.

Castle, N. G. (2006). Measuring staff turnover in nursing homes. *The Gerontologist, 46,* 210.

Centers for Medicare and Medicaid Services (CMS), HHS. (2003). Medicare and Medicaid programs: Requirements for paid feeding assistants in long-term care facilities. Final rule. *Federal Register, 68,* 55528.

Chappell, N. L., & Novak, M. (1992). The role of support in alleviating stress among nursing assistants. *The Gerontologist, 32,* 351.

Charron, M., Fortin, L., & Paquette, I. (1991). De novo mania among elderly people. *Acta Psychiatrica Scandinavica, 84,* 503.

Ciechanowski, P. S., Katon, W. J., & Russo, J. E. (2000). Depression and diabetes: Impact of depressive symptoms on adherence, function, and costs. *Archives of Internal Medicine, 1160,* 3278.

Cohen, C. I., Hyland, K., & Framowitz, I. (1995). *Depression among nursing home residents with dementia: Final report.* Albany, NY: State Department of Health, Bureau of Long-Term Care Services.

Cohen, C. I., Hyland, K., & Magai, C. (1998). Depression among African-American nursing home patients with dementia. *American Journal of Geriatric Psychiatry, 6*, 162.

Cohen-Mansfield, J. (2001). Nonpharmacologic interventions for inappropriate behaviors in dementia: A review, summary, and critique. *American Journal of Geriatric Psychiatry, 9*, 361.

Cohen-Mansfield, J. (2006). Pain assessment in noncommunicative elderly persons—PAINE. *Clinical Journal of Pain, 22*, 569.

Cohen-Mansfield, J., & Marx, M. S. (1993). Pain and depression in nursing home: Corroborating results. *Journal of Gerontology, 48*, 96.

Cohen-Mansfield, J., Marx, M. S., & Werner, P. (1992). Agitation in elderly persons: An integrative report of findings in a nursing home. *International Psychogeriatrics, 4*(Suppl 2), 221.

Cohen-Mansfield, J., Werner, P., & Marx, M. S. (1990). Screaming in nursing home residents. *Journal of the American Geriatrics Society, 38*, 785.

Conwell, Y. (1994). Suicide in the elderly. In L. S. Schneider, C. F. Reynolds, III, B. D. Lebowitz, et al. (Eds.), *Diagnosis and treatment of depression in late life.* Washington, DC: American Psychiatric Press.

Cook, E. A. (1991). The effects of reminiscence on psychological measures of ego integrity in elderly nursing home residents. *Archives of Psychiatric Nursing, 5*, 292.

Crogan, N. L., & Pasvogel, A. (2003). The influence of protein-calorie malnutrition on quality of life in nursing homes. *Journal of Gerontology Series A: Biological Sciences and Medical Sciences, 58*, 159.

Crutchfield, D. B. (2001). The consultant pharmacist's role in identification and management of depression in the long-term care facility resident. *Journal of the American Society of Consultant Pharmacists, 16*(Suppl 3), 1.

Datto, C. J., Oslin, D. W., Streim, J. E., et al. (2002). Pharmacologic treatment of depression in nursing home residents: A mental health services perspective. *Journal of Geriatric Psychiatry and Neurology, 15*, 141.

Depp, C. A., & Jeste, D. V. (2004) Bipolar disorder in older adults: A critical review. *Bipolar Disorders, 6*, 343.

Dobie, D. J. (2002). Depression, dementia, and pseudodementia. *Seminars in Clinical Neuropsychiatry, 7*, 170.

Dorr, D. A., Horn, S. D., & Smout, R. J. (2005). Cost analysis of nursing home registered nurse staffing times. *Journal of the American Geriatrics Society, 53*, 840.

Drevets, W. C. (2003). Neuroimaging abnormalities in the amygdala in mood disorders. *Annals of the New York Academy of Sciences, 985*, 420.

Fenton, J., Raskin, A., & Gruber-Baldini, A. L. (2004). Some predictors of psychiatric consultation in nursing home residents. *American Journal of Geriatric Psychiatry, 12*, 297.

Firbank, M. J., Lloyd, A. J., Ferris, N., et al. (2004). A volumetric study of MRI signal hyperintensities in late-life depression. *American Journal of Geriatric Psychiatry, 12*, 606.

Fiveash, B. (1998). The experience of nursing home life. *International Journal of Nursing Practice, 4*, 166.

Foner, N. (1994). Nursing home aides: Saints or monsters? *Gerontologist, 34*, 245.

Foster, J. R., & Cataldo, J. K. (1993). Prediction of first episode of clinical depression in patients newly admitted to a medical long-term care facility: Findings from a prospective study. *International Journal of Geriatric Psychiatry, 8(4)*, 297–304.

Foster, J. R., Cataldo, J. K., & Boksay, I. J. E. (1991). Incidence of depression in a medical long-term care facility: Findings from a restricted sample of new admissions. *International Journal of Geriatric Psychiatry, 3,* 13.

Frazer, D. W. (1997). Psychotherapy in residential settings: Preliminary investigations and directions for research. In R. L. Rubinstein & M. P. Lawton (Eds.), *Depression in long-term and residential care: Advances in research and treatment.* New York: Springer.

Frederiksen, K., Tariot, P., & De Jonghe, E. (1996). Minimum Data Set Plus (MDS+) scores compared with scores from five rating scales. *Journal of the American Geriatrics Society, 44,* 305.

Frey, D. E., Kelbley, T. J., Durham, L., et al. (1992). Enhancing the self-esteem of selected male nursing home residents. *The Gerontologist, 32,* 552.

Friedman, R., Gryfe, C. I., Tal, D. T., et al. (1992). The noisy elderly patient: Prevalence, assessment, and response to the antidepressant doxepin. *Journal of Geriatric Psychiatry and Neurology, 5,* 187.

Gallo, J., Rabins, P., & Lyketsos, C. (1997). Depression without sadness: Functional outcomes of nondysphoric depression in later life. *Journal of the American Geriatrics Society, 45,* 570.

Gerety, M. B., Williams, J. W., Jr, Mulrow, C. D., et al. (1994). Performance of case-finding tools for depression in the nursing home: Influence of clinical and functional characteristics and selection of optimal threshold scores. *Journal of the American Geriatrics Society, 42,* 1103.

German, P. S., Rovner, B. W., Burton, L. C., et al. (1992). The role of mental morbidity in the nursing home experience. *The Gerontologist, 32,* 152.

Gildengers, A. G., Butters, M. A., Seligman, K., et al. (2004). Cognitive functioning in late-life bipolar disorder. *American Journal of Psychiatry, 161,* 736.

Gold, P. W., & Chrousos, G. P. (2002). Organization of the stress system and its dysregulation in melancholic and atypical depression: High vs. low CRH/NE states. *Molecular Psychiatry, 7,* 254.

Goldfarb, A. I. (1962). Prevalence of psychiatric disorders in metropolitan old age and nursing homes. *Journal of the American Geriatrics Society, 10,* 77.

Goldman, E. B., & Woog, P. (1975). Mental health in nursing homes training project. *The Gerontologist, 15,* 119.

Goldwasser, A. N., Auerbach, S. M., & Harkins, S. W. (1987). Cognitive, affective, and behavioral effects of reminiscence group therapy on demented elderly. *International Journal of Aging and Human Development, 25,* 209 .

Goyal, R., Sameer, M., & Chandrasekaran, R. (2006). Mania secondary to right-sided stroke—responsive to olanzapine. *General Hospital Psychiatry, 28,* 262.

Gruber-Baldini, A. L., Zimmerman, S., Boustani, M., et al. (2005). Characteristics associated with depression in long-term care residents with dementia. *The Gerontologist, 45*(Special issue 1), 50–55.

Gupta, N., & Basu, D. (1997). Mania secondary to alcohol binge. *Indian Journal of Medical Sciences, 51,* 394.

Gurland, B., & Toner, J. (1983). Differentiating dementia from nondementing conditions. *Advances in Neurology, 38,* 1.

Haight, B. K., Michel, Y., & Hendrix, S. (1998). Life review: Preventing despair in newly relocated nursing home residents short- and long-term effects. *International Journal of Aging and Human Development, 47,* 119.

Haight, B. K., Michel, Y., & Hendrix, S. (2000). The extended effects of the life review in nursing home residents. *International Journal of Aging and Human Development, 50,* 151.

Hawes, C. (2002, June 18). Elder abuse in residential long-term care facilities: What is known about prevalence, causes, and prevention. Testimony before the US Senate Committee on Finance. Retrieved July 23, 2006, from http://finance.senate.gov/hearings/testimony/061802chtest.pdf

Hawes, C., Morris, J. N., Phillips, C. D., et al. (1995). Reliability estimates for the Minimum Data Set for nursing home resident assessment and care screening (MDS). *The Gerontologist, 35,* 172.

Heston, L. L., Garrard, J., Markris, L., et al. (1992). Inadequate treatment of depressed nursing home elderly. *Journal of the American Geriatrics Society, 40,* 1117.

Horgas, A. L., & Dunn, K. (2001). Pain in nursing home residents. Comparison of residents' self-report and nursing assistants' perceptions. Incongruencies exist in resident and caregiver reports of pain; therefore, pain management education is needed to prevent suffering. *Journal of Gerontological Nursing, 27,* 44.

Hsu, L. K. G., & Zimmer, B. (1988). Eating disorders in old age. *International Journal of Eating Disorders, 7,* 133.

Hussian, R. A., & Lawrence, P. S. (1981) Social reinforcement of activity and problem-solving training in the treatment of depressed institutionalized elderly patients. *Cognitive Therapy and Research, 5,* 57.

Institute of Medicine. (1986). *Improving the quality of care in nursing homes.* Washington, DC: National Academy Press.

Jiang, J., Tang, Z., Futatsuka, M., et al. (2004). Exploring the influence of depressive symptoms on physical disability: A cohort study of elderly in Beijing, China. *Quality of Life Research, 13,* 1337.

Johnson, J. C. (1990). Delirium in the elderly. *Emergency Medicine Clinics of North America, 8,* 255–265.

Jones, E. D. (2003). Reminiscence therapy for older women with depression: Effects of nursing intervention classification in assisted-living long-term care. *Journal of Gerontological Nursing, 29,* 26.

Jongenelis, K., Pot, A. M., Eisses, A. M., et al. (2004). Prevalence and risk indicators of depression in elderly nursing home patients: The AGED study. *Journal of Affective Disorders, 83,* 135.

Kafonek, S., Ettinger, W. H., Roca, R., et al. (1989). Instruments for screening for depression and dementia in a long-term care facility. *Journal of the American Geriatrics Society, 37,* 29.

Kahn, D. L. (1999). Making the best of it: Adapting to the ambivalence of a nursing home environment. *Qualitative Health Research, 9,* 119.

Katon, W. (1984). Depression: Relationship to somatization and chronic medical illness. *Journal of Clinical Psychiatry, 45,* 4.

Katz, I. R., Lesher, E., Kleban, M., et al. (1989). Clinical features of depression in the nursing home. *International Psychogeriatrics, 1,* 5.

Katz, I. R., & Parmelee, P. A. (1994). Depression in elderly patients in residential care settings. In L. S. Schneider, C. F. Reynolds III, B. D. Lebowitz, & A. J. Freidhoff (Eds.), *Diagnosis and treatment of depression in late life.* Washington, DC: American Psychiatric Press.

Katz, I. R., Simpson, G. M., Curlik, S. M., et al. (1990). Pharmacologic treatment of major depression for elderly patients in residential care settings. *Journal of Clinical Psychiatry, 51*(Suppl), 41.

Kawakami, N., Takatsuka, N., Shimizu, H., et al. (1999). Depressive symptoms and occurrence of type 2 diabetes among Japanese men. *Diabetes Care, 22,* 1071.

Kerstetter, J. E., Holthausen, B. A., & Fitz, P. A. (1992). Malnutrition in the institutionalized older adult. *Journal of the American Dietetic Association, 92,* 1109.

Kiloh, L. G. (1961). Pseudodementia. *Acta Psychiatrica Scandinavica, 37,* 336.

Kivela, S. L., & Pahkala, K. (2001). Depressive disorder as a predictor of physical disability in old age. *Journal of the American Geriatrics Society, 49,* 290.

Koenig, H. G., & Blazer, D. G. (1992). Epidemiology of geriatric affective disorders. *Clinics in Geriatric Medicine, 8,* 235.

Kolcaba, K., & Miller, C. A. (1989). Behavior problems: Geropharmacology treatment: Extend nursing responsibility. *Journal of Gerontological Nursing, 15,* 29.

Krauthammer, C., & Klerman, G. L. (1978). Secondary mania: Manic syndromes associated with antecedent physical illness or drugs. *Archives of General Psychiatry, 35,* 1333.

Kruzich, J. M., Clinton, J. F., & Kleber, S. T. (1992). Personal and environmental influences on nursing home satisfaction. *The Gerontologist, 32,* 342.

Kukull, W. A., Koepsell, T. D., Inui, T. S., et al. (1986). Depression and physical illness among general medical clinic patients. *Journal of Affective Disorders, 10,* 153.

Langer, E. J., & Rodin, J. (1976). The effects of choice and enhanced personal responsibility for the aged: A field experiment in an institutional setting. *Journal of Personality and Social Psychology, 34,* 191.

Larson, S. L., Owens, P. L., Ford, D., et al. (2001). Depressive disorder, dysthymia, and risk of stroke: Thirteen-year follow-up from the Baltimore Epidemiologic Catchment Area Study. *Stroke, 32,* 1978.

Lawton, M. P., Casten, R., Parmelee, P. A., et al. (1998) Psychometric characteristics of the Minimum Data Set II. Validity. *Journal of the American Geriatrics Society, 46,* 736.

Lenze, E. J., Munin, M. C., Skidmore, E. R., et al. (2007). Onset of depression in elderly persons after hip fracture: Implications for prevention and early intervention of late-life depression. *Journal of the American Geriatrics Society, 55,* 81.

Leonard, R., Tinneti, M. E., & Allore, H. G., & Drickamer, M. A. (2006). Potentially modifiable resident characteristics that are associated with physical or verbal aggression among nursing home residents with dementia. *Archives of Internal Medicine, 166*(12), 1295.

Lesperance, F., Frasure-Smith, N., Talajic, M., et al. (2002). Five-year risk of cardiac mortality in relation to initial severity and one-year changes in depression symptoms after myocardial infarction. *Circulation, 105,* 1049.

Lesse, S. (1964). *Masked depression.* New York: Jason Aronson.

Libow, L., & Starer, P. (1989). Care of the nursing home patient. *New England Journal of Medicine, 231,* 93.

Loebel, J. P., Borson, S., Hyde, T., et al. (1991). Relationships between requests for psychiatric consultations and psychiatric diagnoses in long-term care facilities. *American Journal of Psychiatry, 148,* 898.

Loebel, J. P., Loebel, J. S., Dager, S. R., et al. (1991). Anticipation of nursing home placement may be a precipitant of suicide among the elderly. *Journal of the American Geriatrics Society, 39,* 407.

Magai, C., Kennedy, G., Cohen, C. I., et al. (2000). A controlled clinical trial of sertraline in the treatment of depression in nursing home patients with late-stage Alzheimer's disease. *American Journal of Geriatric Psychiatry, 8,* 66.

McCullough, P. K. (1991). Geriatric depressions: Atypical presentations, hidden meanings. *Geriatrics, 46,* 72.

McCurren, C., Dowe, D., Rattle, D., et al. (1999). Depression among nursing home elders: Testing an intervention strategy. *Applied Nursing Research, 12*, 185.

McEwan, B. S. (2003). Mood disorders and allostatic load. *Biological Psychiatry, 54*, 200.

McMurdo, M. E. T., & Rennie, L. (1993). A controlled trial of exercise by residents of old people's homes. *Age and Ageing, 22*, 11.

Mendez, M. F. (2000). Mania in neurologic disorders. *Current Psychiatry Reports, 2*, 440.

Mendez, M. F., McMurtray, A., Chen, A. K., et al. (2006). *Journal of Neurology, Neurosurgery, and Psychiatry, 77*, 4.

Menon, A. S., Gruber-Baldini, A. L., Hebel, J. R., et al. (2001). Relationship between aggressive behaviors and depression among nursing home residents with dementia. *International Journal of Geriatric Psychiatry, 16*, 139.

Michelson, D., Stratakis, C., & Hill, L. (1996). Bone mineral density in women with depression. *New England Journal of Medicine, 335*, 1176.

Miller, D. K., Morley, J. E., Rubenstein, L. Z., et al. (1991). Abnormal eating attitudes and body image in older undernourished individuals. *Journal of the American Geriatrics Society, 39*, 462.

Miller, M. D., & Reynolds, C. F., 3rd. (2007). Expanding the usefulness of Interpersonal Psychotherapy (IPT) for depressed elders with co-morbid cognitive impairment. *International Journal of Geriatric Psychiatry, 22*, 101.

Mirchandani, I. C., & Young, R. C. (1993). Management of mania in the elderly. An update. *Annals of Clinical Psychiatry, 5*, 67.

Moak, G., & Borson, S. (2000). Mental health services in long-term care. *American Journal of Geriatric Psychiatry, 8*, 96–101.

Moran, J. A., & Gatz, M. (1987). Group therapies for nursing home adults: An evaluation of two treatment approaches. *The Gerontologist, 27*, 588.

Morris, P. L. P., Robinson, A. G., Andrezejewski, P., et al. (1993). Association of depression with 10-year post-stroke mortality. *American Journal of Psychiatry, 150*, 124.

Moses, J. (1982). New role for hands-on caregivers: Part-time mental health technicians. *Journal of American Health Care Association, 8*, 19.

Nebes, R. D., Pollock, B. G., Houck, P. R., et al. (2003). Persistence of cognitive impairment in geriatric patients following antidepressant treatment: A randomized, double-blind clinical trial with nortriptyline and paroxetine. *Journal of Psychiatric Research, 37*, 99.

O'Connor, M. K., Knapp, R., Husain, M., et al. (2001). The influence of age on the response of major depression to electroconvulsive therapy: A CORE report. *American Journal of Geriatric Psychiatry, 9*, 382.

Olin, J. T., Katz, I. R., & Meyers, B. S. (2002). Provisional diagnostic criteria for depression of Alzheimer's disease. *American Journal of Geriatric Psychiatry, 10*, 125.

Orten, J. D., Allen, M., & Cook, J. (1989). Reminiscence groups with confused nursing center residents: An experimental study. *Social Work in Health Care, 14*, 73.

Osgood, N. (1992). Environmental factors in suicide in long-term care facilities. *Suicide and Life-Threatening Behavior, 22*, 98.

Oslin, D. W., Streim, J. E., Katz, I. R., et al. (2000). Heuristic comparison of sertraline with nortriptyline for the treatment of depression in frail elderly patients. *American Journal of Geriatric Psychiatry 8*, 141.

Oslin, D. W., Ten Have, T. R., Streim, J. E., et al. (2003). Probing the safety of medications in the frail elderly: Evidence from a randomized clinical trial of sertraline and venlafaxine in depressed nursing home residents. *Journal of Clinical Psychiatry, 64*, 875.

Parmelee, P. A., Katz, I. R., & Lawton, M. P. (1989). Depression among institutionalized aged: Assessment and prevalence estimation. *Journal of Gerontology, 44*, 22.

Parmelee, P. A., Katz, I. R., & Lawton, M. P. (1991). The relation of pain to depression among institutionalized aged. *Journal of Gerontology, 46*, 15.

Parmelee, P. A., Katz, I. R., & Lawton, M. P. (1992a) Depression and mortality among institutionalized aged. *Journal of Gerontology, 47*, 3.

Parmelee, P. A., Katz, I. R., & Lawton, M. P. (1992b). Incidence of depression in long-term care settings. *Journal of Gerontology, 47*, 189.

Parmelee, P. A., Katz, I. R., & Lawton, M. P. (1993a). Anxiety and its association with depression among institutionalized elderly. *American Journal of Geriatric Psychiatry, 1*, 46.

Parmelee, P. A., Lawton, M. P., & Katz, I. R. (1998). The structure of depression among elderly institution residents: Affective and somatic correlates of physical frailty. *Journal of Gerontology Series A: Biological Sciences and Medical Sciences, 53*, 155.

Parmelee, P. A., Smith, B., & Katz, I. R. (1993b). Pain complaints and cognitive status among elderly institution residents. *Journal of the American Geriatrics Society, 41*, 517.

Payne, J. L., Sheppard, J. M. E., Steinberg, M., et al. (2002). Incidence, prevalence, and outcomes of depression in residents of a long-term care facility with dementia. *International Journal of Geriatric Psychiatry, 17*, 247.

Penninx, B. W., Geerlings, S. W., Deeg, D. J., et al. (1999). Minor and major depression and the risk of death in older persons. *Archives of General Psychiatry, 56*, 889.

Pillemer, K., & Bachman, R. (1991). Helping and hurting: Predictors of maltreatment of patients in nursing homes. *Research on Aging, 13*, 74.

Pillemer, K., & Hudson, B. (1993). A model abuse prevention program for nursing assistants. *The Gerontologist, 33*, 128.

Pillemer, K., & Moore, D. W. (1989). Abuse of patients in nursing homes: Findings from a survey of staff. *The Gerontologist, 29*, 314.

Pillemer, K., & Moore, D. W. (1990). Highlights from a study of abuse of patients in nursing homes. *Journal of Elder Abuse and Neglect, 2*, 5.

Poon, L. W. (1992). Toward an understanding of cognitive functioning in geriatric depression. *International Psychogeriatrics, 4*(Suppl 2), 241.

Post, F. (1965). *The clinical psychiatry of late life.* Oxford: Pergamon Press.

Price, W. A., Gianini, A. J., & Collella, J. (1985). Anorexia nervosa in the elderly. *Journal of the American Geriatrics Society, 37*, 184.

Rapp, M. A., Schnaider-Beeri, M., Grossman, H. T., et al. (2006). Increased hippocampal plaques and tangles in patients with Alzheimer disease with a lifetime history of major depression. *Archives of General Psychiatry, 63*, 161.

Rattenbury, C., & Stones, M. J. (1989). A controlled evaluation of reminiscence and current topics discussion groups in a nursing home context. *The Gerontologist, 29*, 768.

Reichman, W. E., Coyne, A., Borson, S., et al. (1998). Psychiatric consultation in the nursing home: A survey of six states. *American Journal of Geriatric Psychiatry, 6*, 320.

Reynolds, C. F., 3rd, Frank, E., Perel, J. M., et al. (1999). Nortriptyline and interpersonal psychotherapy as maintenance therapies for recurrent major depression: A randomized controlled trial in patients older than 59 years. *JAMA, 281*, 39.

Ridman, D., & Feller, A. G. (1989). Protein-calorie undernutrition in the nursing home. *Journal of the American Geriatrics Society, 37*, 173.

Rodin, J., & Langer, E. J. (1977). Long-term effects of a control-relevant intervention with the institutionalized aged. *Journal of Personality and Social Psychology, 35*, 897.

Rojas-Fernandez, C. H., Lanctot, K. L., & Allen, D. D. (2001). Pharmacotherapy of behavioral and psychological symptoms of dementia: Time for a different paradigm? *Pharmacotherapy, 21*, 74.

Roose, S. P., Nelson, J. C., Salzman, C., et al. (2003). Open-label study of mirtazapine orally disintegrating tablets in depressed patients in the nursing home. *Current Medical Research and Opinion, 19*, 737.

Rosen, J., Mulsant, B. H., & Pollock, B. G. (2000). Sertraline in the treatment of minor depression in nursing home residents: A pilot study. *International Journal of Geriatric Psychiatry, 15*, 177.

Rosen, J., Rogers, J. C., Marin, R. S., et al. (1997). Control-relevant intervention in the treatment of minor and major depression in a long-term care facility. *American Journal of Geriatric Psychiatry, 5*, 247.

Rosenblatt, A., Samus, Q. M., Steele, C. D., et al. (2004). The Maryland Assisted Living Study: Prevalence, recognition, and treatment of dementia and other psychiatric disorders in the assisted living population of central Maryland. *Journal of the American Geriatrics Society, 52*, 1618–1625.

Rovner, B. W., Kafonek, S., Filipp, L., et al. (1986). Prevalence of mental illness in a community nursing home. *American Journal of Psychiatry, 143*, 1446.

Rovner, B. W., & Katz, I. R. (1993). Psychiatric disorders in the nursing home: A selective review of studies related to clinical care. *International Journal of Geriatric Psychiatry, 8*, 75.

Rovner, B. W., German, P. S., Brant, L. J., et al. (1991). Depression and mortality in nursing homes. *JAMA, 265*, 993.

Rovner, B. W., Steele, C. D., German, P., et al. (1992). Psychiatric diagnosis and uncooperative behavior in nursing homes. *Journal of Geriatric Psychiatry and Neurology, 5*, 102.

Royall, D. R., Mahurin, R. K., & Gray, K. (1992). Bedside assessment of executive cognitive impairment: The Executive Interview (EXIT). *Journal of the American Geriatrics Society, 40*, 1221.

Rubin, E. H. (1988). Aging and mania. *Psychiatric Developments, 4*, 329.

Ruckdeschel, K., Thompson, R., Datto, C. J., et al. (2004). Using the Minimum Data Set 2.0 mood disturbance items as a self-report screening instrument for depression in nursing home residents. *American Journal of Geriatric Psychiatry, 12*, 43–49.

Sackheim, H. A. (1993). The use of electroconvulsive therapy in late-life depression. In L. S. Schneider, C. F. Reynolds III, B. D. Lebowitz, et al. (Eds.), *Diagnosis and treatment of depression in late life* (pp. 259–277). Washington, DC: American Psychiatric Press.

Salzman, C., Fisher, J., Nobel, K., et al. (1992). Cognitive improvement following benzodiazepine discontinuation in elderly nursing home patients. *International Journal of Geriatric Psychiatry, 7*, 89.

Samuels, S. C., & Katz, I. R. (1995). Depression in the nursing home. *Psychiatric Annals, 25*, 419.

Santmyer, K. S., & Roca, R. P. (1991). Geropsychiatry in long-term care: A nurse-centered approach. *Journal of the American Geriatrics Society, 39*, 156.

Scanlan, J., & Borson, S. (2001). The Mini-Cog: Receiver operating characteristics with expert and naive raters. *International Journal of Geriatric Psychiatry, 16*, 216.

Schleifer, S. J., Keller, S. E., Bond, R. N., et al. (1989). Major depressive disorder and immunity. *Archives of General Psychiatry, 46*, 81.

Schneider, L. S., & Sobin, P. B. (1992). Non-neuroleptic treatment of behavioral symptoms and agitation in Alzheimer's disease and other dementia. *Psychological Bulletin, 28*, 71.

Schnittker, J. (2005). When mental health becomes health: Age and the shifting meaning of self-evaluations of general health. *Milbank Q, 83*, 397.

Schulz, R. (1976). Effect of control and predictability on the physical and psychological well-being of the institutionalized aged. *Journal of Personality and Social Psychology, 33*, 563.

Sengstaken, E. A., & King, S. A. (1993). The problem of pain and its detection among geriatric nursing home residents. *Journal of the American Geriatrics Society, 41*, 541.

Shahpesandy, H. (2005). Different manifestation of depressive disorder in the elderly. *Neuroendocrinology Letters, 26*, 691.

Sheline, Y. (2003). Neuroimaging studies of mood disorder effects on the brain. *Biological Psychiatry, 54*, 338.

Shulman, K. I., Rochon, P., Sykora, K., et al. (2003). Changing prescription patterns for lithium and divalproex in old age: Shifting without evidence. *British Medical Journal, 326*, 960.

Silver, A. J., Morley, J. E., Strome, S., et al. (1988). Nutritional status in an academic nursing home. *Journal of the American Geriatrics Society, 36*, 487.

Slatter, E., & Roth, M. (1977). *Clinical psychiatry* (3rd ed.). London: Bailliere, Tindall and Cassell.

Snow, A. L., O'Malley, K. J., Cody, M., et al. (2004). A conceptual model of pain assessment for noncommunicative persons with dementia. *The Gerontologist, 44*, 807.

Snowden, J. (1986). Dementia, depression, and life satisfaction in nursing homes. *International Journal of Geriatric Psychiatry, 1*, 85.

Snowden, J., & Donnelly, N. (1986). A study of depression in nursing homes. *Journal of Psychiatric Research, 20*, 327.

Snowden, M., Sato, K., & Roy-Byrne, P. (2003). Assessment and treatment of nursing home residents with depression or behavioral disturbances associated with dementia: A review of the literature. *Journal of the American Geriatrics Society, 51*, 1305.

Spector, A., Orrell, M., Davies, S., et al. (2001). Can reality orientation be rehabilitated? Development and piloting of an evidence-based programme of cognition-based therapies for people with dementia. *Neuropsychology Review, 11*, 377.

Starkstein, S. E., Mizrahi, R., & Garau, L. (2005). Specificity of symptoms of depression in Alzheimer's disease. *American Journal of Geriatric Psychiatry, 13*, 802.

Stone, K. (1989). Mania in the elderly. *British Journal of Psychiatry, 155*, 220.

Streim, J. E., Beckwith, E. W., Arapakos, D., et al. (2002). Regulatory oversight, payment policy, and quality improvement in mental health care in nursing homes. *Psychiatric Services, 53*, 1414.

Streim, J. E., Oslin, D. W., Katz, I. R., et al. (2000). Drug treatment of depression in frail elderly nursing home residents. *American Journal of Geriatric Psychiatry, 8*, 150.

Talerico, K. A., Evans, L. K., & Strumpf, N. E. (2002). Mental health correlates of aggression in nursing home residents with dementia. *The Gerontologist, 42*, 169.

Tariot, P. N., Podgorski, C. A., Blazina, L., et al. (1993). Mental disorders in the nursing home: Another perspective. *American Journal of Psychiatry, 150*, 1063.

Teeter, R. B., Garetz, F. K., Miller, W. R., et al. (1976). Psychiatric disturbances of aged patients in skilled nursing care. *American Journal of Psychiatry, 133*, 1430.

Tellis-Nayak, V., & Tellis-Nayak, M. (1989). Quality of care and the burden of two cultures: When the world of the nurse's aide enters the world of the nursing home. *The Gerontologist, 29*, 307.

Teresi, J., Abrams, R., Holmes, D., et al. (2001). Prevalence of depression and depression recognition in nursing homes. *Social Psychiatry and Psychiatric Epidemiology, 36*, 613.

Thomas, A. J., Davis, S., Morris, C., et al. (2005). Increase in interleukin-1beta in late-life depression. *American Journal of Psychiatry, 162*, 175.

Thomas, A. J., Perry, R., Kalaria, R. N., et al. (2003). Neuropathological evidence for ischemia in the white matter of the dorsolateral prefrontal cortex in late-life depression. *International Journal of Geriatric Psychiatry, 18*, 7.

Toseland, R. W., Diehl, M., Freeman, K., et al. (1997). The impact of validation group therapy on nursing home residents with dementia. *Journal of Applied Gerontology, 16*, 31.

Trappler, B., & Cohen, C. I. (1996). Using fluoxetine in "very old" depressed nursing home residents. *American Journal of Geriatric Psychiatry, 4*, 258.

Trappler, B., & Cohen, C. I. (1998). Use of SSRIs in "very old" depressed nursing home residents. *American Journal of Geriatric Psychiatry, 6*, 83.

Unutzer, J., Katon, W., Callahan, C. M., et al. (2002). Collaborative care management of late-life depression in the primary care setting: A randomized controlled trial. *JAMA, 288*, 2836.

Van Wattum, P. J., & Chiles, C. (2001). Rapid response to low dose citalopram in pathological crying. *General Hospital Psychiatry, 23*, 167.

Vilalta-Franch, J., Garre-Olmo, J., Lopez-Pousa, S., et al. (2006). Comparison of different clinical diagnostic criteria for depression in Alzheimer's disease. *American Journal of Geriatric Psychiatry 14*, 589.

Wagenaar, D., Colenda, C. C., Kreft, M., et al. (2003). Treating depression in nursing homes: Practice guidelines in the real world. *Journal of the American Osteopathic Association, 10*, 465.

Warden, V., Hurley, A. C., & Volicer, L. (2003). Development and psychometric evaluation of the Pain Assessment in Advanced Dementia (PAINAD) scale. *Journal of the American Medical Directors Association, 4*, 9.

Weintraub, D., Datto, C. J., Streim, J. E., et al. (2002). Second-generation issues in the management of depression in nursing homes. *Journal of the American Geriatrics Society, 50*, 2100.

Weintraub, D., Streim, J. E., Datto, C. J., et al. (2003). Effect of increasing the dose and duration of sertraline trial in the treatment of depressed nursing home residents. *Journal of Geriatric Psychiatry and Neurology, 16*, 109.

Weissman, M. M., Bruce, M. L., Leaf, P. J., et al. (1991). Affective disorders. In L. N. Robins & D. A. Regier (Eds.), *Psychiatric disorders in America: The Epidemiological Catchment Area Study.* New York: Free Press.

Weverer, S., Schaufele, M., & Zimber, A. (1999). Alcohol problems among residents in old age homes in the city of Mannheim, Germany. *Australian and New Zealand Journal of Psychiatry, 33*, 825.

Whooley, M. A. (2006). Depression and cardiovascular disease: Healing the broken-hearted. *JAMA, 295*, 2874.

Whyte, E., Pollock, B. G., Wagner, W., et al. (2001). Influence of the serotonin transporter-linked region polymorphism on platelet activation in geriatric depression. *American Journal of Psychiatry, 158,* 2074.

Winn, P. A., & Dentino, A. N. (2004). Effective pain management in the long-term care setting. *Journal of the American Medical Directors Association, 5,* 342.

Wulsin, L. R., & Singal, B. M. (2003). Do depressive symptoms increase the risk for the onset of coronary disease? A systematic quantitative review. *Psychosomatic Medicine, 65,* 201.

Young, R. C., Gyulai, L., Mulsant, B. H., et al. (2004). Pharmacotherapy of bipolar disorder in old age. *American Journal of Geriatric Psychiatry, 12,* 342.

Zenmore, R., & Eames, N. (1979). Psychic and somatic symptoms of depression among young adults, institutionalized adults, and noninstitutionalized aged. *Journal of Gerontology, 34,* 716.

Zerhusen, J. D., Boyle, K., & Wilson, W. (1991). Out of the darkness: Group cognitive therapy for depressed elderly. *Journal of Psychosocial Nursing and Mental Health Services, 29,* 16.

5

Anxiety Disorders

Art Walaszek and *Timothy Howell*

Not unlike depression, anxiety may be protean in its many manifestations, varying from mild, fleeting apprehension to immobilizing panic. It may be that the very familiarity with this "all-too-human" emotion sometimes interferes with understanding how anxiety affects patients in long-term care (LTC) settings, thus hindering accurate assessment and treatment. Through misplaced empathy, for example, care providers may place themselves in the shoes of LTC residents in an effort to appreciate their experience of an anxiety-provoking situation. But if they forget to "age themselves" in the process, and adopt the residents' perspectives and values, they may miss the mark. The prospect of arthroplasty may seem much less anxiety-provoking to a younger health professional, for example, than an octogenarian.

Avoiding the hazard of unwittingly trivializing excessive anxiety as "normal" or "expectable under the circumstances" necessitates becoming objectively familiar with the landscape of anxiety. This chapter reviews ways to approach the assessment and treatment of anxiety disorders in LTC patients that can help address the diagnostic and prognostic ambiguities endemic to psychiatric problems with this patient population.

EPIDEMIOLOGY

Several methodologically rigorous studies have explored the prevalence of anxiety in LTC settings (Table 5.1). These studies have found a high rate of both anxiety symptoms (up to 38%) and DSM-based anxiety disorders (up to 20%; *Diagnostic and Statistical Manual of Mental Disorders, DSM*). One can appreciate the findings in LTC by comparing them with findings from community-dwelling elders, where the estimated prevalence of anxiety symptoms is 19% (Mehta et al., 2003) and of specific disorders is as follows: phobias, 4.8% to 8.9%; posttraumatic stress disorder (PTSD), 0.9%; obsessive-compulsive disorder (OCD), 0.8%; and panic disorder (PD), 0.1% (Cohen et al., 2006; Regier et al., 1988; van Zelst et al., 2003). Thus, it appears that the LTC population is at higher risk for both anxiety symptoms and anxiety disorders.

Methodological and clinical issues hamper interpretation of epidemiological studies of late-life anxiety. For example, there are varying approaches to attributing etiology for somatic symptoms of anxiety (e.g., tremor, dry mouth) that

TABLE 5.1. Epidemiology of Anxiety in Long-Term Care

STUDY	SETTING	PARTICIPANTS	PREVALENCE
German et al. (1986)	NH	N = 350	Phobia 2.1%–11.6%
Parmelee et al. (1993)	NH and congregate housing	N = 791, ≥ 61 years old	GAD or PD, 3.5%; anxiety disorders not sufficient for diagnosis, 13.2%
Junginger et al. (1993)	NH	N = 100, without dementia	GAD, 6%; PD, 5%; OCD, 5%; agoraphobia without panic, 4%; phobia, 1%; any anxiety disorder, 20%
Morgan et al. (2001)	AL	N = 2078	Anxiety, 35%–38%
Rosenblatt et al. (2004)	AL	N = 198	anxiety disorder, 13%
Cook et al. (2005)	NH	N = 35 veterans without dementia	PTSD, 9%
Smalbrugge et al. (2005a)	NH	N = 333, MMSE > 14	Phobia, 3.6%; PD, 1.5%; GAD, 1.2%; anxiety symptoms, 29.7%

Note: AL, assisted living, GAD, generalized anxiety disorder, MMSE, Mini-Mental State Examination, NH, nursing home, OCD, obsessive-compulsive disorder, PD, panic disorder, PTSD, posttraumatic stress disorder.

can be caused by either medical or psychiatric conditions. In one study, somatic symptoms were attributed to concurrent medical problems and, thus, omitted (Parmelee et al., 1993). As a consequence, anxiety disorders due to general medical conditions may have been missed and other anxiety disorders underestimated. But the attribution of somatic symptoms to either physical or psychiatric disorders may actually have little effect on the prevalence rates of anxiety disorders. Smalbrugge's group undertook a sensitivity analysis to determine to what degree the validity of their psychiatric instruments may have been compromised by the presence of comorbid physical illnesses in their subjects. In their original study, when the interviewer was unsure of the origin of a somatic symptom, it was coded as due to a physical problem. When they recoded such ambiguous somatic symptoms as instead due to a psychiatric disorder, there was very little change in the prevalence rates: for generalized anxiety disorder (GAD), the rate remained the same, whereas for PD, it increased modestly from 1.5% to 1.8% (Smalbrugge et al., 2005b).

Several of the studies cited in Table 5.1 excluded cognitively impaired subjects, which limits the generalizability of their findings, since the majority of residents of nursing homes have dementia. No mention is made of subjects with dementia in the Junginger study, whereas the Smalbrugge study omitted subjects with more severe cognitive impairment (MMSE scores less than 15; Junginger et al., 1993; Smalbrugge et al., 2005a). The prevalence of clinically significant anxiety is estimated to be 9.7% among community-dwelling elders with dementia and 5% among those with mild cognitive impairment (Lysketsos et al., 2002). The Maryland Assisted Living Study, which did not exclude cognitively impaired residents, found significant overlap between the population of residents with dementia and those with discrete anxiety disorders (Rosenblatt et al., 2004).

Another confounding issue in the epidemiology of anxiety disorders is that anxiety is frequently a prominent component of other psychiatric disorders, including depression, cognitive disorders (as described above), psychosis, adjustment disorders, personality disorders, substance abuse, chronic pain syndromes, and sleep disorders. For example, anxiety and depression are highly comorbid: The Longitudinal Aging Study Amsterdam found that 47.5% of elders with major depressive disorder (MDD) also had an anxiety disorder, whereas 26.1% with anxiety disorders also met criteria for MDD (Beekman et al., 2000). The Smalbrugge group reported that 4.8% of LTC residents had a "pure" anxiety disorder, whereas another 5.1% had comorbid depressive and anxiety disorders (Smalbrugge et al., 2005c).

Because most studies of anxiety in LTC have been cross-sectional, risk factors for anxiety are difficult to determine. Cross-sectional correlates of anxiety include female gender, depression, stroke, impaired vision, pain, functional impairment, lack of social supports, and recent negative life events (Parmelee et al., 1993;

Smalbrugge et al., 2003, 2005a). These studies have yielded contradictory results regarding the correlation between cognitive status and anxiety: Parmelee's group found an association between cognitive impairment and anxiety, whereas Smalbrugge's group (which excluded subjects with severe cognitive impairment) found that MMSE scores greater than 23 were associated with anxiety. In a prospective study set in the community, predictors of developing anxiety included female gender, problems with hearing and vision, adverse life events (typically the death of a partner or partner developing a major illness), and the personality trait of high neuroticism (de Beurs et al., 2000, 2001).

CLINICAL PRESENTATION

The phenomenology of anxiety can usefully be divided into four categories of signs and symptoms: psychological features, psychomotor signs, autonomic signs, and vigilance (see Table 5.2). These many ways in which LTC patients may present with anxiety account for why the diagnosis of an anxiety disorder may be delayed or missed altogether. Anxiety syndromes in late life, particularly among those prone to somatization, can present with confusing sets of complaints that vary, even over very short periods of time. Cultural and subcultural issues markedly influence the symptoms of anxiety and how they are interpreted. In the United States, the open expression of emotions generally tends to

TABLE 5.2. Signs and Symptoms of Anxiety

Psychological features	Dysphoric apprehension or expectation
	Avoidance of anxiety-provoking situations or stimuli
Psychomotor signs	Tremulousness, twitching, feeling shaky
	Muscle tension, aches, soreness
	Restlessness
	Easily fatigued
Autonomic signs	Shortness of breath, "smothering"
	Palpitations, increased heart rate
	Sweating, cold/clammy feeling
	Dry mouth
	Dizziness, light-headedness
	Nausea, vomiting, GI distress
	Flushing, hot flashes, chills
	Frequent urination
	Dysphagia, "lump in throat"
Vigilance	Feeling keyed up, on edge
	Exaggerated startle response
	Poor concentration, "mind goes blank"
	Insomnia
	Irritability

be highly valued. In other cultures and subcultures, however, social harmony and the avoidance of confrontation have a higher priority. Thus, cultural influences may determine not only what constitutes an anxiety-provoking situation and the nature of the anxiety syndrome, but also the ways of coping and seeking help, as well as how others respond (Kirmayer, 2001). For example, it is also possible that the current cohort of older adults in the United States is less comfortable with talking about feelings and hence more likely to focus on somatic symptoms of anxiety. Such a phenomenon could result in more medical evaluations before the anxiety disorder is recognized. Below we describe various manifestations of anxiety in LTC settings.

Situational Anxiety

The most likely precipitant of anxiety for residents of LTC facilities is facing an unfamiliar situation. Examples of such situations include sudden, nonroutine events (e.g., a false fire alarm) or a need to undertake a task that the individual has not had any need to perform or practice for some time (e.g., to balance a financial account or to spell a word backward as part of a mental status exam). If the anxiety response appears excessive in intensity or duration, one should consider the possibility of an underlying anxiety disorder or other disorder. For example, *catastrophic reactions* are intense emotional and behavioral responses precipitated by common tasks with which a patient with dementia no longer has the ability to cope.

Adjustment Disorder with Anxiety

Anxiety that develops in response to a known stressor and is severe enough to interfere with functioning is referred to as an adjustment disorder with anxiety. Stressors may be crises (e.g., LTC placement, illness in family, death of a peer) or less severe (e.g., relocation from one room to another). A new medical problem, even if not severe or disabling, may precipitate anxiety. A precipitating stressor may be acute or chronic (lasting 6 months or longer), though anxiety lasting longer than 6 months should lead one to consider an alternate diagnosis, for example, GAD.

Generalized Anxiety Disorder

GAD is characterized by apprehension that is both persistent (i.e., lasting 6 months or longer) and frequent (i.e., occurring on more days than not), either excessive or unrealistic, and difficult for affected individuals to control. By *DSM-IV-TR* criteria (*DSM*, 4th ed., text revision, American Psychiatric Association, APA, 2000), the diagnosis of GAD requires that patients have at least three of the following six symptoms: restlessness, irritability, muscle tension, disturbed sleep, poor concentration, and easy fatigability. If an LTC resident has another major psychiatric disorder concurrently, the pervasive anxiety of GAD must involve different, unrelated issues. Thus, to qualify for the diagnosis of GAD, someone with a comorbid PD must worry about more than having additional panic attacks, someone with comorbid social phobia must worry about more than public embarrassment, and someone with comorbid OCD must worry about more than contamination. Other exclusion criteria include the anxiety being attributable to a demonstrable organic cause or occurring only in the context of an affective or psychotic disorder.

GAD and MDD are frequently comorbid. Older adults with both have a worse prognosis than those with either alone. For example, Schoevers et al. (2005) found, whereas 48% of subjects with GAD at baseline had remitted at 3-year follow-up, 24% "switched" to MDD and 16% to a mixed anxiety-depression syndrome. Subjects with mixed-anxiety depression had lower remission rates (27%) than those with MDD alone (41%) or GAD alone (48%). Lenze et al. (2005) found that 36% of older adults with GAD have had chronic symptoms (10 or more years), while the mean episode duration was 17 years; their group confirmed that GAD commonly converts to mixed anxiety-depression in late life. Finally, subjects in a pharmacological trial of late-life depression had lower response rates if they had comorbid anxiety (Flint & Rifat, 1997).

Phobias

Phobias are the most common anxiety disorder found in samples of community-dwelling older adults. Phobic anxiety involves a recurrent, disproportionate, almost instantaneous fear of a specific object or situation, sufficiently intense to cause significant subjective distress or avoidant behavior and to interfere with the individual's normal routine or social activities. It may be precipitated by confrontation with the object or situation (i.e., specific phobia) or by a social or performance situation involving unfamiliar people, scrutiny by others, or potential embarrassment (i.e., social phobia). Specific and social phobias are usually lifelong and associated with little impairment. One exception is the fear of falling, which has an estimated prevalence of 12% to 65% in older adults who have not fallen and 29% to 92% in those who have fallen; it is associated with restriction of activities, increased risk of falls, and lower quality of life (Jorstad et al., 2005).

Agoraphobia is characterized by a fear of entering places from which escape could be difficult or embarrassing, or where there would not be any help should symptoms of panic set in. Residents fearful of leaving the LTC facility, or even their rooms, may be manifesting this disorder. Agoraphobia in older adults often starts after the age of 60 and is not infrequently associated with moderate impairment. The association of late-life agoraphobia with the loss of a parent in early life may indicate that such a separation, through death or divorce, is a risk factor (Lindesay, 1991).

Older adults often attribute their phobic anxiety to a distressing medical or social experience and seldom report panic attacks (Burvill et al., 1995). Hence new-onset "phobias" in late life mandate careful assessment since they may not be altogether unwarranted or irrational. For example, LTC residents may become apprehensive about social events due to the onset of incontinence or cognitive impairment. Out of embarrassment, they may not volunteer this information. Or, traumatized by some experience, either recent (e.g., assault) or remote (e.g., war-related), they may exhibit phobic anxiety when encountering a reminder of that trauma (see Posttraumatic Stress Disorder below). Hence, the appearance of a "phobia" may be an indicator of another anxiety problem.

Obsessive-Compulsive Disorder

The presence of obsessions and compulsions is the defining feature of this disorder. Obsessions consist of persistently recurring ideas, images, or impulses that intrude into a patient's consciousness. They seem to make no sense and frequently are either morally or physically repugnant, not only to others but also to the patient as well. Obsessions are usually "ego-dystonic," that is, they are experienced as invasive and not voluntarily originating from the individual's own mental process. Furthermore, they are often refractory to suppression by the patient and can become a source of considerable distress. The most common obsessions in older adults involve contamination, pathological doubt, somatic concerns, and aggression (Kohn et al., 1997). Others include a need for symmetry and intrusive sexual images or impulses (Rasmussen & Eisen, 1992).

Compulsions are actions with the same defining characteristics as obsessions but are the behavioral responses to obsessive thoughts. They involve seemingly purposeful repetitive behaviors, performed according to specific rules or in a stereotypic manner. Compulsions, however, are not ends in themselves but rather the means to bring about or prevent something else. These behaviors provide temporary relief from anxiety, but with the anxiety soon rebuilding, a cycle of obsessions and compulsions is maintained. As with obsessions, affected individuals initially recognize the compulsions to be irrational but feel unable to resist performing them. For example, in order to ward off a calamity (e.g., preventing all the other residents from dying), a patient may be anxiously driven to some meaningless activity (e.g., systematically touching all the doorknobs). The most common compulsions in the elderly are checking, counting, and washing (Kohn et al., 1997). Others include needing to ask or confess something, arranging objects precisely, and hoarding (Rasmussen & Eisen, 1992).

The assessment of OCD in elderly LTC residents may be complicated if their long-standing symptoms cease to be "ego-dystonic." After many years, patients may become relatively used to them, and some may even incorporate them into their sense of identity. No longer experienced as irrational, their obsessions or compulsions may then resemble psychotic symptoms such as thought insertions or delusional behavior. Assessing the individual's earlier history, for example, from collateral sources, may be clarifying. Another variant of this condition is the occurrence of OCD symptoms in the ruminative thinking sometimes seen in depression, and the delusions of psychotic depression can be a diagnostic challenge. Distressing repetitive behaviors associated with dementing conditions, especially frontotemporal dementia, may also mimic OCD.

The initial onset of OCD in late life is quite rare, hence the development of obsessions or compulsions in an LTC resident should lead to a careful exploration of possible medical etiologies. Weiss and Jenike (2000) reported a series of five cases of patients with OCD beginning after the age of 50, four of whom were found to have intracerebral lesions involving the frontal lobes and caudate. In the absence of such lesions, it may be that a combination of anxiety-prone traits (e.g., limited flexibility, meticulousness) and late-life stressors over which the patient has limited control (e.g., severe illness in a spouse) can precipitate symptoms of OCD (Velayudhan & Katz, 2006).

Panic Disorder

PD is characterized by recurrent attacks of acute anxiety that generally arise in an unpredictable fashion. These attacks usually manifest themselves with intense sensations of terror, fear, or doom, which initially occur both suddenly and spontaneously over the space of several minutes. Common somatic symptoms of panic attacks include dyspnea, palpitations, light-headedness, chest pain/pressure, smothering/choking sensations, paresthesias, hot–cold flashes, perspiration, and nausea or other gastrointestinal distress. Psychological symptoms of panic include a sense of being out of control—"going crazy" or "about to die"—as well as anticipatory apprehension of further attacks. Recurrent panic attacks may lead subsequently to the formation of phobias, with patients avoiding, or having to endure, the situations in which they have experienced prior panic attacks.

The onset of PD in late life is rare and, in fact, PD generally appears to be a chronic illness with onset in early life whose symptoms decrease in severity over time (Flint, 1994; Sheikh et al., 2004a). The diagnostic challenge of panic attacks in late life is that they can occur in the context of cardiovascular, pulmonary, and gastrointestinal disorders (Hassan & Pollard, 1994) and may present as possible myocardial infarction, transient ischemic attack, pulmonary embolus, or other acute medical problem. The usual scenario can involve several panic attacks, with negative medical workups (physical exam, laboratory tests) before the psychiatric nature of the problem is established. Elderly patients and their families may be reluctant to accept the diagnosis of PD and thus may require careful counseling. Even with successful treatment of the panic attacks, significant anticipatory anxiety may persist and require considerable reassurance or psychotherapy.

Posttraumatic Stress Disorder

PTSD consists of a cluster of characteristic symptoms which emerge after an extreme, psychologically painful experience. Precipitating events may involve actual or threatened death, serious injury, or destruction of property, as in war, accidents, crimes, or disasters, which engender feelings of intense fear, horror, or helplessness. PTSD symptoms cluster into three categories: reexperiencing, avoidant, and hyperarousal.

Typical reexperiencing symptoms include persistent, intrusive thoughts, memories, dreams, or even flashbacks, through which the traumatic event is relived. These can occur spontaneously or be triggered by everyday events that constitute reminders, through association or similarity, of the initial trauma. When unusually intense, the reexperience of the traumatic event may involve dissociative states.

A consequence of such distressing, unwanted recollections is that individuals with PTSD avoid the thoughts or situations that evoke them and may thereby become withdrawn from significant activities. Other symptoms of avoidance include feelings of estrangement, constriction of affect, or undue pessimism. Characteristic signs of autonomic hyperarousal include insomnia, irritability, hypervigilance, exaggerated startling, and impaired concentration.

Though PTSD is considered to be delayed in onset when it develops more than 6 months after the initial traumatic event, delays may sometimes be measured in years or even decades. Delayed-onset PTSD can be triggered by a late-life stressor, such as retirement, widowhood, or a medical problem (Kaup et al., 1994). Nursing home placement, for example, can precipitate PTSD in a concentration camp survivor (Herrmann & Ergavec, 1994). PTSD in older adults has been associated with higher rates of disability, lower life satisfaction, greater use of medical services and increased rates of prescriptions for benzodiazepines (BZs), a medication class that may be counterproductive in PTSD (van Zelst et al., 2006).

ETIOLOGY AND PATHOPHYSIOLOGY

While traditional theories of the development of anxiety focused on unconscious process, a modern biopsychosocial view includes an understanding of the neural circuitry involved in the production of various symptoms of anxiety (Stahl, 2003). This is especially germane in older adults, who often have disruptions in the functional neuroanatomy of mood regulation because of neurodegenerative and/or cerebrovascular disease. The putative circuitry for anxiety disorders includes the amygdala, which is critical in the coordination of the response to fearful stimuli; the orbitofrontal cortex, which may be involved in the development of obsessive thoughts; and the hippocampus, where abnormalities have been found in those with PTSD. Neuronal pathways utilizing serotonin and GABA have been implicated in the pathophysiology and treatment of anxiety disorders (Stahl, 2003). Genetic factors and gene-environment interactions may also be important. For example, a twin study of GAD among older adults found the heritability of GAD to be 0.27; there was significant overlap between the genetic influences on GAD with those on the personality trait of neuroticism (Mackintosh et al., 2006). Using data from the Longitudinal Aging Study Amsterdam, the de Beurs group has elegantly validated a model whereby vulnerabilities (female gender, high neuroticism, poor physical health) combine with stresses (death of a family member, illness of partner or family member, or conflict with others) to increase the risk of developing an anxiety disorder (with adequacy of emotional supports as a somewhat mitigating factor; de Beurs et al., 2001).

ANXIETY DISORDERS, SUBSTANCES, AND MEDICAL ILLNESS

Medical illness and medications themselves can cause or exacerbate the psychological symptoms of anxiety. Formerly known as "organic anxiety disorders," these conditions are now referred to as anxiety disorders due to a general medical condition and substance-induced anxiety disorders (APA, 2000). Anxiety symptoms may represent a physiological consequence of a medical condition or a side effect of a treatment for a medical condition. Study of medical conditions causing anxiety may also lead to clues about the pathophysiology of anxiety disorders. Attention should be paid to the relationship between caffeine use and anxiety, especially given the availability of coffee and sodas in LTC settings and the role of imbibing these in socialization. The possibility that anxiety is due to alcohol withdrawal should also be considered, especially in new LTC residents who perhaps have been cut off their usual source of alcohol. Table 5.3 summarizes medical problems and substances that should be part of the differential diagnosis of anxiety disorders in LTC residents.

There is growing appreciation of the impact of anxiety (and treatment of anxiety) on medical outcomes. Patients with excessive anxiety are prone to developing a number of cardiovascular disorders, including hypertension, arrhythmias, and

TABLE 5.3. Medical Causes of Anxiety

1. **Cardiovascular disorders**
   Congestive heart failure
   Arrythmias
   Myocardial infarction
   Mitral valve prolapse
   Angina
   Cardiomyopathy
   Syncope
2. **Respiratory disorders**
   Chronic obstructive pulmonary disease
   Pneumonia
   Hypoxia
   Pulmonary embolus
   Sleep apnea
   Asthma
   Pneumothorax
   Pulmonary edema
3. **Endocrine disorders**
   Hyperthyroidism/hypothyroidism
   Cushing's disease
   Hypoglycemia
   Hypocalcemia/hypercalcemia
   Pheochromocytoma
   Carcinoid syndrome
   Hypokalemia
   Insulinoma
4. **Nutritional deficiency**
   Vitamin B_{12}
5. **Neurologic disorders**
   CNS infections
   CNS masses
   Parkinson's disease
   Movement disorders
   Focal seizures
   Postconcussion syndrome
   Toxins
   Multiple sclerosis
   Vertigo
6. **Drugs**
   Anticholinergic toxicity
   Digitalis toxicity
   Excessive thyroid supplementation
   Anithypertensive side effects
   Stimulants
      Amphetamines
      Methylphenidate

Continued

TABLE 5.3. Continued

    Cocaine
    Caffeine
    Steroids
   Sympathomimetics
    Decongestants
    Bronchodilators
   Antidepressants
    Selective serotonin reuptake inhibitors
    Tranylcypromine
    Tricyclics
7. **Other**
   Neuroleptic-induced akathisia
   Withdrawal
    Alcohol
    Sedative hypnotics
   Chronic pain syndromes

---

myocardial ischemia and are subsequently at higher risk of impaired recovery or death from these conditions (Bowen et al., 2000; Kawachi et al., 1994; Moser & Dracup, 1996; Sullivan et al., 1997; van Hout et al., 2004). Two longitudinal studies have independently demonstrated that anxiety is a risk factor for worsening disability (Brenes et al., 2005; de Beurs et al., 1999). Patients treated for anxiety with BZs are at higher risk for cognitive impairment, excess sedation, falls, and hip fractures.

ASSESSMENT AND TREATMENT

Accurate assessment of anxiety requires an understanding of how the patient experiences stressors in terms of her or his own values, perspectives, and history. In addition, because LTC residents can have multiple medical, psychiatric, and social problems contributing to anxiety, clinicians should appreciate anxiety disorders as multifactorial and should therefore be inclusive in their diagnostic approach. However well anxiety may be linkable to a new or recent stressor, one should also consider other factors, such as a concurrent medical problem or medication (Table 5.3) and psychiatric or personality disorders that may be associated with anxiety. Instruments such as the Geriatric Anxiety Inventory, a 20-item self-report or nurse-administered scale, may be useful for identifying LTC residents with possible anxiety disorders (Pachana et al., 2007).

    The Minimum Data Set (MDS) 2.0, completed for all new LTC residents, could serve as a screening tool for anxiety disorders, though no studies have tested this hypothesis. The MDS assesses the following symptoms that may be indicative of anxiety: expressions of what appear to be unrealistic fears, repetitive questions or verbalizations or recurrent statements that something terrible is about to happen, repetitive health complaints or other repetitive anxious concerns, repetitive physical movements and reduced social interaction, persistent anger with self or others, and insomnia (Center for Medicare and Medicaid Services, 2007).

The treatment of anxiety disorders in LTC settings begins with a careful assessment of the biopsychosocial factors that could be contributing to them. A high tolerance of ambiguity helps, given the likelihood with older patients for overlapping situations in which different concurrent problems cause similar symptoms. Initially it may not be clear, for example, how much of a patient's apprehensiveness, tachycardia, chest tightness, and tremulousness involves her angina, painful osteoarthritis, GAD, excessive caffeine use, dependent personality style, cultural heritage, or her brother's recent death. But by addressing each as a potential source of excess morbidity, the overall anxiety can be managed optimally, even though it may be difficult to ascertain how much of the overall anxiety is due to which factor. It is important to attend regularly to patients' cultural identity, their own explanations or models of their illness, and the culturally distinct aspects of their social milieu, as well as the nature of the relationships between individual patients and clinicians within that context (Kirmayer, 2001). Doing so will go a long way toward enhancing the therapeutic alliances that promote successful outcomes. The basic principles of such a biopsychosocial approach are outlined in Table 5.4.

In primary care settings, anxiety, not unlike depression, tends to be undertreated or untreated, especially in older adults. Data taken from a national sample of persons aged 19 to 97 years old, over a 1-year period, revealed that more than 80% of individuals with a probable anxiety disorder were seen by primary care providers. A total of 23% of those with probably anxiety disorders received treatment that was deemed appropriate: 18% received appropriate medications, and 11% received appropriate counseling. Subjects older than 59 were less likely

TABLE 5.4. Biopsychosocial Treatment of Anxiety

A. Eliminate/minimize use of anxiogenic substances
B. Modify medications that may be causative/exacerbating factors
C. Treat underlying acute/chronic medical problems
D. Treat concurrent psychiatric disorders
E. Nonpharmacological approaches:
    1. Psychosocial support—eliminate/modify stressors
    2. Psychotherapy
F. Pharmacological treatment with anxiolytic agents

to get appropriate treatment than those aged 30 to 59 (Young et al., 2001). In the assisted-living setting, inadequate treatment of anxiety disorders is also common (Rosenblatt et al., 2004).

Psychosocial Interventions

Psychological interventions for anxiety include both general support and psychotherapy. Supportive psychotherapy can help patients learn problem-solving techniques and enhance their coping styles. Through cognitive-behavioral therapy (CBT), individuals learn about the ways in which they frame situations and then make incorrect (e.g., overly generalized) assumptions, thus contributing to the generation of anxious feelings. Behavioral therapy includes such techniques as systematic desensitization and progressive relaxation. The latter may be especially helpful where muscular tension is a significant component of a patient's anxiety, whereas the former is effective for agoraphobia and specific phobias. Desensitization therapy consists of exposure to a series of stimuli, each of which more closely resembles the object of the phobia. Through increasing the duration and intensity of the exposure, the patient's anxieties, fears, or compulsions are gradually extinguished (Dar & Greist, 1992).

Wetherell et al. (2005) conducted an evidence-based review of both pharmacologic and nonpharmacologic treatment of geriatric anxiety. Their inclusion criteria required research subjects in published studies that were at least 55 years old, with a principal or coprincipal diagnosis of anxiety disorder according to DSM criteria (III-R or IV), who participated either in a randomized controlled trial (RCT) or in an open trial or case series involving more than five subjects. They also required that data be reported on at least one outcome measure (either self-report or interviewer-rated).

The authors located 13 studies of psychotherapy for late-life anxiety, of which 8 were RCTs, with the number of subjects in each ranging from 8 to 85. All studies involved some form of CBT. The RCTs also utilized supportive counseling, discussion groups, wait lists, medication management, and usual care for the control groups. The number of psychotherapy sessions ranged from 3 to 15 (most 8 to 12) and were either individual ($N = 9$) or group ($N = 4$) in format. Most of the studies focused on GAD or mixed populations that also included PD, social phobia, agoraphobia, or anxiety disorder not otherwise specified. One study was devoted to OCD, but none included PTSD. The authors concluded on the basis of published outcome data that CBT is of potential value, particularly for GAD. They noted, however, the lack of consistent evidence for the superiority of CBT over other psychosocial treatment options, such as supportive therapy, as well as a higher dropout rate in many trials (21%–39%) in contrast to younger adults (about 10%). There was some evidence for better outcomes with individual psychotherapy over group psychotherapy, perhaps due to the former being able to be more specifically tailored to the needs of a heterogeneous population. Two further limitations of the CBT studies were their outcome data being based upon completers, as opposed to an intent-to-treat basis, and the lack of a psychotherapeutic equivalent to a pill placebo for purposes of comparison.

Older adults are high utilizers of BZs, and discontinuing such medications can be particularly challenging because of rebound anxiety. CBT has been found to assist the discontinuation of BZ medications by reducing associated psychological symptoms of dementia, with some treatment benefits maintained at 6-month follow-up (Gorenstein et al., 2005).

Pharmacological Interventions

The use of anxiolytic medication is best reserved for when nonpharmacologic measures fail to adequately treat the symptoms interfering with patients' ability to function, causing them significant subjective distress, or exacerbating their other illnesses. Although BZs continue to be the most common medication class prescribed for anxiety in older adults—ranging from 10% to 12% in those with persistent anxiety (Gleason et al., 1998; Gray et al., 2003; Holmquist et al., 2005)—there are good reasons for them to be used with caution, if not avoided. Good data on their use in elderly patients are limited. In their evidence-based review of pharmacologic treatments for geriatric anxiety, Wetherell et al. (2005) found just three RCTs for the use of BZs in late life. Two focused on GAD, and only one utilized a BZ available in the United States (oxazepam). Although the treatment was generally effective (response rates 57%–83%) in these trials, and attrition rates low (<18%), all the trials were of quite brief duration (3–6 weeks). The use of BZs for long-term treatment of anxiety in late life is best avoided if possible, given the age-related increases of risk for adverse side effects, including cognitive impairment, gait instability (with falls), and increased reaction times (especially when driving or using machinery). Hence, BZs are generally best reserved for brief use in acute clinical situations. When employed, those with short half-lives (e.g., lorazepam, oxazepam) are usually the first choice. Those with long half-lives (e.g., diazepam, clonazepam) are best reserved for use with adherent, stable patients, where cumulative toxicity is less likely and once daily dosing preferable. Alprazolam should be avoided because its short half-life may lead to repeated withdrawal symptoms over the course of each day and because tapering it can be very difficult.

The number of studies on the use of antidepressants for anxiety in late life is starting to grow. Katz et al. (2002) pooled data on the older (60+) participants in five RCTs of venlafaxine for GAD and found significant improvement in those taking the active medication. An 8-week RCT of citalopram 20–30 mg/day for late-life GAD demonstrated a 65% response rate versus 27% for placebo (Lenze et al., 2005). An RCT of CBT versus sertraline versus wait-list control found effect sizes of 0.42 for CBT and 0.94 for sertraline (Schuurmans et al., 2006). Open label trials of imipramine for PD (Sheikh and Swales, 1999), sertraline for PD (Sheikh, Lauderdale, & Cassidy, 2004), fluvoxamine for GAD (Wylie et al., 2000), and buspirone for anxiety (Bohm et al., 1990) yielded favorable response rates; all four studies, however, were quite small in numbers of subjects enrolled. The literature is lacking, however, in medication trials for late-life PTSD or OCD.

In summary, although both CBT and pharmacotherapy appear to be useful in geriatric anxiety, the comparative efficacy of CBT versus other forms of psychotherapy, and of pharmacotherapy versus psychotherapy, and differences in treatment response among various medication classes remain unknown. Given what is known of the side effect profiles of the respective classes of medications, however, selective serotonin reuptake inhibitors and serotonin-norepinephrine reuptake inhibitors are generally considered preferable for longer term use than BZs for anxiety in late life. Medications should of course be started at low doses and titrated slowly, with careful attention paid to the emergence of side effects. (See Chapter 13).

REFERENCES

American Psychiatric Association. (2000). *Diagnostic and statistical manual of mental disorders* (4th ed., text revision). Washington, DC: Author.

Beekman, A. T., de Beurs, E., van Balkam, A. J., et al. (2000). Anxiety and depression in later life: Co-occurrence and communality of risk factors. *American Journal of Psychiatry, 157,* 89–95.

Bohm, C., Robinson, D. S., Gammons, R. E., et al. (1990). Buspirone therapy in anxious elderly patients: A controlled clinical trial. *Journal of Clinical Psychopharmacology, 10*(3 Suppl), 7S–51S.

Bowen, R. C., Senthilselvan, A., & Barale, A. (2000). Physical illness as an outcome of chronic anxiety disorders. *Canadian Journal of Psychiatry, 45,* 459–464.

Brenes, G. A., Guralnik, J. M., Williamson, J. D., et al. (2005). The influence of anxiety on the progression of disability. *Journal of the American Geriatrics Society, 53,* 34–39.

Burvill, P. W., Johnson, G. A., Jamrozik, K. D., et al. (1995). Anxiety disorders after stroke: Results from the Perth Community Stroke Study. *British Journal of Psychiatry, 166,* 328–332.

Center for Medicare and Medicaid Services. (2007). *MDS 2.0 for nursing homes* [Web site]. Retrieved May 8, 2007, from http://www.cms.hhs.gov/NursingHomeQualityInits/20_NHQIMDS20.asp

Cohen, C. I., Magai, C., Yaffee, R., et al. (2006). The prevalence of phobia and its associated factors in a multiracial aging urban population. *American Journal of Geriatric Psychiatry, 14*(6), 507–514.

Cook, J. M., Elhai, J. D., Cassidy, E. L., et al. (2005). Assessment of exposure and post-traumatic stress in long-term care veterans: Preliminary data on psychometrics and posttraumatic stress disorder prevalence. *Military Medicine, 170,* 862–866.

Dar, R., & Greist, J. H. (1992). Behavior therapy for obsessive-compulsive disorder. *Psychiatric Clinics of North America, 15,* 885–894.

de Beurs, E., Beekman, A., Deeg, D. J., et al. (2000). Predictors of change in anxiety symptoms of older persons: Results from the Longitudinal Aging Study, Amsterdam. *Psychological Medicine, 30,* 515–527.

de Beurs, E., Beekman, A., Geerling, S., et al. (2001). On becoming depressed or anxious in late life: Similar vulnerability factors but different effects of stressful life events. *British Journal of Psychiatry, 179,* 426–431.

de Beurs, E., Beekman, A., van Balkom, A. J., et al. (1999). Consequences of anxiety in older persons: Its effect on disability, well-being and use of health services. *Psychological Medicine, 29,* 583–593.

Flint, A. J. (1994). Epidemiology and comorbidity of anxiety disorders in the elderly. *American Journal of Psychiatry, 151,* 640–649.

Flint, A. J., & Rifat, S. L. (1997). Anxious depression in elderly patients: Response to antidepressant treatment. *American Journal of Geriatric Psychiatry, 5,* 107–115.

German, P. S., Shapiro, S., & Kramer, M. (1986). Nursing home study of the eastern Baltimore epidemiological catchment area study. In M. S. Harper & B. D. Lebowitz (Eds), *Mental illness in nursing homes: Agenda for research.* Rockville, MD: National Institute of Mental Health (or DHHS).

Gleason, P. P., Schulz, R., Smith, N. L., et al. (1998) Correlates and prevalence of benzo-diazepine use in community dwelling elderly. *Journal of General Internal Medicine, 13,* 243–250.

Gorenstein, E. E., Kleber, M. S., Mohlman, J., et al. (2005). Cognitive-behavioral therapy for management of anxiety and medication taper in older adults. *American Journal of Geriatric Psychiatry, 13,* 901–909.

Gray, S. L., Eggen, A. E., Blough, D., et al. (2003). Benzodiazepine use in older adults enrolled in a health maintenance organization. *American Journal of Geriatric Psychiatry, 11,* 568–576.

Hassan, R., & Pollard, C. A. (1994). Late-life-onset panic disorder: Clinical and demo-graphic characteristics of a patient's sample. *Journal of Geriatric Psychiatry and Neurology, 7,* 86–90.

Herrmann, N., & Ergavec, G. (1994). Posttraumatic stress disorder in institutionalized World War II veterans. *American Journal of Geriatric Psychiatry, 2,* 324–331.

Holmquist, I. B., Svensson, B., & Hoglund, P. (2005). Perceived anxiety, depression, and sleeping problems in relation to psychotropic drug use among elderly in assisted-living facilities. *European Journal of Clinical Pharmacology, 61,* 215–224.

Jorstad, E. C., Hauer, K., Becker, C., et al. (2005). Measuring the psychological out-comes of falling: A systematic review. *Journal of the American Geriatrics Society, 53,* 501–510.

Junginger, J., Phelan, E., Cherr, K., et al. (1993). Prevalence of psychopathology in elderly persons in nursing homes and the community. *Hospital and Community Psychiatry, 44,* 381–383.

Katz, I. R., Reynolds, C. F., Alexopoulos, G. S., et al. (2002). Venlafaxine ER as a treatment for generalized anxiety disorder in older adults: Pooled analysis of five randomized placebo-controlled clinical trials. *Journal of the American Geriatrics Society, 50,* 18–25.

Kaup, B. A., Ruskin, P. E., & Nymen, G. (1994). Significant life events and PTSD in elderly World War II veterans. *American Journal of Geriatric Psychiatry, 2,* 239–243.

Kawachi, I., Sparrow, D., Vokonas, P. S., et al. (1994). Symptoms of anxiety and risk of Corneille heart disease: The Normative Aging Study. *Circulation, 90,* 2225–2229.

Kirmayer, L. J. (2001). Cultural variations in the clinical presentation of depression and anxiety: Implications for diagnosis and treatment. *Journal of Clinical Psychiatry, 62*(Suppl 13), 22–28.

Kohn, R., Westlake, R. J., Rasmussen, S. A., et al. (1997). Clinical features of obsessive-compulsive disorder in elderly patients. *American Journal of Geriatric Psychiatry, 5,* 211–215.

Lenze, E. J., Mulsant, B. H., Shear, M. K., et al. (2005). Efficacy and tolerability of citalopram in the treatment of late-life anxiety disorders: Results from an 8-week randomized, placebo-controlled trial. *American Journal of Psychiatry, 162,* 146–150.

Lindesay, J. (1991). Phobic disorders in the elderly. *British Journal of Psychiatry, 159,* 531–541.

Lysketsos, C. G., Lopez, O., Jones, B., et al. (2002). Prevalence of neuropsychiatric symptoms in dementia and mild cognitive impairment: Results from the cardiovascular health study. *JAMA, 288,* 1475–1483.

Mackintosh, M. A., Gatz, M., Wetherell, J. L., & Pedrsen, N. L. (2006). A twin study of lifetime GAD in older adults: Genetic and environmental influences shared by neuroticism and GAD. *Twin Research: Human Genetics, 9*(1), 30–37.

Mehta, K. M., Simonsick, E. M., Pennix, B. W., et al. (2003). Prevalence and correlates of anxiety symptoms in well-functioning older adults: Findings from the health aging and body composition study. *Journal of the American Geriatrics Society, 51,* 499–504.

Morgan, L. A., Gruber-Baldini, A. L., & Magaziner, J. (2001). Resident characteristics. In S. Zimmerman, P. D. Sloane & J. K. Eckert (Eds.), *Assisted living* (pp. 144–172). Baltimore: Johns Hopkins University Press.

Moser, D. K., & Dracup, K. (1996). Is anxiety early after myocardial infarction associated with subsequent ischemic and a rhythmic events? *Psychosomatic Medicine, 58,* 395–401.

Pachana, N. A., Byrne, G. J., Siddle, H., et al. (2007). Development and validation of the Geriatric Anxiety Inventory. *International Psychogeriatrics, 19,* 103–114.

Parmelee, P. A., Katz, I. R., & Lawton, M. P. (1993). Anxiety and its association with depression among institutionalized elderly. *American Journal of Geriatric Psychiatry, 1,* 46–58.

Rasmussen, S. A., & Eisen, J. L. (1992). The epidemiology and clinical features of obsessive-compulsive disorder. *Psychiatric Clinics of North America, 15,* 743–758.

Regier, D. A., Boyd, J. H., Burke, J. D., et al. (1998). One-month prevalence of mental disorders in the United States. *Archives of General Psychiatry, 45,* 977–986.

Rosenblatt, A., Samus, Q. M., Steele, C. D., et al. (2004). The Maryland Assisted-Living Study: Prevalence, recognition, and treatment of dementia and other psychiatric disorders in the assisted-living population of central Maryland. *Journal of the American Geriatric Society, 52,* 1618–1625.

Schoevers, R. A., Deeg, D. J., van Tilburg, W., et al. (2005). Depression and generalized anxiety disorder: Co-occurrence and longitudinal patterns in elderly patients. *American Journal of Geriatric Psychiatry, 13*, 31–39.

Schuurmans, J., Comijs, H., Emmelkamp, P. M. G., et al. (2006). A randomized, controlled trial of the effectiveness of cognitive-behavioral therapy and sertraline versus a wait-list control group for anxiety disorders in older adults. *American Journal of Geriatric Psychiatry, 14*, 255–263.

Sheikh, J. I., & Swales, P. J. (1999). Treatment of panic disorder in older adults: A pilot study comparison of imipramine, and placebo. *International Journal of Psychiatry in Medicine, 29*, 107–117.

Sheikh, J. I., Lauderdale, S. A., & Cassidy, E. L. (2004). Efficacy of sertraline for panic disorder in older adults: A preliminary open-label trial. *American Journal of Geriatric Psychiatry, 12*, 230.

Sheikh, J. I., Swales, P. J., Carlson, E. B., et al. (2004). Aging and panic disorder: Phenomenology, comorbidity, and risk factors. *American Journal of Geriatric Psychiatry, 12*, 102–119.

Smalbrugge, M., Pot, A. M., Jongenelis, K., et al. (2003). Anxiety disorders in nursing homes: A literature review of prevalence, course and risk indicators [article in Dutch]. *Tijdschrift voor gerontologie en geriatrie, 34*, 215–221.

Smalbrugge, M., Pot, A. M., Jongenelis, K., et al. (2005a). Prevalence and correlates of anxiety among nursing home patients. *Journal of Affective Disorders, 88*, 145–153.

Smalbrugge, M., Pot, A. M., Jongenelis, K., et al. (2005b). The effect of somatic symptom attribution on the prevalence rate of depression and anxiety among nursing home patients. *International Journal of Methods in Psychiatric Research, 14*, 146–150.

Smalbrugge, M., Pot, A. M., Jongenelis, K., et al. (2005c). Comorbidity of depression and anxiety in nursing home patients. *International Journal of Geriatric Psychiatry, 20*, 218–226.

Stahl, S. M. (2003). Symptoms and circuits, part 2: Anxiety disorders. *Journal of Clinical Psychiatry, 64*(12), 1408–1409.

Sullivan, M. D., La Croix, A. Z., Baum, C., et al. (1997). Functional status in coronary artery disease: A one-year prospective study of the role of anxiety and depression. *American Journal of Medicine, 103*, 348–356.

Van Hout, H. P., Beekman, A. T., de Beurs, E., et al. (2004). Anxiety and the risk of death in older men and women. *British Journal of Psychiatry, 185*, 399–404.

Van Zelst, W. H., de Beurs, E., Beekman, A. T., et al. (2003). Prevalence and risk factors of posttraumatic stress disorder in older adults. *Psychotherapy and Psychosomatics, 72*, 333–342.

Van Zelst, W. H., de Beurs, E., Beekman, A. T., et al. (2006). Well-being, physical functioning, and use of health services in the elderly with PTSD and subthreshold PTSD. *International Journal of Geriatric Psychiatry, 11*, 180–188.

Velayudhan, L., & Katz, A. W. (2006). Late-onset obsessive-compulsive disorder: The role of stressful life events. *International Psychogeriatrics, 18*, 341–344.

Weiss, A. P., & Jenike, M. A. (2000). Late-onset obsessive-compulsive disorder: A case series. *Journal of Neuropsychiatry and Clinical Neurosciences, 12*, 116–118.

Wetherell, J. L., Lenze, E. J., & Stanley, M. A. (2005). Evidence-based treatment of geriatric anxiety disorders. *Psychiatric Clinics of North America, 28*, 871–896.

Wylie, M. E., Miller, M. D., Shear, M. K., et al. (2000). Fluvoxamine pharmacotherapy of anxiety disorders in later life: preliminary open-trial data. *Journal of Geriatric Psychiatry and Neurology, 13,* 43–48.

Young, A., Klap, R., Sherbourne, C. D., et al. (2001). The quality of care for depressive and anxiety disorders in the United States. *Archives of General Psychiatry, 58,* 55–61.

6

Schizophrenia and Other Psychotic Disorders

Gauri N. Savla, Jody DelaPena-Murphy, Daniel D. Sewell,
Daniel S. Kim, and *Dilip V. Jeste*

Long-term care facilities for patients with severe mental illness are an integral part of mental health care. Schizophrenia is a severely disabling mental illness that affects 3 million people aged 18 or older in the United States and contributes to an enormous economic burden in terms of mental health-care costs and loss of productivity (U.S. Census Bureau, 2006). Persons with schizophrenia not only suffer from clinical symptoms such as hallucinations and delusions but also have generalized mild-to-moderate cognitive deficits, which directly impact their quality of life and everyday functioning (Green, 1996). Historically, a diagnosis of schizophrenia was associated with a dire prognosis, with little hope of long-term symptom relief, let alone the possibility that patients may some day be reintegrated into mainstream society. With the conceptualization of schizophrenia as a "dementia praecox" (Kraepelin, 1919) or "precocious dementia" that had its onset in young adulthood (as opposed to "senile dementia," that had its onset at an older age, e.g., Alzheimer's disease [AD]), relegating these patients to state psychiatric facilities for close supervision appeared to be a reasonable option at the time. Research in schizophrenia has come a long way since those early observations, and the more accurate general characterization of the illness has dispelled the notion that schizophrenia is a form of dementia. Furthermore, the introduction of antipsychotic medications and their efficacy on schizophrenic psychopathology heralded the hope that persons with schizophrenia have the potential to benefit from rehabilitation programs in order to live independently, or at least, with minimal supervision. Nonetheless, when the treatment model of long-term inpatient care for schizophrenia was reformed by the Community Mental Health Centers Act in 1963, there were no rehabilitation programs that could help persons with schizophrenia transition into mainstream society. Younger patients needed to be accommodated in "halfway-homes," and older patients were "transinstitutionalized" to nursing homes (Bartels & Dums, 2004). It is estimated that as many as 93% of younger patients with severe mental illness live in community-based residential facilities today (Talbot, 1995), whereas 89% of elderly patients (>65 years of age) with severe mental illness live in nursing homes (Burns, 1991). Recent research efforts are focused on interventions for improving cognition and everyday functioning in patients with schizophrenia (e.g., Green et al., 2004), but in the meanwhile, community-based long-term care facilities continue to remain the mainstay of patients with schizophrenia, where they obtain various levels of supervised care, treatment, and a secure environment.

This chapter aims at characterizing long-term care for schizophrenia and other psychotic disorders, the nature of the patients who use these facilities, and treatment targets and considerations. In the first section, we describe the main types of long-term facilities used by patients with psychotic disorders, i.e., adult residential facilities (ARFs), skilled nursing facilities (SNFs), and state psychiatric hospitals. The next section describes the categories of patients who reside in assisted living facilities and medical comorbidity in patients with psychosis, which may complicate course of illness, treatment, and care. We also discuss available pharmacological and psychosocial treatments and treatment considerations for patients. We conclude with recommendations for better assessment of patients and their symptoms, and potential for rehabilitation, experience with medication including side effects, and suitability for psychosocial/ cognitive intervention programs.

CHARACTERIZATION OF CURRENT LONG-TERM CARE FACILITIES

There are several different types of residential facilities that provide care for individuals with severe mental illness. As mentioned earlier, most patients with schizophrenia live in ARFs, whereas a small minority, typically older and/or more acutely ill, lower functioning patients, live in SNFs or long-stay psychiatric hospitals.

Adult Residential Facilities

ARFs provide 24-h nonmedical care for adults who are unable to provide for their own daily needs. They include group homes, intermediate facilities, wards in the community, board-and-care (B&C) homes, supervised hostels, and sheltered apartments. ARF residents may have physical or mental challenges due to developmental and/or mental disorders. Typically, each ARF is devoted to caring for a specific clinical population, for example, there are facilities designated only for people with developmental disabilities, whereas others may only accommodate persons with severe mental illness. B&Cs, the most common type of ARF, do not require completely independent living but are not as regimented as nursing homes. They are typically privately run, semistructured, secure residences of varying sizes for patients with limited cognitive and functional abilities. They provide lodging, prepared meals, supervision of residents' activities, and management of medications. ARF residents with schizophrenia typically are able to adequately perform activities of daily living (ADLs), such as self-care, but are generally impaired on instrumental activities of daily living (IADLs), such as driving, cooking, financial management, etc. They may also have a more chronic form of the illness, usually characterized by few severe psychotic symptoms, but substantial residual symptoms, and mild-to-moderate generalized cognitive deficits. They may also be relatively more stable on their medications than residents of SNFs or psychiatric hospitals and are also more likely to be ambulatory.

As an illustration of the ARF network, we present data from San Diego County, the 6th largest county in the United States, with a population of 2.9 million (U.S. Census Bureau, 2006). There are approximately 150 B&Cs in San Diego County that accommodate persons with severe mental illness (California Department of Social Services, 2006). The number of residents may range from 6 to10, but some facilities may accommodate as many as 150 residents. In the state of California, licensed B&Cs are required to provide a basic set of services (e.g., boarding and lodging, medication management) at a standard rate, typically afforded by patients whose only source of income is Supplemental Security Income. B&Cs must comply with administrator and personnel requirements and staffing ratios and provide night supervision and transportation to attend community programs. A "needs and services plan" is developed for each resident, which provides an evaluation of his/her physical, mental, and social functioning, and specific objectives and plans for maintenance or improvement of functioning. Each facility must either provide services to meet residents' needs as described in the plan or involve certified consultants. Typically, these outside consultations include routine medication consultations by a psychiatrist (Fleishman, 1989). Primary medical care is usually provided by a team of mobile physicians, whose services include everything that may be expected at a visit to a physician's office, i.e., there are provisions for phlebotomy, X-ray, electrocardiograms, and the like.

Previous research has shown that compared with persons with schizophrenia living independently, residents of B&Cs have an earlier age of onset of illness, more severe negative symptoms, worse cognitive impairment, and poorer health-related quality of well-being but have similar levels of positive and depressive symptoms and take similar doses of antipsychotic medication (Auslander et al., 2001). However, there is also evidence that schizophrenia patients who live in ARFs are likely to more effectively utilize outpatient mental health services than those who live independently, or those who are homeless. Consequently, they received more optimal treatment, have fewer exacerbations of psychoses, and required fewer hospitalizations (Gilmer et al., 2003).

Skilled Nursing Facilities

An SNF is a place of temporary residence for people with at least one skilled nursing need defined by Medicare guidelines (e.g., care of a stage two or greater decubitus ulcer), or who meet Medicare criteria for a specific type of therapy (e.g., physical therapy), which may be provided in an SNF (U.S. Department of Health and Human Services, 2006). Some SNFs have wards or units that provide custodial care for patients. If a facility provides exclusively custodial care, it may be referred to as a nursing facility, which is less expensive to operate for a variety of reasons, including different staffing requirements. In the United States, SNFs are required to have a licensed nurse on duty 24 h a day and a registered nurse at least one shift per day. Medicare does not cover custodial care. Custodial care is covered by Medicaid (called Medi-Cal in California), some long-term insurance plans, or private funding sources. Residents in custodial care typically are low functioning, to the extent that they may have substantial difficulties with ADLs, including self-care skills as basic as eating, showering, and using the toilet independently. Although schizophrenia, per se, is not associated with such kind of impairment (but rather, difficulty with the more cognitively demanding IADLs, such as cooking, driving, etc.; Klapow et al., 1997), there is a small proportion of patients who have more severe overall functional impairment. These patients tend to have psychotic symptoms that may be secondary to a neurologic or systemic medical condition, sensory impairment, cardiovascular event, or even medication side effects (Reichman & Rabins, 1996), and they are more likely to have comorbid medical illnesses. Nearly 20% of newly admitted residents with cognitive impairment have psychotic symptoms, specifically, delusions, which may or may not be attributable to schizophrenia (Chandler & Chandler, 1988).

Psychiatric Hospitals

The first psychiatric hospitals were built on the premise that the most effective treatment for persons with mental illness was isolation from mainstream society and its demands and stresses. Reports estimate that by the year 1950, state psychiatric facilities accommodated over a half million patients with severe mental illness (Fisher et al., 2001). The role of psychiatric hospitalization has greatly changed in keeping with the more accurate characterization of schizophrenia, advancements in treatment, and reforms in managed care so that today only a small minority of the sickest patients requires long-stay institutionalization. Also, many U.S. states today have designated most of their long-stay hospital beds for forensic psychiatry settings, that is, for severely mentally ill persons convicted of a felony. In California, for example, fewer than three hospital beds for every 100,000 of the total population are reserved for nonforensic patients (Lamb & Bachrach, 2001). A recent study of state psychiatric hospitals demonstrated that while patients who require hospitalization are very similar to patients in SNFs, they may, in addition, have substantial behavioral disturbances, including impulsive, self-destructive behaviors that mandate closer supervision, in a more restricted treatment setting (Fisher et al., 2001). A consequence of the reduced number of hospital beds has been that patients who need intensive, supervised treatment, and do not have the resources for nursing home care, are likely to be homeless and destitute, or incarcerated (Lamb & Shander, 1993). For the most part, however, most patients with severe mental illness live in ARFs or SNFs and are likely to be hospitalized only briefly, mostly during the first episode of psychosis or later acute exacerbations of symptoms.

CHARACTERISTICS OF RESIDENTS WITH SCHIZOPHRENIA AND OTHER PSYCHOTIC DISORDERS

Both younger and older patients with schizophrenia reside in long-term care facilities. However, as mentioned earlier, residents tend to be patients with onset of symptoms of schizophrenia at a relatively younger age. Consequently, older residents tend to be those who have suffered from the illness for most of their life, rather than those who had their first episode in later life, i.e., after the age of 60. Only a small proportion of patients in the latter category reside in long-term care facilities; most continue to reside in their own homes and are cared for by their own families. Although late- and early-onset schizophrenia are not distinct psychiatric conditions, and have many similarities, they do have differences in clinical manifestations of illness, nature of cognitive deficits, treatment considerations, and importantly, prognosis. The two categories of patients are described below, followed by a description of patients with other, miscellaneous types of psychoses, who also utilize long-term care facilities.

Early-Onset Schizophrenia

Schizophrenia is a neurodevelopmental, neurocognitive disorder, which can manifest as one of several subsyndromes that may constitute paranoid, disorganized, or catatonic subtypes of the illness. For many years, it was considered a disease that affected mainly the young, and indeed, even today, although onset of illness in later life is acknowledged, the most typical onset of illness is between late adolescence and the mid-thirties (*Diagnostic and Statistical Manual of Mental Disorders*, 4th ed., text revision, *DSM-IV-TR*). The term, "early-onset schizophrenia" is used differently in various contexts: some researchers use it to describe the minority (approximately 4%) of people who develop the illness before the age of 18, or even 12 (e.g., Frangou, 2006); others use it to describe the more typical schizophrenia, i.e., with onset in young adulthood (e.g., Jeste et al., 1995). In this chapter, we will use the term, "early-onset schizophrenia" or EOS to denote the latter population.

Retrospective studies of schizophrenia patients have reported that they may have had subtle cognitive weaknesses, reflected in lower school grades, lower IQ, and learning and attentional difficulties *prior* to the onset of illness (Bilder et al., 2006; Kremen et al., 1998) There is also evidence that preschizophrenic children sometimes show subtle motor difficulties, presumably reflecting early dysregulation of dopamine receptors (Walker, 1994). Most patients may also have a distinct prodrome, characterized by social withdrawal, apathy, and eccentric/odd thinking. The full onset of symptoms includes hallucinations, bizarre delusions, or disorganized thinking and behavior, catatonia, and negative symptoms such as alogia, apathy, or avolition. The clinical presentation of the illness varies widely among patients, and negative symptoms and/ or thought disorder are associated with lower functioning. Although many patients have subtle premorbid cognitive deficits, there is a distinct, substantial drop in overall cognitive function associated with the first episode of illness (Hoff et al., 2005). These mild-to-moderate generalized cognitive deficits can affect multiple cognitive domains, such as attention and working memory, executive function, and verbal and visual anterograde learning (Heinrichs & Zakzanis, 1998). For most patients, these deficits remain stable over time (Heaton et al., 2001), and only a minority of lower functioning, institutionalized patients experience decline in cognition over time (Harvey et al., 1999).

Owing to the early onset of the symptoms, and cognitive and emotional difficulties that precede actual onset, persons with EOS are less likely to have had "normal" periods of psychosocial functioning in their lifetime. Few patients are likely to have held a paying job, and a substantial proportion live in poverty all their life. Patients are also likely to have iatrogenic medical illnesses and/ or comorbid systemic medical conditions, and many have comorbid substance use disorders, with related additional cognitive impairment, and/or infections (e.g., HIV, hepatitis C) caused by intravenous drug use or risky sexual behavior. Furthermore, schizophrenia patients comprise as much as 10% of the total homeless population (Folsom et al., 2005). Given their lifelong lower levels of everyday functioning, it might be expected that such patients have a poor prognosis, with little hope of gaining and maintaining a normal livelihood. That outlook

is now changing with advancements in both pharmacological and psychosocial/
cognitive interventions.

Late-Onset Schizophrenia

Early editions of the most widely used diagnostic classification systems, such as
the *DSM-III* (APA, 1980) specifically mandated onset of symptoms *before age
45 years* for a diagnosis of schizophrenia to be made. Late-onset schizophrenia
(LOS) has only been recognized as "true" schizophrenia in the past 2 decades;
DSM-III-R (APA, 1987) specifically acknowledged LOS, whereas *DSM-IV* (APA,
1994) and its text revision (*DSM-IV-TR*; APA, 2000) do not impose restrictions
on age of onset of illness. It is currently estimated that about 24% of patients
have onset of schizophrenia after age 40 (Jeste, 1988; Jeste et al., 1995). Of note,
observations of schizophrenia onset in older persons were made by Manfred
Bleuler in the 1940s, who also first used the term "late-onset schizophrenia"
(Howard et al., 2000). Kraepelin, too, wrote of "late-paraphrenia," characterized
mainly by hallucinations and delusions (Kraepelin, 1919).

Early arguments against classifying LOS as true schizophrenia arose from
the contention that schizophrenia being a neurodevelopmental condition offered
no explanation as to why LOS patients functioned "schizophrenia-free" for most
of their life (Andreasen, 1999; Green, 1998). LOS is more prevalent in women,
with the paranoid subtype being the most common (Castle & Murray, 1993) and
the symptom picture consisting of hallucinations and delusions, in the absence
of blunted affect, severe thought disorder, and disorganized behavior (Harris &
Jeste, 1988). A study directly comparing LOS with age-comparable EOS confirmed that patients with LOS were more likely to have paranoid schizophrenia
and were also more likely to be married and have better premorbid functioning,
including completion of education, and consistent work histories (Jeste et al.,
1995, 1997). The consistent finding that there is a greater proportion of women
with LOS (whereas, more men than women have EOS) has generated several
hypotheses that consider the role of estrogen depletion in the modulation of
the dopaminergic system implicated in schizophrenia (Seeman, 1996), none of
which have been supported by empirical data.

Schizoaffective Disorder

Schizoaffective disorder is generally conceptualized as schizophrenia with an
affective component. The *DSM-IV-TR* distinguishes between schizoaffective
disorder and mood disorder with psychosis by requiring that for the former
diagnosis there be at least a 2-week period of psychotic symptoms without the
presence of mood symptoms, whereas in the latter, psychotic symptoms occur
exclusively during a mood episode (APA, 2000). Studies have demonstrated

that clinical and cognitive symptoms of schizoaffective disorder substantially overlap with those of schizophrenia (Evans et al., 1999). Patients with schizoaffective disorder also have significant functional deficits and are more likely (than patients with mood disorders without psychosis) to live in long-term care facilities. Some studies have reported that patients with schizoaffective disorder may have a somewhat better prognosis than those with schizophrenia. For all practical purposes, treatment considerations for patients are equivalent to that of schizophrenia, depending upon age, onset of symptoms, severity of symptoms, and response to medication.

Delusional Disorder

The *DSM-IV-TR* characterizes delusional disorder as the presence of nonbizarre delusions, i.e., delusions involving situations that may occur in real life, in the absence of criteria ever having been met for a diagnosis of schizophrenia (APA, 2000). Delusions typically involve a monothematic belief, the most common being the belief that one is being persecuted. Other subtypes include jealous, erotomanic, grandiose, and somatic delusions, and mixed subtypes are also common, in which more than one delusional theme coexists. Apart from the specific focus of the delusion and its ramifications, there is little impact on everyday functioning, and therefore, patients with delusional disorder are rarely seen in clinical settings. Patients with delusional disorders may be rarely encountered in a long-term care facility, but those that do need such care often have comorbid depression and have a poorer prognosis (Fenning et al., 2005).

Psychotic Disorder Not Otherwise Specified

Clinical syndromes that include psychosis (e.g., hallucinations, disorganized speech, etc.) that do not fit any specific diagnostic category of the *DSM-IV-TR* are labeled Psychotic Disorder Not Otherwise Specified (PDNOS). Some examples of *DSM-IV-TR* PDNOS are postpartum psychosis, persistent auditory hallucinations without any other symptoms of schizophrenia, and persistent nonbizarre delusions with overlapping periods of affective symptoms. A study of PDNOS in persons whose first onset of symptoms was after the age of 45 (Lesser et al., 1992) demonstrated that a majority of the study sample had nonspecific structural brain abnormalities, in the absence of dementia or focal neurological findings. Common psychotic symptoms associated with late-onset PDNOS were pure hallucinatory states without delusions; bizarre, elaborate delusions without hallucinations; or both hallucinations and delusions, without substantial impairment in everyday functioning.

Most first psychotic episodes are provisionally labeled PDNOS and subsequently changed to one of the specific diagnostic categories when new information about the illness and its course becomes available. Of note, patients with delusional disorder accompanied by substantial functional impairment are also diagnosed with PDNOS and often need more structured and supervised living conditions such as long-term care facilities.

RELEVANT DIAGNOSTIC CATEGORIES
NOT INCLUDED IN *DSM-IV-TR*

Other psychotic syndromes encountered in older residents of long-term care facilities are psychosis associated with AD and very-late-onset schizophrenia-like psychosis. Neither is a *DSM-IV-TR* category of mental disorder but may be prevalent in residents over the age of 60. It is estimated that 30% to 50% of persons with AD have hallucinations and/or delusions, which may be associated with aggression, agitation, and disruptive behavior (Jeste & Finkel, 2000). Such patients are especially likely to require long-term care in SNFs. There are some reports that persons with AD who have psychotic symptoms may experience more rapid decline (Ropacki & Jeste, 2005), but other reports have also reported that the psychosis may resolve in advanced stages of dementia.

Very-late-onset schizophrenia-like psychosis is only a recently acknowledged category of illness (Howard et al., 2000). Patients who have the first onset of psychotic symptoms after the age of 60 fall into this category; it has been noted that their symptoms are often accompanied by sensory impairment and social isolation. Like LOS, very-late-onset schizophrenia-like psychosis is more prevalent in women, and age of onset is inversely correlated with the level of severity of cognitive impairment, that is, later-onset is associated with milder impairment. Patients are also less likely to have genetic predisposition to schizophrenia or another psychotic disorder. As with patients with LOS, patients with very-late-onset schizophrenia-like psychosis may continue to live in their own homes, unless they have medical or other complications that mandate nursing home care. They are rarely encountered in ARFs.

Psychosis Secondary to Other Medical/Neurological/Psychiatric Conditions

The *DSM-IV-TR* estimates that 20% of persons with untreated endocrine disorders, 15% with systemic lupus erythematosus, and 40% with temporal lobe epilepsy may present with psychotic symptoms (APA, 2000). Whereas most psychoses remit with treatment of the underlying medical condition, some persist or recur with exacerbations of the condition. Patients with persisting psychotic disorder due to general medical condition tend to reside in long-term care facilities. A surprisingly large number of medical conditions must be ruled out as a possible etiology for psychotic symptoms. They include endocrine disorders (e.g., hypothyroidism), metabolic conditions (e.g., hypoxia), electrolyte imbalance, renal disease, autoimmune disorders, and the like. Psychotic symptoms may also be associated with neurologic conditions, such as Huntington's disease, and Lewy body spectrum disorders such as dementia due to Lewy bodies and Parkinson's disease. Psychotic symptoms, such as hallucinations, are also associated with medications used to treat Parkinson's disease, particularly, levadopa, which increases dopamine levels in the brain. Other neurological conditions such as epilepsy, cerebrovascular disease, and multiple sclerosis may also cause psychotic symptoms. Such patients, with psychosis secondary to a medical or neurologic condition, are more likely to be residents of SNFs because their illness may cause moderate-to-severe physical disability, resulting in impairments in ADLs.

MEDICAL COMORBIDITY IN PATIENTS WITH SCHIZOPHRENIA OR OTHER PSYCHOSIS

The NIMH-initiated Clinical Antipsychotic Trials of Intervention Effectiveness (CATIE), a recent nationwide study of antipsychotic medication, reported that nearly 60% of patients with schizophrenia had at least one comorbid medical condition, the most frequent being hypertension, followed by type II diabetes mellitus (Chwastiak et al., 2006). These conditions often have central nervous system effects, resulting in further exacerbations of already existing cognitive deficits in schizophrenia. Many persons with schizophrenia may not have insight into their physical illnesses and therefore may not seek treatment or report symptoms (Jeste et al., 1996). Some studies have reported that certain medical conditions have lower prevalence among older schizophrenia patients than in the general population, particularly, degenerative joint disease, hypertension, and congestive heart failure (Lacro & Jeste, 1994). Nonetheless, given the prevalence of iatrogenic medical conditions, such as neuroleptic-induced tardive dyskinesia (TD), cardiovascular disease, or type II diabetes mellitus (Jeste et al., 1996), patients must be routinely evaluated to screen for such conditions.

PHARMACOLOGICAL TREATMENT AND SIDE EFFECTS

The most commonly used medications for schizophrenia are conventional (typical) and novel (atypical) antipsychotics. The two classes of medications and their potential side effects are described below.

Conventional Antipsychotics

Conventional antipsychotics were introduced with chlorpromazine in the early 1950s. Subclassifications within this broader category of drugs include phenothiazines (e.g., thioridazine), thioxanthenes (e.g., thiothixene), butyrophenones (e.g., haloperidol), and dibenzoxazepines (e.g., loxapine). Although these drugs are highly effective in controlling mainly positive psychotic symptoms caused by any etiology, they have little or no effect on thought disorder or negative symptoms associated with schizophrenia. Furthermore, they have potential side effects, including anticholinergic effects, sedation, acute extrapyramidal symptoms (EPS; e.g., acute dystonia, akathisia, parkinsonism), and TD, which severely limit their utility as effective antipsychotic agents. A rare, but potentially fatal side effect of all antipsychotic medications, but especially of conventional antipsychotics, is neuroleptic malignant syndrome, which clinically presents as muscular rigidity, fever, autonomic instability, and altered mental status, and laboratory findings of elevated creatine kinase. Early detection and treatment can substantially reduce mortality. Though anticholinergic medications (e.g., benztropine) are frequently used to treat EPS, the first step in reducing side effects should be reduction of the antipsychotic dose, as anticholinergics are associated with hyperthermia, sustained tachycardia, constipation, memory impairment, and delirium.

Conventional antipsychotics are most indicated for the treatment of exacerbations of positive psychopathology (hallucinations and delusions), disorganized thoughts and behavior, and catatonic symptoms in patients who have a history of responding well to conventional antipsychotics, respond better to conventional rather than atypical antipsychotics, and have shown reasonable tolerance to side effects of the drugs. They may also be effectively used as maintenance therapy, although a recent meta-analysis showed that about 23% of patients relapse within a year even while they are on medication (Marder & van Kammen, 2005). That number doubles, however, when they are withdrawn from treatment, and it is therefore recommended that patients with chronic schizophrenia who have had multiple prior exacerbations of symptoms continue to be maintained on drug therapy, perhaps on long-acting or depot forms of the drug, for at least 2 to 5 years, but often indefinitely, in the absence of severe side effects. Extra caution must be exercised when prescribing both neuroleptics and anticholinergic medications to older patients, especially those with LOS because they are at greatest risk for neuroleptic-induced side effects, particularly EPS, as well as anticholinergic-related side effects (Sciolla & Jeste, 1998). TD is particularly challenging in older patients due to its notably higher incidence and refractory nature (Jeste et al., 1999). For these reasons, atypical antipsychotics are strongly recommended as the first-line treatment in this population.

Atypical Antipsychotics

Atypical antipsychotic medications available today are clozapine, risperidone, olanzapine, quetiapine, ziprasidone, and aripiprazole. The first atypical antipsychotic, clozapine, was introduced in 1988. Like conventional antipsychotics, the primary action of these medications is the blockade of the D_2 (dopamine) receptors, but in addition, they act at a variety of other sites, e.g., the $5\text{-}HT_{2A}$ (serotonin) receptors, with dramatic reduction in the risk of motor side effects such as EPS and TD and potential improvement in negative symptoms and cognitive deficits. However, side effects such as weight gain, hyperglycemia, diabetes, ketoacidosis, and lipid dysregulation—collectively known as metabolic syndrome—are associated to varying degrees with all of the atypical antipsychotics (most prominently with clozapine and olanzapine, to a lesser degree with risperidone, and least with quetiapine, aripiprazole, and ziprasidone). As a result, current expert consensus guidelines recommend screening patients at baseline for metabolic risk factors: body mass index, waist circumference, blood pressure, fasting blood glucose, and fasting lipids, and then regular monitoring afterward for any significant changes (see ADA, APA, AACE, NAASO Consensus Statement, 2004).

The FDA has also warned that the use of atypical antipsychotic medications in older patients with dementia is associated with a near doubling in the risk of mortality (http://www.fda.gov/cder/drug/advisory/antipsychotics.htm). This is on top of previous warnings by the FDA of the increased incidence of cerebrovascular adverse events such as stroke associated with the use of atypical antipsychotic medications in older patients with dementia. In addition, the results of the CATIE study suggest that although the atypical antipsychotic medications may reduce the behavioral problems of dementia, they are frequently poorly tolerated by patients. Nonetheless, due to the paucity of alternative treatments and the considerable risks associated with conventional antipsychotic medications, up to and including a similar risk of mortality, the atypical antipsychotics continue to be used frequently for the treatment of psychosis and accompanying behavioral disturbances in older patients with dementia. Clinicians must take steps to educate not only the patient but also family of these safety concerns in order to ensure adequate informed consent for treatment with atypical antipsychotic medications.

Due to the varying receptor-binding profiles of the different atypical antipsychotic medications, individual agents have uniquely identifiable clinical uses and concerns. Clozapine is especially effective at managing treatment-resistant schizophrenia and reducing severe EPS and TD (Sajatovic et al., 1998). Clozapine, however, can have some serious side effects, including potentially fatal agranulocytosis, reduced seizure threshold, marked weight gain, and notable anticholinergic side effects, which often limits its tolerability, particularly in older patients. The risk of agranulocytosis can be substantially minimized with routine monitoring of leukocyte counts. Olanzapine, like clozapine, is associated with weight gain and increased metabolic syndrome, though the CATIE study suggests that it may be more effective than most atypical antipsychotics, at least when it comes to rates of discontinuation (Lieberman et al., 2005). Risperidone, when used at the higher dosing range, is associated with increased incidence of EPS and TD, as well as increased prolactin levels, although its long-acting injectable formulation may enhance adherence to treatment. Quetiapine has minimal EPS side effects but is associated with increased sedation and orthostatic hypotension. Ziprasidone and aripiprazole are newer medications, and the only existing data come from clinical reports. Both medications are associated with reduction of psychotic symptoms and a relatively low incidence of EPS, weight gain, and anticholinergic effects (Sable & Jeste, 2002). Ziprasidone, however, is associated with a dose-related prolongation of the QT-interval and is therefore contraindicated in persons with a history of QT-interval prolongation or cardiac arrhythmia, recent myocardial infarction, or uncompensated heart failure.

A general recommendation is that prescription of any antipsychotic medication should begin with the lowest indicated dosage, followed by gradual titration and careful evaluation of dose–response and presence of side effects. This is particularly true for older patients, for whom starting and maximum doses should be lower, and titration increments smaller. Clozapine is typically initiated at 12.5 to 25 mg daily, and titrated by increments of 25 to 50 mg/day to up to a dose of 450 mg daily in divided doses, although increased efficaciousness has been demonstrated with doses up to 600 mg and even 900 mg daily (Davis & Chen, 2004). If clozapine is used with older patients, starting doses are generally cut in half to 6.25 to 12.5 mg daily, titrated no more than 6.25 to 12.5 mg once or twice weekly to 50 to 100 mg daily. Risperidone is usually started at 1 mg twice daily and titrated by 1 mg/day increments to 4 to 8 mg per day, with increased risk of EPS noted at higher doses without notable increase in efficaciousness. In older patients, risperidone should be started at a daily dose of 0.25 to 0.5 mg, titrated more slowly by 0.25 to 0.5 mg/week increments up to a maximum daily dose of 1 to 2.5 mg. Olanzapine is generally started at 5 to 10 mg daily, titrated by 5 mg/week to 20 mg daily; in older patients, it should be initiated at 1 to 5 mg daily, up to a maximum dose of 5 to 15 mg daily. Initial doses of quetiapine typically begin at 25 mg twice daily, with subsequent increases by 25 to 50 mg twice daily to a maximum of 800 mg daily, whereas older patients are typically started at 12.5 to 25 mg daily, with an optimal target of 75 to 125 mg/day in divided doses (Jeste et al., 1999). Ziprasidone should be started 20 mg twice daily, titrated every 2 days up to 80 mg twice daily; the starting dose of aripiprazole is 10 to 15 mg per day, up to a maximum of 30 mg per day. There are limited data on the use of ziprasidone and aripiprazole in older persons, but similar guidelines of reducing starting doses and slower titration schedules should apply. In patients with psychosis associated with dementia, at some point, an attempt should be made to reduce or discontinue antipsychotic medication because as the dementia progresses, the psychotic symptoms may improve substantially, or even resolve. This is particularly appropriate for residents of nursing homes, which are required by the Omnibus Budget Reconciliation Act of 1987 to routinely attempt dosage reductions to deter excessive use of psychotropic medications.

PSYCHOSOCIAL TREATMENTS/COGNITIVE REHABILITATION

Psychosocial interventions serve as an important adjunctive treatment for schizophrenia (Marder, 1996). Research on psychosocial treatments focusing on improving residual clinical and/or cognitive symptoms in schizophrenia, such as Cognitive Behavioral Social Skills Training (CBSST; Granholm et al., 2002; Granholm, McQuaid, et al., 2002), Functional Adaptation Skills Training (FAST), and Cognitive Training (Twamley et al., 2003), is currently underway. A description of these interventions and preliminary findings from the studies are discussed below.

CBSST for psychosis consists of teaching patients with psychosis to challenge false beliefs and to restructure maladaptive beliefs with interpersonal/social problem solving skills. Younger persons with schizophrenia have consistently benefited from similar interventions, and a recently published study in older patients demonstrated that CBSST significantly increased social activities that led to greater insight into maladaptive cognitive processes and improved everyday functioning (Granholm et al., 2005).

Recent studies have consistently demonstrated that cognitive deficits in schizophrenia are stronger predictors of everyday functioning deficits than clinical symptoms (Evans et al., 2003; Green, 1996). The FAST intervention targets everyday living skills that are frequently impaired in schizophrenia patients. Specific skills include medication management, social and communication skills, planning, use of public transportation, and financial management. The 24-week training involves psychoeducation about solutions to everyday functioning problems, practice (including behavioral modeling, role playing, and reinforcement), and homework to facilitate generalizing skills to a real-world setting. A recent study of effectiveness of FAST among older patients with psychotic disorders demonstrated that the intervention was associated with greatly improved financial management skills, ability to use public transportation, and grocery shopping skills, which have implications for improvements in "real-world" outcomes such as employment and independent living. FAST has been culturally adapted to develop the *Programa de Entrenamiento para el Desarrollo de Aptitudes para Latinos* (Program for Training and Development of Skills in Latinos) to meet the needs of Spanish-speaking Latino persons with chronic psychotic disorders in the United States (Patterson et al., 2005). A pilot study of this intervention in older Latino patients indicated that it had some potential to improve patients' independent everyday living skills.

Interventions for cognitive rehabilitation teach strategies to patients with schizophrenia to help them compensate for their cognitive deficits (reviewed by Twamley et al., 2003). Specific interventions such as Cognitive Training (developed by Twamley et al., 2003) include training on the use of mnemonic devices to compensate for learning (encoding) and planning difficulties and/or modification of patients' environment to help accommodate deficit areas.

These interventions can be easily adapted for use in long-term care facilities (in fact, the FAST trials were exclusively carried out in B&C homes in San Diego, with considerable success). The findings from such intervention studies have already begun to generate interest among clinical care providers, and the ultimate goal of disseminating these findings is that they eventually become readily available to all persons with psychosis, including those who reside in long-term care facilities.

TELEPSYCHIATRY

An innovative development in mental health care is telepsychiatry, aimed at providing psychiatric services to patients who live in assisted living facilities in remote geographic locations and have no or little means of commuting to mental health clinics. It involves the use of interactive-video-conferencing to provide mental health services and is currently being explored as a viable alternative to inperson care that can improve patient adherence to appointments as well as increase access to specialized care providers (Hilty et al., 2004). Several studies have demonstrated its reliability in evaluating persons with schizophrenia and found levels of patient satisfaction similar to inperson care (Chae et al., 2000; Zarate et al., 1997). It may also have implications for improving treatment (medication) adherence, which continues to be a problem in persons with schizophrenia (Dolder et al., 2003). Future treatment of persons with serious mental illness will likely include some type of remote clinical assessment of the patient at their place of residence rather than in a clinical setting.

RECOMMENDATIONS FOR ASSESSMENTS AND REHABILITATION

As the primary treatment setting for the majority of patients with severe mental illness, long-term care facilities are gradually evolving as the bridge between symptom stabilization and independent functioning in mainstream society. Therefore, along with the management of patients' symptoms of psychopathology, these facilities, particularly ARFs, could be a useful setting in which to characterize patient's cognitive and functional strengths and weaknesses in order to develop individualized intervention strategies, which could potentially facilitate social and vocational rehabilitation. Core assessments such as evaluation of presence and severity of clinical symptoms, response to medication and side effects, routine screening for comorbid (including iatrogenic) medical conditions may be supplemented with assessments of cognition and everyday functioning abilities. Assessment of real-world functioning is an important and understudied facet of patients' lives. Assessment of abilities such as cooking, cleaning, self-care, driving, using public transportation, interactions with other people are all important functioning of everyday, normal living. Long-term care facilities, such as ARFs, could not only provide opportunities for patients to carry out such functions but also perform routine assessments of their quality and efficiency in order to make accurate predictions about independent living abilities. The refinement of interventions such as CBSST, FAST, and Cognitive Training could play a central role in helping patients cope with their residual deficits; furthermore, vocational rehabilitation programs such Individual Placement Support (Becker & Drake, 1993) help patients find individualized job placements and train them on the job. Others are more conventional vocational rehabilitation programs that first train patients and then help them find jobs. There are ongoing studies comparing the outcomes of both methods. Such interventions and programs, along with the changing role of long-term care facilities, have the potential to facilitate true rehabilitation for a majority of patients with schizophrenia, without the overwhelming need for institutional long-term care as it is defined today.

REFERENCES

American Diabetes Association, American Psychiatric Association, American Association of Clinical Endocrinologists, North American Association for the Study of Obesity. (2004). Consensus development conference on antipsychotic drugs and obesity and diabetes. *Journal of Clinical Psychiatry, 65,* 267–272.

American Psychiatric Association. (1980). *Diagnostic and statistical manual of mental disorders* (3rd ed.). Washington, DC: Author.

American Psychiatric Association. (1987). *Diagnostic and statistical manual of mental disorders* (3rd ed., rev.). Washington, DC: Author.

American Psychiatric Association. (1994). *Diagnostic and statistical manual of mental disorders* (4th ed.). Washington, DC: Author.

American Psychiatric Association. (2000). *Diagnostic and statistical manual of mental disorders* (4th ed., text revision). Washington, DC: Author.

Andreasen, N. C. (1999). I don't believe in late onset schizophrenia. In R. Howard, P. V. Rabins & D. J. Castle (Eds.), *Late-onset schizophrenia* (pp. 111–123). Philadelphia: Wrightson Biomedical.

Auslander, L. A., Lindamer, L. L., Delapena, J., et al. (2001). A comparison of community-dwelling older schizophrenia patients by residential status. *Acta Psychiatrica Scandinavica, 103,* 380–386.

Bartels, S. J., & Dums, A. R. (2004). Mental health policy and financing of services for older adults with severe mental illness. In C. I. Cohen (Ed.), *Schizophrenia in later life* (pp. 269–288). Arlington, VA: American Psychiatric.

Becker, D. R., & Drake, R. E. (1993). *A working life: The Individual Placement Support (IPS) program.* Concord: New Hampshire-Dartmouth Psychiatric Research Center.

Bilder, R. M., Reiter, G., Bates, J., et al. (2006). Cognitive development in schizophrenia: Follow-back from the first episode. *Journal of Clinical and Experimental Neuropsychology, 28,* 270–282.

Burns, B. J. (1991). Mental health services research on the hospitalized and institutionalized CMI elderly. In B. D. Lebowitz & E. Light (Eds.), *The elderly with chronic mental illness* (pp. 207–215). New York: Springer.

Castle, D. J., & Murray, R. M. (1993). The epidemiology of late-onset schizophrenia. *Schizophrenia Bulletin, 19,* 691–700.

Chae, Y. M., Park, H. J., et al. (2000). The reliability and acceptability of telemedicine for patients with schizophrenia in Korea. *Journal of Telemedicine and Telecare, 6,* 83–90.

Chandler, J. D., & Chandler, J. E. (1988). The prevalence of neuropsychiatric disorders in a nursing home population. *Journal of Geriatric Psychiatry and Neurology, 1,* 71–76.

Chwastiak, L. A., Rosenheck, R. A., McEvoy, J. P., et al. (2006). Interrelationships of psychiatric symptom severity, medical comorbidity, and functioning in schizophrenia. *Psychopharmacology Services, 57,* 1102–1109.

Davis, J. M., & Chen, N. (2004). Dose response and dose equivalence of antipsychotics. *Journal of Clinical Psychiatry, 24,* 192–208.

Dolder, C. R., Lacro, J. P., Leckband, S., et al. (2003). Interventions to improve antipsychotic medication adherence. *Journal of Clinical Psychiatry, 23,* 389–399.

Evans, J. D., Heaton, R. K., Paulsen, J. S., et al. (1999). Schizoaffective disorder: A form of schizophrenia or affective disorder? *Journal of Clinical Psychiatry, 60,* 874–882.

Evans, J. D., Heaton, R. K., Paulsen, J. S., et al. (2003). The relationship of neuropsychological abilities to specific domains of functional capacity in older schizophrenia patients. *Bibliotheca Psychiatrica, 53,* 422–430.

Fenning, S., Fotchman, L. J., & Bromet, E. J. (2005). Delusional disorder and shared psychotic disorder. In B. J. Sadock & V. A. Sadock (Eds.), *Kaplan and Sadock's comprehensive textbook of psychiatry* (8th ed.) (pp. 1525–1532). Philadelphia, PA: Lipincott Williams & Wilkins.

Fisher, W. H., Barriera, P. J., Geller, J. L., et al. (2001). Long-stay patients in state psychiatric hospitals at the end of the 20th century. *Psychopharmacology Services, 52,* 1050–1056.

Fleishman, M. (1989). The role of the psychiatrist in board-and-care homes. *Hospital and Community Psychiatry, 40,* 415–418.

Folsom, D. P., Hawthorne, W., Lindamer, L., et al. (2005). Prevalence and risk factors for homelessness and utilization of mental health services among 10,340 patients with serious mental illness in a large public mental health system. *American Journal of Psychiatry, 162*, 370–376.

Frangou, S. (2006). Early onset schizophrenia: Cognitive and clinical characteristics. In T. Sharma & P. D. Harvey (Eds.), *The early course of schizophrenia* (pp. 59–70). New York: Oxford University Press.

Gilmer, T. P., Folsom, D. P., Hawthorne, W., et al. (2003). Assisted living and use of health services among Medicaid beneficiaries with schizophrenia. *Journal of Mental Health Policy and Economics, 6*, 59–65.

Granholm, E., McQuaid, J. R., McLure, F. S., et al. (2005). A randomized, controlled trial of cognitive behavioral social skills training for middle-aged and older outpatients with chronic schizophrenia. *American Journal of Psychiatry, 162*, 520–529.

Green, M. F. (1996). What are the functional consequences of neurocognitive deficits in schizophrenia? *American Journal of Psychiatry, 153*, 321–330.

Green, M. F. (1998). *Schizophrenia from a neurocognitive perspective: Probing the impenetrable darkness.* Boston: Allyn & Bacon.

Green, M. F., Kern, R. S., & Heaton, R. K. (2004). Longitudinal studies of cognition and functional outcomes in schizophrenia: Implications for MATRICS. *Schizophrenic Research, 72*, 41–51.

Harris, M. J., & Jeste, D. V. (1988). Late-onset schizophrenia: An overview. *Schizophrenia Bulletin, 14*, 39–55.

Harvey, P. D., Silverman, J. M., Mohs, R. C., et al. (1999). Cognitive decline in late-life schizophrenia: A longitudinal study of geriatric chronically hospitalized patients. *Bibliotheca Psychiatrica, 45*, 32–40.

Heaton, R. K., Gladsjo, J. A., Palmer, B. W., et al. (2001). Stability and course of neuropsychological deficits in schizophrenia. *Archives of General Psychiatry, 58*, 24–32.

Heinrichs, R. W., & Zakzanis, K. K. (1998). Neurocognitive deficit in schizophrenia: A quantitative review of the evidence. *Neuropsychology, 12*, 426–445.

Hilty, D. M., Marks, S. L., et al. (2004). Clinical and educational telepsychiatry applications: A review. *Canadian Journal of Psychology, 49*, 12–23.

Hoff, A. L., Svetina, C., Shields, G., et al. (2005). Ten year longitudinal study of neuropsychological functioning subsequent to a first episode of schizophrenia. *American Journal of Psychiatry, 157*, 172–178.

Howard, R., Rabins, P. V., Seeman, M. V., et al. (2000). Late-onset schizophrenia and very-late-onset schizophrenia-like psychosis: An international consensus. *American Journal of Psychiatry, 157*, 172–178.

Jeste, D. V., & Finkel, S. I. (2000). Psychosis of Alzheimer's disease and related dementias. Diagnostic criteria for a distinct syndrome. *American Journal of Geriatric Psychiatry, 8*, 29–34.

Jeste, D. V., Gladsjo, J. A., Lindamer, L. A., et al. (1996). Medical comorbidity in schizophrenia. *Schizophrenia Bulletin, 22*, 413–430.

Jeste, D. V., Harris, M. J., Krull, A., et al. (1995). Clinical and neuropsychological characteristics of patients with late-onset schizophrenia. *American Journal of Psychiatry, 152*, 722–730.

Jeste, D. V., Rockwell, E. et al. (1999). Conventional vs. newer antipsychotics in elderly patients. *American Journal of Geriatric Psychiatry, 7*, 70–76.

Jeste, D. V., Symonds, L. L., Harris, M. J., et al. (1997). Nondementia nonpraecox dementia praecox? Late-onset schizophrenia. *American Journal of Geriatric Psychiatry, 5*, 302–317.

Klapow, J. C., Evans, J., Patterson, T. L., et al. (1997). Direct assessment of functional status in older patients with schizophrenia. *American Journal of Psychiatry, 154,* 1022–1024.

Kraepelin, E. (1919). *Dementia praecox and paraphrenia.* Chicago: Chicago Medical Book.

Kremen, W. S., Buka, S. L., Seidman, L. J., et al. (1998). IQ decline during childhood and adult psychotic symptoms in a community sample: A 19-year longitudinal study. *American Journal of Psychiatry, 155,* 672–677.

Lacro, J. P., & Jeste, D. V. (1994). Physical comorbidity and polypharmacy in older psychiatric patients. *Bibliotheca Psychiatrica, 36,* 146–152.

Lamb, H. R., & Bachrach, L. L. (2001). Some perspectives on deinstitutionalization. *Psychiatric Services, 52,* 1039–1045.

Lamb, H. R., & Shander, R. (1993). When there are almost no state hospital beds left. *Hospital and Community Psychiatry, 44,* 973–976.

Lesser, I. M., Jeste, D. V., Boone, K. B. et al. (1992). Late-onset psychotic disorder, not otherwise specified : Clinical and neuroimaging findings. *Bibliotheca Psychiatrica, 31,* 419–423.

Lieberman, J. A., Stroup, T. S., et al. (2005). Effectiveness of antipsychotic drugs in patients with chronic schizophrenia. *New England Journal of Medicine, 353,* 1209–1223.

Marder, S. R. (1996). Management of schizophrenia. *Journal of Clinical Psychiatry, 57,* 9–13.

Marder, S. R., & van Kammen, D. P. (2005). Dopamine receptor antagonists (typical antipsychotics). In B. J. Sadock & V. A. Sadock (Eds.), *Kaplan and Sadock's comprehensive textbook of psychiatry* (8th ed.). Philadelphia: Lippincott Williams & Wilkins.

Patterson, T. L., Bucardo, J., McKibbin, C. L. et al. (2005). Development and pilot testing of a new psychosocial intervention for older Latinos with chronic psychosis. *Schizophrenia Bulletin, 31,* 922–930.

Reichman, W. E., & Rabins, P. R. (1996). Schizophrenia. In W. E. Reichman & P. R. Katz (Eds.), *Psychiatric care in the nursing home* (pp. 109–117). New York: Oxford University Press.

Ropacki, S. A., & Jeste, D. V. (2005). Epidemiology of and risk factors for psychosis of Alzheimer's disease: A review of 55 studies published from 1990 to 2003. *American Journal of Psychiatry, 162,* 2022–2030.

Sable, J. A., & Jeste, D. V. (2002). Antipsychotic treatment for late-life schizophrenia. *Current Psychiatry Reports, 4,* 299–306.

Sajatovic, M., Ramirez, L. F., Garver, D., Thompson, P., Ripper, G., & Lehmann, L. S. (1998). Clozapine therapy for older veterans. *Psychiatric Services, 49,* 340–344.

Sciolla, A., & Jeste, D. V. (1998). Use of antipsychotics in the elderly. *International Journal of Psychiatry in Clinical Practice, 2,* S27–S34.

Seeman, M. V. (1996). The role of estrogen in schizophrenia. *Journal of Psychiatry and Neurosciences, 21,* 123–127.

State of California Department of Social Services Community Care Licensing Division Licensing Information System Directory Report 1–03-06. (2006). Retrieved August 31, 2006, from http://ccld.ca.gov/

Talbot, J. A. (1995). Nursing homes are not the answer. *Hospital and Community Psychiatry, 39,* 115–118.

Twamley, E. W., Jeste, D. V., & Bellack, A. S. (2003). A review of cognitive training in schizophrenia. *Schizophrenia Bulletin, 29,* 359–382.

U.S. Department of Health and Human Services. (2006). Retrieved September 15, 2006, from http://www.cms.hhs.gov/SNFPPS/

U.S. Census Bureau. (2006). Retrieved August 31, 2006, from www.census.gov

Walker, E. F. (1994). Developmentally moderated expression of the neuropathology underlying schizophrenia. *Schizophrenia Bulletin, 20,* 453–480.

Zarate, C. A., Weinstock, L., et al. (1997). Applicability of telemedicine for assessing patients with schizophrenia: Acceptibility and reliability. *Journal of Clinical Psychiatry, 58,* 22–25.

7

Sleep–Wake Disorders

Yohannes W. Endeshaw

Sleep–wake disturbances are common among residents of long-term care (LTC) facilities (Cohen et al., 1983; Fetveit & Bjorvatn, 2002; Jacobs et al., 1989; Rao et al., 2005; Voyer et al., 2006). In fact, sleep–wake disturbance may be one of the major factors that influenced relatives to place their loved one in an LTC facility (Pollak, 1991). Nighttime sleep disturbance (commonly referred to as insomnia) manifests as persistent difficulty with sleep initiation and/or maintenance that occurs despite adequate time and opportunity for sleep and results in impairment of daytime activities (American Academy of Sleep Medicine, 2005a); daytime wake problems manifest as excessive daytime sleepiness.

Insomnia is divided into primary and secondary insomnia. Secondary insomnia is caused by primary sleep disorders (e.g., obstructive sleep apnea, restless legs syndrome [RLS], etc.) and sleep disorders due to medical, neurological, or psychiatric disorders. When insomnia is not caused by any of the conditions mentioned above, it is referred to as primary insomnia. Previous reports have documented that the majority of insomnia in LTC settings is due to secondary insomnia (Voyer et al., 2006). Other important factors that contribute to occurrence of insomnia in LTC facilities are the structural and functional characteristics of these facilities. In this chapter, etiological factors of sleep–wake disorders commonly encountered among LTC residents, and their management will be discussed. To facilitate our understanding of these sleep–wake disturbances, a brief discussion of normal sleep architecture and changes associated with normal aging is presented.

AGE-ASSOCIATED CHANGES IN SLEEP ARCHITECTURE

Sleep consists of two states referred to as nonrapid eye movement (NREM) and rapid eye movement (REM) sleep. NREM sleep comprises four stages, stage 1 through stage 4 sleep. In young and healthy human adults, stage 1 is considered a transitory sleep and comprises only 2% to 5% of the total sleep time (TST); stage 2 comprises 45% to 55% of the TST, whereas stages 3 and 4 (also known as slow wave sleep or deep sleep) comprise about 15% to 20%. REM sleep comprises 20% to 25% of TST, and it is the sleep period when most dreams occur. In addition to decreased responsiveness, REM sleep is also characterized by loss of muscle tone (atonia) in most of the skeletal muscles. This phenomenon is important as it prevents the individual from acting out his or her dream. Sleep is entered through stage 1 and progresses to stages 2, 3, and 4 and then REM sleep. This NREM–REM sleep cycle lasts about 90 to 110 min and repeats itself throughout the sleep period (Carskadon, 2005). Changes in sleep architecture that occur with aging include a decrease in stages 3 and 4, an increase in stages 1 and 2, a decrease in REM sleep and an increase in the number of arousals from sleep (Redline et al., 2004; Ohayon et al., 2004). Older adults spend a longer time in bed without a corresponding increase in TST, and as a result have decreased sleep efficiency (TST/total time in bed). In short, the nighttime sleep of older adults is "lighter" and more fragmented when compared with healthy younger adults.

Another factor that is important in sleep regulation and that shows changes with aging is the circadian timing system (also known as circadian rhythm). The circadian rhythm is a term used to describe the 24-h rhythm in behavior and functions of the body, such as body temperature, secretion of hormones, activities of the cardiovascular system, autonomic nervous system activities, and sleep–wake cycle. The rhythm is generated by a master biological clock that is found in the suprachiasmatic nucleus (SCN) of the hypothalamus (Turek et al., 2005). Although these rhythms can occur freely, they are synchronized to the appropriate 24-h period by environmental cues such as light physical and social activities (Turek et al., 2005). This synchronization of biological rhythms and the environment makes it possible for activities to occur at the appropriate time of the 24-h cycle. The circadian timing system is described to be less robust and shifted to an earlier period (phase advanced) with aging (Monk, 2005; Munch et al., 2005). The phase advance in circadian rhythm is believed to explain the habit of some older adults to go to bed early in the evening and to get up early in the morning.

Although these age-related changes are described in otherwise healthy older adults, their contribution to sleep complaints in general may be limited.

Epidemiological studies have shown that sleep complaints among older adults with no coexisting morbidities are not common, suggesting that primary and secondary sleep disorders are primarily responsible for sleep disturbance in older adults (Foley et al., 1995; Vitiello et al., 2002). It is possible that the changes in sleep architecture that are associated with aging may make older adults more vulnerable to sleep disturbance in the presence of other morbidities.

SLEEP–WAKE PATTERN AMONG NURSING HOME RESIDENTS

Both nighttime sleep problems and excessive daytime sleepiness are common among nursing home residents (Ancoli-Israel et al., 1989; Bliwise et al., 1990a, 1990b; Fetveit & Bjorvatn, 2002; Jacobs et al., 1989; Pat-Horenczyk et al., 1998). One of the factors that impact the occurrence of sleep–wake disturbances among nursing home residents is the suboptimal sleep promoting and wake promoting practices in these facilities. Practices that promote the initiation and maintenance of a good quality of nighttime sleep and daytime alertness include keeping regular sleep time and wake time, restricting the amount of time in bed, avoiding or limiting daytime napping or dozing off, limiting intake of caffeinated beverages and alcohol during evening hours and at night, minimizing exposure to light and noise during the night, and providing exposure to adequate light, physical and social activities during the day (Morin et al., 1999). The realization of these practices in the current nursing home milieu may be a challenge. Previous studies have shown that during the daytime, nursing home residents spend a longtime in bed, stay mostly within the building, do not get sufficient exposure to bright light, and do not engage in an adequate amount of physical and social activities (Shochat et al., 2000). This limited exposure to light and activities reduces the input of the environment to the circadian timing system and may limit the contribution of the circadian system to maintenance of wakefulness during the day (Duffy & Wright, 2005; Mistlberger & Skene, 2005). During the night, there are limited activities in most of these facilities. The residents may go to bed shortly after dinner whether they are ready to go to sleep or not and get out of bed at a specific time in the morning (Schnelle et al., 1998). In short, the sleep–wake schedule is set up to fit the timetable of the facility rather than the sleep–wake pattern of the individual resident. Furthermore, studies have shown that nursing home residents are exposed to excessive noise and light during the night and these exposures are associated with poor sleep (Schnelle et al., 1998). It is interesting to note that the majority of the nighttime noise originated from staff vocalization (26%); television (19%); and intercoms, bells, and alarms (11%; Schnelle et al., 1998). It is imperative that attempts to improve the quantity and quality of sleep in nursing home residents should include interventions to address these factors.

SECONDARY SLEEP DISORDERS

These are sleep disorders caused by medical, neurological, or psychiatric diseases and the medications taken to treat these conditions. Common causes of secondary sleep disorders and their effect on sleep is shown in Table 7.1. In addition, selected secondary sleep disorders are discussed below.

Medications

Polypharmacy is a common occurrence among older adults in general and LTC residents in particular. Reports from nursing homes in the United States and

TABLE 7.1. Sleep Problems Associated with Common Medical, Neurological, and Psychiatric Problems

CONDITION	MECHANISM	SLEEP PROBLEM
Congestive heart failure	Orthopnea Paroxysmal nocturnal dyspnea (sudden awakening from sleep with shortness of breath ± cough, wheezing) Nocturia	Sleep onset insomnia Sleep maintenance insomnia
Osteoarthritis	Pain	Sleep onset insomnia Sleep maintenance insomnia
Chronic obstructive pulmonary disease	Hypoventilation and hypoxemia during sleep (especially REM sleep) Sleep fragmentation	Sleep maintenance insomnia
Gastro-esophageal reflux disease	Epigastric burning, reflux Sleep disruption	Sleep maintenance insomnia
Parkinson's disease	Stiffness, pain (motor symptoms) Associated PLMD, RBD Degeneration of neural structures	Sleep onset insomnia Sleep maintenance insomnia Excessive daytime sleepiness
Dementia	Degenerative CNS changes	Irregular sleep–wake pattern Fragmented nighttime sleep Excessive daytime sleepiness
Seizure disorders	Sleep disruption	Sleep maintenance insomnia
Depression	Physiological arousal, emotional arousal, cognitive arousal, faulty conditioning	Sleep onset insomnia Sleep maintenance insomnia Early morning awakenings Daytime fatigue
Anxiety disorder	Worrying at bedtime Nocturnal panic	Sleep onset insomnia Sleep maintenance insomnia

Europe have indicated that the majority of the residents are taking more than four different scheduled medications per day (Broderick, 1997; Field et al., 2001; Nygaard et al., 2003). These medications given for various medical, neurological, and psychiatric conditions may affect sleep in different ways. Some medications may have wake-promoting effects and if taken in the evening hours may predispose to insomnia (e.g., bupropion prescribed for depression). Other medications may have sleep-promoting (sedating) effects and may result in sleepiness when taken during the day. One example is daytime sleepiness and sleep attacks (sudden onset of sleepiness) caused by dopaminergic drugs given for the treatment of Parkinson's disease (Arnulf, 2005). In addition, some medications have been reported to cause specific side effects such as the nightmares associated with beta-blockers and sleep walking associated with CNS sedating medications. Another important aspect of pharmacotherapy in older adults is the change in pharmacokinetics associated with aging that may result in prolonged half-life of drugs (Cusack, 2004). As a result, the effect of a sedating agent given in the early evening hours may linger into the morning hours of the day. Furthermore, interaction between the different medications (drug–drug interaction; Herrlinger & Klotz, 2001; Zhan et al., 2005) and/or drug–disease interaction (Ferrell et al., 1995; Lindblad et al., 2006) may result in untoward effects that disrupt sleep. For these reasons, careful assessment of medications must be included in the evaluation of LTC residents for sleep–wake problems. In addition, the principle of "start low and go slow" should be observed when prescribing sleep-promoting agents.

Pain

Chronic pain is a common problem among LTC residents and remains underreported, underdiagnosed, and undertreated (Ferrell, 1995; Pilowsky et al., 1985). Underreporting of pain may be even more common among LTC residents with cognitive impairment (Ferrell et al., 1995). The presence of pain interferes with both daytime function and nighttime sleep. Both epidemiological and physiological studies have shown a positive relationship between pain and sleep disturbance (Drewes et al., 1997; Pilowsky et al., 1985). Implementation of pain assessment and management protocols are important measures that should be taken to improve the treatment of pain and associated sleep–wake disturbances.

Nocturia

Nocturia, defined as waking up from sleep at night to urinate (Gentili et al., 1997; Van Kerrebroeck et al., 2002), is a common problem among older adults in general and may be even more common among nursing home residents (Gentili et al., 1997; Ouslander et al., 1993). It is described as one of the most bothersome lower urinary tract symptoms due to the sleep disruption that it causes. Nocturia can be caused by several etiologies, which include

- Problems related to urinary bladder: In these situations there may be inappropriate contraction of the detrusor muscle (over active bladder), inadequate contraction of the detrusor muscle or bladder outlet obstruction causing urinary retention, or a combination of the above. These conditions usually manifest as increased frequency of urination both during the day and the night.
- Problems not related to the bladder: These conditions are usually associated with increased urine production during sleep (nocturnal polyuria; sleep time urine output/24-h urine output > 0.35; Van Kerrebroeck et al., 2002), although the anatomy and physiology of the bladder may be within normal limits. Several disorders as shown below may result in nocturnal polyuria and increased frequency of nocturia.
  - Medical disorders such as congestive heart failure (CHF), use of diuretics, syndrome of inappropriate ADH secretion.
  - Neurological disorders such as Parkinson's disease.
  - Primary sleep disorders such as obstructive sleep apnea.

In some cases, the cause of nocturia may not be related to overactive bladder or nocturnal polyuria. The subjects may wake up due to a sleep disorder such as periodic leg movement disorder (PLMD) or pain and then go to the bathroom to urinate. But this possibility should be entertained only after ruling out the common causes of nocturia mentioned above. Addressing these issues may be important to improve sleep interruption associated with increased nocturia frequency.

Congestive Heart Failure

Shortness of breath in the form of orthopnea and/or paroxysmal nocturnal dyspnea in patients with CHF may result in difficulty initiating or maintaining sleep. Nocturia associated with CHF leads to sleep interruption. This implies that optimal control of CHF is essential for the treatment of sleep disturbance related to this disorder. Furthermore, sleep disorders such as central sleep apnea (CSA) and obstructive sleep apnea and hypopnea (OSAH) are reported to be common among patients with uncontrolled CHF (Bradley & Floras, 2003a, 2003b; Pepin et al., 2006). In addition to disturbing sleep, the hypoxia and hemodynamic changes associated with OSAH and CSA may exacerbate the heart failure. Thus, in this group of patients, optimal management of heart failure requires the treatment of the sleep-related breathing disorders mentioned above.

Dementia

Sleep–wake disturbances are commonly described in patients with dementia (studies examining sleep problems in dementia have primarily included participants with dementia of Alzheimer's type). Older adults with dementia are reported to have nighttime sleep fragmentation (Ancoli-Israel et al., 1989; Bliwise, 1993; Jacobs et al., 1989; Tractenberg et al., 2005). Polysomnographic changes observed in patients with dementia include increased stage 1 and decreased slow wave sleep and increased awakenings in excess of that described in healthy older adults. Decreased time in REM sleep and increased REM sleep latency has also been reported in moderate to severe dementia (Prinz et al., 1982; Vitiello et al., 1984, 1990). During the daytime, patients with dementia are observed to be sleepy, dozing off through out the day (Bliwise et al., 1990a; Pat-Horenczyk, 1998). Figure 7.1 shows the sleep–wake pattern of nursing home residents between the hours of 8:00 and 20:00. The causes of nighttime sleep disturbances in dementia are usually multifactorial and may include primary sleep disorders like obstructive sleep apnea, degeneration of sleep-regulating neural structures , and other accompanying medical and psychiatric disorders (Bliwise et al., 1990b; Stopa et al., 1999; Swaab et al., 1985). Although the cause of daytime sleepiness observed in patients with dementia is believed to be a result of nighttime sleep disruption, in a recent study conducted to determine correlates of daytime sleepiness in nursing home residents with dementia, there

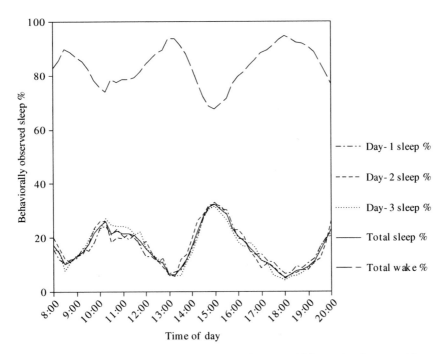

FIGURE 7.1. Percentage of behavioral observations at which nursing home residents were observed asleep during 12 h of observation (8 a.m.–8 p.m.) over a 3-day period (Endeshaw et al. 2007). Note that observed sleepiness was minimal between 8:00 and 9:00 a.m., 12:00 and 1:00 p.m., and 6:00 and 7:00 p.m. corresponding to meal times.

was no significant relationship between quantity of nighttime sleep and daytime sleepiness (Endeshaw et al., 2007). This finding suggests that the etiology of daytime sleepiness in this particular group of study participants may be unrelated to nighttime sleep disturbance, and could be a consequence of degenerative changes in wake-promoting centers of the central nervous system.

Sundowning

Sundowning, also referred to as nocturnal agitation, is reported among patients with dementia and is described as abnormal motor or vocal behavior which usually manifests in the late afternoon or early evening hours. The symptoms may range from simple vocalization to aggressive behavior. The prevalence of sundowning has been reported to range from 12% to 24%, depending on the site of the study, specifically, the proportion of residents with dementia in the facility (Bachman & Rabins, 2006; Bliwise, 1994). The mechanism of sundowning in patients with dementia is not clearly understood. One contributing factor may be "unmet needs." For example, leg discomfort associated with RLS shows a circadian pattern and mostly occurs in the evening hours. Pain due to arthritis has also been shown to show a circadian pattern (Labrecque & Vanier, 1995). It is possible that abnormal behavior observed in the afternoon and evening hours may be a reaction to these painful and uncomfortable conditions as these cognitively impaired individuals are not able to make their complaints known.

Because the abnormal behaviors associated with sundowning are observed to occur at about the same time each day, the possibility that this disorder may be related to disturbance of the circadian rhythm is also considered (Volicer et al., 2001). Accordingly, interventional studies with bright light therapy were conducted in demented patients with nocturnal agitation; however, the results of these studies have not shown a consistent beneficial effect (Forbes et al., 2007).

Management of sundowning in the LTC environment remains a challenge (McGaffigan & Bliwise, 1997). Treatment should be individualized and includes identifying and treating possible precipitating factors (potentially treatable conditions like pain, discomfort, etc.), nonpharmacological behavioral management, and pharmacological treatment when appropriate.

There is no simple solution for the treatment of sleep–wake disturbances in patients with dementia. It involves identifying the specific nocturnal and diurnal problem to be addressed, nonpharmacological interventions (e.g., increased daylight exposure and daytime activity, decreased nighttime noise and light exposure, etc.), and treatment of associated primary and/or secondary sleep problems. Isolated treatment of one aspect of the multifactorial problem may not yield optimal results. For example, inconsistent results were reported after bright light therapy of LTC residents with dementia; one study reporting increased consolidation of nighttime sleep and another study reporting no significant improvement in nighttime sleep (Ancoli-Israel et al., 2003; Dowling et al., 2005; Forbes et al., 2007). Behavioral interventions aimed at improving nighttime sleep, and daytime sleepiness did not show a significant improvement of nighttime sleep, although a modest improvement in daytime activity was reported (Alessi et al., 2005; Ouslander et al., 2006). These findings imply that sleep–wake disturbance in the nursing home residents has a multifactorial etiology and that a similar multifaceted approach should be utilized in its management.

Depression

Sleep complaints are common among patients with depression, and (Buysse et al., 1994; Gerber et al., 1992; Livingston et al., 1993; Roberts et al., 2000) these complaints include difficulty initiating and maintaining sleep, early morning awakenings, not feeling well rested in the morning, and fatigue during the day. In addition, long-term sleep complaints have been reported to predict future development of depression in otherwise nondepressed individuals (Breslau et al., 1996; Ford & Kamerow, 1989; Livingston et al., 1993; Roberts et al., 2000), thus making the relationship between sleep and depression complex. Polysomnographic studies in patients with depression have shown prolonged sleep latency, increased number of arousals, decrease in slow wave sleep, reduced REM latency, and increased REM sleep (Benca, 2005). With a high prevalence rate of depression reported among nursing home residents (Jones et al., 2003; Jongenelis et al., 2004), sleep disturbance secondary to depression may be a major problem.

Sleep disturbance associated with depression usually responds to treatment of depression. However, the sleep effects of antidepressant agents should also be taken into consideration while prescribing these medications. For example, fluoxetine, venlafaxine, and bupropion may have wake-promoting effects and may cause insomnia in some patients. On the other hand, tricyclic antidepressants, trazadone, and mirtazapine may have sedating effects. Although they are potentially useful in depressed patients with insomnia, the possibility of a hangover effect in the morning, especially in frail older adults, should also be considered. Given the different groups of drugs available for treatment of depression, choosing the right antidepressant that is appropriate for the individual patient should be considered. In some patients, sleep complaints may persist despite adequate treatment of depression. It would be prudent to consider the possibility of primary sleep disorders such as SDB, RLS, and PLMD in these patients and refer them for evaluation by a sleep specialist. For example, serotonin reuptake inhibitors are reported to exacerbate or unmask the symptoms of RLS and PLMD (Bakshi, 1996; Dimmitt & Riley, 2000; Hargrave & Beckley, 1998; Picchietti & Winkelman, 2005).

PRIMARY SLEEP DISORDERS

Sleep-Disordered Breathing

Sleep-disordered breathing (SDB) comprises three conditions: OSAH, CSA, and upper airway resistance syndrome. Because upper airway resistance syndrome has not been described in LTC residents, we will limit the discussion to OSAH and CSA. OSAH is characterized by cessation of breathing for ≥ 10 s (apnea) or decrease in airflow during sleep for associated with a decrease in oxygen saturation or arousal from sleep (hypopnea) (American Academy of Sleep Medicine, 1999, 2005b). These apnea and hypopnea events occur as a result of complete or partial obstruction of the upper airway respectively.

Epidemiology. OSAH is common among older adults, with up to 20% reported to have a moderate to severe form of the disorder (Young et al., 2002). The prevalence rate is even higher in nursing home residents with more than a third reported to have a moderate to severe form of the disorder (Ancoli-Israel et al., 1991; Bliwise et al., 1990b; Endeshaw et al., 2007). The rate is reported to be much higher when a mild form of the disorder is included. Traditional risk factors for OSAH include snoring, increased body mass index, increased neck circumference (>17 in males and >16 in females), and craniofacial abnormalities (e.g., micrognathia). But in older adults, OSAH may occur in the absence of these traditional risk factors (Endeshaw, 2006). Changes in the anatomy of the upper airway (e.g., associated with edentulism) and decreased activity of upper airway muscles that keep the airway open during sleep may be major risk factors for OSAH in old age (Malhotra et al., 2006; Martin et al., 1997; Oliven et al., 2001). These changes in the upper airway may be a result of age-related changes in the upper airway muscles (e.g., muscle-mass loss involving the upper airway muscles) or a result of other pathology. Moreover, a significant relationship between the use of dentures and OSAH has been reported, suggesting that changes in the upper airway anatomy associated with edentulism may predispose to development of apnea or hypopnea during sleep (Endeshaw et al., 2004).

Clinical manifestations. In addition to the traditional clinical manifestations like snoring, OSAH in nursing home residents may manifest with unexplained awakenings from sleep, excessive daytime sleepiness (Bliwise et al., 1990b), increased frequency of nocturia (Bliwise et al., 2004; Endeshaw et al., 2004), and cognitive impairment (American Academy of Sleep Medicine, 2005b). Increased cardiovascular and cerebrovascular morbidities including death during sleep has been reported in middle-aged adults with OSAH (Gami et al., 2005; Lavie, 2005; Quan & Gersh, 2004; Yaggi et al., 2005). Whether these complications also occur in nursing home residents with OSAH has not been investigated. Furthermore, the impact of treatment of OSAH on functional and morbidity status, and quality of life of LTC residents is not known.

Laboratory investigation. Clinical suspicion of OSAH is confirmed by monitoring of breathing during sleep. The diagnostic method of choice is polysomnography (PSG). PSG simultaneously monitors brain activity (sleep stages), air flow and oxygenation, and muscle activity during sleep. The results would indicate the number of apneas and hypopneas per hour of sleep (apnea-hypopnea index, AHI), and the severity of oxygen desaturations. The AHI is used to determine the severity of OSAH with an AHI of 5 to14, 15 to29, and ≥30 per hour of sleep indicating mild, moderate, and severe OSAH, respectively (American Academy of Sleep Medicine, 2003; Thorpy et al., 1994).

Other respiration monitoring systems during sleep are also available. These techniques monitor respiratory parameters that include airflow, chest and abdominal movements, and pulse oximetry and determine the AHI and the severity of oxygen desaturation. The advantage of these systems is that the procedure is performed at the patient's living facility and it does not require the presence of a technician during the study. This makes such techniques attractive for use in nursing homes. The results of these tests have been shown to have good correlation when compared with simultaneous PSG recording (Dingli et al., 2003). Overnight monitoring of oxygen saturation with a pulse oximeter has been used as a screening tool for OSA. The obvious shortcoming of this method is that the result does not provide any information about the breathing status (presence of apnea or hypopnea) of the person. For this reason, information obtained using pulse oximetry should be confirmed by more detailed tests before any treatment recommendation is made.

Treatment

Conservative management. In patients who are obese or who have their apnea or hypopnea predominantly in the supine position, weight loss or avoiding the supine position during sleep would be helpful. In addition, drugs that worsen SDB (alcohol, sedative hypnotics) should be avoided.

Continuous Positive Airway Pressure. This is the treatment of choice for SDB. The Continuous Positive Airway Pressure (CPAP) equipment consists of an air blower connected to facemask via a short tube. The machine delivers air to the upper airway via the mask, and this air pressure keeps the upper airway open during sleep. The pressure required to keep the airway open is determined during an overnight CPAP titration study. The question of whether frail older adults would tolerate CPAP has always been a concern. A recent study reported that older adults (mean age 78 years) with mild to moderate Alzheimer's dementia were successfully treated with CPAP for 6 weeks, implying that these patients were able to tolerate such treatment (Ancoli-Israel et al., 2006; Ayalon et al., 2006). As mentioned above, the impact of treatment of LTC facility residents with OSAH has not been systematically investigated and should be addressed in future studies.

Other forms of treatment for OSAH include oral appliances and surgical intervention, but there is no clinical study or experience in the use of these modalities of treatment among LTC residents. More important is the issue of use of dentures during sleep. Most patients who use dentures are advised by their dentists to remove their dentures during sleep. A previous report has indicated that removing dentures during sleep may worsen OSAH (Bucca et al., 1999, 2006). Although it is premature to recommend a change in practice based on the results of a non-randomized study, the practice of removing dentures during sleep may have to be examined further. To date there are no effective medications for the treatment of OSAH (Smith & Lasserson, 2002).

Central Sleep Apnea

CSA is also characterized by cessation of breathing during sleep, but unlike OSAH, the upper airway remains patent and the malfunction is in the respiratory center of the central nervous system. The apnea may be associated with oxygen desaturation and arousals. CSA has been described to occur in patients with CHF, chronic obstructive pulmonary disease, metabolic encephalopathy such as uremia, and stroke. Treatment of CSA is aimed at the optimal management of the underlying medical disorder (Badr, 2005; Bradley & Floras, 2003 ; White, 2005).

Restless Legs Syndrome and Periodic Limb Movement Disorder

RLS is a common sleep disorder characterized by the urge to move the legs, usually associated with leg discomfort (Allen & Earley, 2001; Trenkwalder et al., 2005). The diagnosis is based on diagnostic criteria established by the International Restless Legs Syndrome Study Group (Allen et al., 2003) and include

1. an urge to move the legs, usually accompanied or caused by uncomfortable and unpleasant sensations in the legs (sometimes the urge to move is present without the uncomfortable sensations);
2. the urge to move or unpleasant sensations begin to worsen during periods of rest or inactivity such as lying or sitting;
3. the urge to move or unpleasant sensations are partially or totally relieved by movement, such as walking or stretching as long as the activity continues; and
4. the urge to move or unpleasant sensations are worse in the evening or night than during the day or only occur in the evening or night.

These criteria would be useful in cognitively intact people who can describe their symptoms but may not apply to individuals with cognitive impairment who are not able to communicate. The diagnosis of RLS in LTC residents with cognitive impairment remains a challenge. In patients with cognitive impairment, manifestation of RLS may include difficulty staying in bed at night, walking in the hallway during sleep time, or abnormal behavior during the evening hours and sleep time. Those who are wheelchair bound may continuously move their feet and legs and also manifest abnormal behavior. If these symptoms occur frequently during the evening hours or at night, RLS should be considered a strong possibility.

Epidemiology and pathogenesis

There are no reported prevalence studies of RLS among LTC residents, but among community dwelling older adults, the rate is reported to range from 5% to more than 15%. It is higher in females than in males (Allen et al., 2005; Berger et al., 2004; Garcia-Borreguero et al., 2006; Phillips et al., 2000; Rothdach et al., 2000). RLS occurs in two forms: primary (idiopathic) and secondary. Primary RLS (onset before age 50 years) is common in those with early-onset disease; family history is positive in these individuals in up to 50% of the time (Mata et al., 2006; Trenkwalder et al., 1996). Secondary RLS is more common in individuals with late-onset disease (O'Keeffe, 2005). Secondary causes of RLS include iron deficiency anemia, end stage renal disease, spinal cord lesions, and medications such as selective serotonin reuptake inhibitors and dopamine antagonists (Earley, 2003; Hargrave & Beckley, 1998; Montplaisir et al., 1991; Wetter et al., 2002). The exact mechanism of RLS is not clearly established. The two commonly suggested factors include decreased brain iron and dopamine dysfunction. The brain iron deficiency theory is supported by studies that reported decreased CSF and brain iron levels in patients with RLS (Allen et al., 2001; Connor et al., 2003; Earley et al., 2005). Iron is required in the rate limiting step of conversion of tyrosine to L-hydroxyphenylalanine in dopamine synthesis. The theory of dopamine dysfunction is supported by the therapeutic response to dopaminergic agents (Hening et al., 1999) and exacerbation of RLS with the use of dopamine antagonists (Montplaisir et al 1991, Wetter TC 2002).

Management of RLS involves both conservative and pharmacological treatment. Conservative treatment includes correcting factors that contribute to the occurrence or exacerbation of symptoms and include replacing medications that are known to exacerbate RLS and investigation of the iron and renal function status of the individual. Replacement of iron is recommended when the ferritin level is low (<50 mg/dL).

The drugs of choice for initial treatment of RLS are dopamine agonists such as ropirinole (Requip) and pramipexole (Mirapex). These medications are approved by FDA for this use (Bliwise et al., 2005; Bogan et al., 2006; Hening et al., 1999; Littner et al., 2004; Saletu et al., 2000a, 2000b, 2002). Treatment is started with the lowest dose and titrated up if required. Other medications have also been used off-label for treatment of RLS. These include carbidopa-L-dopa (Sinemet; Littner et al., 2004), benzodiazepines (Chesson et al., 1999; Hening et al., 1999; e.g., clonazepam, temazepam), opiates (Chesson et al., 1999; Hening et al., 1999; Tribl et al., 2005; Walters et al., 2001; e.g., oxycodone, codeine) and gabapentin (Neurontin; Burchell, 2003; Chesson et al., 1999; Happe et al., 2003; Hening et al., 1999; Micozkadioglu et al., 2004). Use of Carbidopa-L-dopa (Sinemet) is associated with recurrence of symptoms more frequently when compared with dopamine agonists (Littner et al., 2004). Benzodiazepines are not a good choice for treatment of RLS in older adults due to their side effects, which include day-time sedation, cognitive impairment, and falls and related injuries (Buffet-Jerrot & Stewart, 2002; Madhusoodanan, & Bogunovic 2004). Furthermore, they may worsen apnea and hypopnea events in subjects with SDB. There is a presumed risk of abuse and addiction with the use of opiates, and for this reason, use of these medications for initial treatment of RLS should be avoided.

Periodic limb movement of sleep (PLMS) is a condition characterized by repetitive movement of the lower extremities (big toe extension, ankle dorsi-flexion, with or without knee and hip flexion), which occur during sleep or relaxed wakefulness and may result in arousals or awakening and daytime sleepiness (Littner et al., 2004). PLMS mostly occur during the NREM sleep cycle. The prevalence of PLMS increases with age, with reported prevalence of 5% of subjects between the age of 30 and 50 years and over 30% of subjects older than 65 years (Hornyak et al., 2006). Up to 80% of patients with RLS symptoms are reported to have PLMS (Hornyak et al., 2006). The diagnosis is based on the number of characteristic leg movements recorded with electromy-ography of the anterior tibialis muscles of both legs during an overnight PSG (Bonnet et al., 1993). Recently, simpler devices that perform home-based multi-ple night recordings have been introduced for the diagnosis of PLMS (Shochat et al., 2003). A PLM index of 5 or more per hour of sleep is considered abnor-mal. These movements may be associated with arousals from sleep, resulting in nocturnal sleep disruption and daytime sleepiness.. Most people with PLMS complain of daytime fatigue or sleepiness and are not aware of the problem, and the diagnosis may be made during an overnight PSG study for suspected SDB. Pharmacologic treatment of PLMS is the same as RLS.

There are two phenomena that have been observed with the use of dopamin-ergic agents. These are rebound of symptoms and augmentation of symptoms (Earley, 2003). Rebound of symptoms occurs when the symptoms of RLS recur (usually 2–6 h after the initial dose) after an initial improvement and corresponds to the duration of action of the drug. Rebound of symptoms occurs less fre-quently with the use of dopamine agonists as compared with levodopa/carbidopa preparations (Comella, 2002). Appropriate scheduling or use of a longer acting drug usually takes care of this problem. Augmentation occurs when after initial improvement of symptoms, which may last from weeks to months, the patient starts to complain of RLS symptoms which may be even more severe than the initial symptoms. The symptoms usually improve with changing to another medication. The mechanism for this phenomenon is not clearly understood.

Drug dosing and scheduling

In general, it is advised to follow the general drug dosing recommendation used in older people, that is, "start low and go slow." The scheduling is best done based on the frequency and timing of symptoms of the individual patient and the drug half-life. As most RLS symptoms start in the evenings, it is recommended that the patient takes the first dose of medication about 45 min before the typical start of symptoms. To prevent rebound and also to treat accompanying PLMS, another dose may be taken at bedtime if the initial dose was taken in the early evening hours. In situations where the symptoms start in the afternoon, appropriate modifications may be made. Table 7.2 shows the dopaminergic agents used for the treatment of RLS.

Rapid Eye Movement Sleep Behavior Disorder

Rapid Eye Movement Sleep Behavior Disorder (RBD) is a condition characterized by "abnormal" behaviors that occur during REM sleep. One of the characteristics of REM sleep is atonia of most of the skeletal muscles and this atonia prevents the physical enactment of dreams. In patients with RBD, there is absence of muscle atonia during REM sleep and as a result the patients act out

TABLE 7.2. Commonly Used Dopaminergic Drugs for Treatment of Restless Legs Syndrome

	DOSE (mg)	HALF-LIFE (h)	COMMENT
Levodopa/carbidopa (Sinemet) 25/100	25/100	1.5	More rebound and augmentation of symptoms reported as compared with dopamine agonists.
Pramiperxole (Mirapex)	0.125	8–12	A one time dose of 0.125 mg may be adequate for frail older adults. Renal excretion is the major route of elimination.
Ropinirole HCL (Requip)	0.25	6	A one time dose of 0.25 mg may be adequate for frail older adults. May potentiate the effect of warfarin. Metabolized by the liver to inactive metabolites.

Note: Half-life may be longer in the elderly.

their dreams. This dream enactment behavior ranges from simple movements of the extremities to activities that could be injurious to self or the bed partner, may include jumping out of bed and punching and kicking the bed partner. The patient may remember the dream content but does not remember acting out his or her dream (Mahowald & Schenck, 2005; Schenck et al., 1986).

Clinical features

RBD is more commonly seen in older adults with a reported mean age of onset of about 60 years and is more common in males (Ohayon et al., 1997; Olson et al., 2000). The disease may present in acute or chronic forms. The acute form of the disease occurs in association with drug withdrawal states, most commonly withdrawal from alcohol (ethanol). It is also described as a side effect of some drugs, such as tricyclic antidepressants, monoamine oxidase inhibitors, fluoxetine, venlafaxine, and excessive caffeine intake (Mahowald et al., 2005). The chronic form of the disease may be idiopathic and appears in apparently healthy individuals or occurs in association with neurological disorders like Parkinson's disease, dementia, and other degenerative central nervous system diseases (Friedman, 2002; Gagnon et al., 2002; Seyd et al., 2003). RBD has been reported by some investigators as a harbinger of neurodegenerative central nervous system disorders preceding the clinical onset of diseases such as Parkinson's disease and dementia (Mahowald, 2006; Turner, 2002). A recent imaging study of cognitively intact RBD patients reported abnormal PET scan findings involving the regions of the brain normally affected by dementia of Alzheimer's type and Lewy body dementia (Caselli et al., 2006). Such observations support the notion that RBD, in otherwise normal people, may indicate the future onset of a neurodegenerative disease. RBD usually has an insidious onset, starting with sleep talking, yelling, and jerking movements of the extremities for years before the violent behavior is manifested. The dream is reported to become more vivid and violent as the disorder progresses.

Patients usually present to the clinic with their bed partners, and a more detailed history of the events is obtained from the bed partner than the patient. Patients may present to physicians with signs of injury (echymoses, lacerations, bruises, etc.) to themselves or their bed partner. Diagnosis is based on history and confirmed by over night PSG with video recording, where increased muscle (electromyographic) activity and abnormal movements are observed during REM sleep period. The differential diagnosis includes nocturnal seizures, sleep walking, sleep terror, and related disorders.

Treatment

Management of RBD includes both nonpharmacological and pharmacological interventions. The nonpharmacological measures are directed at avoiding injury, for example, placing a cushion around the bed, mattress on the floor, low

beds if available, and other related measures. Drugs that are known to exacerbate symptoms of RBD should be replaced when possible. The drug most frequently used to treat RBD is clonazepam. It is given at bedtime, and therapeutic
response is generally reported within the first week (Mahowald MW 2005).
Preliminary clinical studies, including one small randomized controlled trial,
have reported successful use of melatonin for treatment of RBD (Boeve et al.,
2003; Kunz et al., 2006; Takeuchi et al., 2001). Given the side effects associated with the use of a long-acting benzodiazepine like clonazepam, melatonin
may be a safer alternative for frail older adults if the findings of these studies
are confirmed. Other drugs reported to be useful for treatment of RBD include
donezepil (Ringman & Simmons, 2000) and pramipexole (Fantini et al., 2003;
Schmidt et al., 2006). These studies are limited by nonrandom allocation of
treatment and small sample sizes.

USE OF SLEEP-PROMOTING AGENTS IN LONG-TERM CARE

The long-term use of sedative hypnotics in LTC residents remains a controversial issue for many reasons. There is no evidence to guide long-term use of these
medications as all clinical trials involving older adults lasted less than 4 weeks
(Glass et al., 2005). Consequently, information about outcome of treatment
(risk-benefit ratio) is not available. This is in contrast to young and middle-aged
adults with insomnia, in which treatment with eszopiclone (Lunesta) continued
for 6 months showed beneficial effect on nighttime sleep with no significant
adverse effect during the day (Krystal et al., 2003). On the other hand, among
older adults the possibility that these medications may not be effective for long-
term use has been reported (Monane et al., 1996). In addition, use of hypnotics
is reported to be associated with undesired effects such as daytime sleepiness,
cognitive impairment, falls and related injuries, and worsening of undiagnosed
OSAH (Benca, 2005; Buffet-Jerott & Stewart, 2002; Rubenstein et al., 1994;
Toner et al., 2000). A recent meta-analysis has shown that short-term (less than
4 weeks) use of sedative hypnotics, including nonbenzodiazepine hypnotics, are
associated with a small but significant improvement in sleep and also relevant
adverse events (Glass et al., 2005), indicating that even when used for a short
period of time, the use of these medications in the elderly may be associated
with significant adverse effects. But despite the lack of evidence, long-term use
of sedative hypnotics is common among nursing home residents with prevalence
of hypnotic use ranging from 10% to 24% (Gobert & D'Hoore, 2005; James,
1985; Opedal et al., 1998).

Table 7.3 shows selected commonly used FDA-approved hypnotics and their
half-life (Bain, 2006). In general, the use of sedative-hypnotics with long duration of action may be associated with undesired effect the next day and should

TABLE 7.3. Selected FDA-Approved Hypnotics with Their Duration
of Action

MEDICATION	DURATION OF ACTION (H)	MEAN HALF-LIFE (H)
Benzodiazepines		
Estazolam	6–10	15
Flurazepam	10–20	75
Temazepam	6–10	9
Nonbenzodiazepines		
Zolpidem	3–8	2.5
Zolpidem CR	3–8	2.8
Zaleplon	2–4	1
Eszopiclone	5–8	6
Melatonin agonist		
Ramelteon	6–8	2

Source: Bain (2006).

be avoided. On the other hand, the effect of short-acting drugs may wear off
in the middle of the night and may not prevent awakenings from sleep. For
this reason, therapy should be individualized depending on the type and timing
of the sleep related symptom. In addition, long-term use of these medications
should be discouraged until evidence about the risk-benefit ratio is available.

A more recent addition to the list of hypnotics is ramelteon (Rozerem), a
melatonin receptor agonist. This drug has been shown to decrease sleep latency
(time to fall asleep) and increase TST in the elderly, but it had no significant
effect on number of awakenings and difficulty going back to sleep (Roth et al.,
2006). This suggests that the drug may not be suitable for treatment of sleep
maintenance insomnia, a common problem among LTC residents. There are no
published reports on whether ramelteon has any significant effect in shifting the
circadian rhythm.

A readily available and more commonly used sleep aid among older adults is
melatonin. Melatonin is a hormone synthesized and secreted by the pineal gland
and controlled by the suprachiasmatic nuclei. During daylight period, output from
the SCN inhibits melatonin synthesis, whereas secretion is stimulated during the
night (Caustrat et al., 2005). In humans, endogenous melatonin is closely related
to sleep period and is described to promote sleep. Decreased serum levels of
melatonin has been reported in nursing home residents and community dwelling
older adults complaining of insomnia, suggesting that low melatonin level may
contribute to sleep problems in this group of individuals (Haimov et al., 1994).
But the effect of exogenous melatonin on sleep quality in subjects with insomnia

has yielded conflicting results. One meta-analysis reported no beneficial effect of exogenous melatonin on sleep quality (Buscemi et al., 2006), whereas another meta-analysis indicated a modest beneficial effect (Brezinski et al., 2005). These studies included subjects of all ages, and thus the generalizability of these results to LTC facility residents may be questioned. Among older adults with low melatonin level and insomnia complaints, one double-blind placebo-controlled study showed that physiological dose of melatonin (0.3 mg) increased serum melatonin level as well as sleep efficiency (Zhdanova et al., 2001). Another randomized and placebo-controlled study using 2.5 and 10 mg of melatonin in subjects with Alzheimer's disease failed to show significant improvement in sleep quantity and quality (Singer et al., 2003). Overall, because of these conflicting results, there is no consensus on the use of melatonin for treatment of insomnia. But it is possible that older adults with insomnia complaints and low melatonin level may benefit from treatment with physiological dose of melatonin.

One last issue that should be mentioned on the use of sedative-hypnotics among older adults is a recent report in which insomnia, and not hypnotic use was found to be independently associated with falls in nursing home residents (Avidan et al., 2005). This finding suggests that previous reports of associations between sedative-hypnotic use and falls may be confounded by insomnia. The data in this study were obtained from the Minimum Data Set collected in nursing homes in Michigan; and presence or absence of insomnia was determined based on a couple of sleep-related questions in the Minimum Data Set. However, the validity of these sleep relate questions to measure insomnia was not clearly established. For this reason, it is difficult to know to what extent these sleep-related questions measure what they are supposed to measure (insomnia in this case). More research may be required before a definite conclusion can be made on this issue.

USE OF BRIGHT LIGHT THERAPY IN LONG-TERM CARE

Light therapy has been used for treatment of insomnia related to disorders of the circadian rhythm. Under normal circumstances, light from the environment activates the melanopsin photoreceptors in the retina, which then discharge impulses to the suprachiasmatic nuclei via the retino-hypothalamic tract (Peirson & Foster, 2006). This input is important in synchronizing and consolidating the activity of the SCN and the circadian rhythm (Monk & Welsh, 2003). In addition, light exposure can also advance (shift to earlier period) or delay (shift to a later period) the circadian rhythm according to the time of light exposure. For example, light exposure during early evening period delays the circadian rhythm, whereas light exposure during the early morning hours advances the rhythm. Accordingly, bright light treatment is indicated for subjects who have advanced sleep phase or delayed sleep phase syndrome (Cheeson et al, 1999).

Bright light therapy has also been used for improving sleep and behavioral problems among patients with dementia, but the results have not shown consistent beneficial effects. Exposure to bright light may also improve the sleep-wake pattern of nursing home residents who are not exposed to adequate bright light during the day (Chesson et al., 1999). In general, a minimum of 2500 lux bright light for 3 to 4 h is recommended. However, treatment of LTC facility residents with bright light therapy has not shown beneficial effect consistently across studies as described earlier in the chapter. Factors that may contribute to these conflicting results may include differences in the dose, time, and duration of light therapy used in the different studies, as well as ocular lens and retinal pathology in some subjects that may interfere with light transmission. Further research is needed to standardize light therapy in long-term facility settings and evaluate its effects on the quantity and quality of sleep.

In summary, sleep–wake disturbance is common among LTC residents with multifactorial etiology, and its successful management requires a multifaceted approach, which include

- Improving the LTC facility environment: Instituting sleep and wake promoting conditions and practices in the LTC facility such as adequate daytime light exposure, ample physical and social activities, limiting noise and light during the night, improving sleep hygeine of LTC facility residents by avoiding staying in bed for a long time, and establishing reasonable bedtime and wake time schedules that would take into consideration the needs of LTC facility administration as well as the residents.
- Comprehensive evaluation of sleep complaints to identify the possible cause or causes of sleep related problems. This would require training of physicians, nurses and nursing assistants on recognizing the manifestations of common sleep disorders and management of these disorders. Appropriate referral to a sleep specialist may be necessary in selected cases.
- Judicious use of hypnotics for short term treatment of insomnia.

Successful implementation of a multi-faceted approach to the management of sleep-wake problems entails active participation of the administrative and nursing staff as well as the treating physician. Educational sessions for the administrative and the nursing staff about the importance of sleep problems in general and the approach to their management in LTC facilities would go a long way in making this plan a reality.

REFERENCES

Alessi, C. A., Martin, J. L., Webber, A. P., Cynthia Kim, E., Harker, J. O., & Josephson, K. R. (2005). Randomized, controlled trial of a nonpharmacological intervention to improve abnormal sleep/wake patterns in nursing home residents. *Journal of the American Geriatrics Society, 53,* 803–810.

Allen, R. P., Barker, P. B., Wehrl, F., Song, H. K., & Earley, C. J. (2001). MRI measurement of brain iron in patients with restless legs syndrome. *Neurology, 56,* 263–265.

Allen, R. P., & Earley, C. J. (2001). Restless legs syndrome: A review of clinical and pathophysiologic features. *Journal of Clinical Neurophysiology, 18,* 128–147.

Allen, R. P., Picchietti, D., Hening, W. A., et al. (2003). Restless legs syndrome: Diagnostic criteria, special considerations, and epidemiology: A report from the restless legs syndrome diagnosis and epidemiology workshop at the National Institutes of Health. *Sleep Medicine, 4,* 101–119.

Allen, R. P., Walters, A. S., Montplaisir, J., et al. (2005). Restless legs syndrome prevalence and impact: REST general population study. *Archives of Internal Medicine, 165,* 1286–1292.

American Academy of Sleep Medicine. (2003). Sleep-related breathing disorders in adults: Recommendations for syndrome definition and measurement techniques in clinical research. *Sleep, 22,* 667–689.

American Academy of Sleep Medicine. (2005a). *Insomnia. International classification of sleep disorders* Diagnostic and Coding Manual. Westchester, IL: 2005.

American Academy of Sleep Medicine. (2005b). *Obstructive sleep apnea syndromes. The international classification of sleep disorders. Diagnostic and coding manual.* Westchester, IL: 2005.

American Academy of Sleep Medicine Task Force. (1999). Sleep-related breathing disorders in adults: Recommendations for syndrome definition and measurement techniques in clinical research. The report of an American Academy of Sleep Medicine Task Force. *Sleep, 22,* 667–689.

Ancoli-Israel, S., Gehrman, P., Martin, J. L., et al. (2003). Increased light exposure consolidates sleep and strengthens circadian rhythms in severe Alzheimer's disease patients. *Behavioral Sleep Medicine, 1,* 22–36.

Ancoli-Israel, S., Klauber, M. R., Butters, N., Parker, L., & Kripke, D. F. (1991). Dementia in institutionalized elderly: Relation to sleep apnea. *Journal of the American Geriatrics Society, 39,* 258–263.

Ancoli-Israel, S., Palmer, B., Loredo, J., Corey-Bloom, J., Marler, M., & Greenfield, G. (2005). CPAP improves cognitive function in Alzheimer's disease patients with sleep apnea: Preliminary results. *Sleep, 28,* A110 (0325; Abstract supplement).

Ancoli-Israel, S., Parker, L., Sinaee, R., Fell, R. L., & Kripke, D. F. (1989). Sleep fragmentation in patients from a nursing home. *Journal of Gerontology, 44,* 18–21.

Arnulf, I. (2005). Excessive daytime sleepiness in Parkinsonism. *Sleep Medicine Reviews, 9,* 185–200.

Avidan, A. Y., Fries, B. E., James, M. L., Szafara, K. L., Wright, G. T., & Chervin, R. D. (2005). Insomnia and hypnotic use, recorded in the minimum data set, as predictors of falls and hip fractures in Michigan nursing homes. *Journal of American Geriatric Society, 53,* 955–962.

Ayalon, L., Ancoli-Israel, S., Stepnowsky, C., et al. (2006). Adherence to continuous positive airway pressure treatment in patients with Alzheimer's disease and obstructive sleep apnea. *American Journal of Geriatric Psychiatry, 14,* 176–180.

Bachman, D., & Rabins, P. (2006). "Sundowning" and other temporally associated agitation states in dementia patients. *Annual Review of Medicine, 57,* 499–511.

Badr, M. S. (2005). Central sleep apnea. Primary care. *Clinics in Office Practice, 32,* 361–374.

Bain, K. T. (2006). Management of chronic insomnia in elderly persons. *American Journal of Geriatric Pharmacotherapy, 4,* 168–192.

Bakshi, R. (1996). Fluoxetine and restless legs syndrome. *Journal of Neurological Sciences, 142,* 151–152.

Barriere, G., Cazalets, J. R., Bioulac, B., Tison, F., & Ghorayeb, I. (2005). The restless legs syndrome. *Progress in Neurobiology, 77,* 139–165.

Benca, R. M. (2005). Mood disorders. In M. H. Kryger, T. Roth, & W. C. Dement (Eds.), *Principles and practice of sleep medicine* (pp. 1315–1316). Philadelphia: Elsevier Saunders.

Benca, R. M. (2005). Diagnosis and treatment of chronic insomnia: A review [see comment]. *Psychiatric Services, 56,* 332–343.

Berger, K., Luedemann, J., Trenkwalder, C., John, U., & Kessler, C. (2004). Sex and the risk of restless legs syndrome in the general population. *Archives of Internal Medicine, 164,* 196–202.

Bliwise, D. L. (1993). Sleep in normal aging and dementia. *Sleep, 16,* 40–81.

Bliwise, D. L. (1994). What is sundowning? *Journal of the American Geriatrics Society, 42,* 1009–1011.

Bliwise, D. L., Adelman, C. L., & Ouslander, J. G. (2004). Polysomnographic correlates of spontaneous nocturnal wetness episodes in incontinent geriatric patients. *Sleep, 27,* 153–157.

Bliwise, D. L., Bevier, W. C., Bliwise, N. G., Edgar, D. M., & Dement, W. C. (1990a). Systematic 24-hr behavioral observations of sleep and wakefulness in a skilled-care nursing facility. *Psychology and Aging, 5,* 16–24.

Bliwise, D. L., Carroll, J. S., & Dement, W. C. (1990b). Predictors of observed sleep/wakefulness in residents in long-term care. *Journal of Gerontology, 45,* 126–130.

Bliwise, D. L., Freeman, A., Ingram, C. D., Rye, D. B., Chakravorty, S., & Watts, R. L. (2005). Randomized, double-blind, placebo-controlled, short-term trial of ropinirole in restless legs syndrome. *Sleep Medicine, 6,* 141–147.

Boeve, B. F., Silber, M. H., & Ferman, T. J. (2003). Melatonin for treatment of REM sleep behavior disorder in neurologic disorders: Results in 14 patients. *Sleep Medicine, 4,* 281–284.

Bogan, R. K., Fry, J. M., Schmidt, M. H., Carson, S. W., Ritchie, S. Y., & Group TRUS. (2006). Ropinirole in the treatment of patients with restless legs syndrome: A US-based randomized, double-blind, placebo-controlled clinical trial. *Mayo Clinic Proceedings, 81,* 17–27.

Bonnet, M., Carley, D., Carskadon, M., et al. (1993). Recording and scoring leg movements. The Atlas Task Force. *Sleep, 16,* 748–759.

Bradley, T. D., & Floras, J. S. (2003a). Sleep apnea and heart failure: Part I: Obstructive sleep apnea. *Circulation, 107,* 1671–1678.

Bradley, T. D., & Floras, J. S. (2003b). Sleep apnea and heart failure: Part II: Central sleep apnea. *Circulation, 107,* 1822–1826.

Breslau, N., Roth, T., Rosenthal, L., & Andreski, P. (1996). Sleep disturbance and psychiatric disorders: A longitudinal epidemiological study of young adults. *Biological Psychiatry, 39,* 411–418.

Brezinski, A., Vangel, M. G., Wurtman, R. J., Norrie, G., Zhdanova, I., Ben-Shushan, B., et al. (2005). Effects of exogenous melatonin on sleep: A meta analysis. *Sleep Medicine Reviews, 9,* 41–50.

Broderick, E. (1997). Prescribing patterns for nursing home residents in the US. The reality and the vision. *Drugs and Aging, 11,* 255–260.

Bucca, C., Carossa, S., Pivetti, S., Gai, V., Rolla, G., & Preti, G. (1999). Edentulism and worsening of obstructive sleep apnoea. *Lancet, 353,* 121–122.

Bucca, C., Cicolin, A., Brussino, L., et al. (2006). Tooth loss and obstructive sleep apnea. *Respiratory Research, 7,* 8.

Buffett-Jerrott, S. E., & Stewart, S. H. (2002). Cognitive and sedative effects of benzodiazepine use. *Current Pharmaceutical Design, 8,* 45–58.

Burchell, B. J. (2003). Treatment of restless legs syndrome with gabapentin: A double-blind, cross-over study. *Neurology, 60,* 1558.

Buscemi, N., Vandemeer, B., Hooton, N., et al. (2006). Efficacy and safety of exogenous melatonin for secondary sleep disorders and sleep disorders accompanying sleep restriction: Meta-analysis. *BMJ, 332,* 385–393.

Buysse, D. J., Reynolds, C. F., 3rd, Kupfer, D. J., et al. (1994). Clinical diagnoses in 216 insomnia patients using the International Classification of Sleep Disorders (ICSD), *DSM-IV* and ICD-10 categories: A report from the APA/NIMH *DSM-IV* Field Trial. *Sleep, 17,* 630–637.

Carskadon, M. W. D. (2005). Normal human sleep. In M. H. Kryger, T. Roth, & W. C. Dement (Eds.), *Principles and practice of sleep medicine* (pp. 13–24). Philadelphia: Elsevier Saunders.

Caselli, R. J., Kewel, C., Bandy, D., et al. (2006). A preliminary fluorodeoxyglucose positron emission tomography study in health adults reporting dream-enactment behavior. *Sleep, 29,* 927–933.

Caustrat, B., Brun, J., & Chazot, G. (2005). The basic physiology and pathophysiology of melatonin. *Sleep Medicine Reviews, 9,* 11–24.

Cheeson, A. L., Littner, M., Davila, D., et al. (1999). Practice parameters for the use of light therapy in the treatment of sleep disorders. *Sleep, 22,* 641–660.

Chesson, A. L., Jr., Wise, M., Davila, D., et al. (1999). Practice parameters for the treatment of restless legs syndrome and periodic limb movement disorder. An American Academy of Sleep Medicine report. Standards of Practice Committee of the American Academy of Sleep Medicine. *Sleep, 22,* 961–968.

Cohen, D., Eisdorfer, C., Prinz, P., Breen, A., Davis, M., & Gadsby, A. (1983). Sleep disturbances in the institutionalized aged. *Journal of the American Geriatrics Society, 31,* 79–82.

Comella, C. L. (2002). Restless legs syndrome: Treatment with dopaminergic agents. *Neurology, 58*(4 Suppl 1), S87–S92.

Connor, J. R., Boyer, P. J., Menzies, S. L., et al. (2003). Neuropathological examination suggests impaired brain iron acquisition in restless legs syndrome. *Neurology, 61,* 304–309.

Cusack, B. J. (2004). Pharmacokinetics in older persons. *American Journal of Geriatric Pharmacotherapy, 2,* 274–302.

Dimmitt, S. B., & Riley, G. J. (2000). Selective serotonin receptor uptake inhibitors can reduce restless legs symptoms. *Archives of Internal Medicine, 160,* 712.

Dingli, K., Coleman, E. L., Vennelle, S. P., et al. (2003). Evaluation of a portable device for diagnosing the sleep apnea/hypopnea syndrome. *European Respiratory Journal, 21,* 253–259.

Dowling, G. A., Mastick, J., Hubbard, E. M., Luxenberg, J. S., & Burr, R. L. (2005). Effect of timed bright light treatment for rest-activity disruption in institutionalized patients with Alzheimer's disease. *International Journal of Geriatric Psychiatry, 20,* 738–743.

Drewes, A. M., Nielsen, K. D., Arendt-Nielsen, L., Birket-Smith, L., & Hansen, L. M. (1997). The effect of cutaneous and deep pain on the electroencephalogram during sleep—an experimental study. *Sleep, 20,* 632–640.

Duffy, J. F., & Wright, K. P., Jr. (2005). Entrainment of the human circadian system by light. *Journal of Biological Rhythms, 20*, 326–338.

Earley, C. J. (2003). Clinical practice. Restless legs syndrome. *New England Journal of Medicine, 348*, 2103–2109.

Earley, C. J., Connor, J. R., Beard, J. L., Clardy, S. L., & Allen, R. P. (2005). Ferritin levels in the cerebrospinal fluid and restless legs syndrome: Effects of different clinical phenotypes. *Sleep, 28*, 1069–1075.

Endeshaw, Y. (2006). Clinical characteristics of obstructive sleep apnea in community dwelling older adults. *Journal of the American Geriatrics Society, 54*, 1740–1744.

Endeshaw, Y., Katz, S., & Ouslander, J. B. D. (2004). Association between sleep-disordered breathing and denture use. *Journal of Public Health Dentistry, 64*, 181–183.

Endeshaw, Y., Ouslander, J., Schnelle, J., & Bliwise, D. (2007). Polysomnographic and clinical correlates of behaviorally observed daytime sleep in nursing home residents. *Journal of Gerontology Medical Sciences, 62A*, 55–61.

Endeshaw, Y. W., Johnson, T. M., Kutner, M. H., Ouslander, J. G., & Bliwise, D. L. (2004). Sleep-disordered breathing and nocturia in older adults. *Journal of the American Geriatrics Society, 52*, 957–960.

Fantini, M. L., Gagnon, J. F., Filipini, D., & Montplaisir, J. (2003). The effects of pramipexole in REM sleep behavior disorder. *Neurology, 61*, 1418–1420.

Ferrell, B. A. (1995). Pain evaluation and management in the nursing home. *Annals of Internal Medicine, 123*, 681–687.

Ferrell, B. A., Ferrell, B. R., & Rivera, L. (1995). Pain in cognitively impaired nursing home patients. *Journal of Pain and Symptom Management, 10*, 591–598.

Fetveit, A., & Bjorvatn, B. (2002). Sleep disturbances among nursing home residents. *International Journal of Geriatric Psychiatry, 17*, 604–609.

Field, T. S., Gurwitz, J. H., Avorn, J., et al. (2001). Risk factors for adverse drug events among nursing home residents. *Archives of Internal Medicine, 161*, 1629–1634.

Foley, D. J., Monjan, A. A., Brown, S. L., Simonsick, E. M., Wallace, R. B., & Blazer, D. G. (1995). Sleep complaints among elderly persons: An epidemiologic study of three communities. *Sleep, 18*, 425–432.

Forbes, D., Morgan, D. G., Bangma, J., Peacock, S., & Adamson, J. (2007). Light therapy for managing sleep, behaviour, and mood disturbances in dementia. *Cochrane Database Systemic Review, 1*.

Ford, D. E., & Kamerow, D. B. (1989). Epidemiologic study of sleep disturbances and psychiatric disorders. An opportunity for prevention? *JAMA, 262*, 1479–1484.

Friedman, J. H. (2002). Presumed rapid eye movement behavior disorder in Machado-Joseph disease (spinocerebellar ataxia type 3). *Movement Disorders, 17*, 1350–1353.

Gagnon, J. F., Bedard, M. A., Fantini, M. L., et al. (2002). REM sleep behavior disorder and REM sleep without atonia in Parkinson's disease. *Neurology, 59*, 585–589.

Gami, A. S., Howard, D. E., Olson, E. J., & Somers, V. K. (2005). Day-night pattern of sudden death in obstructive sleep apnea. *New England Journal of Medicine, 352*, 1206–1214.

Garcia-Borreguero, D., Egatz, R., Winkelmann, J., & Berger, K. (2006). Epidemiology of restless legs syndrome: The current status. *Sleep Medicine Reviews, 10*, 153–168.

Gentili, A., Weiner, D. K., Kuchibhatil, M., & Edinger, J. D. (1997). Factors that disturb sleep in nursing home residents. *Aging-Clinical and Experimental Research, 9*, 207–213.

Gerber, P. D., Barrett, J. E., Barrett, J. A., et al. (1992). The relationship of presenting physical complaints to depressive symptoms in primary care patients. *Journal of General Internal Medicine, 7*, 170–173.

Glass, J., Lanctot, K. L., Herrmann, N., Sproule, B. A., & Busto, U. E. (2005). Sedative hypnotics in older people with insomnia: Meta-analysis of risks and benefits. *BMJ, 331,* 1169.

Gobert, M., & D'Hoore, W. (2005). Prevalence of psychotropic drug use in nursing homes for the aged in Quebec and in the French-speaking area of Switzerland. *International Journal of Geriatric Psychiatry, 20,* 712–721.

Haimov, I., Laudon, M., Zisapel, N., et al. (1994). Sleep disorders and melatonin rhythms in elderly people. *BMJ, 309,* 167.

Happe, S., Sauter, C., Klosch, G., Saletu, B., & Zeitlhofer, J. (2003). Gabapentin versus ropinirole in the treatment of idiopathic restless legs syndrome. *Neuropsychobiology, 48,* 82–86.

Hargrave, R., & Beckley, D. J. (1998). Restless leg syndrome exacerbated by sertraline. *Psychosomatics, 39,* 177–178.

Hening, W., Allen, R., Earley, C., Kushida, C., Picchietti, D., & Silber, M. (1999). The treatment of restless legs syndrome and periodic limb movement disorder. An American Academy of Sleep Medicine review. *Sleep, 22,* 970–999.

Herrlinger, C., & Klotz, U. (2001). Drug metabolism and drug interactions in the elderly. *Best Practices and Research. Clinical Gastroenterology, 15,* 897–918.

Hornyak, M., Feige, B., & Riemann, D. U. V. (2006). Periodic leg movements in sleep and periodic leg movement disorder: Prevalence, clinical significance and treatment. *Sleep Medicine Reviews, 10,* 169–178.

Jacobs, D., Ancoli-Israel, S., Parker, L., & Kripke, D. F. (1989). Twenty-four-hour sleep-wake patterns in a nursing home population. *Psychology and Aging, 4,* 352–356.

James, D. S. (1985). Survey of hypnotic drug use in nursing homes. *Journal of the American Geriatrics Society, 33,* 436–439.

Jones, R. N., Marcantonio, E. R., & Rabinowitz, T. (2003). Prevalence and correlates of recognized depression in U.S. nursing homes. *Journal of the American Geriatrics Society, 51,* 1404–1409.

Jongenelis, K., Pot, A. M., Eisses, A. M. H., Beekman, A. T. F., Kluiter, H., & Ribbe, M. W. (2004). Prevalence and risk indicators of depression in elderly nursing home patients: The AGED study. *Journal of Affective Disorders, 83,* 135–142.

Krystal, A. D., Walsh, J. K., Laska, E., et al. (2003). Sustained efficacy of eszopiclone over 6 months of nightly treatment: Results of randomized, double blind, placebo-controlled study in adults with chronic insomnia. *Sleep, 26,* 793–799.

Kunz, D. B. F., Mueller, C., & Mahberg, R. (2006). A controlled clinical trial of melatonin in RBD patients. *Sleep, 29*(Abstract suppl.), 0795–0270.

Labrecque, G., & Vanier, M. C. (1995). Biological rhythms in pain and in the effects of opioid analgesics. *Pharmacology and Therapeutics, 68,* 129–147.

Lavie, L. (2005). Sleep-disordered breathing and cerebrovascular disease: A mechanistic approach. *Neurologic Clinics, 23,* 1059–1075.

Lindblad, C. I., Hanlon, J. T., Gross, C. R., et al. (2006). Clinically important drug–disease interactions and their prevalence in older adults. *Clinical Therapeutics, 28,* 1133–1143.

Littner, M. R., Kushida, C., Anderson, W. M., et al. (2004). Practice parameters for the dopaminergic treatment of restless legs syndrome and periodic limb movement disorder. *Sleep, 27,* 557–559.

Livingston, G., Blizard, B., & Mann, A. (1993). Does sleep disturbance predict depression in elderly people? A study in inner London. *British Journal of General Practice, 43,* 445–448.

Madhusoodanan, S., & Bogunovic, O. J. (2004). Safety of benzodiazepines in the geriatric population. *Expert Opinion on Drug Safety, 3,* 485–493.

Mahowald, M. (2006). Does "idiopathic" REM sleep behavior disorder exist? *Sleep, 29,* 874–875.

Mahowald, M. W., & Schenck, C. H. (2005). REM sleep parasomnias. In M. H. Kryger, T. Roth, & W. C. Dement (Eds.), *Principles and practice of sleep medicine* (4th ed., pp. 897–916). Philadelphia: Elsevier Saunders.

Malhotra, A., Huang, Y., Fogel, R., et al. (2006). Aging influences on pharyngeal anatomy and physiology: The predisposition to pharyngeal collapse. *American Journal of Medicine, 119,* 72.e9–72.e14.

Martin, S. E., Mathur, R., Marshall, I., & Douglas, N. J. (1997). The effect of age, sex, obesity and posture on upper airway size. *European Respiratory Journal, 10,* 2087–2090.

Mata, I. F., Bodkin, C. L., Adler, C. H., et al. (2006). Genetics of restless legs syndrome. *Parkinsonism Related Disorders, 12,* 1–7.

McGaffigan, S., & Bliwise, D. L. (1997). The treatment of sundowning. A selective review of pharmacological and nonpharmacological studies. *Drugs and Aging, 10,* 10–17.

Micozkadioglu, H., Ozdemir, F. N., Kut, A., Sezer, S., Saatci, U., & Haberal, M. (2004). Gabapentin versus levodopa for the treatment of restless legs syndrome in hemodialysis patients: An open-label study. *Renal Failure, 26,* 393–397.

Mistlberger, R. E., & Skene, D. J. (2005). Nonphotic entrainment in humans? *Journal of Biological Rhythms, 20,* 339–352.

Monane, M., Glynn, R. J., & Avorn, J. (1996, January). The impact of sedative-hypnotic use on sleep symptoms in elderly nursing home residents. *Clinical Pharmacology and Therapeutics, 59,* 83–92.

Monk, T. H. (2005). Aging human circadian rhythms: Conventional wisdom may not always be right. *Journal of Biological Rhythms, 20,* 366–374.

Monk, T. H., & Welsh, D. K. (2003). The role of chronobiology in sleep disorders medicine. *Sleep Medicine Reviews, 7,* 455–473.

Montplaisir, J., Lorrain, D., & Godbout, R. (1991). Restless legs syndrome and periodic leg movements in sleep: The primary role of dopaminergic mechanism. *European Neurology, 31,* 41–43.

Morin, C. M., Mimeault, V., & Gagne, A. (1999). Nonpharmacological treatment of late-life insomnia. *Journal of Psychosomatic Research, 46,* 103–116.

Munch, M., Knoblauch, V., Blatter, K., et al. (2005). Age-related attenuation of the evening circadian arousal signal in humans. *Neurobiology of Aging, 26,* 1307–1319.

Nygaard, H. A., Naik, M., Ruths, S., & Straand, J. (2003). Nursing-home residents and their drug use: A comparison between mentally intact and mentally impaired residents. The Bergen District Nursing Home (BEDNURS) study. *European Journal of Clinical Pharmacology, 59,* 463–469.

Ohayon, M. M., Carskadon, M. A., Guilleminault, C., & Vitiello, M. V. (2004). Meta-analysis of quantitative sleep parameters from childhood to old age in healthy individuals: Developing normative sleep values across the human lifespan [see comment]. *Sleep, 27,* 1255–1273.

Ohayon, M. M., Caulet, M., & Priest, R. G. (1997). Violent behavior during sleep. *Journal of Clinical Psychiatry, 58,* 369–376.

O'Keeffe, S. T. (2005). Secondary causes of restless legs syndrome in older people. *Age and Ageing, 34,* 349–352.

Oliven, A., Carmi, N., Coleman, R., Odeh, M., & Silbermann, M. (2001). Age-related changes in upper airway muscles morphological and oxidative properties. *Experimental Gerontology, 36,* 1673–1686.

Olson, E. J., Boeve, B. F., & Silber, M. H. (2000). Rapid eye movement sleep behaviour disorder: Demographic, clinical and laboratory findings in 93 cases. *Brain, 123*(Pt 2), 331–339.

Opedal, K., Schjott, J., & Eide, E. (1998). Use of hypnotics among patients in geriatric institutions. *International Journal of Geriatric Psychiatry, 13*, 846–851.

Ouslander, J. G., Connell, B. R., Bliwise, D. L., Endeshaw, Y., Griffiths, P., & Schnelle, J. F. (2006). A nonpharmacological intervention to improve sleep in nursing home patients: Results of a controlled clinical trial. *Journal of the American Geriatrics Society, 54*, 38–47.

Ouslander, J. G., Palmer, M. H., Rovner, B. W., & German, P. S. (1993). Urinary incontinence in nursing homes: Incidence, remission and associated factors. *Journal of the American Geriatrics Society, 41*, 1083–1089.

Pat-Horenczyk, R., Klauber, M. R., Shochat, T., & Ancoli-Israel, S. (1998). Hourly profiles of sleep and wakefulness in severely versus mild-moderately demented nursing home patients. *Aging-Clinical and Experimental Research, 10*, 308–315.

Peirson, S., & Foster, R. G. (2006). Melanopsin: Another way of signaling light. *Neuron, 49*, 331–339.

Pepin, J. L., Chouri-Pontarollo, N., Tamisier, R., & Levy, P. (2006). Cheyne-Stokes respiration with central sleep apnoea in chronic heart failure: Proposals for a diagnostic and therapeutic strategy. *Sleep Medicine Reviews, 10*, 33–47.

Phillips, B., Young, T., Finn, L., Asher, K., Hening, W. A., & Purvis, C. (2000). Epidemiology of restless legs symptoms in adults. *Archives of Internal Medicine, 160*, 2137–2141.

Picchietti, D., & Winkelman, J. W. (2005). Restless legs syndrome, periodic limb movements in sleep, and depression. *Sleep, 28*, 891–898.

Pilowsky, I., Crettenden, I., & Townley, M. (1985). Sleep disturbance in pain clinic patients. *Pain, 23*, 27–33.

Pollak, C. P., & Perlick, D. (1991). Sleep problems and institutionalization of the elderly. *Journal of Geriatric Psychiatry and Neurology, 4*, 204–210.

Prinz, P. N., Peskind, E. R., Vitaliano, P. P., et al. (1982). Changes in the sleep and waking EEGs of nondemented and demented elderly subjects. *Journal of the American Geriatrics Society, 30*, 86–93.

Quan, S. F., Gersh, B. J., National Center on Sleep Disorders Research, National Heart, Lung, and Blood Institute. (2004). Cardiovascular consequences of sleep-disordered breathing: Past, present and future: Report of a workshop from the National Center on Sleep Disorders Research and the National Heart, Lung, and Blood Institute. *Circulation, 109*, 951–957.

Rao, V., Spiro, J. R., Samus, Q. M., et al. (2005). Sleep disturbances in the elderly residing in assisted living: Findings from the Maryland Assisted Living Study. *International Journal of Geriatric Psychiatry, 20*, 956–966.

Redline, S., Kirchner, H. L., Quan, S. F., Gottlieb, D. J., Kapur, V., & Newman, A. (2004). The effects of age, sex, ethnicity, and sleep-disordered breathing on sleep architecture. *Archives of Internal Medicine, 164*, 406–418.

Ringman, J. M., & Simmons, J. H. (2000). Treatment of REM sleep behavior disorder with donepezil: A report of three cases. *Neurology, 55*, 870–871.

Roberts, R. E., Shema, S. J., Kaplan, G. A., & Strawbridge, W. J. (2000. Sleep complaints and depression in an aging cohort: A prospective perspective. *American Journal of Psychiatry, 157*, 81–88.

Roth, T., Seiden, D., Sainati, S., Wang-Weigand, S., Zhang, J., & Zee, P. (2006). Effects of ramelteon on patient-reported sleep latency in older adults with chronic insomnia. *Sleep Medicine, 7*, 312–318.

Rothdach, A. J., Trenkwalder, C., Haberstock, J., Keil, U., & Berger, K. (2000). Prevalence and risk factors of RLS in an elderly population: The MEMO study. Memory and morbidity in Augsburg elderly. *Neurology, 54*, 1064–1068.

Rubenstein, L. Z., Josephson, K. R., & Robbins, A. S. (1994). Falls in the nursing home. *Annals of Internal Medicine, 121*, 442–451.

Saletu, M., Anderer, P., Saletu, B., et al. (2000a). Sleep laboratory studies in restless legs syndrome patients as compared with normals and acute effects of ropinirole. 2. Findings on periodic leg movements, arousals and respiratory variables. *Neuropsychobiology, 41*, 190–199.

Saletu, M., Anderer, P., Saletu-Zyhlarz, G., Hauer, C., & Saletu, B. (2002). Acute placebo-controlled sleep laboratory studies and clinical follow-up with pramipexole in restless legs syndrome. *European Archives of Psychiatry and Clinical Neuroscience, 252*, 185–194.

Saletu, B., Gruber, G., Saletu, M., et al. (2000b). Sleep laboratory studies in restless legs syndrome patients as compared with normals and acute effects of ropinirole. 1. Findings on objective and subjective sleep and awakening quality. *Neuropsychobiology, 41*, 181–189.

Schenck, C. H., Bundlie, S. R., Ettinger, M. G., & Mahowald, M. W. (1986). Chronic behavioral disorders of human REM sleep: A new category of parasomnia. *Sleep, 9*, 293–308.

Schmidt, M. H., & Koshal, V. B., & Schmidt, H. S. (2006). Use of pramipexole in REM sleep behavior disorder: Results from a case series. *Sleep Medicine, 7*, 418–23.

Schnelle, J. F., Cruise, P. A., Alessi, C. A., Ludlow, K., al-Samarrai, N. R., & Ouslander, J. G. (1998). Sleep hygiene in physically dependent nursing home residents: Behavioral and environmental intervention implications. *Sleep, 21*, 515–523.

Shochat, T., Martin, J., Marler, M., & Ancoli-Israel, S. (2000). Illumination levels in nursing home patients: Effects on sleep and activity rhythms. *Journal of Sleep Research, 9*, 373–379.

Shochat, T., Oksenberg, A., Hadas, N., Molotsky, A., & Lavie, P. (2003). The KickStrip: A novel testing device for periodic limb movement disorder. *Sleep, 26*, 480–483.

Singer, C., Tractenberg, R. E., Kaye, J., et al. (2003). A multicenter, placebo-controlled trial of melatonin for sleep disturbance in Alzheimer's disease. *Sleep, 26*, 893–901.

Smith, I., & Lasserson, T. J. W. (2002). Drug treatments for obstructive sleep apnea. *Cochrane Database of Systematic Reviews, 4*.

Stopa, E. G., Volicer, L., Kuo-Leblanc, V., et al. (1999). Pathologic evaluation of the human suprachiasmatic nucleus in severe dementia. *Journal of Neuropathology and Experimental Neurology, 58*, 29–39.

Swaab, D. F., Fliers, E., & Partiman, T. S. (1985). The suprachiasmatic nucleus of the human brain in relation to sex, age and senile dementia. *Brain Research, 342*, 37–44.

Syed, B. H., Rye, D. B., & Singh, G. (2003). REM sleep behavior disorder and SCA-3 (Machado-Joseph disease). *Neurology, 60*, 148.

Takeuchi, N., Uchimura, N., Hashizume, Y., et al. (2001). Melatonin therapy for REM sleep behavior disorder. *Psychiatry and Clinical Neurosciences, 55*, 267–269.

Thorpy, M., Chesson, A., Ferber, R., et al. (1994). Practice parameters for the use of portable recording in the assessment of obstructive sleep apnea. *Sleep, 17*, 372–377.

Toner, L. C., Tsambiras, B. M., Catalano, G., Catalano, M. C., & Cooper, D. S. (2000). Central nervous system side effects associated with zolpidem treatment. *Clinical Neuropharmacology, 23,* 54–58.

Tractenberg, R. E., Singer, C. M., & Kaye, J. A. (2005). Symptoms of sleep disturbance in persons with Alzheimer's disease and normal elderly. *Journal of Sleep Research, 14,* 177–185.

Trenkwalder, C., Paulus, W., & Walters, A. S. (2005). The restless legs syndrome. *Lancet Neurology, 4,* 465–475.

Trenkwalder, C., Seidel, V. C., Gasser, T., & Oertel, W. H. (1996). Clinical symptoms and possible anticipation in a large kindred of familial restless legs syndrome. *Movement Disorders, 11,* 389–394.

Tribl, G. G., Sycha, T., Kotzailias, N., Zeitlhofer, J., & Auff, E. (2005). Apomorphine in idiopathic restless legs syndrome: An exploratory study. *Journal of Neurology, Neurosurgery, and Psychiatry, 76,* 181–185.

Turek, F., Dugovic, C., & Laposky, A. (2005). Master circadian clock, master circadian rhythm. In M. H. Kryger, T. Roth, & W. C. Dement (Eds.), *Principles and practice of sleep medicine* (pp. 318–321). Philadelphia: Elsevier Saunders.

Turner, R. S. (2002). Idiopathic rapid eye movement sleep behavior disorder is a harbinger of dementia with Lewy bodies. *Journal of Geriatric Psychiatry and Neurology, 15,* 195–199.

Van Kerrebroeck, P., Abrams, P., Chaikin, D., et al. (2002). The standardization of terminology in nocturia: Report from the standardization subcommittee of the International Continence Society. *BJU International, 90*(Suppl 3), 11–15.

Vitiello, M. V., Bokan, J. A., Kukull, W. A., Muniz, R. L., Smallwood, R. G., & Prinz, P. N. (1984). Rapid eye movement sleep measures of Alzheimer's-type dementia patients and optimally healthy aged individuals. *Biological Psychiatry, 19,* 721–734.

Vitiello, M. V., Moe, K. E., & Prinz, P. N. (2002). Sleep complaints cosegregate with illness in older adults: Clinical research informed by and informing epidemiological studies of sleep. *Journal of Psychosomatic Research, 53,* 555–559.

Vitiello, M. V., Prinz, P. N., Williams, D. E., Frommlet, M. S., & Ries, R. K. (1990). Sleep disturbances in patients with mild-stage Alzheimer's disease. *Journal of Gerontology, 45,* 131–138.

Volicer, L., Harper, D. G., Manning, B. C., Goldstein, R., & Satlin, A. (2001). Sundowning and circadian rhythms in Alzheimer's disease. *American Journal of Psychiatry, 158,* 704–711.

Voyer, P., Verreault, R., Mengue, P. N., & Morin, C. M. (2006). Prevalence of insomnia and its associated factors in elderly long-term care residents. *Archives of Gerontology and Geriatrics, 42,* 1–20.

Walters, A. S., Winkelmann, J., Trenkwalder, C., et al. (2001). Long-term follow-up on restless legs syndrome patients treated with opioids. *Movement Disorders, 16,* 1105–1109.

Wetter, T. C., Brunner, J., & Bronisch, T. (2002). Restless legs syndrome probably induced by risperidone treatment. *Pharmacopsychiatry, 35,* 109–111.

White, D. (2005). Central sleep apnea. In M. H. Kryger, T. Roth, & W. C. Dement (Eds.), *Principles and practice of sleep medicine* (pp. 969–982). Philadelphia: Elsevier Saunders.

Yaggi, H. K., Concato, J., Kernan, W. N., Lichtman, J. H., Brass, L. M., & Mohsenin, V. (2005). Obstructive sleep apnea as a risk factor for stroke and death. *New England Journal of Medicine, 353,* 2034–2041.

Young, T., Shahar, E., Nieto, F. J., et al. (2002). Predictors of sleep-disordered breathing in community-dwelling adults: The Sleep Heart Health Study. *Archives of Internal Medicine, 162,* 893–900.

Zhan, C., Correa-de-Araujo, R., Bierman, A. S., et al. (2005). Suboptimal prescribing in elderly outpatients: Potentially harmful drug–drug and drug–disease combinations. *Journal of the American Geriatrics Society, 53,* 262–267.

Zhdanova, I. V., Wurtman, R. J., Regan, M. M., Taylor, J. A., Shi, J. P., & Leclair, O. U. (2001). Melatonin treatment for age-related insomnia. *Journal of Clinical Endocrinology and Metabolism, 86,* 4727–4730.

8

Sexual Disorders

Peggy A. Szwabo

A decline in sexual functioning is associated with aging, but sexual activity and interest continue into older age (Busse & Maddox, 1998). The elderly lose much with aging: decline in their senses, health, mobility, and independence. With admission to nursing homes, further loss occurs when the intimacy needs of the resident and their partner are often overlooked and ignored. This omission is resultant of society's stereotypical and prejudicial thinking of the elderly as asexual or the sexual activity of older persons as perverse. Intimacy and touching are the last pleasurable things an elderly person gives up. The person who is denied touch, affection, or connection with another human being slowly deteriorates and dies physically and emotionally.

About 1.6 million persons live in approximately 20,000 nursing homes in the United States. Many remain in the nursing home for the rest of their lives (Richardson & Lazur, 1995). For these individuals, long-term-care facilities serve less as medical facilities than as homes. Health-care providers in nursing homes should strive to provide a homelike atmosphere for these elderly persons. The challenge for long-term-care settings is to overcome barriers that deny intimate caring relationships. This includes assessing and managing the sexual needs of the men and women living in long-term-care facilities (Richardson & Lazur, 1995). Wallace (2003) insists that sexual needs be evaluated with the same thoroughness as other basic needs, such as nutrition, hydration, and mobility.

INTIMACY AND SEXUALITY

Intimacy is a lifelong need. All people have the need for love, to be touched, and desire companionship and intimacy. Sensuality, sexuality, and intimacy are integral parts of one's life. The desire for sex is one of the basic human drives, whereas sexual behavior generally involves physical aspects of anatomy, the genitalia, and erogenous zones. More important, sexuality is much broader and involves sexual behaviors, emotions, beliefs, attitudes, capacities, and relationships. Sexuality has biologic, affective, cognitive, and motivational components. Society is recognizing the multidimensional nature of sexuality and intimacy and is giving attention to the added aspects of touch, love, companionship, caring, play, and trust. The need to be touched, to be an object of affection, to care about, and to be cared for is perhaps the most basic human need (Avis, 2000; Duffy, 1998; Hellie Huyck, 2001; Kliger & Nedelman, 2006; Silverstone & Kandel Hayman, 1992; Wallace, 1992; Wallerstein & Blakesless, 1995; Zeiss & Kasl-Godley, 2001).

Several authors have found a relationship between unmet intimacy and sexual needs of aging persons with reports of increased loneliness, aggression, medical and psychiatric symptoms, and increased use of sedatives (Ginsberg et al., 2005; Hellie Huyck, 20001; Miles & Parker, 1999). In contrast, Duffy (1998) suggests that sex has a restorative function and enhances healing and energy.

AGING AND SEXUALITY

In recent years, the subject of sexuality and aging has gained prominence in treating older adults. But stereotypes and myths still prevail that older adults are sexless and loveless or laughingly described as "dirty old men" if sexually active. Kass (1981) presents a theory describing "geriatric sexuality breakdown syndrome" where the older adult internalizes the negative attitudes of society and perceive themselves as nonsexual. She also emphasizes that this syndrome can be treated with education and developing ways to cope with negative attitudes. Contrary to the stereotypes, myths, and societal ignorance, older adults remain sexual beings with desires, fantasies, and active sex lives. In an American Association for Retired Persons (AARP)/Modern Maturity (1999) mail survey of sexuality in 1382 older adults, the survey found that 67% of men and 57% women indicated that satisfying sex is an important part of their lives. Of men and women 45 to 69 years of age, 6 out of 10 men and women have sex once a week. A slight decline occurs in the 60- to 74-year-old group, with 30% of men and 24% of women reporting sex once weekly. Of those 75 years and older, one out of four continues to have sex weekly. Those surveyed viewed health problems and lack of a partner as major obstacles to continued sexual health and functioning. As important, 9 of 10 men and women indicated a good relationship with their partner was important to their quality of life. And contrary to societal myths, many older couples found their mates more attractive as they aged (Tallmer, 1996; Wallerstein & Blakesless, 1995). Like their younger counterparts, older adults find that sexual activity provides pleasure and release of sexual tension. Sex for the older adult may fulfill additional needs of self-esteem and self-worth. Although these studies were of community dwelling older adults, the results can be applied to long-term-care settings. Of concern is that the elderly themselves are a product of their own history and may have limited knowledge of their own sexuality. Their ability to discuss sexual topics may be hampered and their beliefs may impede healthy sexual functioning.

Intimacy and sexuality is an integral part of human behavior that cannot be overlooked by those who care for nursing home residents. Nursing home residents continue to have an interest in sexual expression regardless of age (Bullard-Poe et al., 1994; Messinger-Rapport et al., 2003; Miles & Parker, 1999; Wallace, 1992, 2003). A study of sexuality among 40 elders (17 men and 23 women) in a Canadian long-term-care facility found infrequent sexual activity with reports of higher sexual desire in men than in women. For women, lack of a functioning partner equates to loss of sexual activity (Spector & Fremuth, 1996). For men, age, poor health, medication, and erectile dysfunction (ED) all impact upon sexual activity. Self-efficacy related to sex correlated positively with sexual desire (Messinger-Rapport et al., 2003; Spector & Fremuth, 1996). Ginsberg et al. (2005) conclude that the elderly surveyed wanted to maintain sexual relationships including touching and kissing and they would like to have more sexual experiences than they have available. Further, the elderly wanted to have sexual activities more often than they did.

SEXUAL CHANGES WITH AGING

A review of the physiologic changes of aging that alter sexual response in the elderly can help health-care professionals deal more effectively with this issue (Messinger-Rapport et al., 2003; Richardson & Lazur, 1995; Wallace, 2003). Physiological changes to sexual response change with age for both men and women. There are four stages of sexual response (excitement, plateau, orgasm, and resolution). Both sexes are affected by age-related changes, which in turn affect sexual response. The following changes in response occur: the excitement phase takes longer for both the male and female, and more stimulation is needed for both partners to reach orgasm. Both have decreased lubrication. After orgasm, the refractory time is longer.

Butler and Lewis (2002) note that men begin to worry about sexual aging in their thirties and these worries accelerate through the decades peaking in their sixties as they notice definite sexual changes. Aging males have to contend with the public view that they will be sexually impaired. These beliefs have psycho-social consequences affecting performance and self-concept. Erection and ejac-ulation remain, but erections are not as firm and ejaculation is not as forceful. The quantity of sperm declines as men age and seminal fluid often becomes thinner.The older male experiences a shorter period of awareness before ejacula-tion. In some there is no awareness at all. Orgasm is less explosive and contrac-tions are less. Older men often lose their erection quickly after orgasm. None of these physiological changes, however, prevent the older male from experiencing satisfaction. It is critical that older men know that satisfying sexual experiences are not dependent upon ejaculation. Men may have frequent sexual intercourse and may ejaculate only half of the time. By delaying ejaculation, the older male may be able to become erect repeatedly and have intercourse and its pleasurable feelings. As men age, it takes longer to develop an erection. Greater stimulation of the penis is often necessary to develop and maintain erection and a greater time interval is necessary between one erection and the next (refractory period). The time that it takes a male to regroup (refractory period) can take anywhere from 12 to 24 h or longer before he can achieve another orgasm. This period increases as the male becomes older.

Decline in testosterone is a consequence of male aging. Andropause or male menopause results in physical, sexual, and psychological symptoms as a result of decreased testosterone (Messinger-Rapport et al., 2003; Morley et al., 2000). These symptoms include decreased muscle and muscle strength, decreased bone mass, sleep disturbance, and loss of sexual interest and emotional well-being. Male hormone treatment is an option for some.

Masturbation or self-stimulation is recognized as normal sexual activity that usually begins in childhood. Previously, masturbation had been viewed as inap-propriate and the cause of both mental and physical diseases. Self-stimulation provides an outlet for people who do not have partners, either being single or with ill or unavailable partners, as well as those who use masturbation in addi-tion to sexual intercourse. Some people begin to masturbate later in life because they have no partner or are too incapacitated for intercourse (Butler & Lewis, 2002; Miles & Parker, 1999; Richardson & Lazur, 1995).

A common sexual impairment is ED. It is the temporary or permanent inability to have an erection strong enough to have intercourse. ED has a higher incidence with aging but may be more related to the number of health problems the male is experiencing than as a result of aging per se (Butler & Lewis, 2002). Each man has his own pattern of frequency of erection and length of time an erection is maintained. Evaluation of ED must thus take into account each indi-vidual's history of performance.

To treat ED, underlying medical conditions need to be ruled out. Numerous endocrine, vascular, and neurological disorders may interfere in sexual function, as well as many medications and surgery. Drugs that affect the autonomic nervous system may interfere with sexual function. Many medications that older people use, such as antihypertensives, antidepressants, tranquilizers, and certain high blood pressure drugs, can adversely affect erectile function and libido. Further, obesity, alcohol intake, smoking, hypercholesterolemia, and lack of physical activity have been linked to ED (Morley et al., 2000; Wise & Crone, 2006).

There are several treatment options for ED. Three medications are available: sildenafil, vardenil, and tadalafil. This class of drugs acts on the penile vascular system to allow improved tumescence by fostering blood flow and to relax the smooth muscle in the penile vasculature. These drugs are essentially the same except for their individual half-life. The major contraindication is in using in combination with nitrates for angina. Other treatments available include penile implants and transurethral and injectible prostaglandin E_1, which require more in-depth evaluation and may be less convenient (Morley et al., 2000; Wise & Crone, 2006).

Menopause is the defining event that impacts female sexuality on several levels. Stereotypes abound as a loss or end of sexuality and the beginning of troubling symptoms such as hot flashes and irritability. The more positive reaction is that it is a sexually freeing experience. Avis (2000) found that other factors, overall health, marital status, smoking, and mental health, impact sexual functioning more so than menopause. Many women experience a variety of menopausal symptoms but approximately 15% do not (Butler & Lewis, 2002).

The loss of hormones causes an overall drying and thinning of the vaginal walls. This thinning can result in bleeding, dysparunia, and irritation during intercourse. Vaginal muscle weakening can cause urinary incontinence during intercourse and stress incontinence, a source of embarrassment, avoidance, and restriction of social activities. Lack of vaginal lubrication is the result of both loss of estrogen, which is needed to produce secretions and vaginal wall changes through which the secretions ooze. Pain occurs if intercourse is of long duration, there is poor lubrication, or if intercourse is resumed after a long period of abstinence. Information and education about lubrication, topical ointments, and suppositories are indicated. Hormone replacement therapy is controversial but needs to be evaluated as an option (Butler & Lewis, 2002; Messinger-Rapport et al., 2003).

IMPACT OF ILLNESS

Health changes affect sexuality. As well as aging physiologic changes, medical conditions have an impact on one's sexual needs and activity. Many chronic illnesses affect sexual health. Cardiovascular disease and diabetes may cause impotence because of altered circulation to the genitalia. Medications for both these conditions may add to impotence and cause fatigue. Individuals that have angina or myocardial infarction may be leery of resuming sexual activities. Stroke with one-sided weakness or paralysis can physically and psychologically inhibit sexual activities. Incontinence, previously mentioned, may cause avoidance because of embarrassment. Emotional problems and depression can affect desire and response, and the medications used to treat these conditions can have sexual side effects. Many surgical procedures can affect sexual response, such as prostatectomy, which can cause ED, or a mastectomy, which may affect response and feelings of desirability. In addition, rectal and gastrointestinal surgeries resulting in ostomies can be embarrassing and require one to work through their own feelings and perceptions of other's attitudes. Butler and Lewis (2002) estimate that it takes up to a year to make a comfortable adjustment to an ostomy. Postsurgically, patients should be prepared that their stamina and vitality may be reduced for a time and encouraged to ask questions and keep an open dialogue concerning their situation and their assumptions about sexual activity.

Messinger-Rapport et al. (2003) discuss the impact of catheterization upon sexual functioning. Those requiring self-catheterization change the function of the bed from association with pleasure to medical procedure. Individuals with indwelling catheters often remain silent about their sexual concerns.

Arthritis and other painful conditions can impair comfort and lead to avoidance. Physical issues such as pain, mobility, and limited range of motion are possible concerns or deterrents to a previously active sex life. A frank discussion of new positions or activities can be helpful and identifying times of the day when pain is less or after pain medication has been taken is useful.

Hypersexual behavior occurs rarely in the elderly. Paraphilias or pathological hypersexuality is usually related to neurological and cognitive disorders, such as dementia and levodopa treatment in Parkinson's diseases. Philpot (2003) describes paraphilics in a broader more historical context. She notes that paraphilics are preoccupied with persistent, unconventional, highly erotic thoughts throughout their lifetime and not as a result of aging or illness pathology. These thoughts may occur in more routine sexual behaviors or to the more extreme. These fantasies are related to arousal. They become aroused at erotic thoughts. Arousal leads to orgasm, which is achieved by masturbation. In the privacy of one's home, this may not be problematic, but in a nursing home, can be catastrophic. Once the diagnosis has been made, treatment consists of medication review to ascertain if any drugs, drug interactions, or medical conditions are exacerbating the problem. Treatment consists of medication and behavioral interventions. Antipsychotic medications, antiandrogens, estrogens, gonadrotrophin-releasing hormone analogues, and serononergic medications have been used successfully (Philpot 2003; Wallace, 2003).

Knowledge of the sexual side effects of medications is a crucial part of an intimacy assessment and often overlooked unless the patient requests it. Common medications with sexual side effects are antihypertensives and serotonin reuptake inhibitors, which can cause anorgasmia, loss of libido, and ED. ACE inhibitors and calcium channel blockers may result in impotence. A frank discussion of the impact of illness, medications, and surgical procedures and their impact on one's sexual desires and ability is warranted by the clinician. Under stress of coping with illnesses, the older adult or their partner may not initiate questions about sexual activities (Bullard-Poe et al., 1994; Butler & Lewis, 2002; Ginsberg et al., 2005; Messinger-Rapport et al., 2003; Wallace, 1992, 2008; Wise & Crone, 2006).

PSYCHOLOGICAL ISSUES

Gross (2000) identified four positive emotional responses that older couples faced with ill health demonstrated when forced to change sexual habits. Older couples voiced an emotional commitment. They are married for "keeps." There was an acceptance of aging; they learned to accept change and to strive for a sense of shared normalcy. They were more adaptable. Historically, husbands initiated sex but were not forceful if their partner was ill or not encouraging. These male partners sought to fight the effects of aging, whereas others accepted health problems and substituted other forms of sexual contact if conventional ones were not possible. Last, protectiveness was the mutual sense of caring and sensitivity to each other's needs and seemed to transcend their physical problems with sex.

Other common emotional problems affecting sexual functioning are anxiety, fear, and any troubling life events, such as death, moves, stress, and relationship issues. Anxiety, fear, depression, and anger were associated with loss of an erection. Lack of orgasm may cause anxiety and fear in some. Some women have been brought up that sex is a duty and may affect relationships and closeness. A major emotional problem for women is the likelihood of being alone. This generation of women was raised to consider themselves dependent upon men. When alone, this may cause a variety of emotional responses. Aging itself may stimulate beliefs that they are old, ugly, or undesirable. These beliefs may limit options and express this negativity in hostility and anger, thus limiting contact and relationships. Guilt and shame may limit sexual behavior. Preconceived ideas, misinformation, and religious beliefs repress sexuality. Issues in dating and sexual relations outside of marriage may inhibit or produce guilt (Butler & Lewis, 2002; Kliger & Nedelman, 2006; Starr & Weiner, 1981). Open discussion, education, and possible referral to a mental health specialist can resolve these feelings and responses.

SAFE SEX

Today's sexually active older adults who are dating and seeking a sexually intimate relationship require information about safe sex practices. Many older adults have been sexually monogamous and may be unaware or naïve regarding sexually transmitted diseases and HIV/AIDS. Risky sexual behaviors need to be addressed. HIV/AIDS is not a disease that is restricted to a younger, gay person (HIV Over Fifty, 2002). The National Institute of Aging (HIV Over Fifty, 2007) estimates 19% of HIV individuals are over the age of 50. Of this group women are more susceptible because of the thinning of the vaginal walls, which increases the risk of transmission.

It is very possible for a naive older adult who resumes dating in later life to contact HIV/AIDS by having unprotected sex. Especially, this is an issue in long-term care, with the cognitively impaired sexually active resident. Safety of the persons involved in the sexual activity and protection from communicable diseases needs to be addressed.

HIV/AIDS needs to be assessed in gay and lesbian residents also. Anderson (2005) found that there are increasing numbers of over 50 individuals with HIV/AIDS due to successful treatment regimes. This is an additional challenge for long-term-care staff. If HIV/AIDS is a reality, support is available through the Gay and Lesbian network and through the national organization, HIV Over Fifty. These organizations provide information and support groups and resources locally, nationally, and from their Web sites.

GAYS AND LESBIANS

Gays and lesbians have unique concerns. These specific issues are complicated and may require more intensive support from a mental health specialist or from a specialty support group. Weg (1996) found that overall, gay older men have fewer partners, do less cruising, and maintain longer relationships. In the few studies that have been done on older gays and lesbians, the findings noted high levels of satisfaction and acceptance of aging. Other research reported greater flexibility in gender roles throughout life, which may contribute to positive aging role changes (Gay older men, 2002; Weg, 1996). Gays experience similar issues including the loss of a partner, fear of losing a younger partner, and fears of being excluded if long-term care is needed. There are real concerns and fears of their partner being excluded in end-of-life planning issues and health-care issues when there is no "legal" relationship. There are realistic fears that the person they trust may be usurped for a more traditional and legally defined responsible person.

BARRIERS TO SEXUALITY IN LONG-TERM-CARE RESIDENTS

Placement in a long-term-care facility should not mean that one's sex life is over. The challenge is to incorporate and discuss healthy attitudes about sexual behavior wherever the older adult resides and to insure accommodations are in place to meet those needs.

Environmental Barriers

Little has been written about the physical environmental barriers to intimacy. With some thought, issues in addressing the "right" environment could enhance intimacy needs among the elderly and prevent uncomfortable and embarrassing situations that are mentioned throughout the literature (Hajjar et al., 2003; Nagarathnam & Gayagay, 2002). As with any positive experience, administration and staff need to address privacy issues and how to insure that these needs are openly and comfortable addressed. Wallace (2003) suggests privacy may be achieved by keeping the roommate busy or finding a common room for private visits. She recommends that staff address safety issues, including call lights close at hand and adaptive equipment such as, trapezes and side rails. Staff will need to demonstrate the proper use of such equipment for the older couple. Hajjar and Kamel (2003) note the need for beauty salons and access to cosmetics be offered on site. Facilities may need to consider offering lubricants and condoms where cosmetics are sold.

Staff Attitudes

In nursing home environments, Nagarathnam and Gayagay (2002) found that the freedom of elderly people to move on from acceptable behaviors (e.g., caressing and touching) to greater physical intimate relationships between residents was often inhibited and discouraged by staff, who would intervene when they perceived behaviors to be unacceptable and inappropriate. In these settings, the concerns of staff and their abilities to handle the sexual expressions were more important considerations in determining whether older peoples' desires and wishes to express themselves sexually should be recognized, acknowledged, and met.

An understanding of how residential home care staff respond and interpret older people's sexual acts would be important, particularly when staff plays a prime role in facilitating what and how sexuality of older people should be expressed in the home. Although Nagarathnam and Gayagay's (2002) review highlighted issues of staff responses to older residents' sexual expression and

strategies to address sexual needs, these have largely been the subject of specu-
lation and opinion, with little research-based findings. More recently, however,
there has been an interest to examine strategies to assist staff to make decisions
about handling ethical dilemmas concerning sexuality of institutionalized elders
with dementia (Ehrenfeld et al., 1997). Ideally, strategies that address the cognitively impaired and inappropriate sexual behaviors can be used as a discussion
to develop staff education and approaches to raise sensitivity and creativity in
enhancing intimacy needs among their residents.

Despite the fact that some sexual behaviors are easier to accept than others,
sexuality of older people emerges as a concern and a burden to staff. Consistently
the literature supports the limited insights and vague understanding of residential care home staff in handling older residents' sexual acts—often construing
sexual behaviors as behavioral problems, rather than elders' expressions for
love and intimacy (Miles & Parker, 1999). Against a set of negative attitudes
reported by staff, earlier studies found that older people's sexual expressions
were met with apprehension, disapproval, judged as misbehavior, and punished
using restraints or segregation (Butler & Lewis, 2002). It was not unusual for
staff to feel threatened, awkward, and uncomfortable and to react by ignoring
the expressions.

Kass (1978) compared the sexual attitudes of nursing home staff with those
of nursing home residents. Interviewing nursing staff, Kass identified why many
nurses avoid the topic of sexuality. Discussions, even intervention based, are
difficult because of personal reluctance and discomfort and lack of knowledge.
She notes that ageist assumptions leave older adults in great need of information and neglect to provide comprehensive, holistic care. Katz (2005) observed
that nurses may feel that questions about sex may invade the older adult's privacy, though others found that patients wanted to discuss these feelings with a
health-care professional (AARP, 1999). Another concern Katz (2005) identified
was fear of legal ramifications and fear that questions about sexuality could be
considered inappropriate particularly when interviewing patients of the opposite
sex. Similarly, Ehrenfeld et al. (1997) demonstrated that staff expressed mixed
emotions of confusion, embarrassment, and helplessness when older people
acted sexually. In making sense of the negative reactions of staff, a categoriza-
tion system was developed to help staff understand different sexual expressions
displayed by older people (Ehrenfeld et al., 1997). It was found that staff were
able to accept and support loving and caring behaviors but were hostile, angry,
and disgusted when older people's behaviors were openly erotic.

In addition, sexual behaviors that were linked to romance brought on reactions of humor, ridicule, and teasing from staff (Bauer, 1999; Ehrenfeld et al.,
1997). Using humor as a strategy, Bauer (1999) found that humor enabled staff to
communicate about sexuality easily by first relieving the stress of the situation,
then understanding the meaning behind the situation, and identifying their role

in the situation. If used with understanding and sensitivity, humor is a useful strategy to safely deal with emotional and socially unacceptable incidents (Katz, 2005; Robinson, 1983).

The lack of knowledge and experience of staff in handling sexuality in old age is one of the main reasons for not being able to promote awareness of older people's sexuality in residential care homes (Lyder, 1994). Undoubtedly, the attitude and mind-set of staff continue to be an influential factor inhibiting sexual expression of older people. This is particularly the case when staff cannot comfortably talk about sexuality, hesitate venturing into intimate discussions with older people, and hesitate dealing with their sexual expressions. If older people are discouraged from expressing sexual interests and activities, this can impede them from becoming fully accepted into residential living. Those elders who choose to lead a relatively active sexual life will continue to conceal their true sexual needs and desires.

Resident Attitudes

Sadly, Kass (1981, 1978) reported that residents were more likely than staff to agree that sex is not needed for women after menopause or for men after age 65. This finding is likely a result of stereotypical beliefs. Sixty-one percent of residents did not feel sexually attractive and did not think they would enjoy sexual activity if they had a partner. Nursing home residents reported masturbating some of the time. Lack of privacy was the most frequent reason given, by both residents and staff, for lack of sexual activity. In contrast, the Starr-Weiner (1981) report of 800 people, 60 to 91 years of age across the United States, found that the frequency of sexual activity did not necessarily decline with age as long as opportunity existed for its expression. They summarize that sexual activities among older persons remain pretty much the same as in their youth unless some outside event occurs such as health problems, loss of a spouse, impotence, or boredom.

Role Change

Prior to admission many family caregivers may be exhausted from the tasks of providing care. Providing physical caregiving can change one's view of their partner as a "patient" rather than a lover. Simple suggestions for changing roles from caregiver back to partner or lover can be helpful. A simple example would be visiting, providing privacy, encouraging massage, and snuggling activities.

Special Needs

Special intimacy and sexual functioning issues need to be routinely addressed but are often overlooked or seem unimportant in providing day-to-day medical treatment. There are many unvoiced concerns on how to have an intimate relationship when one's partner is in a nursing home. Many nursing home staff do an excellent job of assisting couples ensuring and encouraging their private time together. The staff help orchestrate sensitive and caring discussions on how to meet these important needs. Unfortunately, other nursing home staff are uncomfortable, ignore, and even discourage intimacy. Incorporating sexual health education into nursing home in-service training can begin to offer healthier environments for both older adults and the staff providing their care.

Cognitive impairment or dementing illnesses poses significant concerns for couples and for staff. For partners of people with cognitive impairment, the long course of the illness and anticipatory bereavement challenges their capacity to meet intimacy needs. Couples who struggle with dementia have unasked and unanswered questions about intimacy. Often the topic is too private and too sensitive to discuss openly. Dementia initially puts these needs on the back burner; however, as the days of caregiving increase, the lack of intimacy and loss of companionship become major stressors. These losses affect both the person with dementia and the partner (Wright, 1993). Many couples need to know that previously desirable, sexual behaviors can continue through the disease. Residing in a nursing home poses additional logistical problems in privacy and requesting privacy for both partners requires frank and open discussion with staff regarding possibilities to ensure continued intimate times together.

For the person with dementia, sexual and intimate behaviors can range from appropriate to more disturbing and impulsive behaviors. An open discussion of appropriate and desirable behaviors as well as prediction of potentially disturbing sexual behaviors is necessary for the clinician working with a person with dementia. The desirable behaviors that may need to be reviewed and encouraged include hugging, touching, voicing loving comments, using terms of endearment, and sexual activity that continues to be pleasing to both partners. It is important to acknowledge that sexual behaviors can be pleasing and desirable, as well as inappropriate and disturbing, depending upon when, where, with whom, and how often the behaviors occur. The unimpaired partner needs to feel that he or she can contact staff if these behaviors occur and that they will be addressed.

Problematic sexual behavior is exhibited in about 25% of nursing home residents (Ehrenfeld et al., 1997; Hajjar & Kamel, 2003). Researchers suggest that 7% to 17% of persons with dementia have sexual disinhibition including touching, fondling others' genitalia (both staff and other residents), public masturbation, disrobing, and sexual requests. These behaviors are very troublesome for health-care professionals and are difficult to manage. Wallace (2003) observed that some inappropriate sexual behavior is related to staff's perceptions and lack of privacy. Although these behaviors are often viewed as manipulative and attention seeking, she cautions these behaviors will not disappear without interventions that both set limits and fulfill the sexual needs underlying the behavior.

Institutionalization brings about another potential sexual crisis for the healthy or unimpaired partner. Questions arise for the healthy partner: Is abstinence a reality or a desire? Is masturbation an acceptable alternative? Is dating or being with someone else a source of conflict? The AARP study (1999) reports that the younger older adult is more accepting of sex outside of marriage, whereas for over half of the 75-year-old plus group this is still taboo. Issues of this nature need referral to a therapist for more in-depth discussion (HIV Over Fifty, 2002; Johnson, 1997; Wallerstein & Blakeless, 1995). Some families would be supportive if mom or dad dated while aware that their spouse/partner was unavailable and the course of illness was long and drawn out, whereas other families would find this situation to be very difficult. Dating sometimes arises out of the need for companionship and may begin at a support group talking with other adults who are living with similar losses and problems. This situation may give rise to guilt and conflict and need to be referred to help the individual sort out what is best for his/her situation (Rosenthal, 2001; Silverstone & Kandel Hayman, 1992).

A very difficult challenge facing nursing home staff and families of residents is in the area of consent with the cognitively impaired. A priority for staff is the need to protect the vulnerable from public and inappropriate sexual behavior. Determination of consent in participating in sexual activities for the cognitively impaired requires staff education and sensitivity, involvement of the family, and/ or a surrogate manager. Family responses can vary, and they may have their own issues and judgments about their loved ones' sexual activity. Families may need referral for counseling in dealing with sexual activities of their loved ones. Wallace (2003) recommends addressing the following questions: Is the resident's behavior consistent with previous behaviors, values, and religious beliefs? Is the resident delusional, acting out the belief that the other person is a spouse? Cognitively impaired individuals can make decisions to participate in sexual activities but these issues need to be addressed to help determine if the resident is safe to go forward with a relationship that can possibly enhance quality of life (Gaile & Henderson, 2004).

Assessment and Counseling

In long-term-care facilities, there is opportunity for clinicians and staff to assess and address the intimacy needs of their residents. Assessment of sexuality should incorporate structured and open-ended questions. Concerns and questions regarding sexuality and functioning need to be raised by their clinicians. Because sexual information is rarely volunteered, questions about intimacy and sexuality need to be addressed by the clinician. Table 8.1 outlines communication strategies for health-care providers to discuss sexual concerns with their residents/patients. Even basic information that sexual activity takes

TABLE 8.1. Guidelines for Health-Care Providers for Discussing Sexuality

---

For the patient
  Spend time with the older adult
  Actively listen and be attentive
  Use plain everyday language
  Allow time for question and answers
  Help break the ice and introduce the topic
  Give permission to express feelings
  Help the patient feel comfortable asking questions
  Ask to write down their concerns between visits

For the health-care provider
  Learn about sexuality
  Treat older adults as sexual beings
  Incorporate as part of standard assessment
  Be prepared to listen
  Do not avoid the subject
  Ask direct questions; probe if necessary
  Let patient talk
  Develop handouts
  Develop referral sources (therapists, other clinicians, support groups, information)

Source: Adapted from Johnson (1997).

longer and requires more foreplay or preparation is not routinely shared with the elderly. The elderly may be reluctant to ask their health-care clinician about these concerns.

Assessment includes three overlapping areas that include prevention or education, treatment or intervention, and special needs. Table 8.2 was designed to assist the provider in incorporating intimacy questions into their existing assessment. To assist nurses in discussing their patient's sexual needs, Wallace (2008) developed Annon's PLISSIT (1976) model of sexuality assessment for older adults. This model begins with permission (P) of the older adult for a sexual discussion. Permission to discuss can be easily incorporated into routine assessment or visit. The next step is to give limited information (LI) to the older adult. This could be general information such as aging-related sexual changes. The SS of the model refers to specific suggestions to help the older adult fulfill their sexuality. An example would be the impact of a medical condition or concerns about an existing relationship. Medication review is an opportune teaching moment to address sexual changes and potential sexual side effects. Suggestions for lubricants and "how to"s may be offered.

In treatment planning with the patient, an open and frank discussion of how certain medical conditions can affect sexual functioning and any precautions that the couple may need to take needs to be addressed. It is desirable to discuss when to resume intercourse after a heart attack, identifying position changes for intercourse when arthritis or pain is a problem and how long after

TABLE 8.2. Assessment of Sexual Relationships in the Elderly

I. Assessment of sexual function and desire
A. Physical assessment and history
　1. Past sexual history and functioning
　2. Current sexual activity
　　a. Desire for sexual intimacy
　3. Past difficulties experienced
　4. Presence of sexually transmitted diseases or HIV
　5. Presence of medications or medical conditions that inhibit sexual functioning
　　a. Antidepressants, tranquilizers
　　b. Antihypertensives
　　c. Antipsychotics, phenothiazines
B. Assess desire to participate in a sexual relationship
　1. Maintain open communication
　2. Identify current levels of sexuality and how maintained
　3. Ask about problems and concerns
　4. Listen for nonverbal attempts to talk about

II. Management of sexual relationships
A. HCP's knowledge and comfort level
B. Identify ways to compensate for physical changes
　1. Provide ongoing teaching on normal changes of anatomy and physiology, functioning, desires, impact of intimacy needs on both partners
　2. Provide teaching and resources about artificial lubricants
　3. Identify and treat causes of ED
　4. Discuss the risks and benefits of hormone replacement therapy
　5. Discuss other noncoital ways of achieving satisfaction
C. Teach safe sex and specific information about HIV and STDs
D. Provide psychological support and refer for therapy when needed
E. Redesign existing assessment and evaluation tools to incorporate sexual functioning and intimacy needs

---

surgery to wait before resuming sexual activity and how much activity would be appropriate to attempt. Clinicians should point out that physical weakness may hinder usual sexual activity and "going slow" may be the operative approach; giving a concrete example, such as, "If you can walk a flight of stairs without shortness of breath" can be helpful. With mutilative surgery, mastectomy, or ostomies, clinicians should address concerns of physical discomfort and also need to respond to patient fears of rejection because of drastic changes in body image. The healthy partner may be reluctant to discuss feelings of revulsion or contagion. Referrals to a therapist and support groups offered by the American Cancer Society and ostomy groups can provide support and guidance (Carlton, 1994; Healing Well; Steinke, 2000; United Ostomy Association Web site).

The last part of the model is intensive therapy, which would be provided for any issues that arise from the assessment. This may include sexual abuse, fears, or inhibitions. Problems identified should be referred for more in-depth counseling. These guidelines are suggestions to initiate and incorporate discussions of sexuality as a matter of routine. Katz (2005) discusses how nurses can become more comfortable including sexual questions in the daily encounter with residents. She offers another model, The Better Model of Treatment (Mick et al., 2003), which was designed to assess sexuality in cancer patients. The acronym BETTER includes Bringing up the topic; Explaining that sex is a part of life and normal; Telling about available resources; Timing of the intervention, plant the seed of information, and leave the contact information; Education regarding sexual side effects of treatments; and Record the results of the discussion. Katz (2005) further notes that staff's personal barriers and discomfort need to be addressed at in-services, workshops, and observations of experts in action.

THE CHALLENGE

Sexuality is an integral part of human behavior but is often overlooked in residents in long-term-care facilities. The elderly continue to have interests in sexual expression regardless of age. Staff and family should expect sexual behaviors to occur and be ready to respond appropriately. The challenge is to be proactive and create an environment where all aspects of life are nurtured.

Nursing home staff have multiple responsibilities in the domain of intimacy and sexuality in the elderly. The administration and staff need to view sexual and intimacy needs as important as any others in planning for care and quality of life. The approach is multidimensional incorporating the following: personal self-awareness; professional education and discussion; incorporation of intimacy and sexual functioning into assessments and in therapeutic conversations; development of an overall facility philosophy; expansion of safety protocols to include safe sex practices, risk assessment, and interventions for inappropriate sexual behaviors. Miles and Parker (1999) stress that encouragement and accommodation of intimate behaviors enhance life satisfaction and psychological well-being. Further, the failure to accommodate intimate relationships in nursing homes could cause poor quality of life, poor adjustment to nursing homes, aggression, confusion, feelings of confinement and abandonment, decision-making difficulties, and greater use of medical and psychiatric care and sedation.

The challenge remains for long-term care to set the standards of care for the elderly in providing for their sexual needs in a knowledgeable and caring environment.

REFERENCES

AARP/Modern Maturity Sexuality Survey. (1999, September/October). *Modern maturity*, 57–69.

Anderson M. (2005, May). HIV/AIDS and the elderly. Available at www.final call.com/ artman/publisher/printer_2010.shtml

Annon, J. (1976). The PLISSIT model: A proposed conceptual scheme for the behavioral treatment of sexual problems. *Journal of Sex Education Therapy, 2*(2), 1–15.

Avis, N. (2000). Sexual function and aging in men and women: Community and population-based studies. *Journal of Gender Specific Medicine, 3*(2), 37–41.

Bauer, M. (1999). The use of humor in addressing sexuality of elderly nursing home residents. *Sexuality and Disability, 17*(2), 147–155.

Bullard-Poe, L., Powell, C., & Mulligan, T. (1994). The importance of intimacy to men living in a nursing home. *Archives of Sexual Behavior, 23*(2), 231–236.

Busse, E., & Maddox, G. (1998). *The Duke longitudinal studies of normal aging (1955–1980)*. New York: Springer.

Butler, R., & Lewis, M. (2002). *The new love and sex after sixty* (Rev. ed.). New York: Ballantine.

Carlton, L. (1994). *Sex, love, and chronic illness*. Miami, FL: National Parkinson Foundation.

Duffy, L. (1998). Lovers, loners and lifers: Sexuality in the older adult. *Geriatrics, 53*(1), 566–569.

Ehrenfeld, M., Tabak, N., Bronner, G., & Bergman, R. (1997). Ethical dilemmas concerning sexuality of elderly patients suffering dementia. *International Journal of Nursing Practice, 3*(4), 225–259.

Gaile, S., & Henderson, R. (2004). Consensual sexual activity: Guidelines for assessment of capacity. In P. R. Katz, M. D. Mezey, & M. B. Kapp (Eds.), *Vulnerable populations in the long term care continuum* (pp. 57–72). New York: Springer.

Gay older men. (2002). Harvard Medical School consumer information. Available at www.health-harvard.edu.

Ginsberg, T., Pomerantz, S., & Kramer-Feeley, V. (2005). Sexuality in older adults: Behaviours and preferences. *Age and Ageing, 34*, 447–480.

Gross, H. (2000). *Seasons of the heart*. Navato, CA: New World Library.

Hajjar, H., & Kamel, H. (2003, August). Sex and the nursing home. *Clinical Geriatric Medicine, 19*(3), 575–586.

Healing Well. A resource directory for Crohn's disease and ostomies. Available at www. Healingwell.com

Hellie Huyck, M. (2001, Summer). Romantic relationships in later life. *Generations Journal of the American Society on Aging, 25*(20), 9–17.

HIV Over Fifty. (2002) Available at www.HIVoverfifty.org

HIV Over Fifty. (2007). NIA publication. Available at www.niapublications.org/agepage/ aids.asp

Johnson, B. (1997). Older adults suggestions for health care providers regarding questions of sex. *Geriatric Nursing, 18*, 65–67.

Kass, M. (1981). Geriatric sexuality breakdown syndrome. *International Journal of Aging and Human Development, 13*, 71–77.

Kass, M. (1978). Sexual expression of the elderly in nursing homes. *The Gerontologist, 18*, 372–378.

Katz, A. (2005, July). Do ask, do tell—why so many nurses avoid the topic of sexuality. *American Journal of Nursing, 105*(7), 66–68.

Kliger, L., & Nedelman, D. (2006). *Still sexy after all these years.* New York: Berkley.

Lyder, C. (1994). The role of the nurse practitioner in promoting sexuality in the institution-alized elderly. *Journal of the American Academy of Nursing Practice, 6*(2), 61–63.

Messinger-Rapport, B., Sandhu, S., & Hujer, M. (2003, October). Sex and sexuality: Is it over after 60? *Clinical Geriatrics, 11*(10), 45–55.

Mick, J., Hughes, M., & Cohen, M. (2003). Sexuality and cancer: How oncology nurses can address it better [Abstract 180]. *Oncology Nursing Forum, 30*(2 Suppl.), 152–153.

Miles, S., & Parker, K. (1999, Spring). Sexuality in the nursing home: Iatrogenic loneli-ness. *Generations Journal of the American Society on Aging, 23,* 36–43.

Morley, J. F., Charlton, E., Patrick, P., et al. (2000, September). Validation of a screening questionnaire for androgen deficiency in aging males. *Metabolism, 49*(9), 1239–1242.

Nagarathnam, N., & Gayagay, G. (2002). Hypersexuality in nursing home facilities: A descriptive study. *Archives of Gerontology and Geriatrics, 35*(3), 195–203.

National Institute of Aging (2007). Available at nia.nih.gov/healthinformation/publica-tion/hiv-aids.htm

Philpot, C. (2003, August). Paraphilia and aging. *Clinics in Geriatric Medicine, 19*(3), 629–636.

Richardson, J., & Lazur, A. (1995). Sexuality in the nursing home patient. *American Family Physician, 5*(1), 121–124.

Robinson, V. (1983). Humor and health. In P. McGee & J. Goldstein (Eds.), *Handbook of humor research* (Vol. 2, pp. 109–128). New York: Springer-Verlag.

Rosenthal, A. (2001). Geriatric care management with families. In C. Cressy (Ed.), *Handbook of geriatric care management* (pp. 149–170). Gaithersburg, MD: Aspen.

Silverstone, B., & Kandel Hayman, H. (1992). *Growing older together.* New York: Pantheon.

Spector, I., & Fremuth, S. (1996). Sexual behaviors and attitudes of geriatric residents in long-term care facilities. *Journal of Sex and Marital Therapy, 22*(4), 235–246.

Starr, B., & Weiner, M. (1981). *The Starr–Weiner report on sex and sexuality in the mature years.* New York: Stein & Day.

Steinke, E. (2000). Sexual counseling after myocardial infarction. *American Journal of Nursing, 100*(12), 38–44.

Tallmer, M. (1996). Questions and answers about sex in later life. Philadelphia, PA: Charles Press, 1–9.

Tallmer, M., & Kutshcer, L. (1984). *Sex and life-threatening illness.* Springfield, IL: Thomas.

United Osotomy Association, a national support group for individuals with ostomies. www.uoa.org, 1–800-826-0826

Wallace, M. (1992). Management of sexual relationships among elderly residents of long-term care facilities. *Geriatric Nursing, 11*(12), 308–311.

Wallace, M. (2003, February). Sexuality in long-term care. *Annals of Long-Term Care, 11*(2), 53–59.

Wallace, M. (2008). Assessment of Sexual Health in older adults. *AJN, American Journal of Nursing, 108*(7), 52–60. Available online at www.GeroNurseOnline.org

Wallerstein, J., & Blakesless, S. (1995). *The good marriage: How and why love lasts.* New York: Houghton Mifflin.

Weg, R. (1996). Sexuality, sensuality, and intimacy. In J. Birren (Ed.), *Encyclopedia of gerontology* (Vol. 2, pp. 479–487). San Diego, CA: Academic Press.

Wise, T., & Crone, C. (2006). Sexual functioning in the geriatric patient. *Clinical Gerontology, 14*(12), 17–26.

Wright, L. (1993). *Alzheimer's disease and marriage.* Newbury Park, CA: Sage.

Zeiss, A. & Kasl-Godley, J. (2001). Sexuality in older adults' relationship. *Generations, 25*(2), 18–25.

9

Personality Disorders

Marc E. Agronin

Clinicians often underestimate the role of both personality and personality disorders (PDs) in long-term care (LTC) settings, focusing instead on more immediate concerns—agitation, psychosis, depression—and other major psychiatric conditions. Sooner or later, however, PDs emerge as some of the most recalcitrant psychopathologic symptoms, exerting a disproportionately disruptive effect on staff and milieu. PDs are defined in the *Diagnostic and Statistical Manual of Mental Disorders,* fourth edition, text revision (*DSM-IV-TR*) by an enduring and pervasive pattern of inflexible and maladaptive inner experiences and behaviors, which deviate from cultural expectations, and lead to significant disruptions in areas of cognitive interpretation and perception, affective expression, interpersonal relations, and impulse control (American Psychiatric Association, APA, 2000). According to official diagnostic criteria, PDs typically manifest in early adulthood, although their roots may be found in childhood. In LTC settings, however, distant history is by necessity less important than more recent personality patterns and the impact of brain injury from a host of factors, most notably dementia. This chapter will review the basic characteristics of PDs in late life, and focus on unique manifestations in LTC settings and how they can be managed with both pharmacologic and nonpharmacologic approaches.

DEFINITIONS AND DIAGNOSIS

DSM-IV-TR posits ten categorical PDs under axis II that are grouped into three clusters ("odd," "dramatic," and "anxious") based on similar phenomenology. There is also a "not otherwise specified (NOS)" category for PDs with features that don't fit into any existing category, or that represent criteria of several disorders. Passive-aggressive and depressive PDs are listed in the appendix of *DSM-IV-TR* since they have not yet accumulated sufficient empirical evidence to become official disorders. All 12 disorders are described in Table 9.1, along with late-life characteristics seen in LTC settings (Agronin, 2006; Zweig &

TABLE 9.1. *DSM-IV-TR* Personality Disorders and Late-Life Features in LTC

PERSONALITY DISORDERS	FEATURES IN LATE-LIFE AND LTC SETTINGS
Paranoid	Suspicious and distrustful of others. May become rageful, agitated, and even transiently psychotic when interacting with other residents and staff, especially when needs are not met.
Schizoid	Isolative, aloof, eccentric, with few if any friendships and little desire for socializing. Often avoids contacts with other residents and staff, and can be difficult to engage in activities and treatment.
Schizotypal	Odd, bizarre, eccentric beliefs, appearance, or speech. Detached from and uncomfortable with social relationships. Other residents and staff may be uncomfortable with their odd appearance and statements, leading to further isolation or even anger and social ostracism directed toward them. LTC placement may prompt resistant and belligerent behaviors.
Antisocial	Aggressive, reckless, impulsive, and deceitful, without regard for social norms. Lack of conscience for behavior. Frequent history of criminal behaviors and substance abuse. Late-life presentation often with depression and ongoing substance abuse. In LTC settings, may be aggressive, assaultive, reckless, and inappropriate, sometimes prompting expulsion.
Borderline	Impulsive, self-injurious, rageful, with unstable interpersonal relationships and poor self-image. Emotional lability and impulsive behaviors may prompt crises and conflicts with residents and staff. Depression is common endpoint.
Histrionic	Overly extroverted and provocative; sometimes in a sexually inappropriate manner. Emotionally shallow and attention seeking. Such behaviors may exhaust staff and provoke hostility or ostracism from other residents. May resemble frontal lobe disinhibition, hypomania, or even ADHD.

Continued

TABLE 9.1. Continued

PERSONALITY DISORDERS	FEATURES IN LATE-LIFE AND LTC SETTINGS
Narcissistic	Arrogant, entitled, and grandiose, with little regard for others. May react with anger, paranoia, and indignation to LTC placement. Age-associated losses can prompt rage, depression, and paranoia. Frequently in conflict with LTC staff over personal demands and complaints.
Avoidant	Timid, socially inhibited, and fearful of rejection. Loss of long-held social contacts after LTC placement can be devastating. Anxiety and depression are common after placement.
Dependent	Clinging, needy, and dependent on others for decisions. May tax and even exhaust staff with neediness, sometimes reacting with anger and panic when needs are not met. Comorbid anxiety and depression is common.
Obsessive-compulsive	Preoccupied with orderliness and perfectionism, coupled with a rigid and overly conscientious approach to activities. LTC placement may increase rigidity and prompt resistance and belligerence when demands are not met. Major depression is common.
Passive-aggressive	Resistant to demands and responsibilities, noncompliant, hostile to authority. May agree to but then resist daily care needs, medications, and other treatments, prompting conflict with LTC staff.
Depressive	Gloomy and pessimistic, poor self-esteem, and overly critical attitudes. In LTC often resistant to and pessimistic about care. Condition often difficult to distinguish from major depression, and may occur simultaneously.

Agronin, 2006). In late life, mixed or unspecified PDs are more common than pure categorical diagnoses. For example, one study of elderly psychiatric outpatients found that nearly 50% met criteria for two or more PDs, and another 12% were best described as PD, NOS (Agronin & Orr, 1998).

Given this clinical heterogeneity, the diagnosis of PDs in LTC can be difficult. First of all, there are 12 possible disorders, each with multiple criteria that can be met in any combination above a certain threshold. Most clinicians would need to review these criteria or conduct a lengthy structured interview in order to accurately make a PD diagnosis, and this simply does not occur routinely in LTC settings. Even when clinicians are diligent about reviewing and then applying current *DSM* criteria, they are hampered by the fact that many criteria do not apply to older individuals (Agronin & Maletta, 2000). In addition, PD diagnoses require significant longitudinal history that is not always available in typical nursing home charts, and may not be accurately obtained by the affected individuals and their informants. Reported history may be distorted by recall bias (the tendency to present more socially desirable traits), memory impairment, or the very PD in question. For instance, paranoid individuals may provide guarded responses, or refuse to answer, whereas schizoid or schizotypal individuals may respond in vague or bizarre ways.

Clinicians must also try to discern the role of both normal and pathologic personality traits from comorbid psychiatric conditions that can significantly distort the clinical presentation, such as dementia, psychosis, and depression. For example, the odd thinking and unusual perceptual experiences seen in schizotypal PD may resemble a psychotic disorder, whereas the emotional lability seen in borderline or histrionic PDs may mimic a disinhibited or hypomanic state. Chronic or reactive depressive symptoms seen in several PDs can be extremely difficult to distinguish from symptoms of major mood disorders, perhaps making it impossible to make a valid diagnosis of PD during a major depressive episode (Scott et al., 1992). Many elderly psychiatric patients also have chronic medical conditions that will interfere with diagnosis. Alzheimer's disease and other types of dementia may cause or exacerbate many of the maladaptive behaviors seen in PDs, especially when frontal or temporal regions of the brain are involved. Chronic pain and disability can lead to excessive patterns of dependent or avoidant behaviors that resemble those seen in PDs.

Finally, the clinician's own bias may interfere with diagnosis, in which maladaptive personality traits are too often considered normal in late life. Put together, these diagnostic barriers often lead clinicians to either defer PD diagnoses or to simply lump difficult individuals into a "PD, NOS" category.

There are several clinical guidelines that can aid diagnosis. Clinicians should, first of all, obtain as much longitudinal information as possible on what the individual was like as a person for several years prior to placement, and then decades earlier. Look for a history of disrupted, unstable relationships such as multiple marriages (or never being married) or estrangement from children. Inquire about reckless behaviors, criminal history, substance abuse, and poor work history. Paranoid, schizoid, and schizotypal individuals typically appear odd and isolative and have few informants or social contacts. Borderline, narcissistic, and antisocial characters may initially present in a benign or even charming manner, but their history will reveal a lot of interpersonal conflict. Anxious, dependent, and avoidant individuals are typically already diagnosed as depressed and anxious, but these symptoms persist despite attempts at treatment. Obsessive-compulsive symptoms may be less pronounced, and only emerge in caregiving relationships where schedules, hygiene, and organization are the focus. Histrionic and passive-aggressive individuals are more difficult to identify in LTC as the pathology can be subtle, or may be seen as simply a natural reaction to placement. For example, the older histrionic woman is often quite successful at engaging clinicians in discussion, and manifestations of provocative or seductive behaviors can be such a contrast to other residents that they are viewed as charming or entertaining. The ageist bias here is clear, however, since similar behaviors in a younger woman would be viewed in a more negative manner. Depressive individuals are almost always diagnosed as having a mood disorder instead of a PD, in part due to lack of clinical understanding of the criteria (Agronin, 1999a).

EPIDEMIOLOGY

In community epidemiologic studies, the prevalence of PDs in individuals 65 years or older ranges from 5% to 13% (Abrams & Horowitz, 1996; Agronin & Maletta, 2000). In comparison, epidemiologic studies of younger adults have found prevalence rates ranging from 10% to 18% (Phillips & Gunderson, 1994; Weissman, 1993). A recent large epidemiologic study that assessed a representative sample of over 43,000 individuals in the United States found an overall prevalence rate of PDs of 14.79% (Grant et al., 2004). In elderly psychiatric patients, studies have found the prevalence of PDs to range from less than 5% to over 50%, depending on inpatient versus outpatient setting, comorbid diagnoses, and diagnostic method (Agronin, 1994). One study of 546 elderly psychiatric inpatients found a 13% prevalence rate of PDs (Kunik et al., 1993). Of the 154 patients in the study suffering from major depression, the prevalence rate of PDs increased to 24%. The most common PDs seen in elderly individuals across several studies have been avoidant, dependent, obsessive-compulsive, and paranoid (Agronin, 1994; Agronin & Orr, 1998). These rates will vary widely depending on the clinical setting, comorbid diagnoses, and gender of the subjects.

Few studies have looked specifically at LTC populations. Using clinical interviews, Teeter and colleagues (1976) found that 10.8% of a nursing home sample ($N = 78$) had a primary or secondary diagnosis of PD. A review of nursing home psychiatric referrals found that 15% were for unspecified personality problems (Margo et al., 1980), although this rate likely overestimates the actual number who had true PDs. A third study that looked at mentally retarded individuals older than 40 years admitted to an LTC setting found that slightly over 11% had a PD (Day, 1985). The relative rates of specific PDs in LTC settings have not been established. However, in the author's own experience as a psychiatrist at a large LTC facility, the most common PDs seen for consultation include narcissistic, depressive, paranoid, borderline, and passive-aggressive. Other PDs may actually be more common, such as avoidant or obsessive-compulsive, but they do not come as often to psychiatric attention.

LONG-TERM COURSE

A number of longitudinal studies have found gradual improvement of several PDs in middle age, most notably borderline PD (McGlashan, 1986; Paris et al., 1987) and antisocial PD (Blazer et al., 1985; Robins et al., 1984). These findings may serve to confirm the beliefs of many clinicians that PDs tend to burn out in late life. However, it is clear that individuals with PDs remain at risk for comorbid psychiatric conditions such as depression, anxiety, and substance abuse (Black et al., 1995), and may demonstrate reemergent symptoms in late life (Agronin, 1994; Agronin & Maletta, 2000; Rosowsky & Gurian, 1992). Some individuals with a previous history of stability can decompensate in response to specific age-related stressors. When this occurs, the clinical manifestations of PDs may be modified by the presence of comorbid medical or psychiatric illnesses, disability, dementia, and by age-related changes in behavior. For example, Rosowsky and Gurian (1992) have suggested that elderly borderline individuals display less impulsivity, self-mutilation, and risk-taking, but more age-appropriate symptoms such as anorexia, polypharmacy, and noncompliance with treatment. Similarly, antisocial individuals may be less impulsive and their aggressivity may be limited by physical disability, but their disregard for safety or certain rules of conduct can persist. As a result, clinicians often see the initial presentation of certain symptom constellations in late life.

ACUTE COURSE IN THE LTC SETTING

The reemergence of PD-related dysfunctional inner experiences or behaviors is a common reaction to the unique stresses of LTC placement, and may be what led to the placement in the first place. Many of these individuals arrive at facilities having suffered recent medical illness and/or psychosocial losses that can easily overwhelm brittle and maladaptive coping styles. Complicating the picture is that individuals with poor or volatile interpersonal skills must try to deal with forced contacts with roommates and staff, and those with rigid or idiosyncratic habits must adjust to institutional schedules and rules. The loss of a familiar environment, personal items, privacy, and the control over one's schedule can lead to intense anxiety or anger and a sense of disorganization. Resultant inappropriate, odd, or disruptive behaviors can interfere with caregiving; promote conflict with family, other residents, and staff; and even trigger psychiatric crises. For example, an obsessive-compulsive individual may attempt to maintain a sense of control by demanding rigid adherence to schedules and rules of hygiene. Dependent individuals may feel helpless and panicked without enough attention to their needs, and respond with clinging behaviors and excessive questions or requests for assistance. Paranoid, antisocial, and borderline patients may aggravate staff by refusing to cooperate with treatment plans or institutional rules. Without careful and thoughtful assessment and management, individuals with PDs often become viewed as intolerably hateful, demanding, or strange, leading sometimes to neglect, inappropriate medicating, and even attempts to eject them from the LTC facility. Appropriate management approaches will be discussed later in this chapter.

Not all individuals in LTC settings with apparent personality dysfunction will have a longstanding history of similar symptoms or a formal diagnosis of a PD, and their symptoms may have a more recent onset. Keep in mind, first, that the stresses inherent in LTC placement and daily life can lead to adjustment disorders and associated behavioral changes that may mimic PDs, but without the defining pervasiveness and enduring quality that is necessary for diagnosis. Recent onset personality dysfunction may also have an organic etiology. The term *organic personality disorder* that appeared in earlier diagnostic schemes is now referred to as *personality change due to a general medical condition or dementia* in the *DSM-IV-TR*, with common etiologies such as traumatic brain injury (TBI), stroke, endocrine dysfunction, encephalitis, and Alzheimer's disease (AD). AD, for example, has been associated with apathy (withdrawal, passivity, decreased interest and initiative), egocentricity, and increased irritability, aggression, and impulsivity (B¢zzola et al., 1992; Petry et al., 1988; Rubin et al., 1987). Specified types of personality change disorder include labile, disinhibited, aggressive, apathetic, and paranoid.

TREATMENT STRATEGIES

Management of PDs in LTC settings is challenging, and typically results in improvement without resolution. Given the chronic and pervasive nature of PDs, the overall goal is not to cure the disorder, but to decrease the frequency and intensity of disruptive behaviors. Management strategies should draw upon the efforts of multidisciplinary staff working together to identify comorbid medical and psychiatric disorders as well as psychological and environmental stressors that may be exacerbating disruptive behaviors. Some of the biggest offenders include pain, depression, and conflict with roommates. It is important for the mental health clinician to provide a comprehensive psychiatric diagnosis as well as a practical case formulation that explains underlying personality dynamics. When staff members understand these deficits in personality functioning, they are less apt to blame themselves or overreact to outrageous behaviors, and are more able to have empathy for the individual. When possible, it is important to clarify the presence of a PD or disruptive personality traits prior to admission, and to anticipate what institutional stresses might be most noxious. When current and antecedent stressors have been identified, staff can work to manipulate the milieu to accommodate the patient. Disruptive behaviors can sometimes be traced to particular activities or staff interactions, which can be adapted as part of an overall treatment strategy. Sometimes, disengagement from patients will reduce the intensity of disruptive interactions. In other situations, continuity of staffing and daily schedules are critical.

A staff meeting or case conference often provides the best forum to discuss the formulation, and to coordinate a consistent treatment plan. Treatment plans should be well documented and communicated to the patient and involved family members and caregivers. Sometimes a written contract, signed by all parties, is needed to eliminate ambiguity. All plans must provide appropriate limits to ensure the safety of patients and staff. Although it is important to involve family members in the treatment plan, clinicians must recognize that patients with PDs often have conflictual relationships with them. Attention should also be given to individual staff members who must work with difficult patients. They need opportunities to vent feelings of anxiety and frustration, and to feel acknowledged and supported by administrative staff.

Individual psychotherapy can be useful when a patient is willing to engage in a therapeutic relationship, especially for borderline, histrionic, narcissistic, dependent, and obsessive-compulsive individuals. The success of therapy depends, however, on the availability of a psychotherapist to visit the institution on a consistent basis in order to provide an enduring therapeutic relationship, and not just occasional, brief contacts. Cognitive-behavioral treatments tend to be the most practical in LTC settings, especially when they can be adapted and applied by hands-on caregiving staff. For example, a cognitively intact individual with borderline PD who refuses to cooperate with certain nurses during caregiving can be educated about the consequences of her refusal (e.g., angry staff, poor hygiene, increased risk of infection) and rewarded with some desired perk for more cooperative behaviors (e.g., staff 1:1 time for a walk outside, or some small goodie from a local store). Behavior plans that aim to reshape disruptive behaviors require coordination amongst nursing, medical, mental health, and social work staff, as well as any involved family members and other caregivers.

One of the most useful therapeutic approaches to treating PDs is dialectical behavior therapy or DBT (Robins & Chapman, 2004). Although DBT was developed initially for borderline PD, it has been adapted for other PDs and for elderly individuals with depression and comorbid PD (Lynch, 2000). The goal of DBT is to train the patient to be more aware of both adaptive and maladaptive behaviors, to understand and learn to modulate the consequences of their behaviors, and to identify and avoid triggers (Lively, 2002). In adults, DBT has been shown to reduce the incidence of self-injurious and suicidal behaviors, decrease the degree of depression, anxiety, and hopelessness; and decrease the number and length of hospitalizations (Linehan et al., 1991; Robins, 2002). Unfortunately, the use of a specialized psychotherapy such as DBT may be limited in LTC facilities by the unavailability of trained therapists, or by the high frequency of cognitive and functional decline associated with comorbid medical and psychiatric conditions, especially severe depression and dementia.

In addition, antisocial, paranoid, schizoid, and schizotypal individuals are often incapable or unwilling to form strong therapeutic relationships, and may not agree to participate in treatment.

In LTC settings, then, pharmacologic therapy often becomes the most practical and quickest way to reduce the frequency and severity of disruptive behaviors associated with PDs. It is important to recognize, however, that there are no pharmacologic panaceas for PDs, and clinicians must be clear about selecting realistic target symptoms. Such symptoms may include paranoia and transient psychosis, impulsive aggression, rage attacks, self-injurious behaviors, hypochondriasis, and depressed or anxious moods. Reviews of pharmacologic treatment of PDs in adults and in late life indicate that the entire range of agents have been utilized, selected on the basis of target symptoms and not the PDs themselves (Agronin, 1999b; Markovitz, 2004). In addition to treating symptoms of anxiety and depression, antidepressant agents can reduce impulsive aggressive behaviors in some patients. Mood stabilizers and antipsychotics can also treat symptoms of aggression and impulsivity, whereas antipsychotics alone are best used for transient states of psychosis as well as behavioral crises. In any LTC setting, the use of pharmacologic agents must comply with OBRA guidelines, and should be minimized or even avoided when there is noncompliance, reckless or abusive use of medications, or med-seeking behaviors that serve to exacerbate maladaptive personality traits (Agronin, 1999b). Detailed pharmacologic and nonpharmacologic approaches to select target symptoms are outlined in Table 9.2.

TABLE 9.2. Target Symptoms and Treatment Approaches

TARGET SYMPTOMS/PDS	MANAGEMENT STRATEGIES
Paranoid stance/symptoms	
Common in paranoid, narcissistic, borderline, and schizotypal PDs	Rule out frank psychosis Do not challenge paranoia; empathize with and offer help for underlying fear and emotional upset Atypical antipsychotics can reduce paranoia and associated agitation (Adityanjee & Schulz, 2002; Rocca et al., 2002; Koenigsberg et al., 2003)
Impulsive aggression	
Common in antisocial and borderline PDs	Ensure the safety of residents and staff first; this may require involvement of security staff, weapons search, chemical or physical restraints, and acute psychiatric hospitalization Rule out mania, frontal lobe impairment, dementia, occult substance abuse, pharmacologic overstimulation, hyperthyroidism, delirium

Continued

TABLE 9.2 Continued

TARGET SYMPTOMS/PDS	MANAGEMENT STRATEGIES
	Active limit setting prescribed, when necessary, by LTC administrative staff
	Increase involvement in daily exercise, physical therapy, or other therapeutic programming
	Serotonergic antidepressants (Coccaro et al., 1989, 1990; Kavoussi et al., 1994; Markowitz et al., 1991; Rinne et al., 2002; Zanarini et al., 2004)
	Atypical antipsychotics (Hirose, 2001; Rocca et al., 2002; Zanarini et al., 2004; Zanarini & Frankenberg, 2001)
	Divalproex sodium (Frankenberg & Zanarini, 2002; Stein et al., 1995; Wilcox, 1995)
Rage attacks	
Common in antisocial, borderline, and narcissistic PDs	See guidelines for impulsive aggression
Self-injurious behaviors	
Common in borderline PD	Rule out imminent threat to health; medical treatment is first priority
	Assess for suicidality; remove any implements that can be used for self-injury
	SSRI antidepressants (Rinne et al., 2002; Salzman et al., 1995)
	Atypical antipsychotics (Changappa et al., 1999; Frankenberg & Zanarini, 1993; Khouzam & Donnelly, 1997; Rocca et al., 2002; Zanarini et al., 2004)
	Divalproex sodium (Stein et al., 1995; Wilcox, 1995; Frankenberg & Zanarini, 2002)
Hypochondriacal complaints	
Common in histrionic, obsessive-compulsive, dependent, and depressive PDs	Identify underlying anxiety or depression
	SSRI antidepressants (Demopulos et al., 1996)
Medication abuse, nonadherence, or excessive and unusual side effects	Do not allow self-administration of medication
	Minimize the use of PRN ("as needed") dosing strategies
Common in borderline, antisocial, dependent, and passive-aggressive PDs	Simplify regimens, especially if multiple sedative-hypnotics or pain medications are being prescribed
	Reassess appropriateness of even using psychotropic medications; perhaps the best strategy is not to prescribe
Mood and anxiety symptoms	Treat these as with any other similar symptoms in non-PD patients, using appropriate anxiolytic or antidepressant medications
Common in all PDs	

CASE STUDIES

The following case studies look at the clinical presentation, assessment, case formulation, and management of several individuals with PDs in LTC settings.

Case 1

Mrs. Silver was a 70-year-old woman admitted to a nursing home after a stroke left her unable to walk. Extensive interview of her daughter indicated that Mrs. Silver had lived in a spare bedroom of her daughter's house for 5 years after her husband died. During that period of time the relationship with her daughter was severely strained by Mrs. Silver's frequent rages and obscenity-laced screaming. On several occasions, Mrs. Silver had threatened to kill herself after having a fight with her daughter. She would often say, "What's the use, you're going to abandon me anyway!" Sometimes she would refuse meals or medications. Mrs. Silver was calm and charming when visited by a psychiatrist from a local mental health center, but then refused to take the recommended medication or attend a day program.

In the 6 months that she had lived at the nursing home, Mrs. Silver was described by staff as difficult, hateful, and vicious. She would scream at aides and tell them that they were "fired" when she was unhappy with their care. She had constant complaints about the food and cleanliness of the ward. She didn't tolerate her first roommate, and accused her second roommate of stealing from her. Her behavior escalated when she was moved unexpectedly to another floor: she spent her days wheeling up and down the hallways and yelling at other residents about how "terrible" the staff was. She began to throw her linens into the hallway each day after her bed was made. After an angry confrontation with her physician, Mrs. Silver threatened to jump out of the window. She was transferred to an inpatient psychiatric ward, with the expressed hope that an alternate placement could be found.

Case Formulation and Treatment: During the assessment it was learned that Mrs. Silver had a previous history of similar disruptive behaviors since her early 20s, pointing to a likely diagnosis of borderline PD. Following LTC placement, she alienated family, other residents, and staff, and was unable to adapt to the demands of institutional living, such as having to accept the help of aides, or live in close proximity with a roommate. An abrupt change in her environment overwhelmed her brittle coping style, and made a bad situation much worse. In this case, a psychiatric crisis erupted and resulted in discharge before a coherent plan could be implemented. If Mrs. Silver has been treated prior to LTC placement, she might have had a more successful admission. Not surprisingly, after being stabilized in the hospital on an SSRI antidepressant and on a low-dose antipsychotic, she was much calmer, less rageful, and less impulsive, and was able to return to the same institution, but on a different unit. In addition to regular medication management, Mrs. Silver was enrolled in a structured group therapy program for 2 months in order to increase and improve her socialization with other residents and to form some gratifying bonds with clinical staff. Once she was less fearful of abandonment and began to trust staff, her behaviors improved significantly.

Case 2

Mr. Wilson was a 68-year-old single man who was admitted to a Veteran's Administration (VA) nursing home rehabilitation unit for treatment of a chronic leg ulcer. Prior to admission, Mr. Wilson had lived by himself in a rundown house in a small, rural town. Ever since his mother died 10 years ago, he had spent all of his time alone, and had infrequent contact with several neighbors. His social worker learned that Mr. Wilson had never had any close friends or romantic relationships, and had never married. Following a psychiatric hospitalization in the early 1950's for an unspecified "nervous condition," Mr. Wilson had been unemployed and on disability. His mother took care of managing meals, household duties, and finances, and Mr. Wilson in turn helped out around the house. Fortunately, he was able to assume most of the household responsibilities when she died. In the last several years, he spent all of his holidays alone, but stated that he wasn't bothered by this. However, a judge had mandated his placement and assigned a temporary guardian after county social workers reported that Mr. Wilson was refusing to allow visiting nurses to enter his house. This was apparently due to his faithful adherence to instructions his mother had left before her death not to let anyone in the house.

Nursing staff at the rehab unit described Mr. Wilson as a nervous and odd individual, who would never make eye contact. He kept to himself, often spending time in the bathroom. He was timid when approached by staff, and spoke in a soft, high-pitched voice. His affect was flat, and he demonstrated odd hand posturing and facial tics. He told a psychiatric consultant that he was "nervous around people," and worried that his whiskers made him look "awful." Mr. Wilson caused no problems for his primary nurses, and over time they felt that they were able to establish some rapport with him. He worked with the unit social worker to obtain his disability benefits at the VA hospital, and on one occasion a hospital official forgot to send him a receipt. Instead of contacting the social worker directly, Mr. Wilson paced quietly outside of her office for several hours until she emerged, and then timidly reported the missing receipt.

Case Formulation and Treatment: The assessment revealed that Mr. Wilson demonstrated a variety of long-standing, maladaptive traits. Avoidant traits included his timidness and social inhibitions, and lack of social or occupational pursuits, due to fear of exposure and rejection. He also demonstrated many schizoid traits, including a flat, detached affect, solitary pursuits, and a genuine disinterest in relationships. He had a pronounced dependency on his parents when they were living, but had managed to adapt to more independent living. Mr. Wilson was started on an SSRI antidepressant to treat his social anxiety and rejection sensitivity, and within several weeks he demonstrated significantly less anxiety in social interactions. He was able to establish relationships with several nurses as he became more familiar and comfortable with their presence. These nurses were sensitive to his fears, and maintained regular, friendly contacts with Mr. Wilson without being intrusive or critical. After several weeks of successfully residing on the unit, he agreed to remain voluntarily as a permanent resident in the facility.

Case 3

Mr. Peres was a 74-year-old widowed man admitted to a nursing home after being asked to leave an assisted living facility due to verbally abusive behaviors. He suffered from mild cognitive impairment and coronary artery disease, and was ambulatory and relatively independent on the unit. He quickly began getting into fights with other residents and staff, accusing nurses and aides of "incompetence" and "stupidity" and chastising other residents for being afraid to speak up to nursing staff. One night he got into an argument with a nurse and raised his cane toward her, threatening to hit her if she didn't get his sleeping pill immediately.

An emergency meeting of the facility's abuse committee was convened the next day. The psychiatrist who interviewed Mr. Peres noted that he had a 1-year history of mild short-term memory impairment, without previous work-up. His previous psychiatric history was notable for untreated alcohol abuse, although Mr. Peres was reportedly sober for the last 2 years. During the interview he demonstrated an irritable and depressed affect, a grandiose and entitled demeanor, but no evidence of psychosis, suicidality, or homicidality. According to his daughter, Mr. Peres had been married four times, and was estranged from two children from his first marriage. The daughter who served as an informant was from his second marriage, and she described him as an arrogant and a verbally abusive man throughout her life. In fact, when she visited him he would yell at her and berate her in front of staff. When the committee met with Mr. Peres, he denied ever having threatened a nurse, and responded with a list of demands, including wanting a personal aide to take him to movies and shopping.

Case Formulation and Treatment: Clinical assessment of Mr. Peres revealed narcissistic and antisocial personality traits, associated with depression and past substance use. His abusive behaviors were worsened by the narcissistic blow of being asked to leave one facility, and being placed in a nursing home with individuals who were older and more cognitively impaired. His arrogance and lack of empathy for anyone left him without any meaningful relationships except his daughter. Mr. Peres did agree to meet with a psychologist to discuss his stress level, and he was also started on a sedating antidepressant to improve his mood, impulsive aggression, and insomnia. The consistent relationship with an empathetic but very strict female psychotherapist helped contain his behaviors, and the antidepressant significantly reduced his impulsive aggression and underlying depression. He became less abusive, although still was demanding of staff. Later that year he was elected president of the resident's council, which was an extremely gratifying experience for him, and served to further ameliorate his hostile demeanor. His personality dysfunction remained, but at a more manageable level.

Acknowledgment   Several sections of the chapter are based upon or were taken from other writings of the author, including Agronin (2006) and zweig and Agronin (2006).

REFERENCES

Abrams, R. C., & Horowitz, S. V. (1996). Personality disorders after age 50: A meta-analysis. *Journal of Personality Disorders, 10*(3), 271–281.

Adityanjee, A. & Schulz, S. C. (2002). Clinical uses of quetiapine in disease states other than schizophrenia. *Journal of Clinical Psychiatry, 63,* 32–38.

Agronin, M. E. (1994). Personality disorders in the elderly: An overview. *Journal of Geriatric Psychiatry, 27*(2), 151–191.

Agronin, M. E. (1999a, March 16). *Depressive personality disorder in late life: A descriptive study of 11 cases.* Poster and abstract presented at the annual meeting of the American Association for Geriatric Psychiatry in New Orleans, LA.

Agronin, M. E. (1999b). Pharmacologic treatment of personality disorders in late life. In E. Rosowsky, R. C. Abrams, & R. A. Zweig (Eds.), *Personality disorders in older adults* (pp. 229–254). Mahwah, NJ: Lawrence Erlbaum.

Agronin, M. E. (2006). Personality disorders. In D. V. Jeste & J. H. Friedman (Eds.), *Psychiatry for neurologists* (pp. 105–124). Totowa, NJ: Humana Press.

Agronin, M. E., & Maletta, G. (2000). Personality disorders in late life: Understanding and overcoming the gap in research. *American Journal of Geriatric Psychiatry, 8,* 4–18.

Agronin, M. E., & Orr, W. B. (1998, March 8–11). Personality disorders in a geriatric psychiatry outpatient clinic. American Association for Geriatric Psychiatry— abstracts. Annual meeting, San Diego, CA.

American Psychiatric Association. (2000). *Diagnostic and statistical manual of mental disorders* (4th ed., text revision). Washington, DC: Author.

Black, D. W., Baumgard, C. H., & Bell, S. E. (1995, March/April). A 16- to 45-year follow-up of 71 men with antisocial personality disorder. *Comprehensive Psychiatry, 36*(2), 130–140.

Blazer, D. G., George, L. K., Landerman, R., et al. (1985). Psychiatric disorders, a rural/urban comparison. *Archives of General Psychiatry, 42,* 651–656.

Bezzola, F. G., Gorelick, P. B., & Freels, S. (1992). Personality changes in Alzheimer's disease. *Archives of Neurology, 49,* 297–300.

Chengappa, K. N. R., Ebeling, T., Kang, J. S., et al. (1999). Clozapine reduces severe self-mutilation and aggression in psychotic patients with borderline personality disorder. *Journal of Clinical Psychiatry, 60,* 477–484.

Coccaro, E. F., Astill, J. L., Herbert, J. A., et al. (1990). Fluoxetine treatment of impulsive aggression in *DSM-III-R* personality disorder patients. *Journal of Clinical Psychopharmacology, 10,* 373–375.

Coccaro, E. F., Siever, L. J., Klar, H. M., et al. (1989). Serotonergic studies in patients with affective and personality disorders: Correlates with suicidal and impulsive aggressive behavior. *Archives of Geriatric Psychiatry, 46,* 587–599.

Day, K. (1985). Psychiatric disorders in the middle-aged and elderly mentally handicapped. *British Journal of Psychiatry, 147,* 553–558.

Demopulos, C., Fava, M., McLean, N. E., et al. (1996). Hypochondriacal concerns in depressed outpatients. *Psychosomatic Medicine, 58*(4), 314–320.

Frankenburg, F. R., & Zanarini, M. C. (1993) Clozapine treatment of borderline patients: A preliminary study. *Comprehensive Psychiatry, 34*(6), 402–405.

Frankenberg, F. R., & Zanarini, M. C. (2002). Divalproex sodium treatment of women with borderline personality disorder and bipolar II disorder: A double-blind, placebo-controlled pilot study. *Journal of Clinical Psychiatry, 63,* 442–446.

Grant, B. F., Hasin, D. S., Stinson, F. S., et al. (2004). Prevalence, correlates, and disability of personality disorders in the United States: Results from the national epidemiologic survey on alcohol and related conditions. *Journal of Clinical Psychiatry, 65*(7), 948–958.

Hirose, S. (2001). Effective treatment of aggression and impulsivity in antisocial personality disorder with risperidone. *Psychiatry and Clinical Neurosciences, 55,* 161–162.

Kavoussi, R. J., Liv, J., & Coccaro, E. F. (1994). An open trial of sertraline in personality disorder patients with impulsive aggression. *Journal of Clinical Psychology, 55,* 137–141.

Khouzam, H. R., & Donnelly, N. J. (1997). Remission of self-mutilation in a patient with borderline personality during risperidone therapy. *Journal of Nervous and Mental Disease, 185*(5), 348–349.

Koenigsberg, H. W., Reynolds, D., Goodman, M., et al. (2003). Risperidone in the treatment of schizotypal personality disorder. *Journal of Clinical Psychiatry, 64,* 628–634.

Kunik, M. E., Mulsant, B. H., Rifai, A. H., et al. (1993). Personality disorders in elderly inpatients with major depression. *American Journal of Geriatric Psychiatry, 1*(1), 38–45.

Linehan, M. M., Armstrong, H. E., Suarez, A., et al. (1991). Cognitive-behavioral treatment of chronically suicidal borderline patients. *Archives of General Psychiatry, 48,* 1060–1064.

Livesley, W. J. (2002). Treating the emotional dysregulation cluster of traits. *Psychiatric Annals, 32*(10), 601–607.

Lynch, T. R. (2000). Treatment of elderly depression with personality disorder comorbidity using dialectical behavior therapy. *Cognitive and Behavioral Practice, 7,* 447–456.

Margo, J. L., Robinson, J. R., & Corea, S. (1980). Referrals to a psychiatric service from old people's homes. *British Journal of Psychiatry, 136,* 396–401.

Markowitz, P. J. (2004). Recent trends in the pharmacotherapy of personality disorders. *Journal of Personality Disorders, 18*(1), 90–101.

Markowitz, P. J., Calabrese, J. R., Schulz, S. C., et al. (1991). Fluoxetine treatment of borderline and schizotypal personality disorders. *American Journal of Psychiatry, 148,* 1064–1067.

McGlashen, T. H. (1986). The Chestnut Lodge follow-up study: III. Long-term outcome of borderline personalities. *Archives of General Psychiatry, 43,* 20–30.

Paris, J., Brown, R., & Nowlis, D. (1987). Long-term follow-up of borderline patients in a general hospital. *Comprehensive Psychiatry, 2,* 530–535.

Petry, S., Cummings, J. L., Hill, M. A., & Shapira, J. (1988). Personality alterations in dementia of the Alzheimers type. *Archives of Neurology, 45,* 118–190.

Phillips, K. A., & Gunderson, J. G. (1994). Personality disorders. In R. E. Hales, S. C. Yudofsky, & J. A. Talbott (Eds.), *Textbook of psychiatry* (2nd ed.). Washington DC: American Psychiatric Press.

Rinne, T., Van den Brink, W., Wouters, I., & van Dyck, R. (2002). SSRI treatment of borderline personality disorder: A randomized, placebo-controlled clinical trial for females with BPD. *American Journal of Psychiatry, 159,* 2048–2054.

Robins, C. J. (2002). Dialectical behavior therapy for borderline personality disorder. *Psychiatric Annals, 32*(10), 608–616.

Robins, C. J., & Chapman, A. L. (2004). Dialectical behavior therapy: Current status, recent developments, and future directions. *Journal of Personality Disorders, 18*(1), 73–89.

Robins, L. N., Helzer, J. E., Weissman, M. M., et al. (1984). Lifetime prevalence of specific psychiatric disorders in three sites. *Archives of General Psychiatry, 41,* 949–958.

Rocca, P., Marchiaro, L., Cocuzza, E., & Bogetto, E. (2002). Treatment of borderline personality disorder with risperidone. *Journal of Clinical Psychiatry, 63,* 241–244.

Rosowsky, E., & Gurian, B. (1992). Impact of borderline personality disorder in late life on systems of care. *Hospital and Community Psychiatry, 43*(4), 386–389.

Rubin, E. H., Morris, J. C., & Berg, L. (1987). The progression of personality changes in senile dementia of the Alzheimer's type. *Journal of the American Geriatrics Society, 35,* 21–25.

Salzman, C., Wolfson, A. N., Schatzberg, A., et al. (1995). Effect of fluoxetine on anger in symptomatic volunteers with borderline personality disorder. *Journal of Clinical Psychopharmacology, 15*(1), 23–29.

Scott, S., Simons, A. D., Thase, M. E., & Pilkonis, P. (1992). Are personality assessments valid in acute major depression? *Journal of Affective Disorders, 24,* 281–290.

Stein, D. J., Simeon, D., Frenkel, M., et al. (1995). An open trial of valproate in borderline personality disorder. *Journal of Clinical Psychology, 56*(11), 506–510.

Teeter, R. B., Garetz, F. K., Miller, W. R., & Heiland, W. F. (1976). Psychiatric disturbances of aged patients in skilled nursing homes. *American Journal of Psychiatry, 133,* 1430–1434.

Weissman, M. M. (1993). The epidemiology of personality disorders: A 1990 update. *Journal of Personality Disorders, 7,* 44–62.

Wilcox, J. A. (1995). Divalproex sodium as a treatment for borderline personality disorder. *Annals of Clinical Psychiatry, 7*(1), 33–37.

Zanarini, M. C., & Frankenberg, F. R. (2001). Olanzapine treatment of female borderline patients: A double-blind, placebo-controlled pilot study. *Journal of Clinical Psychiatry, 62,* 849–854.

Zanarini, M. C., Frankenberg, F., & Parachini, E. A. (2004). A preliminary, randomized trial of fluoxetine, olanzapine, and the olanzapine- fluoxetine combination in
women with borderline personality disorder. *Journal of Clinical Psychiatry, 65*(7),
903–907.

Zweig, R., & Agronin, M. E. (2006). Personality disorders in late life. In M. E. Agronin
& G. J. Maletta (Eds.), *Principles and practice of geriatric psychiatry* (pp. 449–470).
Philadelphia: Lippincott Williams & Wilkins.

10

Mental Retardation

C. Michael Henderson

This chapter will introduce nursing home clinicians to the patient population that has mental retardation (MR). Although MR is not a psychiatric disorder, patients with MR by definition have impairment of intellectual ability and therefore may present with atypical rates or presentations of medical/psychiatric conditions and challenges. Clinical problems may arise directly from intellectual impairment in persons with MR via limited language skills to report symptoms, or can occur due to associated syndromic disorders or other developmental disabilities. These clinical problems, along with philosophies of care and legal/regulatory issues that pertain to people with MR, make the relatively small number of nursing home patients with MR an important and well-defined population.

In this review of selected topics on MR in long-term care, MR will be defined and described. Legal/regulatory issues that pertain to patients in nursing homes with MR will be briefly discussed. Selected important clinical topics such as pain assessment, health-care decision-making capacity, and health and age status of people with MR in nursing homes will be presented. Although psychiatric disorders are an extremely important clinical area in the population with MR, constituting a veritable subspecialty in psychiatry, this area will be briefly touched on in the contexts of Alzheimer's disease in persons with Down syndrome and the diagnosis of depression in older adults with MR.

Much of the research that has been done in the field of developmental medicine has been directed toward children; work with adults has been largely done
in countries outside of the United States. This point is reflected by the majority
of literature citations referenced in this chapter, and constitutes a problem in
generalizing to the adult population with MR in the United States. Because a
continuum of supportive residential settings are provided in the MR service sector (ranging from "supported" apartments to group homes to group residences
with nursing support (ICF/MR homes), this review will be directed to people
with MR in the context of the general nursing home setting.

NOMENCLATURE

The term "mental retardation" is now felt by many to be pejorative and efforts
are under way to use alternative terms to describe global cognitive/intellectual
disability that is acquired during the developmental period (The Arc, 2004). The
term "developmental disability" is not specific as it can refer to both intellectual
and physical impairments. The term *intellectual disability* has been proposed to
replace the term mental retardation. As there is no definite consensus for new
terminology in the United States, and to preserve clarity, the term mental retardation (MR) will be used in this review.

Habilitation refers to clinical or educational interventions to enable individuals to attain new (as opposed to lost) capabilities.

DEFINITIONS

Mental retardation is not a psychiatric illness. Several definitions of MR have
been provided by federal law and professional organizations. Federal legislation, such as Developmental Disabilities Assistance and Bill of Rights Act
of 2000 (P.L. 106–402), stipulates that developmental disabilities are mental
or physical impairments that have an age of onset before 22 years and that
confer three or more limitations in major life activities. Specified life activities include self-care, receptive and expressive language, learning, mobility,
self-direction, capacity for independent living, and economic self-sufficiency.
This legal definition reflects affected individuals' needs and entitlements for
a personalized array of services provided simultaneously or sequentially to
lessen disability.

The American Association on Mental Retardation (2002) defines MR using
three criteria: (1) limitations in intellectual functioning based on standardized
intelligence test scores, (2) limitations in one or more adaptive skills areas,

and (3) onset prior to age 18 years. The intellectual impairment is defined as a full-scale IQ score on a standardized intelligence test of approximately 70 or below (two or more standard deviations below the mean IQ in a defined population). Impairment in adaptive skills is based on objective measures of deficits in performance of conceptual (i.e., receptive and expressive language), social (i.e., interpersonal skills), and practical (personal activities of daily living) areas. A score less than two standard deviations below the mean in one of the three adaptive areas, or on the overall score of all three areas, constitutes the adaptive skills criterion.

Although the *Diagnostic and Statistical Manual of Mental Disorders*, fourth edition, text revision (*DSM-IV-TR*; APA, 2000) classifies MR as an axis II disorder, diagnostic criteria largely reflects components (IQ, adaptive skills, and age of onset) presented by the American Association on Mental Retardation. Criteria from the *DSM-IV-TR* are generally used to provide a clinical diagnosis of MR. *Although there are differences in these definitions, the overall implication is the identification and provision of needed supports and services that address the specific functional impairments of individuals with MR.*

A number of standardized IQ tests—such as the WAIS III (The Psychological Corporation, 1997) and the Stanford-Binet 5 (Roid, 2003a) are currently used for the IQ test criterion. Validated and reliable standardized adaptive skills measures—such as the AAMR Adaptive Behavioral Scales—Residential and Community Edition (Nihira et al., 1993) are available.

SEVERITY OF MR

There are four degrees of MR severity: (1) mild: IQ range of 70 to 55, (2) moderate: IQ range of 35 to 54, (3) severe: IQ range of 20 to 34, and (4) profound: IQ of below 20. Adults with mild MR may have reading and numerical skills at the 1st to 6th grade level, social and community interests, and capabilities for significant self direction including complete independence with jobs in the competitive economy. People who have mild MR severity can be expected to learn an array of new skills and fulfill all adult expectations. In general, adults who have moderate MR can attain functional language skills, perform self-care skills, and work in supervised settings. People with moderate MR cannot attain independence, and will require lifelong supervision and supports. Adults with severe MR may be able to perform self-care skills, develop peer and friendship social relationships, and acquire some language skills (receptive skills are usually better developed than expressive language). Profound MR confers a spectrum of disability that ranges from lack of all self-care and language skills to extremely limited development of these adaptive areas (Jacobson & Mulick, 1996). It is important that nursing home clinicians do not overestimate the disability of patients with mild or moderate MR. The AAMR definition of MR emphasizes that the majority of persons with MR have some capability for lifelong learning (AAMR, 2002).

Capute and Accardo (1991) conceptualized a continuum of associated developmental disabilities that is directly related to the severity of the causative brain insult. In this model, persons with severe MR are more likely to have other neurological conditions, such as epilepsy, or other developmental disabilities, such as cerebral palsy or autism. Severe MR has an impact on function that is often closely related to the presence of other developmental disabilities or associated comorbid conditions. An analysis of a register of persons with MR in Finland revealed that, out of 461 subjects with severe MR, 91.5% had between one and six associated impairments. In addition, significant congenital birth defects that can cause premature mortality during childhood were relatively common in subjects in the population sample (Arvio & Sillanpana, 2003). Persons with MR with severe intellectual impairment, and with other developmental disabilities or neurological disorders such as cerebral palsy and epilepsy, have been documented to have decreased life expectancy compared to those who have higher functional capabilities and fewer comorbid conditions directly related to the causative CNS insult (Chaney & Eyman, 2000).

CAUSES OF MR

There are a multitude of conditions that have a deleterious effect on the developing brain. Etiologies are classified by the AAMR (2002) by prenatal, perinatal, and postnatal causes. Subcategories of prenatal causes include chromosomal disorders, genetic/syndromic causes, inborn errors of metabolism, developmental disorders of brain development, and environmental causes. Perinatal causes include intrauterine and neonatal disorders, and postnatal causes encompass traumatic brain injury, infections, toxins, neurodegenerative disorders, and other conditions sustained during infancy or childhood.

A total of 290 genes are associated with MR clinical phenotypes and syndromes, and an analysis of the Online Mendelian Inheritance in Man revealed more than 1000 entries for MR (Chelly et al., 2006). Persons with mild MR are less likely to have clearly identifiable causes of their intellectual disability. Stromme (2000) performed clinical evaluations on 178 Norwegian children with MR, and identified biopathological etiologies in 68% of those with mild MR, and 96% of subjects with severe MR. Conditions that can commonly cause MR and that may be (relatively) commonly encountered by nursing home clinicians include (1) Down syndrome—which is present in 0.92% of infants (MMWR, 1994), (2) Fragile X syndrome—an X chromosome-linked MR disorder that is found in 1 out of 3847 males (Beckett et al., 2005), and (3) Fetal Alcohol

Syndrome—estimated to be present in 0.5 to 2 per 1000 newborns in the United States (May & Gossage, 2001).

PREVALENCE OF MR AMONG AGE GROUPS

Based on IQ score criteria for MR (two or more standard deviations below the mean), the expected prevalence of persons with MR is approximately 2.5% of the general population. However, in-depth investigations have revealed lower prevalence rates. Leonard and coworkers (2003) in Australia documented a 1.57% prevalence of MR in Australian children—subjects with mild-to-moderate MR were noted to be 10 times more common than those with severe MR. In Ontario, Canada the prevalence of MR in teenagers was found to be 0.72% (Bradley et al., 2002). Older data presented in the MMRW (1995) documented that, in 1993, U.S. national prevalence rates of MR were 1.14% of children aged 6 to 17 years, and 0.66% of adults aged 18to 64 years. More recently, Bhasin and colleagues (2006), showed that the overall prevalence of MR in children in Atlanta, Georgia aged 8 years was 1.2% in 2000; of these, 61% had mild MR. The findings of rates of varying MR severity and lower than expected prevalence rates in the countries cited above may reflect differing diagnostic methods as well as real variance due to the contribution of various socioeconomic and educational factors, and attrition of severely affected infants and children (see below).

Several comments can be made about the U.S. findings. The approximately 50% greater prevalence of MR in children compared to adults in 1993 (MMRW, 1995) may be attributed to several factors that are related to premature mortality in this population. One is based on the decreased longevity of persons with MR who resided in large institutions (resulting in a cohort effect in the present population of older adults with MR). Another is related to the continuum model of developmental disability that confers early mortality in severely affected children. However, Janicki and coworkers (1999) found that, although longevity differences were decreasing, adults with MR age 40 years and older in New York State had lower life expectancies (average age at death 66.1 years) than adults in the general population. In this study, causes of death were similar in the two populations suggesting that discrepancies in health-care delivery/practices and not purely biological effects were playing roles in the longevity difference.

LAW AND POLICY RELEVANT TO NURSING HOMES

The vast majority of persons with MR do not live in nursing homes. A variety of federal and state funding sources assist individuals with MR to receive services from state and private agencies that enable adults with MR to live by themselves, with their families, or in agency-provided residences (foster family care providers, group homes, ICF/MRs) within the general community.

Several laws and policies are highly relevant to the provision of clinical services to people with MR who reside in Medicaid certified nursing homes. The Nursing Home Reform Act (OBRA 1987, P.L. 100–203) and the OBRA '90 (P.L. 101–508), mandate an evaluation (Pre-Admission Screening and Resident Review, or PASRR) of all nursing home applicants and residents. The PASRR is waived in the following scenarios: (1) individuals admitted directly from a hospital after receiving acute inpatient care and who need nursing home services for the condition that prompted hospital admission, *and* whose attending physicians certify will likely need less than 30 days of nursing home care, (2) readmission of individuals to nursing home from after an acute care hospital stay, and (3) transfer of individuals from one nursing home to another nursing home (the transferring nursing home must provide the most recent PASRR information). The nursing home and (if applicable) the hospital conduct Level I screens for nonexempted new resident-applicants. If Level I screens indicate that nursing home applicants have MR, then independent state-appointed agents conduct Level II subsequent reviews to determine the appropriateness of nursing home admissions. Evaluated applicants who have MR and who do not require nursing services are directed to alternative community-based services. In addition, the care plans of *existing* residents with documented MR are periodically reviewed to ensure that their clinical status continues to require supports provided by nursing homes. New instruments—such as the Supports Intensity Scale (Thompson et al., 2004)—have been designed to determine the nursing and other supportive care needs of persons with MR.

In the Olmstead decision of 1999 (*Olmstead v. L.C. and E.W., 119 S.Ct. 2176*) the U.S. Supreme Court stated that the ADA (Americans with Disabilities Act 1990, P.L 101–333) requires that individuals with MR receive community-based and not nursing home residential services if an integrated community setting is the most appropriate one for their needs.

In the Rolland decision in 2003 (*Rolland v. Romney, 318 F.3d 42 1stCir.*), the U.S. Court of Appeals for the First Circuit reviewed the Commonwealth of Massachusetts's claim that nursing homes were not obligated to provide specialized services to residents with MR who were determined to require nursing home care. The decision found that Massachusetts was in violation of both the ADA and the NHRA. Nursing home residents with MR are deemed to have rights to receive individual-specific specialized services to address their habilitative needs.

These laws and legal case decisions can be summarized as follows: (1) persons with MR can be placed and continue to reside in nursing homes only if their physical (with an exception being dementia) health needs cannot be addressed in less restrictive community-based settings, and (2) persons with MR residing in nursing homes are entitled to individual-based specialized services to maximize their capabilities.

Prevalence and Characteristics of Persons with MR in Nursing Homes

People with MR constitute a small number of total nursing home residents. In 1985, data from the National Nursing Home Survey indicated that there were 83,200 residents with a diagnosis of MR out of a national nursing home census of 974,300 (Strahan, 1991). By 1997, out of a total nursing home population of 1,608,700, there were 14,900 nursing home residents, or approximately 1% of the total nursing home census—who had a primary diagnosis of MR both at the time of admission and at the time of survey. Individuals who had MR in all-listed diagnoses numbered 35,400. Approximately half of the individuals with a primary diagnosis of MR were less than 65 years old (compared to 9.4% of the general nursing home population). The physical care needs of the residents with MR were high, with almost all requiring assistance with bathing and dressing (Gabriel & Jones, 2000).

A national study was conducted using the MDS and other available scales data to further examine the characteristics of patients residing in nursing homes in 1994 to 1996 (Fries et al., 2005). This study confirmed earlier findings regarding nursing home residents with MR (Gabriel & Jones, 2000) and added more detailed information. Subjects were 665,494 total nursing home residents in nine states. Persons under age 65 years accounted for approximately 10% of the total subjects. Thirteen "diagnostic clusters" accounted for 85% of all nursing home residents. Patients with MR and other developmental disabilities with or without spastic quadraparetic cerebral palsy (MR/DD) accounted for high percentages of the younger resident age segments. For example, in the 0 to 4 years, 5 to 14 years, and 15 to 24 years of age segments, total subjects with MR/DD accounted for 54%, 82%, and 42% in these respective age groups. After age 25 years and up to 64 years, subjects with MR accounted for 25% to 35% of the total nursing home residents. In this study, after age 65 years, subjects with MR/DD accounted for only 8% of total residents. In addition, individuals with MR/DD in the younger age brackets exhibited high rates of severe cognitive and physical disability and required extremely high levels of staff interventions such as tube feeding, oxygen and physical therapy/occupational therapy services. If one extrapolates from mortality data (Janicki et al., 1999), then it is likely that older adults with MR had older-age related conditions that conferred disability—such as stroke or late-stage neoplastic disease—requiring nursing home supports.

Clinical Issues Relevant to Persons with MR Living in Nursing Homes

Pain assessment in persons with MR

Pain is now considered the "fifth vital sign" and is a critical component of nursing assessment, physician diagnosis of acute medical disorders, and determination of the adequacy of palliative care in persons who have a terminal illness. Persons with mild or with the upper level of moderate MR can likely use language to convey information about their experience of pain. Little is known about the palliative care needs of persons with more severe MR; expressive language barriers can interfere with interpretation of symptoms and the timely diagnosis of illnesses (Tuffrey-Wijne, 2003). Preliminary work has approached this concern using a number of methodologies. Using heat-pain threshold measures taught to subjects with MR, combined with reaction time to determine the pain threshold of the subjects with MR, there was indication that subjects with MR were more pain sensitive than controls (Defrin et al., 2004). In another study, children with MR and with or without other developmental disorders were evaluated for the number, severity, and duration of painful episodes during a set time period. The episodes, severity, and duration measures were based on caregiver observations. During a 4-week period, it was found that subjects had multiple and prolonged painful episodes—subjects with the lowest cognitive capabilities suffered from the highest burdens of pain (Breau et al., 2003).

Preexisting clinical factors, such as epilepsy and nonverbal status, that convey risk for painful episodes in children with MR due to accidental injury, seizures, and infrequent medical monitoring, were described by Breau and colleagues (2004). These clinical risk factors tend to be more specific than sensitive and therefore are more likely to be helpful in preventing or ruling out potential causes of pain. A questionnaire evaluated nurses' methods to assess pain in persons with severe and profound MR (Zwakhalen et al., 2004). Nurses reported that behavioral specific observations often directed to painful anatomic areas—moaning, crying, grimacing with manipulation of a body part or refusal to use or normally move the affected body part—were important in determining the presence, location, and intensity of pain in persons with severe MR who had limited or no language skills. In addition, "physiological" indicators of pain (i.e., changes in vital signs) were rated as important pain indicators in persons with profound MR. The Pain and Discomfort Scale (PADS) is a multidimensional instrument that uses a combination of physiological and behavioral indicators to measure pain (Norden et al., 1991). Investigators used the PADS to detect pain during dental scaling in subjects with MR; scores were significantly higher during this procedure than when obtained during nonpainful interventions (Phan et al., 2005).

A number of nonverbal pain report methods are available and can be used in a developmentally appropriate way to detect pain in nursing home patients who cannot readily verbalize their discomfort. Examples used to determine pain severity in children include facial expression scales and visual analogue scales (Champion et al., 1998), and the Poker Chip Scale (Hester, 1990). Completion of the modified McGill Pain Questionnaire (Melzack, 2005) is within the capacity of many people with mild MR. Individually appropriate pain assessment tools should be incorporated in the nursing care plans of nursing home patients who have MR.

Determination of capacity to make informed health-care decisions

Biessart and Hubben (1999) used a questionnaire format to examine attitudes regarding the capacity of adults with MR to make health care and other decisions in three groups of subjects: (1) relatives of the subjects with MR, (2) clinicians and administrators who provided oversight and services to the subjects with MR, and (3) adult subjects with MR. Analysis revealed that subjects with MR self-rated themselves as having relatively high rates of capacity, followed by the administrator/clinician subjects, with relatives giving the least endorsement for decision-making capacity. Interestingly, a retrospective analysis revealed that, in previous scenarios involving decision-making, clinician/administrator practices were discordant with the study results, with less actual decision-making input incorporated for the subjects with MR than suggested from the questionnaire results (Biesaart & Hubben, 1999). Gunn and coworkers (1999)—in a study of health-care decision-making capacity in subjects without mental impairment, subjects with mental illness, and subjects with MR—identified several key issues in health-care capacity assessment. They noted that health-care decision-making incapacity can be reversible with therapeutic attention to the presence of active mental illness or health-care knowledge deficits. In addition, they emphasized the context of informed health-care decision-making. Although incapacity may be reversible for some individuals with MR, decisions are made within a clinical and medical-legal context. In addition, it was posed that a need for rapid and complex decision-making might make it difficult or impossible to reverse incapacity in specific decisions for individuals with MR. Fisher (2002) posed that to optimize accuracy of assessments of health-care decision-making capacity, adults with MR may benefit from attention to the way that relevant information is presented. This may include the presence of specific trusted people, the sequential delivery of small amounts of information that describe the clinical problem and the proposed intervention, and the avoidance of medical jargon.

Applebaum and Grisso (1988) proposed a model to determine health-care decision-making capacity in persons with mental impairment. Determination of capacity is based on abilities in four areas: (1) ability to indicate a choice, (2) demonstrated knowledge of the basic factual aspects of the decision, (3) social context, and (4) rational manipulation of information (culminating in weighed risk-benefit judgments). In adults who have MR, social context may include relatives or other caregivers of the adult with MR who have strong opinions about specific decisions. The assessment of social context in adults with MR may involve a determination that the individual is making the decision based on his or her own wishes, and not to placate others. This is potentially important, since a study of adults with MR revealed that 50% of those with mild and 20% of those with moderate MR demonstrated the capacity to make informed health-care decisions including weighed risk/benefit calculations (Cea & Fisher, 2003).

Alzheimer's disease and Down syndrome

Alzheimer's disease is found in relatively high rates in older persons who have Down syndrome. Research findings in the Down syndrome population have yielded information about several potential causes of Alzheimer's disease including the amyloid cascade (Head & Lott, 2004), oxidative stress (Lee et al., 2006; Lott & Head, 2001), and cerebrovascular disease (Lott & Head, 2005) hypotheses.

Even though neuropathology in relatively young adults with Down syndrome is consistent with Alzheimer's disease (Lai, 1992; Wisniewski et al., 1994), not all individuals with Down syndrome will develop clinical dementia (Zigman et al., 1996); there are individual protective factors that influence the occurrence of the disease (Schupf & Sergievsky, 2002). However, the onset of dementia in persons with Down syndrome occurs at ages approximately 20 to 30 years younger than in the general population. Holland and colleagues (Holland et al., 1998) found that 10% of subjects with Down syndrome at age 40 to 49 years and 40% of subjects at age 50 to 59 years had evidence of dementia based on in-depth cognitive measures. The mean age of onset of Alzheimer's disease in individuals with Down syndrome has been found to be about 55 years (Tyrrell et al., 2001; the life expectancy of persons with Down syndrome who develop Alzheimer's disease is 4.6 years (Lai & Williams, 1989). Alzheimer's disease in those with Down syndrome progresses from personality changes and executive dysfunction (Ball et al., 2006) to include aberrant behaviors such as aggression (Haveman et al., 1994), weight loss (Prasher et al., 2004), and seizures and myoclonus (Menendez, 2005). Eventually, there is significant memory impairment with an inability to learn new skills, recall recent events, remember the names of familiar people, and maintain orientation within familiar settings. In the late stages of Alzheimer's disease in adults with Down syndrome, aphasia, agnosia, and apraxia occur and are associated with death (Oliver et al., 1998). Several instruments are available to screen for the presence and monitor the progression of Alzheimer's disease in persons who have Down syndrome (Gedye, 1995; Prasher et al., 2004).

Ongoing health screening and intervention of older persons with Down syndrome with or without dementia needs to account for a number of conditions that are common in this population. Some of these conditions are reversible and can cause cognitive and behavioral disorders that mimic Alzheimer's disease. Weight loss should prompt an evaluation for celiac sprue as this disorder is common in persons with Down syndrome (Book et al., 2001) and can manifest with neurological changes (Voknin et al., 2004). Older persons with Down syndrome acquire a large number of health comorbidities including acquired heart disease, uncorrected congenital heart disease with resulting pulmonary artery hypertension, osteoarthritis, osteoporosis with history of fracture, and recurrent respiratory infections (van Allen et al., 1999). Hypothyroidism due to autoimmune thyroiditis is common in adults with Down syndrome (Prasher, 1999), and subclinical hypothyroidism can worsen cognition in persons with Down syndrome and should be identified and treated (Prasher, 1990). Extremity weakness or dysfunction should prompt an evaluation for cervical spondylotic myelopathy (Bosma, 1999). Adults with Down syndrome are at relative risk for the early-age onset of presbyacusis and significant hearing loss (Buchanan, 1990; Evenhuis, 1992). Visual impairment rates are high in adults with Down syndrome (Evenhuis et al., 2001) and can be due to refractive errors, cataracts, and corneal disease (van Splunder et al., 2004). Finally, depression can cause functional decline both in persons who have Down syndrome with and without dementia (Tsiouris & Patti, 1997); depression can mimic the presentation of dementia in older persons with Down syndrome (Chicoine et al., 1999). If depression is suspected, then antidepressant therapy is recommended and a positive response may have both diagnostic and therapeutic utility (Geldmacher et al., 1997).

The specific recommended medical treatment for Alzheimer's disease in persons with Down syndrome mirrors that for the general population (Prasher, 2004). In those individuals who develop epilepsy, phenytoin should probably be avoided, as one case series documented abrupt severe cognitive decline in persons with Down syndrome and Alzheimer's disease who received this medication; valproic acid is an effective, alternate anticonvulsant medication (Tsiouris et al., 2002).

The diagnosis of depression in older adults who have MR

Ascertaining the prevalence of mental health disorders in older persons with MR has been problematic. Research studies in this area have been under way for only two decades. There is great diversity in the functional and especially language capabilities of the population with MR. Prospective longitudinal studies that address the incidence and duration of psychiatric illness have been lacking. An array of psychiatric diagnostic methods has been used without a clear consensus on "gold standard" practices (Jacobson, 2003). However, data does exist on the prevalence of psychiatric disorders in adults with MR. Jacobson and Harper (1989) studied a sample of older persons with MR living in a variety of residential settings and with differing levels of MR. From age 55 years upward, approximately 20% of subjects had identifiable psychiatric disorders (as opposed to higher rates of aberrant behaviors seen in younger subjects). Lund (1985) found that in the age group 45 to 64 years, psychosis, schizophrenia, neurosis, and depression were present in 12% of subjects. Sansom and colleagues (1994) used *DSM-III-R* criteria to examine adults older than 60 years and found a prevalence of mood disorders in 8.9% and schizophrenia in 6.5% of subjects. More recently, investigators in Australia (White et al., 2005) found that 8% of adults with MR had >6 months of symptoms consistent with depression (ICD-10 criteria). A review of studies of psychopathology prevalence in older persons with MR noted that, compared to the general population, there is a relatively high prevalence of specific psychiatric disorders, and this prevalence increases with attainment of older age (Tyrrell & Dodd, 2003). Depression was found to be underdiagnosed in one study of adults with MR (Gustavson et al., 2005).

Day (1985), and Patel and coworkers (1993), looking specifically for *depression* in *older adults* with MR, described prevalence rates of approximately 5% of subjects. Subpopulations of older individuals with MR who are at specific biological risk for depression include those with Down syndrome (Tsiouris & Patti, 1997) and Fragile X syndrome (Tranebjaerg & Orum, 1991).

Janowsky and Davis (2005) propose that *DSM-IV* criteria can be used to diagnose depression in people who have mild-moderate MR. Various depression screening instruments have been developed for people with MR based on self-report such as the Self Report Depression Questionnaire (SRDQ) (Esbensen et al., 2005) and a broader diagnostic self-report questionnaire for psychopathology, the Psychiatric Assessment Schedule for Adults with Developmental Disability (PAS-ADD; Costello et al., 1997). Informal caregiver report has been questioned as a method to diagnose depression in persons with MR and expressive language skills, with self-report and structured clinical interviews showing more convergence (Bramston & Fogarty, 2000). Diagnostic checklists based on the PAS-ADD have been designed for caregivers (Moss et al., 1998). Cognitive variables associated with depressed mood have been described in adults with MR such as automatic thoughts, negative attributions, hopelessness, and poor self esteem (Esbensen & Benson, 2005). Suicidal ideation has been described in some adults with MR (Lunsky, 2004).

Life scenarios have been explored to ascertain needs for the proactive monitoring of adults with MR to make early diagnoses of depression. Bereavement symptoms such as crying, fatigue, sleep deprivation, loss of appetite, were described in one case series of adults with MR, and the researchers questioned how many subjects had clinical depression (Harper & Wadsworth, 1993.) Dodd and coworkers (2005), in a review of bereavement in adults with MR, posed that more research needs to be done to determine how bereavement may evolve into depression and other psychiatric disorders in persons with MR. Analysis of life events has been studied (Esbensen & Benson, 2006) to correlate with or predict the development of depressive symptoms; a variety of significant or sequential negative life events were found to be linked to depressive symptoms.

The diagnosis of depression in persons with severe-profound MR and little or no expressive language skills is controversial (McBrien, 2003). Current diagnostic methods have poor reliability and validity in persons with severe MR, with many clinicians using aberrant behaviors as surrogate affective observations (Ross & Oliver, 2003). One group of investigators noted a decrease in aggression in adults with severe MR after use of SSRI antidepressants in an open-label, naturalistic trial (Janowsky et al., 2005). However, Tsiouris and colleagues in (2003) cautioned that aggression and other challenging behaviors should not be considered as depressive equivalents—the diagnosis of depression should be based on directly observed or extrapolated *DSM-IV* criteria. In a review of depression in older persons with MR, Prasher (2003) drew upon multiple studies to delineate the common clinical symptoms of major depression in adults and older persons with MR. Very common signs/symptoms included low mood, irritability, anhedonia, decreased appetite, changes in motor activity, sleep disturbances, fatigue, decreased concentration, social withdrawal, aggression, tearfulness, loss of interest in activities, and declines in social skills. Common findings included weight loss, guilt feelings, somatic complaints, self-injury, property destruction, diurnal variation of mood, loss of confidence, constipation, anxiety, and obsessions/compulsions. In older adults with severe MR, there will be a paucity of subjective symptoms, and more observational signs of depression such as psychomotor agitation, irritability, and behavioral disturbances. If depression is diagnosed in older adults who have MR, expert consensus treatment guidelines exist to guide the use of pharmacological and psychotherapeutic interventions (Special Issue Expert Consensus Guidelines Series: Treatment of Psychiatric and Behavioral Problems in Mental Retardation, 2000).

SUMMARY

MR is not a medical diagnosis; rather, MR is conceptualized as a type of disability that is constituted by measured and decreased cognitive and adaptive capabilities relative to age-related norms in the general population, with an age of onset in the developmental period. The prevalence of MR in the United States varies between age groups and from one geographic area to another and ranges within a range of 0.66% to 1.2% of the general population; most people who have MR are young and have milder manifestations of disability. More severe MR roughly correlates to with the presence of other neurological or developmental disorders such as epilepsy and cerebral palsy. Relatively high rates of MR have been documented among children and young adults living in nursing homes. These younger residents with MR require high levels of care due to the presence of associated neurological or other medical disorders. Federal regulations and court decisions mandate that people with MR be admitted to nursing homes solely on the basis of physical care needs. The provision of appropriate, individual-specific habilitative services must be provided to nursing home residents with MR. Nursing home residents with MR with severe language impairment pose special challenges in the determination of the capacity to make informed health-care decisions and diagnosing the presence of pain and depression. However, guidelines and techniques exist that can assist clinicians in addressing these problems. There is a strong association between Down syndrome and Alzheimer's disease; however, this correlation even in older adults is not 100%. A thorough diagnostic work-up needs to be conducted to rule out reversible causes of functional decline in nursing home residents with MR and with or without Down syndrome.

REFERENCES

American Association on Mental Retardation. (2002). *Mental retardation: Definition, classification, and systems of supports* (10th ed.). Washington, DC: Author.

American Psychiatric Association. (2000). *Diagnostic and statistical manual of mental disorders* (4th ed., text revision, pp. 41–49). Washington, DC: Author.

Applebaum, P. R., & Grisso, T. (1988). Assessing patient's capacities to consent to treatment. *New England Journal of Medicine, 319*, 1635–1638.

Arvio, M., & Sillapan, M. (2003). Prevalence, aetiology and comorbidity of severe and profound intellectual disability in Finland. *Journal of Intellectual Disability Research, 47*(Pt 2), 108–112.

Ball, S. L., Holland, A. J., Hon, J., Huppert, F. A., Treppner, P., & Watson, P. C. (2006). Personality and behavioral changes mark the early stages of Alzheimer's disease in adults with Down syndrome: Findings from a prospective population-based study. *International Journal of Geriatric Psychiatry, 21*(7), 661–666.

Beckett, L., Qilu, Y., & Long, A. N. (2005, September). The numbers behind Fragile X: Prevalence and economic impact. *National Fragile X Foundation Quarterly, 21*, 18–22.

Bhasin, T., Brockson, S., Avchen, R. N., & Van Naarden Braun, K. (2006). Prevalence of four developmental disabilities among children aged 8 years- metropolitan Atlanta Developmental Disabilities Surveillance Program, 1996 and 2000. *MMWR Surveillance Summaries, 55*(SS01), 1–9.

Biesaart, M. C., & Hubben, J. H. (1999) Incompetence in practice of health care in the Netherlands: Report of a study. *Journal of Intellectual Disability Research, 43*(Pt 6), 454–460.

Book, L., Hart. A., Black, J., Feolo, M., Zone, J. J., & Neuhausen S. L. (2001). Prevalence and characteristics of celiac disease in Down syndrome in a US study. *American Journal of Medical Genetics, 98*(1), 70–74.

Bosma, G. P., van Buchem, M. A., Voormolen, J. H., & van Biezen, O. F. (1999). Cervical spondylarthrotic myelopathy with early onset in Down's syndrome: Five cases and a review of the literature. *Journal of Intellectual Disability Research, 43*(Pt 4), 283–288.

Bradley, E. A., Thompson, A., & Bryson, S. E. (2002). Mental retardation in teenagers: Prevalence data from the Niagara region, Ontario. *Canadian Journal of Psychology, 47*(7), 652–659.

Bramston, P., & Fogarty, G. (2000). The assessment of emotional distress experienced by people with an intellectual disability: A study of different methodologies. *Research in Developmental Disabilities, 21*(6), 487–500.

Breau, L. M., Camfield, C. S., McGrath, P. J., & Finley, G. A. (2003). The incidence of pain in children with severe cognitive impairments. *Archives of Pediatrics and Adolescent Medicine, 157*(12), 1219–1226.

Breau, L. M., Camfield, C. S., McGrath, P. J., & Finley, G. A. (2004). Risk factors for pain in children with severe cognitive impairments. *Developmental Medicine and Child Neurology, 46*(6), 364–371.

Buchanan, L. H. (1990). Early onset of presbyacusis in Down syndrome. *Scandinavian Audiology, 19*(2), 103–110.

Capute, A. J., & Accardo, P. J. (1991). A neurodevelopmental perspective on the continuum of developmental disabilities. In A. J. Capute & P. J. Accardo (Eds.), *Developmental disabilities in infancy and childhood* (pp. 7–41). Baltimore, MD: Paul H. Brookes.

Cea, C. D., & Fisher, C. B. (2003). Health care decision-making by adults with mental retardation. *Mental Retardation, 41*(2), 78–87.

Celly, J., Khelfaoui, M., Francis, F., Cherif, B., & Bienvenu, T. (2006) Genetics and pathophysiology of mental retardation. *European Journal of Human Genetics, 14*(6), 71–713.

Champion, G. D., Goodenough, B., von Bayer, C., & Thomas, W. (1998). Measurement of pain by self-report. In G. A. Finley & P. J. McGrath (Eds.), *Measurement of pain in infants and children* (pp. 123–160). Seattle, WA: IASP Press.

Chaney, R. H., & Eyman, R. K. (2000). Patterns in mortality over 60 years among persons with mental retardation in a residential facility. *Mental Retardation, 38*(3), 289–293.

Chicoine, B., McGuire, D., & Rubin, S. S. (1999). Specialty clinic perspectives. In M. P. Janicki & A. J. Dalton (Eds.), *Dementia, aging, and intellectual disabilities: A handbook* (pp. 278–293). Philadelphia: Brunner/Mazel.

Costello, H., Moss, S., Prosser, H., & Hatton, C. (1997). Reliability of the Psychiatric Assessment Scale for Adults with Developmental Disability (PAS-ADD). *Social Psychiatry and Psychiatric Epidemiology, 32*(6), 339–343.

Day, K. (1985). Psychiatric disorder in the middle-aged and elderly mentally handicapped. *British Journal of Psychiatry, 147*, 660–667.

Defrin, R., Pick, C. G., Peretz, C., & Carmeli, E. (2004). A quantitative somatosensory testing of pain threshold in individuals with mental retardation. *Pain, 108*(1–2), 58–66.

Dodd, P., Dowling, S., & Hollins, S. (2005). A review of the emotional, psychiatric and behavioral responses to bereavement in people with intellectual disabilities. *Journal of Intellectual Disability Research, 49*(Pt 7), 537–543.

Esbensen, A. J., & Benson, B. A. (2005). Cognitive variables and depressed mood in adults with intellectual disability. *Journal of Intellectual Disability Research, 49*(Pt 7), 481–489.

Esbensen, A. J., Seltzer, M. M., Greenberg, J. S., & Benson B. A. (2005). Psychometric evaluation of self-report measure of depression for individuals with mental retardation. *American Journal of Mental Retardation, 100*(6), 469–481.

Evenhuis, H. M., Theunissen, M., Denkers, I., Verschuure, H., & Kemme, H. (2001). Prevalence of visual and hearing impairment in a Dutch institutionalized population with intellectual disability. *Journal of Intellectual Disability Research*, *45*(Pt 5), 457–464.

Evenhuis, E. M., van Zanten, G. A., Brocaar, M. P., & Roerdinkholder, W. H. (1992). Hearing loss in middle-age persons with Down syndrome. *American Journal of Mental Retardation*, *97*(1), 47–56.

Fisher, C. B. (2002). A goodness-of-fit ethic for informed consent. *Fordham Urban Law Journal*, *30*(1), 159–176.

Fries, B. E., Wodchis, W. P., Blaum, C., Buttar, A., Drabek, J., & Morris J. N. (2005). A national nursing home study showed that diagnoses varied by age group in nursing home residents under age 65. *Journal of Clinical Epidemiology*, *58*, 198–205.

Gabriel, C., & Jones, A. (2000). The National Nursing Home Survey: 1997 Summary. National Center for Health Statistics. *Vital Health Statistics*, *13*(147), 29.

Gedye, A. (1995). *DSDS dementia scale for Down's syndrome. Manual.* Vancouver, British Columbia: Geyde Research and Consulting.

Geldmacher, D. S., Lerner, A. J., Voci, J. M., Noekler, E. A., Sompler, L. C., & Whitehouse, P. J. (1997). Treatment of functional decline in adults with Down syndrome using selective serotonin-reuptake inhibitor drugs. *Journal of Geriatric Psychiatry and Neurology*, *10*(3), 99–104.

Gunn, M. J., Wong, J. G., Clare, I. C., & Holland, A. J. (1999). Decision-making capacity. *Medical Law Review*, *7*(3), 269–306.

Gustavson, K. H., Umb-Carlsson, O., & Sonnander, K. (2005). A follow-up of mortality, health conditions, and associated disabilities of people with developmental disabilities in a Swedish county. *Journal of Intellectual Disability Research*, *49*(Pt 12), 905–914.

Harper, D. C., & Wadsworth, J. S. (1993). Grief in adults with mental retardation: Preliminary findings. *Research in Developmental Disabilities*, *14*(4), 313–330.

Haveman, M. J., Maaskant, M. A., van Schrojenstein, Lantman, H. M., Urlengs, H. F., & Kessels, A. G. (1994). Behavior problems correlate with dementia onset in Down syndrome. *Journal of Intellectual Disability Research*, *38*(Pt 3), 341–355.

Head, E., & Lott, I. T. (2004). Down syndrome and beta-amyloid deposition. *Current Opinion in Neurology*, *17*(2), 95–100.

Hester, N. O., Foster, R., & Kristenson, K. (1990). Measurement of pain in children: Generalizability of the validity of the pain ladder and the poker chip tool. In D. C. Tyler & E. J. Krane (Eds.), *Pediatric pain* (pp. 179–198). New York: Raven Press.

Holland, A. J., Hon, J., Huppert, F. A., Stevens, F., & Watson, P. (1998). Population-based study of the prevalence and presentation of dementia in adults with Down's syndrome. *British Journal of Psychiatry*, *172*, 493–498.

Jacobson, J. (2003). Prevalence of mental and behavioral disorders. In P. W. Davidson, V. P. Prasher, & M. P. Janicki (Eds.), *Mental health, intellectual disabilities, and the aging process* (pp. 9–21). Oxford: Blackwell.

Jacobson, J. W., & Harper, M. S. (1989). Mental health status of older persons with mental retardation in residential care settings. *Australia and New Zealand Journal of Developmental Disabilities*, *15*, 301–310.

Jacobson, J. W., & Mulick, J. A. (1996). Definition of mental retardation. In J. W. Jacobson & J. W. Mulick (Eds.), *Manual of diagnosis and professional practice in mental retardation* (pp. 13–53). Washington, DC: American Psychological Association.

Janicki, M. P., Dalton, A. J., Henderson, C. M., & Davidson, P. W. (1999). Mortality and morbidity among older adults with intellectual disability; health services considerations. *Disability and Rehabilitation*, *21*(5–6), 284–294.

Janowsky, D. S., & Davis, J. M. (2005). Diagnosis and treatment of depression in patients with mental retardation. *Current Psychiatric Reports, 7*(6), 421–428.

Janowsky, D. S., Shetty, M., Banhill, J., Elamir, B., & Davis, J. M. (2005). Serotonergic antidepressant effects on aggressive, self-injurious, and destructive/disruptive behaviors in intellectually disabled adults: A retrospective, open-label, naturalistic trial. *International Journal of Neurology, 8*(1), 37–48.

Lai, F., & Williams, R. S. (1989). A prospective study of Alzheimer disease in Down syndrome. *Archives of Neurology, 46*(8), 849–853.

Lee, H. G., Zhu, X., Nunomura, A., Perr, G., & Smith, M. A. (2006). Amyloid beta: The alternative hypothesis. *Current Alzheimer Research, 3*(1), 75–80.

Leonard, H., Petterson, B., Bower, C., & Sanders, R. (2003). Prevalence of intellectual disability in Western Australia. *Pediatric and Perinatal Epidemiology, 17*(1), 58–67.

Lott, I. T., & Head, E. (2005). Alzheimer disease and Down syndrome: Factors in pathogenesis. *Neurobiology of Aging, 26*(3), 383–389.

Lund, J. (1985). The prevalence of psychiatric morbidity in mentally retarded adults. *Acta Psychiatrica Scandinavica, 72*, 563–570.

Lunsky, Y. (2004). Suicidality in a community sample of adults with mental retardation. *Research in Developmental Disabilities, 25*(3), 231–243.

May, P. A., & Gossage, J. P. (2001). Estimating the prevalence of fetal alcohol syndrome: A summary. *Alcohol Research and Health, 25*(3), 159–167.

McBrien, J. A. (2003). Assessment and diagnosis of depression in people with developmental disability. *Journal of Intellectual Disability Research, 47*(Pt 1), 1–13.

Menendez, M. (2005). Down syndrome, Alzheimer's disease and seizures. *Brain and Development, 27*(4), 246–252.

MMWR. (1994). Down syndrome prevalence at birth—United States, 1983–1990. *43*(33), 617–622.

MMWR. (1994). State-specific rates of mental retardation—United States, 1993. *43*(33), 61–65.

Moss, S., Prosser, H., Costello, H., et al. (1998). Reliability and validity of the PAS-ADD checklist for detecting psychiatric disorders in adults with intellectual disability. *Journal of Intellectual Disability Research, 42*(Pt 2), 173–183.

Nihira, K., Leland, H., & Ladine, W. (1993). AAMR Adaptive Behavior Scales—residential and community edition (2nd ed.). Austin, TX: Pro-Ed.

Norden, J., Hannallal, R., & Geston, P. (1991). Reliability of an objective pain scale in children. *Journal of Pain and Symptom Management, 6*, 196.

Oliver, C., Crayton, L., Holland, A. J., Hull, S., & Bradley, J. (1998). Four year prospective study of age-related cognitive changes in adults with Down syndrome. *Psychological Medicine, 28*(6), 1365–1377.

Patel, P., Goldsberg, D., & Moss, S. (1993). Psychiatric morbidity in older people with moderate and severe learning disability II: The prevalence study. *British Journal of Psychiatry, 163*, 481–491.

Phan, A., Edwards, C. L., & Robinson, E. L. (2005). The assessment of pain and discomfort in individuals with mental retardation. *Research in Developmental Disabilities, 26*(5),433–439.

Prasher, V. P. (1990). Subclinical hypothyroidism may contribute to cognitive impairment in Down syndrome with Alzheimer disease. *American Journal of Medical Genetics, 36*(2), 148–154.

Prasher, V. P. (1999). Down syndrome and thyroid disorders: A review. *Down's Syndrome, Research and Practice, 6*(1), 25–42.

Prasher, V. P. (2003). Depression in aging individuals with intellectual disabilities. In P. W. Davidson, V. P. Prasher, & M. P. Janicki (Eds.), *Mental health, intellectual disabilities, and the aging process* (pp. 51–66). Oxford: Blackwell.

Prasher, V. P. (2004). Review of donepezil, vivastigmine, galantamine, memantine in Alzheimer's disease in adults with Down syndrome: Implications for the intellectual disability population. *International Journal of Geriatric Psychiatry, 19*(6), 509–515.

Prasher, V. P., Farooq, A., & Holder, R. (2004). The Adaptive Behavior Dementia Questionnaire: Screening for dementia in Alzheimer's disease in persons with Down syndrome. *Research in Developmental Disabilities, 25*(4), 385–397.

Prasher, V. P., Metseaghorun, T., & Hague, S. (2004). Weight loss in adults with Down syndrome and with dementia in Alzheimer's disease. *Research in Developmental Disabilities, 25*(1), 1–7.

Roid, G. H. (2003a). *Stanford-Binet Intelligence Scales* (5th ed.). Itasca, IL: Riverside.

Ross, E., & Oliver, C. (2003). The assessment of mood in adults who have severe or profound mental retardation. *Clinical Psychological Review, 23*(2), 225–245.

Sansom, D. T., Singh, I., Jawed, S. H., & Mukherjee, T. (1994). Elderly people with learning disabilities in hospital: A psychiatric study. *Journal of Intellectual Disability Research, 38*, 45–52.

Schupf, N., & Sergievsk, G. H. (2002). Genetic and host factors for dementia in Down syndrome. *British Journal of Psychiatry, 180*, 405–410.

Special Issue Expert Consensus Guidelines Series: Treatment of psychiatric and behavioral problems in mental retardation. (2000). *American Journal on Mental Retardation, 105*(3): 159–228.

Strahan, G. W. (1991). Mental illness in nursing homes. 1985. National Center for Health Statistics. *Vital Health Statistics, 13*(105): 3–4.

Stromme, P. (2000). Aetiology in severe and mild mental retardation; a population based survey of Norwegian children. *Developmental Medicine and Child Neurology, 42*(2), 76–86.

The Arc. (2004). *Introduction to mental retardation.* Available at www.thearc.org

The Psychological Corporation. (1997). *Wechsler Adult Intelligence Scale* (3rd ed.). San Antonio, TX: Author.

Thompson, J. R., Bryant, B., Campbell, E. M., et al. (2004). *Support Intensity Scale.* Washington, DC: American Association on Mental Retardation.

Tranebjaerg, L., & Orum, A. (1991). Major depressive disorder as a prominent but underestimated feature of Fragile X syndrome. *Comprehensive Psychiatry, 45*, 115–120.

Tsiouris, J. A., & Patti, P. J. (1997). Drug treatment for depression associated with dementia or presented as "pseudodementia" in older adults with Down syndrome. *Journal of Applied Research in Intellectual Disabilities, 10*, 312–322.

Tsiouris, J. A., Mann, R., Patti, P. J., & Sturmsky, P. (2003). Challenging behaviors should not be considered as depressive equivalents in individuals with intellectual disabilities. *Journal of Intellectual Disability Research, 47*(Pt 1), 14–21.

Tsiouris, J. A., Patti, P. J., Tipu, O., & Ragthu, S. (2002). Adverse effects of phenytoin given for late-onset seizures in adults with Down syndrome. *Neurology, 59*(5), 779–780.

Tuffrey-Wijne, I. (2003). The palliative care needs of people with intellectual disabilities: A literature review. *Palliative Medicine, 17*(1), 55–62.

Tyrell, J., & Dodd, P. (2003). Psychopathology in older age. In P. W. Davidson, V. P. Prasher, & M. P. Janicki (Eds.), *Mental health, intellectual disabilities, and the aging process* (pp. 22–37). Oxford: Blackwell.

Van Allen, M. I., Fung, J., & Jurenka, S. B. (1999). Health concerns and guidelines for adults with Down syndrome. *American Journal of Medical Genetics, 89*(2), 100–110.

Van Splunder, J., Stilma, J. S., Bernsen, R. M., & Evenhuis, H. M. (2004). Prevalence of ocular diagnosis found on screening in 1539 adults with developmental disabilities. *Ophthalmology, 111*(8), 1457–1463.

Voknin, A., Eliakim, R., Ackerman, Z., & Steiner, I. (2004). Neurological abnormalities associated with celiac disease. *Journal of Neurology, 251*(11), 1393–1397.

White, P., Chant, D., Edwards, N., Townsend, E., & Wagborn, G. (2005). Prevalence of intellectual disability and comorbid mental illness in an Australian community sample. *Australia and New Zealand Journal of Psychiatry, 39*(5), 395–400.

Wisnieski, H. M., Silverman, W., & Weigel, J. (1994). Aging, Alzheimer disease and mental retardation. *Journal of Intellectual Disability Research, 38*(Pt 3), 233–239.

Zigman, W. B., Schupf, N., Sersen, F., & Silverman, W. (1996). Prevalence of dementia in adults with and without Down syndrome. *American Journal of Mental Retardation, 11*(4), 403–412.

Zwakhalen, S. M., van Dongen, K. A., Hamers, J. P., & Abu-Saad, H. H. (2004). Pain assessment in intellectually disabled people: Non-verbal indicators. *Journal of Advanced Nursing, 45*(3), 236–245.

11

Substance Use Disorders

Kenneth Schwartz

Substance abuse is often overlooked as a relevant clinical issue despite being a significant cause of medical and psychiatric illness and disability in nursing home residents. The nonspecificity of alcohol- or drug-related presentations in the elderly coupled with a lack of adequate training of health-care professionals in the area may lead to signs of alcoholism or drug abuse being mistaken for age-related changes. Furthermore, physicians seldom screen for problems.

The American Psychiatric Association's *Diagnostic and Statistical Manual of Mental Disorders,* fourth edition, text revision (*DSM-IV-TR*; APA, 2000) outlines criteria for five categories of substance use disorders. Older adults are considered to be engaging in hazardous, harmful, or abusive use of alcohol or other substances when their use has either already resulted in adverse physical, psychological, occupational, or social problems or greatly increases the risk of occurrence of these problems. The criteria for alcohol dependence also include a loss of control, preoccupation with the substance or physiological symptoms such as tolerance and withdrawal. However, studies establishing the diagnostic criteria for substance abuse were developed and validated in young and middle-aged samples and may have only limited utility among the elderly (Miller et al., 1991). These criteria may not apply to older adults because of changing life circumstances, changing roles, and differing health circumstances (O'Connell et al., 2003). The emphasis on a failure to fulfill major obligations at work, school, or home and alcohol-related legal problems is not as applicable to an older population, especially a nursing home population. With respect to dependence, increased tolerance requiring greater quantities of alcohol to get "high" may not apply to older adults because pharmacokinetic changes in the elderly may be associated with decreased tolerance which may lead to decreased consumption with no apparent reduction in intoxication (Patterson & Jeste, 1999). As a result of these differences, the definition of substance abuse disorders that will be used in this chapter is defined as frequent but not necessarily daily use of a potentially addicting substance that is associated with either biomedical, psychological, or social consequences or puts the patient at risk for developing symptoms of withdrawal (Solomon & Shackson, 1996).

Alcoholism is the third most common psychiatric disorder among older adults (Campbell, 2004). However, the importance of alcoholism as a mental disorder in the elderly is still not recognized (Hirati et al., 2001). The use of illegal drugs similarly continues to be considered a problem primarily among the young (Schlerth, 2007). In addition to a growing older population, the number of older adults who misuse or abuse illicit drugs or alcohol is expected to increase because younger birth cohorts are showing higher rates of use of these substances (Substance Abuse and Mental Health Services Administration, SAMHSA, 2006). More older adults will then experience medical or mental health problems that result from or are worsened by alcohol and drugs increasing the likelihood of admission to a nursing home or assisted living facility. These facilities are potentially well positioned to be a significant component in the provision of health services, both to residents with chronic illnesses requiring long or more permanent stays and to the growing but still smaller number of residents requiring postacute care or rehabilitation. However, the need for improved access to medically necessary psychiatric care in nursing homes remains substantial (Streim et al., 2002). Nursing home and other long-term setting administrators and staff who fail to implement an alcohol policy and inadvertently provide alcohol without much regard for the health history of residents may turn a blind eye to those with substance abuse problems until the problems become too great to ignore (Schwartz & Lasky, 2002).

Lack of recognition of continued substance misuse in long-term care settings may lead to residents experiencing unnecessary adverse interactions with medications; unanticipated withdrawal; or worsening of depression, medical, or behavioral problems (Atkinson, 1991). Comorbidities of alcohol such as cognitive impairment and neurological impairment may impede rehabilitation (Joseph et al., 1995a).

EPIDEMIOLOGY

The issue of substance abuse in nursing homes, aside from prescription medication abuse, has been almost entirely neglected (Joseph & Harvath, 1998). The limited published information on the prevalence of current or lifetime alcohol problems yields varying results depending on the setting characteristics and methods of case definition and time frame (Joseph, 1995). In the 1985 National Nursing Home Survey, the presence of alcohol problems, identified by staff report of current alcohol abuse or dependence, reported a low prevalence of 2.2% among community nursing home residents (National Center for Health Statistics, NCHS, 1989). Studies such as this that employ provider diagnosis versus structured interviews consistently report significantly lower prevalence rates of alcoholism (Joseph, 1995). The highest prevalence rates are found in Veterans Affairs (VA) nursing homes that house primarily male residents and have a rehabilitation focus favoring a younger age of admission (Joseph et al., 1995a). For example, 49% of short-term rehabilitation residents had a lifetime diagnosis of alcohol abuse or dependence, with 18% reporting active symptoms of abuse or dependence within 1 year of admission to a VA nursing home (Joseph et al., 1995b). Similarly, in another study of residents of a VA nursing home, 29% of residents had a lifetime diagnosis of alcohol abuse or dependency with 10% of the residents meeting criteria for abuse or dependence within 1 year of admission (Oslin et al., 1997).

There is a lack of research on illicit drug use in older adults (Schlaerth, 2007). The Epidemiological Catchment Area Study reported that it was much less frequent than problem drinking with lifetime prevalence rates of drug abuse and dependence for individuals 60 and over to be 0.12% for elderly men and 0.06% for elderly women, with the lifetime history of illicit drug use being 2.88% and 0.66%, respectively (Anthony & Helzer, 1991). The 1985 National Nursing Home Survey reported a prevalence of drug abuse or dependence in 0.9% of nursing home residents, with a 2.7% prevalence found among men less than 64 years of age and a 0.7% and 0.8% prevalence for men and women aged 65 and older who make up the majority of residents in community nursing homes (NCHS, 1989). In a VA study, illicit drug abuse or dependence was listed among the diagnoses of 1.2% of nursing home admissions over 50 (Joseph, 1995). Older individuals who meet lifetime criteria for alcohol dependence are most likely to have a diagnosis of illicit drug dependence, which is consistent with the view that it is found only among special populations not in the mainstream of society (Rosenberg, 1995). Hence, the drop-off of drug addicts after age 36 (maturing out) described many years ago (Winick, 1962) is questioned by some as an artifact of treatment centers to not attract aging addicts, the ability of the elderly to maintain their drug habits without much attention from others, and the reluctance of the criminal justice system to prosecute the elderly (Schlaerth, 2007).

Dependence on nicotine was once so much a part of every day life of nursing homes that it was only briefly mentioned in the nursing home literature (Barker et al., 1994). However, the prevalence of smoking has been declining and the segment of the adult population less likely to smoke is older adults (Walker & Whitson, 2007). Residents' safety and health were the greatest concerns for administrators and nurses of VA nursing home care units. These concerns coupled with society's increasing restrictions of smoking in public places has led to an increasing number of nursing homes and assisted living facilities becoming smoke-free despite concerns regarding resident autonomy, quality of life, and limited effectiveness of smoking cessation programs.

Older adults are the largest users of prescription medications in the United States. Most studies suggest that between 55% and 75% of nursing home residents have at least one prescription for a psychotropic medication (Conn, 2007). Factors explaining these variations include differences in prevalence and severity of disorders, levels of physical disability, prescribing habits of physicians, involvement by pharmacists, number of untrained staff, size and design of institutions, funding and type of institutions, socioeconomic background of the residents, and policies regarding admission (Snowden, 1993). In contrast to illicit drug abuse, the duration of a prescribed drug's use is greatly influenced by the directives and attitudes of the physician (Damestroy et al., 1999).

Concerns about the use of psychotropic medications, especially the use of antipsychotic drugs and benzodiazepines, include the lack of a documented diagnosis, the high risk of complications such as falls, fractures, and movement disorders, that physician characteristics (rather than those of patients) predict drug dosage, and that mental health consultation is lacking for nursing home residents (Conn, 2007). These concerns about inappropriate and unnecessary prescribing of psychotropics, as well as other concerns about psychiatric care of nursing home residents led to federal regulations in the United States called the "Omnibus Budget Reconciliation Act of 1987" (OBRA-87). This legislation established strict prescribing guidelines for psychotropic medications. A 10-year review of the effect of OBRA-87 in an academic nursing home showed a decrease in the use of psychotropic medications (Lantz et al., 1996).

RISK FACTORS FOR SUBSTANCE ABUSE
IN NURSING HOME PATIENTS

Most elderly patients admitted to nursing homes have not been recognized as having substance abuse disorders, so they are at risk of continuing or even increasing their consumption. Older women, in particular, are underscreened and underdiagnosed with respect to alcohol and nonprescribed drug use (Campbell, 2004). This is unfortunate as older adults incur problems at lower levels of alcohol consumption because of age-related physiological changes, declining health and functional status, and medication use (Fink et al., 2002). Physiological changes associated with aging include an alteration of body fat–body water ratio (Boxer & Shorr, 2004). Similarly, changes in liver and kidney function decrease the ability of the elderly to process alcohol resulting in a buildup of alcohol and exacerbated effects even without a change in the amount of alcohol consumed (Klein & Jess, 2002). Central nervous sensitivity to alcohol increases with age because of an increased permeability of the blood-brain barrier (Luggen, 2007). Such altered pharmacokinetics and pharmacodynamics place older adults at risk for more frequent and severe adverse drug reactions, especially because testing of medications for safety are mostly conducted with younger populations.

Genetic predisposition to alcoholism is estimated to account for 40% to 60% of alcoholism (Campbell, 2004). Psychiatric diagnoses that have been associated with drug dependence include personality disorder, somatoform disorder, anxiety, sleep, and adjustment disorder (Finlayson & Davis, 1994).

Being an older male is a risk factor for alcohol dependency, especially if single, separated, divorced, with few supports, with lower income, with tobacco dependency and depressive symptoms (Joseph et al., 1995a). Veterans with more intense combat stress or a history of head injury associated with loss of consciousness are shown to have higher prevalences of alcohol abuse (Herrmann & Eryavec, 1996). Older women with alcohol dependence are more likely to be married to men with the same illness, be victims of domestic violence, and have comorbid psychiatric disorders including depression and anxiety (Wiseman, 2003). Being an older female is a risk factor for abuse of prescription medications, especially if white, less-educated, separated or divorced, having experienced a greater number of negative life events, and having a psychiatric diagnosis (Swartz et al., 1991).

Prior to implementation of OBRA-87, several critics asserted that residents in some nursing homes were at greater risk of receiving inappropriate medications because psychotropic medications were used less for the treatment of ailing residents than for the treatment of the ailing institution (Waxman et al., 1985).

For over 40 years, it has been customary that some nursing homes provide cocktail or "happy hours" as an opportunity for social interaction among residents and to recognize that alcohol consumption is a normal part of adult social life in the United States (Klein & Jess, 2002). However, alcohol problems for some residents may be unintentionally exacerbated through these programs that provide opportunities, if not encouragement, for alcohol consumption (Joseph et al., 1995a). Overprescribing of minor tranquillizers for anxiety or sleep may lead to the development of a new psychological dependence (Solomon & Shackson, 1996).

CLINICAL EVALUATION AND PRESENTATION

Traditionally, physicians are taught to ask questions about frequency and quantity of alcohol use to acquire information (Curtis et al., 1989). Although such questions may detect alcohol misuse in those with an admitted high level of use, self-reported consumption is considered generally not reliable enough in detecting alcoholism (Greenberg et al., 2004). This is consistent with the observation that a definition of alcoholism includes among its symptoms "distortions in thinking, notably denial" (Callahan & Tierney, 1995). Physicians and other health-care providers must also be honest with themselves and put aside their own biases that substance abuse in old age is rare and inconsequential because without a proper assessment and diagnosis, prevention and treatment will not occur.

The accurate diagnosis of a substance abuse disorder in the nursing home resident relies on a complete clinical evaluation, including medical history, physical and mental status exams, and collateral history (Solomon & Shackson, 1996). It is suggested to integrate clinical questions about alcohol use into the interview so that these questions follow inquiry about less sensitive habits. For example, it is recommended to begin by saying, "We have talked about your usual diet and your smoking. Can you tell me how you use alcoholic beverages?" (Fingerhood, 2000). For those patients who describe present or past use of alcohol, screen for evidence of alcoholism by asking, "Has your use for alcohol caused any kinds of problems for you?" or "Have you ever been concerned about your drinking?" (Fingerhood, 2000). When dealing with patients who seem to be reporting in a manner that focuses on convincing the physician that there is no problem, the clinician is recommended to be direct and firm and use only highly specific and factual questions that make it difficult to answer evasively (Solomon & Shackson, 1996).

The history at the time of nursing home admission needs to check for signs of the biopsychosocial consequences of alcohol or drug use in the context of the resident's past life. As physicians tend to refill prescriptions for older adults more easily than for younger patients, an older individual may not need to resort to "doctor-shopping" in order to refill a benzodiazepine prescription (Voyer & Préville, 2007). A recent onset or change in the frequency of falls, mental status, anxiety, depression, activities of daily life, or aggressive behavior are clues that should raise the physician's index of suspicion (Solomon & Shackson, 1996). The social consequences of an addict's life may demonstrate itself by isolation and estrangement. Residents with alcohol use disorders use more mental health services than do residents without alcohol use disorders, perhaps as a consequence of having poor-quality social relationships, necessitating professional help with adjustment to life in a nursing home (Brennan, 2005).

Since the majority of nursing home residents are admitted from another health-care facility, serious alcohol withdrawal is likely not to be encountered as frequently in the nursing home as in an acute care hospital (Rubinstein et al., 1988). However, the initial signs of withdrawal symptoms may occur during the first few days of admission as residents who are not properly diagnosed suddenly go without the addicting drug or markedly cut down its use (Solomon & Shackson, 1996). Similarly, elderly individuals requiring opioid medications to control pain may meet criteria for the diagnosis of opioid dependence and be at risk of developing withdrawal symptoms after abrupt dosage reduction (Wiseman, 2003).

Alcohol withdrawal symptoms are more severe with age and with increasing doses of alcohol; the risk starts with five to six drinks per day (Luggen, 2007). Severe withdrawal reactions, especially in those with a history of previous withdrawal and coexisting medical problems must be detoxified in hospital due to high morbidity. Such reactions are characterized by hallucinations, delirium, seizures, or coma. Other substances of abuse such as longer-acting benzodiazepines or opioids have distinct withdrawal symptoms that are also potentially life threatening (Oslin, 2005). Less severe withdrawal from alcohol or some medications, such as shorter-acting benzodiazepines, demonstrate withdrawal symptoms that are usually milder and may be misdiagnosed as anxiety, dysphoria, or sleep disorders. These more minor withdrawal symptoms may be managed in the nursing home.

The medical complications of alcohol abuse are many and include liver disease, pancreatitis, gastrointestinal bleeding, cancer, cardiomyopathy, malnutrition, and susceptibility to infections. End-of-dose anxiety or the "clock-watching" syndrome is present in residents addicted to shorter-acting benzodiazepines or opioid pain medications (Solomon & Shackson, 1996). Insomnia, a common complaint of addicts, can take the form of medication-seeking behavior or as a result of dependence on a hypnotic medication (Solomon & Shackson, 1996). Neurological problems include an increased risk of strokes, cognitive difficulties, gait disturbance, peripheral neuropathy, Wernicke Korsakoff syndrome, and alcohol-related dementia. The odds of a fall injury are between 1.5 and 4.5 times greater for those elderly with mental health and substance abuse issues (Finklestein et al., 2007).

Physical and mental status exams and lab tests should focus on detecting evidence of liver disease, neurological problems, sequelae of poor self-care or nutrition, and cognitive or psychiatric difficulties. There is no lab test with reasonable sensitivity and specificity for the detection of alcoholism (Campbell, 2004). Family or friends may wrongly attribute falls or accidents, confusion, adverse drug reactions, labile emotions, and malnutrition to age, leading to a delay of appropriate treatment (Wiseman, 2003).

ALCOHOL POLICIES

A survey of 167 long-term care facilities in Canada regarding residents' alcohol use showed a wide variation of attitudes and policies from complete prohibition to permissive consumption with common sense parameters (Spencer, 2002). A more restrictive approach in facilities was adopted when there was concern about alcohol-drug interactions because a higher percent of residents were on psychoactive medications (Spencer, 2002). In contrast, two common reasons for adopting permissive approaches were wishing to respect the personal autonomy of residents and the belief that the actual level of alcohol consumption in these facilities was not high (Spencer, 2002).

A semistructured telephone interview examined the alcohol-related policies and practices of 111 intermediate care facilities and elderly people in the northeastern part of the United States (Klein & Jess, 2002). The authors found that despite the problems reported in these facilities, assessment and treatment of alcohol problems and training of staff were not adequate.

It is recommended that long-term care administrators address the following questions prior to implementing a plan or policy regarding alcohol use in their facilities. First, what are the facility characteristics? Are alcohol problems prevalent among the residents? Are there state or federal regulations that must be satisfied? Second, how will alcohol be provided to residents? Will the facility furnish alcoholic beverages or simply allow residents to keep their own supply? Will a physician's order be required? Third, how will adverse effects such as resident intoxication and/or behavioral problems be handled? Finally, if alcohol consumption is not allowed, how will this rule be enforced (Joseph & Harvath, 1998)?

Alcohol in long-term care settings, as well as in the rest of society, is a psychoactive substance and social beverage (Klein & Jess, 2002). Understanding this permits these settings to draft written policies governing alcohol use in their facilities that address assessment, treatment, ethical, and legal concerns (Schwartz, 2007). Drinking limit recommendations regarding the daily use of alcohol for older adults varies. The recommendations of no more than one standard drink daily and on any one day no more than four drinks have been endorsed by both the National Institute of Alcohol Abuse and Alcoholism (NIAAA, 1995) and The Center for Substance Abuse Treatment, Treatment Improvement Protocol (Blow, 1998). These recommendations are in line with the present evidence for the beneficial health effect of low-risk drinking (Klatsky & Armstrong, 1993). Alternatively, it is suggested that two drinks per day for older men and one drink per day for older women is appropriate (McCance & Roberts, 2004). Nursing homes should carefully consider residents' histories of alcohol in formulating alcohol policies because of the high use of medical services in residents with alcohol use disorders (Brennan & Greenbaum, 2005). There are no accepted safe limits for the use of nicotine, marijuana, or other illicit drugs (Oslin, 2006).

SCREENING

A panel of experts in geriatrics and alcohol research agree that to screen for alcohol use, history regarding quantity and frequency, health, use of medications, and functioning must be obtained (Moore et al., 2004). Nursing homes and other long-term care settings ideally should incorporate screening or other measures into an alcohol policy that quickly and accurately identifies any new residents with alcohol problems. The goal of screening for alcoholism is to be confident that one has detected alcoholism, ruled out alcoholism, or must continue to consider alcoholism as a possible diagnosis (Fingerhood, 2000).

The use of formal screening tests pertaining to the effect of alcohol in the individual's life, health, and behavior increases their detection of alcoholism and performs well among older adults with drinking problems in an ambulatory medical clinic (Buchsbaum et al., 1992). Both the CAGE and MAST-G screening questionnaires have a high sensitivity and specificity with respect to a nursing home population (Joseph et al., 1995b). The CAGE screening instrument (Mayfield et al., 1974) is the most widely used screening tool in the elderly because it is simple, easy to administer, and is brief consisting of only four questions that could be easily incorporated into the interview (Ewing, 1984; Table 11.1).

The CAGE does not distinguish between active and inactive drinking so that patients should be given the CAGE questionnaire only after determining if they have had a drink within the past year (Buschsbaum et al., 1992). Any one "yes" answer increases the identification of potential problems and should lead to suitable prevention or treatment interventions. Diagnostic certainty can be increased in those who answer "yes" to any of the four questions by the use of follow-up questions or referral to an alcoholic treatment center (Reid & Anderson, 1997). An intervention, if two or more "yes" answers are obtained, may be more appropriate for a population with a lower percentage of drinking problems (Buschsbaum et al., 1992).

The Short Michigan Alcoholism Screening Test-Geriatric Version (SMAST-G) is a screening tool used in a variety of settings to help detect alcohol abuse or dependence in the elderly (Blow et al., 1998; Table 11.2). It may be superior to other screening tools for the identification of elderly individuals with alcohol abuse or dependence (Oslin, 2004).

Another screening tool for problem drinking, the Alcohol Use Disorders Identification Test (AUDIT), developed by the World Health Organization, focuses on consumption (Snowden, 1993). However, in a study comparing the

TABLE 11.1. CAGE Questionnaire

1. Have you ever felt that you should cut down on your drinking?	C
2. Have people annoyed you by criticizing your drinking?	A
3. Have you ever felt bad or guilt about your drinking?	G
4. Have you ever had a drink first time in the morning just to steady your nerves or get rid of a hangover (eye opener)?	E

Source: Mayfield et al. (1974).

TABLE 11.2. Short Michigan Alcohol Screening Test-Geriatric (SMAST-G)

	YES	NO
When talking with others, do you ever underestimate how much you actually drink?	(1)	(0)
After a few drinks, have you sometimes not eaten or been able to skip a meal because you didn't feel hungry?	(1)	(0)
Does having a few drinks help decrease your shakiness or tremors?	(1)	(0)
Does alcohol sometimes make it hard for you to remember parts of the day or night?	(1)	(0)
Do you usually take a drink to relax or calm your nerves?	(1)	(0)
Do you drink to take your mind off your problems?	(1)	(0)
Have you ever increased your drinking after experiencing a loss in your life?	(1)	(0)
Has a doctor or nurse ever said they were worried or concerned about your drinking?	(1)	(0)
Have you ever made rules to manage your drinking?	(1)	(0)
When you feel lonely, does having a drink help?	(1)	(0)
Total SMAST-G score (0–10)		
A score of 3 or more is indicative of problem drinking		

Source: Reprinted with permission of the University of Michigan Alcohol Research Center. © The Regents of the University of Michigan, 1991.

CAGE, the MAST-G, and the AUDIT for detecting alcoholism in 120 male veterans, 65 years or older, the CAGE and the MAST-G were superior (Morton et al., 1996).

A combination of screening tools such as the CAGE and/or SMAST-G, when accompanied by follow-up questions about consequences and social and family issues, can best identify alcohol use disorders in residents. However, as important as screening is, it is insufficient in ensuring if care is provided (Oslin, 2005). For example, a recent multisite VA Ambulatory Care Quality Improvement Program found low rates of implementation of brief alcohol counseling even after routine screening (Burman et al., 2004). Consequently, the U.S. Preventive Services Task Force (USPSTF, 2004) recommends routine alcohol screening followed by assessment and brief alcohol counseling in appropriate patients.

TREATMENT

Nursing homes can expect to treat two groups of problem drinkers (Liberto & Oslin, 1997). Early-onset alcoholism is more common among lifelong drinkers who are more likely to drink to intoxication; to have been in an alcoholic treatment program in the past; more likely to have legal, financial, or job problems; and less likely to have social support (Brennan & Moos, 1990). They are also at more risk to pursue early discharge in order to return to abusive drinking patterns or to have behavioral problems that contribute to a lengthened nursing home stay (Brennan, 2005). There are several scenarios for the development of late-onset alcoholism. For example, long-standing "functional" alcoholics may develop functional or cognitive impairment unrelated to alcohol use and become unable to function normally if they continue to drink; or with aging, social drinkers become increasingly vulnerable to the effects of alcohol, even if the quantity or frequency of their drinking does not change (Fingerhood, 2000). Social drinkers may increase their quantity or frequency of drinking after a stressor such as loss of spouse, retirement, health, or independence. Lifelong nondrinkers can also develop late-onset alcoholism.

Treatment of alcohol abuse is considered complete for residents with significant cognitive impairment when the residents are medically stable and not drinking. Patients with a history of alcohol dependence should be administered thiamine. If there is coexisting depression, agitation, or psychosis, suitable medications should be administered once it is shown that these psychiatric problems are not present just because of the use or abuse of alcohol (Solomon & Shackson, 1996).

More cognitively intact residents should be offered a full range of individualized treatment options even though treatment of the elderly alcoholic remains a challenge. The presence of a dual disorder of substance abuse and depression in these cognitively intact residents merits special consideration because some residents may use drugs to cope with their psychiatric disorders, others may initially misuse their medications resulting in abuse, and others' abuse of drugs may be associated with psychiatric relapse (Allen & Landis, 1997).

The traditional approach to treatment of alcoholism continues to emphasize abstinence. Forced abstinence associated with a VA nursing home or rehabilitation placement has led to improvements in activities of daily living, alcohol-related cognitive impairment, and discharge back to a community setting (Oslin et al., 1997).

In the nursing home setting, besides appropriate treatment of any comorbid disorder, it is suggested that individual psychotherapy based on the 12-step model advocated by Alcoholics Anonymous (AA) be used to break down the resident's denial, minimization, defocusing, rationalization, and the family's enabling behaviors (Solomon & Shackson, 1996). Nursing home residents, even if so inclined, are unlikely to attend community AA meetings because of transportation issues or physical and mental health problems.

There are now a number of treatment interventions that emphasize controlled drinking as its goal rather than abstinence. Brief techniques, typically refer to 10 to 15 min of counseling patients about setting a goal for a reduction of drinking and ways to achieve that goal (Saitz, 2005). The USPSTF recommends the "Five As" approach (ask, assess, advise, agree, assist; USPSTF, 2004).

General components of successful brief interventions are described using the acronym FRAMES (Miller & Rollnick, 2002). They include Feedback on drinking, Reinforcing the patient's responsibility for changing behavior, Advice about changing behavior, discussing a Menu of options to change behavior, Expressing empathy for the patient, and Support of the patient's self-efficacy. The ultimate path to recovery is one which results from a negotiation between the possibilities put forward by the therapist and the feasibilities chosen by the patient (Judson, 2007). Although not tested in the nursing home population, brief interventions employing motivational-interviewing approaches, which emphasize empathic listening and the autonomy of patients in their own decision making and encourage individuals to identify their own reasons for change, have been shown to be more effective in decreasing drinking than confrontational counseling, which imposes the clinician's view of the patient, minimizes the patient's perspective, and forces the patient to admit to having a problem (Miller & Rollnick, 2002).

More recent evidence-based interventions for controlled drinking include behavioral self-control training, moderation-oriented alcohol exposure, a brief cognitive-behavioral guided self-change motivational treatment, and harm reduction that attempts "to meet people where they are" with respect to motivation (Saladin & Santa Ana, 2004). In practice, however, it is likely more realistic to reserve the goal of controlled drinking for the problem drinker than the dependent alcoholic (Luggen, 2007). In the nursing home, addressing family, social, and interpersonal problems with individual or group therapy, along with medication for any coexisting psychiatric conditions, will also likely decrease the incidence of problem drinking residents (Zimberg, 1978). Encouragement of these residents to engage in healthy alternate activities facilitates the process.

Individuals with alcohol dependence who are more resistant to these measures are best referred to specialists in the field who may recommend the use of medications. However, alcohol dependence is still difficult to treat with medication. Until 1995, disulfiram was the only agent approved for the treatment of alcohol dependence, but the medical problems found in older adults often precluded its safe use (Schukit, 1990). Naltrexone, an opioid-receptor antagonist, makes drinking less pleasurable and reduces cravings. When used in conjunction with a psychosocial rehabilitation treatment program, it has been reported to significantly reduce relapse to heavy drinking among alcohol-dependent veterans aged 50 to 70 years (Oslin et al., 1997). A study testing the efficacy of naltrexone combined with sertraline, a selective serotonin reuptake inhibitor antidepressant for the treatment of older adults with depression, underscores the importance of addressing alcohol use in the context of treating late-life depression (Oslin, 2005). Acamprosate is another alcohol abstinence medication used in the treatment of alcohol dependence. However, there are no studies of its efficacy or safety among older adults (Oslin, 2006). Similarly, topiramate recently produced significant and meaningful improvement in several drinking outcome measures in patients with alcohol dependence aged 18 to 65 years (Johnson et al., 2007). When used, these medications should be combined with counseling or behavioral support to improve their effectiveness (Luggen, 2007). A recent study suggests that quetiapine, an atypical antipsychotic, may be useful in the treatment of alcohol dependence, specifically in Type B alcoholics characterized by an early onset of problem drinking, high severity of dependence, increased psychopathology, and treatment resistance (Kampman et al., 2007). In contrast, sertraline, when used with a 14-week-trial of counseling, helped achieve total abstinence in Type A alcoholics characterized by a late onset of alcoholism, low severity of dependence, few alcohol-related problems, little associated psychopathology, and a relatively promising treatment response with traditional alcoholism treatment (Pettanati et al., 2000).

As is the case with treatment of alcohol problems, brief clinical interventions in smoking cessation are effective and should follow the approach of the five As: ask about smoking at every opportunity, advise all smokers to stop, assess their willingness to stop, assist the smoker to stop, and arrange follow-up (Fiore et al., 2000). Pharmacological options include nicotine replacement therapy, bupropion, and varenicline, a novel nicotine receptor agonist/antagonist (Le Foll & George, 2007). However, there have been few studies of smoking cessation focused on the elderly (Oslin, 2005). Younger adults with moderate-to-severe tobacco dependence reportedly respond best to these three types of pharmacotherapy, with the choice based on the patient's preference and the presence of contraindications (Le Foll & George, 2007).

ETHICAL AND LEGAL CONCERNS

Nursing homes and other long-term care settings are expected to treat a resident's health-care needs, including those related to substance use or misuse. At the same time, preserving the dignity of dependent adults is increasingly being raised by professionals and caregivers alike (Silberfeld, 2007). Research indicates that when older adults feel more in control of some areas of their lives, they are often inclined to make other changes, such as the moderation or elimination of alcohol (Christie, 1997). Therefore, if residents are still competent to determine their own interests, the principle of autonomy must override the nursing home's determination of what is best for those residents because decisions regarding care should be guided by the resident's need, not the home's interest (Priester, 1990). The safe use of alcohol may be indeed meeting a number of the resident's emotional and social needs.

Nursing homes require rules and regulations in order to ensure the safety and well-being of all residents. Those who view drinking as a social issue and not a medical one may question a physician's right to write an order to determine who can drink how much and who cannot drink. On the other hand, for those who view alcohol as a psychoactive drug of abuse, drinking is a medical issue. The establishment of drinking rules is a challenge because nursing homes and other long-term care settings house both social and problem drinkers. This was similarly the case with smoking, but society has changed its rules about smoking in a far broader way than alcohol where the main emphasis currently is on drinking and not driving.

Nursing homes also have a legal duty to exercise reasonable care, although what is reasonable varies with residents' abilities to look after their own safety (Priester, 1990). This can be interpreted to allow nursing homes the right to use discretion in implementing individualized care. Occasionally, legal "waivers of liability" are used so that in optimizing a resident's quality of life, the facility is also protecting itself from being sued if problems occur.

PREVENTION

As elderly abusers have a high use of general medical services, health-care professionals can play a vital role in identifying those in need of treatment and providing appropriate interventions based on clinical need (Coulehan et al., 1987). Coupled with an aging population, nursing homes will house more of these residents who will be triply stigmatized by aging, institutional living, and substance abuse. Public awareness of this anticipated increase of elderly abusers must be raised through education of both health-care professionals and the public. Clinicians working with elderly drug addicts believe treatment will remain hampered until research addresses the physical, medical, and social complications of this neglected population (Rosenberg, 1995). Epidemiological research is important as it improves the understanding of the scope and impact of a disease, as well as being a vital component during the planning stage for new services (Johnson, 2000). Treatment studies testing medications for addictions should begin to include more patients over 65 years of age.

Problematic substance use, misuse, or abuse in the nursing home may be initiated by residents themselves, as in the case of alcohol, tobacco, or illicit drugs, or may occur due to collusion of family or staff. More effective treatment programs emphasizing education, counseling, and addressing interpersonal issues can be implemented after nursing homes take the first important step to identify residents with a drinking or drug problem. Attention needs to be paid to ensure residents are not hiding bottles or arranging for certain staff to sign for the receipt of alcohol from a delivery company (Schwartz & Lasky, 2002). Physicians must be more vigilant in deciding who is allowed to drink during "happy hours" while mindful of residents' autonomy and rights. Reviewing the need for psychotropic medication at regular intervals will decrease inappropriate prescriptions and lessen the risk of psychological dependence on benzodiazepines.

Some family members choose to continue supplying their loved ones with alcoholic drinks, not wanting to deprive them of what they believe is one of their last pleasures in life (Klein & Jess, 2002). These family members could be referred to the social worker for education and help with psychological or emotional issues of anger, guilt, or other feelings related to past or continued use of alcohol by the family member. An approach that describes the impact of the drug on the resident's health or functional status and makes the drug the enemy, not necessarily the behavior, may increase empathy for the family member, leading to more cooperation from the family (Schmader & Moore, 2003). A referral to Alanon is sometimes necessary.

Older alcoholics in nursing homes have some unique needs, which differ from those of the younger alcoholic. Identifying these needs could lead to different treatment strategies, such as groups which particularly address the lack of control, demoralization, and isolation that many elderly problematic drinkers or drug seekers in these facilities experience (Schwartz et al., 2001).

The more inflexible the rules and structure of nursing homes, the more it will be experienced as an institution whose residents will likely experience less connection to the facility, staff, and their previous selves. Such environments increase the likelihood of self-medication or substance abuse. On the other hand, nursing homes that provide a combination of good programming and policies, an attentive staff respectful of the autonomy of residents, and an administration that is genuinely interested in hearing from residents can help improve the quality of life for residents to the point where they engage in less substance misuse or abuse.

REFERENCES

Allen, D. N., & Landis, R. K. B. (1997). Substance abuse in elderly individuals. In P. D. Nussbaum (Ed.), *Handbook of neuropsychology and aging: Critical issues in neuropsychology* (pp. 111–140). New York: Plenum.

American Psychiatric Association. (2000). *Diagnostic and statistical manual of mental disorders* (4th ed., text revision). Washington, DC: Author.

Anthony, J. C., & Helzer, J. E. (1991). Syndromes of drug abuse and dependence. In L. N. Robins & D. A. Regler (Eds.), *Psychiatric disorders in America: The epidemiologic Catchment Area Study* (pp. 116–154). New York: Free Press.

Atkinson, R. W. (1991). Alcohol and drug abuse in the elderly. In R. Jacoby & C. Oppenheimer (Eds.), *Psychiatry in the elderly* (pp. 819–851). Oxford: Oxford University Press.

Barker, J. C., Mitteness, L. S., & Wolfson, C. R. (1994). Smoking and adulthood: Risky business in a nursing home. *Journal of Aging Studies, 8*(3), 309–326.

Blow, F. (1991). *Michigan Alcoholism Screening Test—Geriatric version (MAST-G).* Ann Arbor: University of Michigan Alcohol Research Center.

Blow, F., Gillespie, B., Barry, K., et al. (1998). Brief screening for alcohol problems in Screening Test—Geriatric Version (SMAST-G). *Alcoholism, Clinical and Experimental Research, 22*(Suppl), 131A.

Boxer, R., & Shorr, R. (2004). Principles of drug therapy: Changes with aging, polypharmacy, and drug interaction. In C. S. Landefeld, R. M. Parker, M. A. Johnson, et al. (Eds.), *Current geriatric diagnosis and treatment* (pp. 421–435). New York: McGraw-Hill.

Brennan, P. L. (2005). Functioning and health service use among elderly nursing home residents with alcohol use disorders: Findings from the National Nursing Home Survey. *American Journal of Geriatric Psychiatry, 13*(6), 475–483.

Brennan, P., & Greenbaum, M. (2005). Functioning, problem behaviour and health services use among nursing home residents with alcohol-use disorders. Nationwide data from the VA minimum data set. *Journal of Studies on Alcohol, 66,* 395–400.

Brennan, P. L., & Moos, R. H. (1990). Life stressors, social resources, and late-life problem drinking. *Psychology and Aging, 5,* 491–501.

Buchsbaum, R. G., Buchanan, R. G., Walsh, J., et al. (1992). Screening for drinking disorders in the elderly using the CAGE questionnaire. *Journal of the American Geriatrics Society, 40,* 662–665.

Burman, M., Buchbinder, M., Kivlahan, D., et al. (2004). Alcohol-related advice for VA primary care patients: Who gets it, who gives it? *Journal of Studies on Alcohol, 65*(5), 621–630.

Callahan, C., & Tierney, W. (1995). Health services use and mortality among older primary patients with alcoholism. *Journal of the American Geriatrics Society, 43,* 1378–1383.

Campbell, J. W. (2004). Use of alcohol, tobacco and nonprescribed drugs. In C. S. Landefeld, R. M. Parker, M. A. Johnson, et al. (Eds.), *Current geriatric diagnosis and treatment* (pp. 407–413). New York: McGraw-Hill.

Christie, D. (1997). Alcohol abuse in the elderly: Making a difference. *Canadian Journal of Continuing Medical Education, 9,* 101–114.

Conn, D. K. (2007). Optimizing the use of psychotropic medications. In D. K. Conn, N. Herrmann, A. Kaye, et al. (Eds.), *Practical psychiatry in the long-term care home* (pp. 203–216). Cambridge, MA: Hogrefe.

Coulehan, J., Zettler-Segal, M., Block, M., et al. (1987). Recognition of alcoholism and substance abuse in primary care patients. *Archives of Internal Medicine, 147,* 349–352.

Curtis, J. R., Geller, G., Stokes, E. J., et al. (1989). Characteristics, diagnosis and treatment of alcoholism in elderly patients. *Journal of the American Geriatrics Society, 37*(4), 310–316.

Damestroy, N., Collin, J., & Lalande, R. (1999). Prescribing psychotropic medication for elderly patients: Some physicians' perspectives. *CMAJ, 13,* 243–250.

Ewing, J. A. (1984). Detecting alcoholism. The CAGE questionnaire. *JAMA, 252,* 1905–1907.

Fingerhood, M. (2000). Substance abuse in older people. *Journal of the American Geriatrics Society, 48,* 985–995.

Fink, A., Morton, S. C., Beck, J. C., et al. (2002). The alcohol-related problems survey: Identifying hazardous and harmful drinking in older primary care patients. *Journal of the American Geriatrics Society, 50,* 1717–1722.

Finklestein, E., Prabbhu, M., & Chen, H. (2007). Increased prevalence of falls among elderly individuals with mental health and substance abuse conditions. *American Journal of Geriatric Psychiatry 15*(7), 611–620.

Finlayson, R. E., & Davis, L. J. (1994). Prescription drug dependence of the elderly population: Demographic and clinical features of 100 in patients. *Mayo Clinic Proceedings, 69,* 1137–1145.

Fiore, M. C., Bailey, W. C., Cohen, S. J., et al. (2000). *Treating tobacco use and dependence. Clinical practice guidelines.* Rockville, MD: U.S. Department of Health and Human Services, Public Health Service.

Greenberg, D. M., Lee, J. W. Y., & Lautenschlager, N. T. (2004). Management and treatment of psychotic manifestations in older patients with alcoholism: Part I. *Clinical Geriatrics, 12*(4), 33–40.

Herrmann, N., & Eryavec, G. (1996). Lifetime alcohol abuse in institutionalized World War II veterans. *American Journal of Geriatric Psychiatry, 4,* 39–45.

Hirati, E. S., Almeida, O. P., Feinari, R. R., et al. (2001). Validity of the Michigan Alcoholism Screening Test (MAST) for the detection of alcohol-related problems among male geriatric outpatients. *American Journal of Geriatric Psychiatry, 9*(1), 30–34.

Hughes, J. R., Stead, L. F., & Lancaster, T. (2007). Antidepressants for smoking cessation. *Cochrane Database of Systematic Reviews, 1.*

Johnson, B. A., Rosenthal, N., Capece, J. A., et al. (2007). Topiramate for treating alcohol dependence: A randomized controlled trial. *JAMA, 298*(44), 1641–1651.

Johnson, I. (2000). Alcohol problems in old age: A review of recent epidemiological research. *International Journal of Geriatric Psychiatry, 15,* 575–581.

Joseph, C. J. (1995). Alcohol and drug misuse in the nursing home. *International Journal of the Addictions, 30,* 1953–1984.

Joseph, C. J., & Harvath, T. (1998). Alcohol and drug misuse in the nursing home. *Journal of Mental Health and Aging, 4*(2), 251–269

Joseph, C. L., Atkinson, R. M., & Ganzini, L. (1995a). Problem drinking among residents of a VA nursing home. *International Journal of Geriatric Psychiatry, 10,* 243–248.

Joseph, C. L., Ganzini, L., & Atkinson, R. M. (1995b). Screening for alcohol use disorders in the nursing home. *Journal of the American Geriatrics Society, 43,* 368–373.

Judson, M. (2007). Substance abuse: Treating an illness. *Canadian Journal of Continuing Medical Education, 19*(7), 35–37.

Kampman, K. M., Pettinatti, H. M., Lynch, K. G., et al. (2007). A double-blind, placebo-controlled pilot trial of Quetiapine for the treatment of type A and type B alcoholism. *Journal of Clinical Psychopharmacology, 27*(4), 344–351.

Klatsky, A. L., & Armstrong, A. (1993). Alcohol use, other traits and risk of unnatural death: A prospective study. *Alcoholism, Clinical and Experimental Research, 17,* 1156–1162.

Klein, W. C., & Jess, C. (2002). One last pleasure: Alcohol use among elderly people in nursing homes. *Health and Social Work, 27*(3), 193–203.

Lantz, M. S., Giambanco, V., & Buchalter, E. N. (1996). A ten-year review of the effect of OBRA-87 on psychotropic prescribing practices in an academic nursing home. *Psychiatric Services, 47*(9), 951–955.

Le Foll, B., & George, T. P. (2007). Treatment of tobacco dependence: Integrating recent progress into practice. *CMAJ, 170*(11), 1373–1380.

Liberto, J. G., & Oslin, D. W. (1997). Early versus late onset of alcoholism in the elderly. In A. M. Gurnak (Ed.), *Older adults' misuse of alcohol, medicines and other drugs: Research and practice issues* (pp. 94–112). New York: Springer.

Luggen, A. S. (2007). Unhealthy alcohol intake among older adults. *Geriatrics and Aging, 10*(6), 347–360.

Mayfield, D. G., McLeod, G., & Hall, P. (1974). The CAGE questionnaire: Validation of a new alcoholism screening treatment. *American Journal of Psychiatry, 131,* 1121–1123.

McCance, K. L., & Roberts, L. K. (2004). Biology of cancer. In K. L. McCance & S. E. Huether (Eds.), *Pathophysiology* (4th ed., pp. 290–333). St. Louis, MO: Mosby.

Miller, N., Belkin, B., & Gold, M. (1991). Alcohol and drug dependence among the elderly: Epidemiology, diagnosis and treatment. *Comprehensive Psychiatry, 32,* 153–165.

Miller, W. R., & Rollnick, S. (2002). *Motivational interviewing: Preparing people for change* (2nd ed.). New York: Guildford Press.

Moore, A. A., Morton, S. C., Beck, J. C., et al. (1999). A new paradigm for alcohol use in older persons. *Medical Care, 37*(2), 165–179.

Morton, J. L., Jones, T. V., & Manganaro, B. S. (1996). Performance of elderly questionnaires in elderly veterans. *American Journal of Medicine, 101,* 153–159.

National Center for Health Statistics. (1989). *Nursing home utilization by current residents.* 102 Vital and Health Statistics.

National Institute of Alcohol Abuse and Alcoholism. (1995, October). Diagnostic criteria for alcohol abuse. *Alcohol Alert,* 30(PH 359), 1–6.

O'Connell, H., Chin, A., Cunningham, C., et al. (2003). Alcohol use disorders in elderly people-redefining an age-old problem in old age. *BMJ, 327,* 664–667.

Oslin, D. W. (2004). Late-life alcoholism: Issues relevant to the geriatric psychiatrist. *American Journal of Geriatric Psychiatry, 12*(6), 571–583.

Oslin, D. W. (2005). Evidence-based treatment of geriatric substance abuse. *Psychiatric Clinics of North America, 28*(4), 897–911.

Oslin, D. W. (2006). The changing face of substance misuse in older adults. *Psychiatric Times, 23*(13), 41–44.

Oslin, D. W., Streim, J. E., Parmalee, P., et al. (1997). Alcohol abuse. A source of reversible functional disability among residents of a VA nursing home. *International Journal of Geriatric Psychiatry, 12,* 825–832.

Patterson, T. L., & Jeste, D. V. (1999). The potential impact of the baby-boom generation on substance abuse among elderly persons. *Psychiatric Services, 50*(9), 1184–1188.

Pettinati, H. M., Volpicelli, J. R., Kranzler, H. R., et al. (2000). Sertraline treatment for alcohol dependence: Interactive effects of medication and alcoholic subtype. *Alcoholism, Clinical and Experimental Research, 24,* 1041–1049.

Pipe, A. (2007). Smoking cessation: Practical tips on how to help your patients quit. *Parkhurst Exchange, 15*(10), 27.

Priester, R. (1990). Leaving homes: Residents on their own recognizance. In R. A. Kane & A. L. Caplan (Eds.), *Everyday ethics: Resolving dilemmas in nursing homes* (pp. 155–164). New York: Springer.

Reid, M. C., & Anderson, P. A. (1997). Alcohol and other substance abuse. *Medical Clinics of North America, 81*(4), 999–1016.

Rosenberg, H. (1995). The elderly and the use of illicit drugs: Sociological and epidemiological considerations. *The International Journal of the Addictions, 30*(13–14), 1925–1951.

Rubenstein, L. Z., Ouslander, J. G., & Wieland, D. (1988). Dynamics and clinical implications of the nursing home-hospital interface. *Clinical Geriatric Medicine, 4,* 471–491.

Saitz, R. (2005). Unhealthy alcohol use. *NEJM, 352,* 596–607.

Saladin, M. E., & Santa Ana. E. J. (2004). Controlled drinking: More than just a controversy. *Current Opinion in Psychiatry, 17,* 175–187.

Schlaerth, K. R. (2007). Older adults and illegal drugs. *Geriatrics and Aging, 10*(6), 361–364.

Schmader, K. E., & Moore, A. A. (2003). Misadventures with drugs and alcohol in the older patient: Alcohol use, misuse, and abuse in older persons. *Annals of Long-Term Care, 11*(8), 37–42.

Schuckit, M. A. (1990). Introduction: Assessment and treatment strategies with the late-life alcoholic. *Journal of Geriatric Psychiatry, 23*(2), 83–89.

Schwartz, K. (2007). Alcohol use and misuse. In D. K. Conn, N. Herrmann, A. Kaye, et al. (Eds.), *Practical psychiatry in the long-term care home: A handbook for staff* (3rd rev., exp. ed., pp. 155–167). Cambridge, MA: Hogrefe.

Schwartz, K. M., & Lasky, N. (2002). The development and implementation of an alcohol policy in a nursing home: Overcoming denial. *Journal of Geriatric Psychiatry, 35*(2), 151–167.

Schwartz, K. M., Lasky, N., & Schendel, S. (2001). Alcohol use by residents: What to do. *Long-Term Care, 11*(4), 25–28.

Silberfeld, M. (2007). Legal and ethical dimensions. In D. K. Conn, N. Herrmann, A. Kaye, et al. (Eds.), *Practical psychiatry in the long-term care home: A handbook for staff* (3rd rev., exp. ed., pp. 311–322). Cambridge, MA: Hogrebe.

Snowden, J. (1993). Mental health in nursing homes. Perspectives on the use of medication. *Drugs and Aging, 3*, 122–130.

Solomon, K., & Shackson, J. B. (1996). Substance abuse disorders. In W. E. Reichman & P. R. Katz (Eds.), *Psychiatric care in the nursing home* (pp. 165–187). New York: Oxford University Press.

Spencer, C. (2002). Establishing alcohol protocols in LTC facilities. *Canadian Nursing Home, 13*(1), 23–26.

Streim, J. E., Beckwith, E. W., Arapakos, D., et al. (2002). Regulatory oversight, payment policy, and quality improvement in mental health care in nursing homes. *Psychiatric Services, 53*, 1414–1418.

Substance Abuse and Mental Health Services Administration results from the 2005 National Survey on Drug Use and Health in National Findings. (2006). Rockville, MD: Office of Applied Studies, SMA 06-4194.

Swartz, M., Landerman, R., George, R. K., et al. (1991). Benzodiazepine agents: Prevalence and correlates of use in a southern community. *American Journal of Public Health, 81*, 592–596.

U.S. Preventive Services Task Force. (2004). Screening and behavioral counseling interventions in primary care to reduce alcohol misuse: Recommendation strategies. *Annals of Internal Medicine, 140*, 554–556.

Voyer, P., & Préville, M. (2007). Insomnia and benzodiazepine dependency among older adults. *Geriatrics and Aging, 10*(6), 369–375.

Walker, V. A., & Whitson, H. E. (2007). Smoking cessation in older adults: A review. *Geriatrics and Aging, 10*(6), 365–368.

Waxman, H. M., Klein, M., & Carner, E. A. (1985). Drug misuse in nursing homes: An institutional addiction? *Hospital and Community Psychiatry, 36*(8), 886–887.

Winick, C. (1962). Maturing out of narcotic addiction. *Bulletin on Narcotics, 14*, 1–7.

Wiseman, E. J. (2003). Drug and alcohol abuse. In B. J. Sadock & V. A. Sadock (Eds.), *Kaplan and Sadock's comprehensive textbook of psychiatry* (3rd ed., Vol. 2, pp. 3711–3716). Philadelphia, PA: Lippincott Williams & Wilkins.

Zimberg, S. (1978). Treatment of the elderly alcoholic in the community and in the institutional setting. *Addictive Diseases, 3*(3), 417–422.

PART II

PSYCHIATRIC INTERVENTIONS

12

General Approaches
to Behavioral Disturbances

Lisa L. Boyle, Anton P. Porsteinsson,
and *Pierre N. Tariot*

Careful surveys have documented that 90% or more of nursing home patients have at least one form of behavioral disturbance, with as many as half exhibiting four or more (Rovner et al., 1986; Tariot et al., 1993). In some cases, the severity of these behavioral syndromes is equivalent to that encountered among psychiatric inpatients (Tariot et al., 1993). Despite the complexity of these problems, most caregivers have little or no mental health training; indeed, most are nonprofessionals. The frequency and severity of behavioral disturbances, combined with the lack of preparedness in most nursing homes, are sufficient justification for devoting an entire textbook to the subject.

There are other important reasons for addressing behavioral disturbance in the nursing home. The kinds of psychological symptoms seen are undoubtedly distressing to those experiencing them, such as frightening hallucinations or delusions, abiding depression, sleeplessness, or anxiety of phobic proportions. The term "Behavioral and Psychological Symptoms of Dementia" (BPSD) has been adopted to label these symptoms when associated with dementia (Finkel, 2000). In addition, a variety of adverse consequences can ensue from disturbed behaviors, including violent interactions with others, inappropriate use of psychotropic medications and physical restraint (Tariot & Blazina, 1993), and functional disability (Schultz et al., 2003). Caregivers can suffer serious psychological and physical consequence from their attempts to deal with these behaviors

(Chenoweth & Spencer, 1986; Colerick & George, 1986; Deimling & Blass, 1986; Rabins et al., 1982). Whereas relief of these symptoms can promote increased function, autonomy, and improved quality of life for the patient as well as others, unattended behavioral pathology can lead to greater distress for all concerned.

This chapter proposes a systemic general approach to the evaluation and management of behavioral disturbances in the nursing home, summarized in Table 12.1. The approach is grounded in traditional medical and psychiatric principles of diagnosis and therapy and builds on earlier proposals (American Geriatrics Society & American Association for Geriatric Psychiatry, AAGP & AGS, 2003; Doody et al., 2001; Leibovici & Tariot, 1988; Lyketsos et al., 2006). It is easy for these traditional principles to get lost in the face of the extremely

---

TABLE 12.1. General Approach to Behavioral Disturbance

---

1. **Define target symptoms**
   Elicit data from multiple sources.
   Arrive at a consensus about target symptoms and aggravating and ameliorating factors.
2. **Establish or revisit medical diagnoses**
   Perform traditional evaluation.
   Rule out delirium.
   Rule out other medical diagnoses.
   Assess for associated excess disability (e.g., pain).
   Treat medical disorders specifically.
   Monitor target symptoms.
3. **Establish or revisit neuropsychiatric diagnoses**
   Make traditional evaluation.
   Rule out depression.
   Rule out other discrete disorders.
   Rule out organic mental disorder such as dementia.
   Watch for interacting medical/psychiatric variables.
   Treat specific syndromes when present.
4. **Assess and reverse aggravating factors**
   Sensory impairment.
   Environmental disturbance.
5. **Adapt to specific cognitive deficits**
   Is busy area vs. quiet sport better?
   Pictures or labels can help.
   Place important objects or memory book in room to help orient.
   Simplify environment.
   Provide cues for activities.
   Allow pacing, wandering.
6. **Identify relevant psychosocial factors**
   Allow for adjustment at admission.
   Perceived or real loss of support can lead to systematic behaviors.
   Support, validation, and reminiscences are helpful.

Continued

TABLE 12.1. Continued

Psychotherapy is sometimes indicated.
Optimize physical and social stimulation.
7. **Educate caregivers**
Review evaluation, outline further diagnostic steps.
Summarize functional and cognitive status.
Redefine target symptoms.
Support caregivers.
Educate the system.
8. **Employ behavior management principles**
Staff behavior has a major effect.
9. **Use psychotropics for specific syndromes**
Treat primary syndromes specifically.
If a syndrome is superimposed upon an organic disorder, treat the syndrome first.
10. **Symptomatic pharmacotherapy**
For severe, acute problems, consider hospitalization or neuroleptics.
For the rest, develop "psychobehavioral metaphor": fit target symptoms into a syndrome known to be drug responsive, such as depressive, manic, psychotic, anxious, or vegetative.
11. **The process of treatment**
Assess risk/benefit ratio.
Start low, go slow.
Use lowest effective dose.
In the absence of prompt efficacy, maintain subtoxic dose for an appropriate period, then withdraw.
Perform trial in reverse. Watch for flare of behavioral problems.
Subsequent trials may be in order.
Even effective medications should be empirically withdrawn.
Medications do not always work: go back to step 1!

complex, atypical behavioral disturbances that are so common in the nursing home. Nonetheless, returning to basics pertains for these atypical problems as well as any other medical problem. Thoughtful application of diagnostic and therapeutic principles is, in itself, therapeutic in settings involving multiple disciplines, yet where many of the caregivers may have minimal medical or psychiatric expertise.

A GENERAL APPROACH

Define Target Symptoms

The term "behavioral disturbance" refers to a behavioral or psychological syndrome or pattern associated with subjective distress, functional disability, or impaired interactions with others or the environment (Tariot & Blazina, 1993). An important first step is to delineate the patterns carefully; they will have diagnostic and therapeutic implications that will help the caregiver to succinctly summarize the "target symptoms"; for instance, "bangs on table repeatedly, calls out loudly, resists care, cries intermittently, expresses self-deprecatory ideation, doesn't complete meals without cueing, attempts to leave with apparent purpose in mind," and so on. Characterizing antecedent triggers to the behavioral disturbance can also help to guide interventions. Since many behaviors are ephemeral, it is helpful to elicit observations from the multiple sources that are available in the nursing home: aides, nursing staff, social workers, dietary staff, clergy, and physical, occupational, and recreational therapists, looking for "ground swells" of opinion that particular patterns do or do not exist.

Establish or Revisit Medical Diagnoses

The next step is a comprehensive medical evaluation. It is not unusual for a behavioral disturbance to be the proximate cause for the first detailed medical evaluation: in many cases, preexisting neuropsychiatric diagnoses, for instance, have been undetected. A complete evaluation includes a full medical history, review of medication, physical examination, laboratory testing, and assessment of cognitive and functional performance.

Although behavioral problems can occur by themselves, they often indicate that the patient has one or more treatable medical disorders that are causing the disturbed behavior. These must be established or revisited. The most dreaded is delirium. One of the truisms of geriatrics is to presume that the new onset of disturbed behavior results from delirium until proved otherwise since virtually any behavioral symptoms or syndrome can result from delirium. It has been observed in 6% to 7% of nursing home residents and can present as an acute, subacute, or even chronic picture (Rovner et al., 1986, 1990). While psycho-active medications are the most common culprit, intercurrent infectious processes, dehydration, electrolyte disturbance, and trauma are other precipitants of delirium (See Chapter 3 for a thorough discussion of delirium.).

Other medical disorders, by themselves, can cause behavioral symptoms in the absence of delirium. The classic examples are the "depressive" manifestations of thyroid disease, infections, head injury, sedating medication, and so forth. In addition, medical disorders can result in behavioral symptoms as a result of secondary disability such as constipation or fecal impaction, pain, sensory impairment, disrupted sleep, or physical limitation.

When medical problems or metabolic abnormalities are present, treatment should be directed toward correcting them and the patient should be monitored for his or her response. The same principle holds for associated secondary consequences of medical disorders: they should be corrected where possible or at least accommodated.

Establish or Revisit Neuropsychiatric Diagnoses

It is possible that the disturbed behavior is a consequence of a long-standing, chronic, or recurrent psychiatric disorder, or it could be the initial presentation of a new psychiatric disorder. Establishing the presence of a psychiatric diagnosis entails evaluation of current symptomatology, response to therapy, and family history. Perhaps the most important psychiatric diagnosis in the nursing home, in terms of prevalence and likelihood of therapeutic success, is depression. The prevalence of major depression among cognitively intact nursing home residents has been estimated to be as high as 25% (Parmelee et al., 1992), a figure an order of magnitude higher than that found in the community, whereas the incidence of depression in institutionalized dementia patients has been estimated to be approximately 6% per year (Payne et al., 2000). Physical and verbal aggression and attention-seeking behaviors have been associated with severe depression in nursing home residents (Heeren et al., 2003). The crucial role of drug therapy in the treatment of major depression has been emphasized in the practice guidelines developed by the Agency for Health Care Policy and Research and the American Psychiatric Association. The efficacy and safety of treatment of depression in the elderly is relatively well established, although there are uncertainties about the applicability of carefully done research studies in depressed subjects to frail elderly patients in the nursing home setting (Katz et al., 1990). The evidence is substantial, however, that the value of such treatment is extremely high. Treatment of an underlying depressive disorder may correspond with reduced levels of associated behavioral symptoms. (See Chapter 4 for a complete discussion of depression and Chapter 13 for psychopharmacological considerations.)

Surveys have also indicated a substantial proportion of other psychiatric disorders in the nursing home, such as mania (Chapter 4), anxiety disorders (Chapter 5), schizophrenia (Chapter 6), and substance abuse (Chapter 11; Rovner et al., 1986, 1990; Tariot et al., 1993). In all instances where these are presumed to be the primary etiology of the distributed behavior, specific appropriate therapy should be applied and the response monitored. Adjustment disorders are worth special mention recognizing that admission to a nursing home will be a significant stressor. Recognizing this may helpfully focus attention on needs that will diminish over time.

In fact, a very large proportion of nursing home patients will suffer from dementia (Chapter 2) or some other organic mental disorder in fact, these are the most prevalent neuropsychiatric diagnoses in the nursing home (Rovner et al., 1986, 1990; Tariot et al., 1993), with dementia affecting approximately 50% of nursing home residents (Magaziner et al., 2000). It is obvious that the etiology of the organic mental impairment must be established as it may offer clues to definitive therapy for the behavioral problem. Likewise, it is also perhaps obvious that a patient with an organic mental impairment may suffer a superimposed medical illness, which, while benign in itself, produces unusual behavioral disturbance in the vulnerable patient. Patients with such organic mental disorders can also experience concomitant discrete psychiatric disorders. In residents of care facilities, BPSD were associated with stage of dementia, with depression more common in patients with mild dementia, delusional symptoms more common in moderate dementia, and aberrant motor behavior more common in advanced dementia (Margallo-Lana et al., 2001). Since behavioral disturbances in such patients can occur for either reason (organic mental disorder or discrete psychiatric disorders), it is important to try and make the distinction. It is especially helpful to describe and categorize the target symptoms, as alluded to previously. This will facilitate monitoring and can guide symptomatic pharmacotherapy. Where a syndromal psychiatric disorder is superimposed upon an organic mental disorder, the syndrome should be treated first.

Assess and Reverse Aggravating Factors

Whether psychiatric or medical pathology is present, it is also important to bear in mind other factors that can precipitate or aggravate behavioral disturbance. First among these is sensory impairment. It is unfortunately common to observe health professionals who fail to recognize that a patient cannot see or hear well or cannot use assistive devices properly because of cognitive impairment. For such patients, simplification and clarification of communication is essential. This includes making one's face fully visible to facilitate lipreading, experimenting with different volumes of speech, inserting or adjusting hearing aids, using amplifiers, reducing communication to simple phrases or words, communicating by writing or letter board, and so on. As a related issue, English is a second language for many, and interpreters can be very helpful.

Environmental disturbances such as excessive heat or cold during unusual climate changes, noise from construction or other disruptive residents, or altered daily routines can lead to discomfort that is expressed only by disturbed behavior such as calling out or other apparently purposeless efforts to leave or remedy the problem. Adjustments in light, noise, temperature, or change in room or roommate can sometimes be helpful. Music may help relax certain patients.

Adapt to Specific Cognitive Deficits

In some cases, "problem" behaviors can be better understood as well intentioned but perhaps confused or disruptive efforts to communicate or adapt

(Cohen-Mansfield, 1992). Impaired communication has been associated with all forms of aggression in a sample of nursing home residents with dementia (Talerico et al., 2002). For instance, pacing may reflect a need for stimulation, "wandering" may result from an incorrect belief that the patient needs to get to another place, and verbally disruptive behaviors may represent efforts to obtain assistance.

Suspiciousness may occur when impaired comprehension leads to the understandable perception that the environment or another person is threatening. A host of behaviors may be understandable as "environmentally dependent." This occurs typically in an organically impaired patient with executive control dysfunction (Lezak, 1983). It is common for such patients to react to what is in front of them: an open door prompts passage through it (perhaps into another's room); a visible overcoat is put on, triggering the desire to leave; any food item in view is eaten; and so forth.

A variety of interventions may be designed according to a patient's particular pattern of cognitive impairment. Patients with disorientation but some ability to interpret pictures or words may respond to pictures or labels identifying their room, possessions, family members, activities for the day, and so on. Some will benefit by being in a quiet location, whereas others may enjoy being in a busy public area. Some patients find it helpful to be "anchored," more firmly aware of their personal history, by important possessions such as pieces of furniture or art as well as family photos. A "memory book" can be considered for certain confused patients, consisting of an album of photos and phrases to help remind them of important events, places, and relationships. Patients can also be helped by reducing clutter in their environment or reducing the number of environmental cues to which they might respond inappropriately. On the other hand, those who need to be engaged in a physical activity can respond to cues from the environment (and staff) about this. These could range from simply having magazines available to provide repetitive tasks that patients are capable of completing (e.g., counting, folding, and so on). It may be valuable to create a physical environment where it is possible for patients to stimulate themselves by walking and exploring, such as circular corridors and safe outdoor walking areas, or to design visual or physical barriers to reduce the changes of unsafe egress.

Identify Relevant Psychosocial Factors

Anger, sadness, and even denial can accompany nursing home admission. Once admitted, the patient may experience loss of contact with others through death, a move, or simply a vacation taken by an important other, resulting in a temporary but frequently significant sense of loss or abandonment. A variety of other psychological themes are common and may respond to opportunities to speak of them without requiring psychotherapy. Such themes can include loss of health, function, autonomy, privacy, possessions, and intimacy. Reviewing and acknowledging these losses and stressors can help reduce feelings of sadness and anxiety. It is also important to support those patients who are striving to make healthful adaptations—to accommodate new realities without resigning themselves to despair. Encouragement and validation, and ongoing efforts to reclaim positive memories and experiences from one's prior life, are basic therapeutic tools. It is also obvious, and often overlooked, that the patient's personality plays a major role in determining adaptation to the nursing home setting. How has he or she historically coped with loss, transition, and interaction with others? A developmental history that includes this information should be a part of every patient's database. In some cases, it is desirable to obtain a consultation regarding the utility of psychotherapy, although this is not a generally available option. (The reader is referred to Chapters 14 and 15 for discussions of psychotherapy in the nursing home.)

It is almost always desirable to optimize physical activity and social stimulation. This entails working collaboratively with nurses, clergy, social workers, and physical and recreational therapists to clarify what "mix" of activities is best for the particular patient. Are there appropriate group therapeutic activities? Are religious activities important and available? Are there existing social activities that are well suited to a given patient's temperament? Is it medically safe to go on picnics, shopping trips, or overnight passes?

Educate Caregivers

Education of staff, families, and patients is essential. This typically entails a review of the medical and psychiatric evaluation as it stands and possible further diagnostic steps, a summary of functional and cognitive deficits, a concise summary of disturbed behaviors (target symptoms), and consideration of possible aggravating and ameliorating factors. This first step demonstrates that the team's response to the behavior will be logical, thorough, and thoughtful. This reassuring message is initially established by the manner in which the case is summarized. This feedback phase provides all concerned with an improved and specific behavioral lexicon, which is also reassuring and facilitates improved communication and monitoring of the subsequent course. Clarification of the prognosis and of therapeutic options also helps caregivers and patients cope. It is reassuring to know that there can be discernible and predictable patterns, that "confused" behaviors can actually have understandable origins, and that certain frightening behaviors are a manifestation of a pathological substrate rather than an emotionally laden personal attack. Such knowledge allows caregivers, some of whom have limited experience and training, to interact more helpfully and specifically with their patients. Finally, it is important to emphasize the value of the clinician's ongoing presence during efforts to manage a disruptive patient. Relatively brief visits can bolster staff and patient morale considerably, as can explicit validation of the demanding nature of caring for such patients.

Similar messages can have great impact on family and friends. They may learn how certain of their behaviors are either proactive or helpful. They may be able to appreciate that, although the patient may be aphasic, the perceived abandonment at the time of a vacation can lead to distress that could be ameliorated by asking other friends or family members to help out temporarily by visiting more frequently. At the same time, family and friends may have valuable information and suggestions to offer the multidisciplinary care team regarding optimal care of the patient.

At a broader level, education of the larger system beyond the health-care team can be considered as well. Adequate recognition of behavioral disturbances in the nursing home would lead to sensible implementation of educational programs for all caregivers, thoughtful development of appropriate policies and procedures, establishment of mental health consultation recourses in the facility, and ties to the acute care system for those patients requiring inpatient management.

Employ Behavior Management Principles

The fundamental principles of behavior management are quite relevant to the nursing home without invoking rigorous behavior modification programs. It is easy for staff to underestimate the extent to which their own behavior can influence the behavior of patients, particularly those who are organically impaired. When staff behave in a calm, reassuring manner and are confident in their approach, most patients will respond with reduced fear and anxiety and improved ability to cooperate with care. Conversely, sudden or apparently aggressive approaches or obvious fearfulness are likely to provide an unsettled response. Patients who call out or grab at caregivers repeatedly may do so less often if they are approached at times when they are not calling out, eventually learning that they do not have to send out distress signals in order to have their needs adequately met. Some patients benefit considerably from the brief moments (even a few seconds) of social contact offered repeatedly, as often as every few minutes. A gentle touch can also go a long way. Staff must understand that approaches such as this are very effective but require consistent application over sustained periods.

Use Psychotropics for Specific Syndromes

As in the treatment of any psychiatric disorder, psychosocial and environmental interventions such as those outlined above should be considered first and may be effective by themselves. In other cases, they serve as necessary and helpful adjuncts to psychopharmacological treatment.

For behaviors that remain disturbed despite interventions such as those identified above, there is a legitimate role for psychotropic medication. As emphasized previously when a specific diagnosable syndrome is present, this syndromal diagnosis should determine the treatment plan. Where the syndromal diagnosis is superimposed upon an organic mental disorder, that syndromal diagnosis should also determine the initial treatment plan. For instance, if a nursing home patient with dementia is referred for evaluation of pacing and is found to have features of a concomitant major depressive disorder, the depressive syndrome should become the focus of the treatment, even if the pacing is mild and manageable. An adequate trial of antidepressant treatment can determine the extent to which the depressive syndrome is contributing to the patient's cognitive and functional disability. Similarly, if the patient is found to have either a delusional disorder or a diagnosable anxiety disorder, treatment should be initiated with medications known to be effective for these conditions. The decision about treatment should be based on estimates of the extent to which the syndrome is associated with the behaviors in question as well as on impaired function.

Symptomatic Pharmacotherapy

It should be recognized, however, that many patients with organic mental impairment and behavioral disturbance do not have a specific diagnosable syndrome. For these patients, intervention directed toward symptom reduction is necessary. The most common set of problems is usually referred to loosely as "agitation" (Cohen-Mansfield et al., 1992). The choice of medication in such patients may be influenced by the urgency of the situation. If rapid control of grossly disturbed or unsafe behavior is necessary, neuroleptics are frequently used first or the patient may be admitted to an acute care hospital. In recent years, the use of atypical antipsychotic drugs in vulnerable seniors with dementia has been associated with potential increased risk for adverse outcomes, including death (Gill et al., 2007; Schneider et al., 2005). Since the 2005 U.S. Food and Drug Administration's black box warning about using atypical antipsychotic drugs for patients with dementia, it becomes more imperative that potential benefits be weighed against potential risks and that the informed consent process is followed (AAGP, 2005). Recent studies suggest that increased risk of death is associated also with the use of conventional antipsychotics (Wang et al., 2005), and the risk may be even higher compared with the atypical agents (Gill et al., 2007). Atypical antipsychotic medications have been preferred over conventional agents in the treatment of dementia and its behavioral disturbances (Alexopoulos et al., 2005).

In most cases, however, the choice of drugs and optimization of therapy may involve a lengthier process of trial and error. There is remarkable little empirical evidence to guide decision-making. In view of this, a rational approach has been proposed. An initial step in this process is to develop a "psychobehavioral metaphor" (Leibovici & Tariot, 1988). The term "metaphor" is used to emphasize the heuristic and tentative nature of the process. The aim is to formulate a working hypothesis regarding the nature of the patient's psychopathology that is to be tested in a carefully monitored trial of drug treatment. The clinician obtains information derived from multiple sources, emphasizes the most salient features, and attempts to define a pattern (that well may be fragmented) roughly analogous to a more typical drug-responsive syndrome. Although this process is logical and valid on its face, the clinical evidence in its favor is not strong since choice of medication is derived primarily from case reports, open studies, and extrapolations from studies in other populations. A more detailed discussion of psychopharmacologic therapy will follow in Chapter 13.

The Process of Treatment

An aphorism in the field is that every psychotropic trial in this population is an experiment with an n of 1. This reflects the confusing heterogeneity among patients resulting from variable etiology of behavioral disturbance, medical and psychiatric comorbidity, age, phenomenology, history of prior illness and treatment, vulnerability to adverse effects, and so forth. Concern abut the magnitude of the danger resulting from drug therapy is well justified. The balance between risk and benefit is improved if the process for initiating treatment follows the principles outlined above and if the patient is monitored on a regular basis with honest assessment of benefit as well as toxicity. In the absence of benefit at appropriate doses, or if there are significant adverse affects, the medication should obviously be decreased or discontinued.

Another general principal is "start low, go slow." Medications should generally be started at low doses and increased gradually, with ongoing monitoring for adverse effects as well as efficacy. Dose increases should be planned to allow for the assessment of both and should allow time for input from multiple members of the treatment team. In some cases, standardized rating scales, such as the Cohen-Mansfield Agitation Inventory (Cohen-Mansfield et al., 1989) or the Neuropsychiatric Inventory—Nursing Home version (Wood et al., 2000), can be useful for tracking behavioral change and documenting efficacy. Doses should generally be titrated upward until there is evidence of either clear benefit or early toxicity. In some cases, medications permit measurements of plasma levels, which can serve to guide treatment (e.g., nortriptyline). In other cases, a "subtoxic" dose (i.e., that below which mild adversity occurs) can be maintained for a period of weeks before concluding that a trial has been ineffective.

Where a medication appears ineffective, it is reasonable to perform the empirical trial in reverse, tapering the medication and watching for problems during withdrawal, such as unmasking of behavioral problems that were actually better during the treatment period. Assuming that symptoms are still present and that the patient does deteriorate, a trial with a second, presumably different class of medication can be undertaken. In especially difficult cases, this process is repeated several times. Although there are instances where no agent appears to be helpful, these are fortunately uncommon.

When a treatment trial is positive, it is reasonable to continue treatment for a period of weeks or months and at some point to taper the medication and reevaluate symptoms, once again performing the clinical trial in reverse. There is almost no evidence guiding decision-making in this regard. The usual factors taken into account include the severity of symptoms, prior history of relapse, stability of other relevant variables, and adequacy of monitoring capability—in addition to the duration of treatment. (See Chapter 13 for additional techniques and pharmacotherapy.)

SUMMARY

Many of the key points of this chapter were highlighted in the 2003 position statement of the American Geriatrics Society and American Association for Geriatric Psychiatry, which is paraphrased here (AGS & AAGP, 2003). The basic principles underlying the treatment of psychiatric disorders and behavioral problems in the nursing home are identical to those for the treatment of geriatric patients in other settings. The initial step in evaluation of any psychiatric disorder or behavioral symptom is to establish whether the symptoms result from a medical illness, previously diagnosed or undiagnosed. The next step is to establish or revisit psychiatric disorders. Comprehensive treatment planning takes into account both pharmacological and nonpharmacological interventions. The latter may include modifications of sensory, environmental, or psychosocial variables; education and support of patients as well as families; staff support of behavioral management; or psychotherapy. Despite concerns about overuse of psychotropic medications in the nursing home, they are of value for the treatment of behavioral disturbances and should be applied specifically where possible. Empirical trials of symptomatic pharmacotherapy can be aided by the use of therapeutic metaphors, that is, subtyping behavioral syndromes according to target symptoms that might be suggestive of a good response. Whenever psychotropics are used, the patient should be monitored for reduction of target symptoms that might be suggestive of a good response as well as undesired effects. Useless medications should be stopped and even effective medications may be successfully withdrawn after a period of treatment. This will help to assure that the patient will be neither over- nor undertreated.

REFERENCES

AAGP. (2005, July 13). Comment on the U.S. Food and Drug Administration's (FDA) advisory on off-label use of atypical antipsychotics in the elderly. Accessed January 25, 2008, from http://www.aagponline.org/prof/antipsychstat_0705.asp

American Geriatrics Society & American Association for Geriatric Psychiatry. (2003). Consensus statement on improving the quality of mental health care in U.S. nursing homes: Management of depression and behavioral symptoms associated with dementia. *Journal of the American Geriatrics Society, 51*, 1287–1298.

Alexopoulos, G. S., Jeste, D. V., Chung, H., et al. (2005). The expert consensus guideline series: Treatment of dementia and its behavioral disturbances. *Postgraduate Medicine Special Report*, 6–22.

Chenoweth, B., & Spencer, B. (1986). Dementia: The experience of family caregivers. *Journal of Gerontology, 26*, 267–272.

Cohen-Mansfield, J., Marx, M. S., & Rosenthal, A. S. (1989). A description of agitation in a nursing home. *Journal of Gerontology, 44*, 77–84.

Cohen-Mansfield, J., Marx, M. S., & Werner, P. (1992). Agitation in elderly persons: An integrative report of findings in a nursing home. *International Psychogeriatrics/ IPA, 4*(Suppl 2), 221–240.

Colerick, E., & George, L. (1986). Predictors of institutionalization among caregivers of patients with Alzheimer's disease. *Journal of the American Geriatrics Society, 34*, 493–498.

Deimling, G., & Blass, D. (1986). Symptoms of mental impairment among elderly adults and their effects of family caregivers. *Journal of Gerontology, 41*, 778–784.

Doody, R. S., Stevens, J. C., Beck, C., et al. (2001). Practice parameter: Management of dementia (an evidence-based review). Report of the Quality Standards Subcommittee of the American Academy of Neurology. *Neurology, 56*, 1154–1166.

Finkel, S. (2000). Introduction to behavioural and psychological symptoms of dementia (BPSD). *International Journal of Geriatric Psychiatry, 15*, 2–4.

Gill, S. S., Bronskill, S. E., Normand, S. T., et al. (2007). Antipsychotic drug use and mortality in older adults with dementia. *Annals of Internal Medicine, 146*, 775–786.

Heeren, O., Borin, L., Raskin, A., et al. (2003). Association of depression with agitation in elderly nursing home residents. *Journal of Geriatric Psychiatry and Neurology, 16*, 4–7.

Katz, I. R., Simpson, G. M., Curlik, S. M., et al. (1990). Pharmacologic treatment of major depression for elderly patients in residential care settings. *Journal of Clinical Psychiatry, 51*(Suppl), 41–47.

Leibovici, A., & Tariot, P. N. (1988). Agitation associated with dementia: A systematic approach to treatment. *Psychological Bulletin, 24*, 49–53.

Lezak, M. D. (1983). Executive functions and motor performance. In M. D. Lezak (Ed.), *Neuropsychological assessment* (2nd ed., pp. 507–532). New York: Oxford University Press.

Lyketsos, C. G., Colenda, C. C., Beck, C., et al. (2006). Position statement of the American Association for Geriatric Psychiatry regarding principles of care for patients with dementia resulting from Alzheimer disease. *American Journal of Geriatric Psychiatry, 14*, 561–572.

Magaziner, J., German, P., Zimmerman, S. I., et al. (2000). The prevalence of dementia in a statewide sample of new nursing home admissions aged 65 and older: Diagnosis by expert panel. Epidemiology of dementia in Nursing Homes Research Group. *Gerontologist, 40*, 663–672.

Margallo-Lana, M., Swann, A., O'Brien, J., et al. (2001). Prevalence and pharmacological management of behavioural and psychological symptoms amongst dementia sufferers living in care environments. *International Journal of Geriatric Psychiatry, 16*, 39–44.

Parmelee, P. A., Katz, I. R., & Lawton, M. P. (1992). Depression and mortality among institutionalized aged. *Journal of Gerontology, 47*, 3–10.

Payne, J. L., Sheppard, J. E., Steinberg, M., et al. (2000). Incidence, prevalence, and outcomes of depression in residents of a long-term care facility with dementia. *International Journal of Geriatric Psychiatry, 17*, 247–253.

Rabins, P., Mace, N., & Lucas, M. (1982). The impact of dementia on the family. *JAMA, 248*, 333–335.

Rovner, B. W., German, P. S., Broadhead, J., et al. (1990). The prevalence and management of dementia and other psychiatric disorders in nursing homes. *International Psychogeriatrics/IPA, 2*, 13–24.

Rovner, B. W., Kafonek, S., Filipp, L., et al. (1986). Prevalence of mental illness in a community nursing home. *American Journal of Psychiatry, 143*, 1446–1449.

Schneider, L. S., Dagerman, K. S., & Insel, P. (2005). Risk of death with atypical antipsychotic drug treatment for dementia. Meta-analysis of randomized placebo-controlled trials. *JAMA, 294*, 1934–1943.

Schultz, S. K., Ellingrod, V. L., Turvey, C., et al. (2003). The influence of cognitive impairment and behavioral dysregulation on daily functioning in the nursing home setting. *American Journal of Psychiatry, 160*, 582–584.

Talerico, K. A., Evans, L. K., & Strumpf, N. E. (2002). Mental health correlates of aggression in nursing home residents with dementia. *Gerontologist, 42*, 169–177.

Tariot, P., & Blazina, L. (1993). The psychopathology of dementia. In J. Morris (Ed.), *Handbook of dementing illnesses* (pp. 461–475). New York: Marcel Dekker.

Tariot, P. N., Podgorski, C. A., Blazina, L., et al. (1993). Mental disorders in the nursing home: Another perspective. *American Journal of Psychiatry, 150*, 1063–1069.

Wang, P. S., Schneeweiss, S., Avorn, J., et al. (2005). Risk of death in elderly users of conventional vs. atypical antipsychotic medications. *New England Journal of Medicine, 353*, 2335–2341.

Wood, S., Cummings, J. L., Hsu, M. A., et al. (2000). The use of the neuropsychiatric inventory in nursing home residents: Characterization and measurement. *American Journal of Geriatric Psychiatry, 8*, 75–83.

13

Principles of Geriatric Psychopharmacology

Adrian Leibovici

As shown in Chapter 1 of this book, the prevalence and incidence of mental problems in nursing homes is very high. About 80% of residents in nursing homes suffer with a psychiatric disorder according to studies conducted in different types of nursing homes, in different geographic locations, and utilizing different methodologies (Tariot et al., 1993). Many such psychiatric problems as depression, psychosis, agitation, or cognitive loss are amenable to pharmacological interventions.

The use of psychotherapeutic drugs in nursing home residents though, has been the object of public, regulatory, and scientific scrutiny and controversy for close to three decades now. Concern with adverse effects in this very vulnerable population, the high cost of newer agents, and steady progress in our knowledge and awareness of psychopathology in the elderly, have all shaped the dynamics of the debate. This chapter will review the classes of medications used in treating commonly encountered psychiatric problems in nursing home residents and some of the specific problems associated with psycho-pharmaco-therapy in long-term care.

PSYCHOTHERAPEUTIC AGENTS USED
IN LONG-TERM-CARE FACILITIES

Antidepressants

Depression is very common in nursing homes. About 15% of residents have major depression and up to 50% have some form of depressive syndrome (Katz & Parmelee, 1994). The full phenomenological and etiological spectrum of depressive illness is present: early versus late onset, unipolar versus bipolar, "major" versus "minor," acute versus chronic, isolated versus comorbid with neurodegenerative conditions like dementia or Parkinson's disease. Along with nonspecific support and engagement in rewarding activities and standardized group or individual psychotherapies (interpersonal, cognitive, life review, etc.), antidepressant medication can be very effective in decreasing symptoms and improving the quality of life of depressed nursing home residents. Several classes of agents are available.

Selective Serotonin Reuptake Inhibitors

Since the first edition of this text, selective serotonin reuptake inhibitors (SSRIs) have replaced tricyclic antidepressants as first-line antidepressants. Starting with fluoxetine and continuing with sertraline, paroxetine, fluvoxamine, citalopram, and escitalopram these medications have been perceived as safer than tricyclics and reasonably effective in the treatment of geriatric depression (Solai et al., 2001). Comorbid dementia significantly lowers response rates (Trappler & Cohen, 1998). Unlike previously used antidepressants they do not have significant cardiovascular effects and notwithstanding paroxetine's weak anticholinergic action, prescribers do not have to worry about the consequences of muscarinic blockade like dry mouth, constipation, urinary retention, or acute confusion. There is little evidence that any one of these agents is significantly superior in efficacy to the others. Escitalopram 5 to 10 mg, sertraline 25 to 50 mg or fluoxetine 10 to 20 mg are reasonable starting daily doses in this population. Sometimes, much higher doses are needed before response occurs (Table 13.1). Their effectiveness in most severe forms of depression is thought by some to be inferior to drugs such as tricyclics or SNRIs (see section on tricyclic below; Oslin et al., 2000). Initially marketed as antidepressants, there is increasing awareness of their anti-anxiety potential both in typical anxiety disorders (Panic Disorder, Obsessive-Compulsive Disorder, Generalized Anxiety Disorder) and in mixed states like anxious depression or anxiety associated with dementia.

Despite their overall better tolerability, SSRIs have sometimes limiting side effects. Dyspepsia and appetite loss have been cited just as often as increased appetite and weight gain. Hyponatremia and intestinal bleeding, although not frequent, are potentially serious. Occasionally, restlessness and a sense

TABLE 13.1. Antidepressants for Nursing Home Residents

CLASS	GENERIC NAME	BRAND NAME	GERIATRIC DOSE
SSRIs	Fluoxetine	Prozac	10–40
	Sertraline	Zoloft	25–100
	Paroxetine	Paxil	10–40
	Fluvoxamine	Luvox	100–200
	Citalopram	Celexa	20–60
	Escitalopram	Lexapro	5–30
"Dual action"	Venlafaxine	Effexor, Effexor	75–225
antidepressants		XR	
	Mirtazapine	Remeron	15–45
	Duloxetine	Cymbalta	20–60
Tricyclics	Amitryptiline	Elavil	50–150
	Imipramine	Tofranil	50–150
	Doxepin	Sinequan, Adapin	50–150
	Desipramine	Norpramin	50–150
	Nortriptyline	Pamelor, Aventyl	25–75
	Protriptyline	Vivactil	15–30
	Maprotylin	Ludiomil	25–100
MAOIs	Isocarboxazid	Marplan	10–30
	Phenelzine	Parnate	10–30
	Tranyilcipromine	Nardil	15–60
	Seligiline	Emsam	6 mg/24 h
Dopaminergic	Bupropion	Wellbutrin,	100–300
Noradrenergic		Wellbutrin SR,	
		Wellbutrin XL	
Tetracyclics	Trazadone	Desyrel	50–150
	Nefazodone	Serzone	150–600

of unpleasant activation when first starting the medication, although usually transient, can dissuade a patient or caregiver to allow treatment to continue. Rarely, SSRIs have been associated with increased apathy and extrapyramidal side effects. A discontinuation syndrome is more common and severe with short half-life agents especially paroxetine. The "serotonin syndrome"—a heterogenous set of autonomic, cognitive, and somatic symptoms like shivering, nausea, tachycardia, hyperreflexia, tremor, myoclonus, agitation, confusion—is of concern and probably under-recognized in nursing home patients who take multiple medications competing for the hepatic P450 enzyme system. Until recently very expensive, the advent of generics and slow release forms has widened the availability, affordability, and versatility of this class of medications.

Dual Action Antidepressants (Serotonerigic and Noradrenergic)

These are medications that enhance synaptic presence of both serotonin and norepinephrin: duloxetine and venlafaxine inhibit the reuptake of both transmitters (SNRIs), whereas mirtazapine utilizes a different mechanism involving presynaptic auto-receptors. At therapeutic doses SNRIs are more activating and possibly advantageous in severe, treatment-resistant depression and have analgesic properties (White et al., 2004). Venlafaxine is initiated at 37.5 mg/day and increased to at least 112.5 mg before a full antidepressant effect is expected. Probably doses above 225 mg in this population, even if tolerated, would not show additional therapeutic yield. Duloxetine can be initiated at 20 or 30 mg daily. A maximum geriatric dose should not exceed 60 mg/day. Mirtazapine can improve insomnia at even lower doses soon after initiation of treatment and 7.5 to 15 mg is the usual starting dose; 45 mg daily is a maximum for most patients. Overall tolerability in this group of medications is superior to older agents. Diastolic hypertension is a common dose-dependent side effect of both venlafaxine and duloxetine, whereas night sweats, nightmares, and weight gain are frequent with mirtazapine.

Interestingly SSRIs but not SNRIs were associated with increased risk of falls in older institutionalized patients (Kallin et al., 2004).

Bupropion

This agent was found to be effective and well tolerated in the elderly (Steffens et al., 2001). Although its mechanism of action is still not fully understood, it probably involves dopaminergic and noradrenergic pathways that might explain its stimulant-like properties. This is both an advantage and a disadvantage in the nursing home patient: on the one hand, use of the agent is being advocated in patients with loss of motivation, many of whom do not have depression. On the other hand, it is more likely to cause toxic psychosis and delirium as a consequence of its effect on limbic dopaminergic neurons. Bupropion has been associated with a higher incidence of seizures compared with other antidepressants. It is contraindicated in patients with seizures, although most bupropion-related seizures have been associated with doses of more than 400 mg daily, whereas therapeutic doses range between 100 and 300 mg. The lack of cardiovascular toxicity is an advantage in the elderly, although the activating effect can cause insomnia especially with afternoon administration. Once a day Extended Release dosing is now available. The starting dose can be as low as 75 to 100 mg in the morning and sometimes it is sufficient to energize an apathetic resident whether depression is present or not.

Trazodone

Originally marketed as an antidepressant, trazodone is virtually never used as such, especially in the nursing home setting due to its dose-dependent, sedative effect. In small doses of 25 to 100 mg, it can be helpful as a hypnotic, and if effective, it is preferable to benzodiazepines and other hypnotics for tolerability and lack of habituation. Trazodone has also been advocated in the pharmacological treatment of agitated dementia, especially when perseveration is the major problem (Lebert et al., 2004). Gradually incremental doses reaching sometimes 300 mg/day have been used for this indication.

Tricyclics

Once the first-line agents among antidepressants, these drugs are often avoided because of their side effects: tachycardia, orthostatic hypotension, quinidine-like cardiac conduction delay, dry mouth, constipation, urinary retention, and confusion. These adverse effects are common and especially of concern in frail nursing home residents with preexistent comorbidities easily exacerbated by such effects. On the positive side, drugs like nortriptyline are highly effective, can be monitored with plasma levels, and are significantly more affordable than newer agents. The nursing home environment is controlled and knowledge of expected side effects coupled with diligent monitoring for their emergence can allow for the safe use of such medications in elderly residents (Streim et al., 2000).

Monoamine oxidase inhibitors

Monoamine oxidase activity in the brain is increased with age and dementia (Alexopoulos et al., 1987). Monoamine oxidase inhibitors (MAOIs) are effective and generally safe in geriatric depression (Georgotas et al., 1986). In reality they are not prescribed much in the elderly: the multitude of drug interactions and incompatibilities, dietary constraints, the rare but serious danger of hypertensive crisis or serotonin syndrome, and the rather common occurrence of orthostatic hypotension combine to limit their use. The recent approval of a selegiline patch for treatment of depression has spurred renewed interest in this first ever class of antidepressants, but geriatric studies and especially nursing home studies are still to be conducted.

Antipsychotics

They are also referred to as neuroleptics or major tranquilizers and their wide and indiscriminate use in agitated nursing home residents in the 1970s and 1980s prompted regulation and scrutiny responsible for many of today's practice guidelines.

Drugs in this broad class have the ability to decrease the severity and frequency of psychotic symptoms like delusions, hallucinations, and thought disorganization. They also have a calming, sedative action, which in the nursing home resident can be either a desired target or a disabling side effect. The therapeutic effects, as well as many of the side effects of all drugs in this class, are linked to their antagonism of dopamine-2 receptors in different areas of the brain. The newer drugs in this class known as "atypical antipsychotics" (clozapine, risperidaone, olanzapine, quetiapine, ziprasidone, and aripiprazole) have a more complicated effect on different neurotransmitter systems, most importantly inhibition of the 5H2 serotonin receptor subtype. This mechanism is offered by some as explanation for the atypicals' favorable side effect profile and their weak ability to improve so-called negative symptoms such as apathy and affective blunting.

The advent of atypical antipsychotics led to new hope that safer, better tolerated, and more effective agents were becoming available in treating psychosis and agitation in nursing home residents. Controlled clinical trials with risperidone, olanzapine, and aripiprazole showed modest superiority over placebo (Schneider et al., 2006), whereas quetiapine was effective in open label but not placebo controlled trials (Tariot et al., 2006). They were endorsed as a first line of treatment for dementia-related psychobehavioral abnormalities by experts (Alexopoulos et al., 2005), but review articles have doubted their usefulness (Sink et al., 2005). It is common practice that a resident with agitation, aggression, or discrete psychotic symptoms like delusions or hallucinations would be started on risperidone 0.25 mg once or twice daily, olanzapine 2.5 to 5 mg at bed time or equivalent low doses of quetiapine or aripiprazole (Table 13.2). Based on clinical experience and results of clinical trials, the dose of risperidone is increased gradually to a daily maximum of 2 mg (10 mg for olanzapine, 200 mg for quetiapine, 20 mg for aripiprazole, etc.). The atypicals have all but replaced older drugs; although, when treating delirium or acute dangerous agitation; haloperidol in oral or injectable form (doses ranging from 0.25 to 3 mg are common) is still widely used. Atypicals are not devoid of side effects. Sedation,

TABLE 13.2. Antipsychotics for Elderly Nursing Home Residents

CLASS	GENERIC	BRAND	GERIATRIC DOSE	CHLORPROMAZINE EQUIVALENT
Low potency	Chlorpromazine	Thorazine	25–200	100
	Thioridazine	Mellaril	10–100	95
	Mesoridazine	Serentil	10–100	50
Intermediate potency	Molindone	Moban	5–50	10
	Loxapine	Loxitan	5–50	10
	Perphenazine	Trilafon	4–32	8
	Thiotixene	Navane	2–20	5
	Trifluoperazine	Stelazine	2–20	5
High potency	Fluphenazine	Prolixin	0.25–2	2
	Haloperidol	Haldol	0.25–2	2
"Atypical"	Clozapine	Clozaril	12.5–200	?
	Risperidone	Risperidal	1–2	2?
	Olanzapine	Zyprexa	2.5–10	?
	Quetiapine	Seroquel	25–200	?
	Ziprazidone	Geodon	40–120	?
	Aripiprazole	Abilify	5–20	?

can interfere with nighttime sleep. (3) Have problems like sleep apnea or sleep interruption due to medical illness been addressed?

The most common chemical remedy for insomnia in the nursing home is a benzodiazepine receptor agonist. For sleep induction needs, as in initial (sleep-onset) insomnia, zaleplon 5 to 20 mg with a short half-life of 1 to 2 h or zolpidem 5 to 10 mg with a half-life of 2 to 3 h should suffice. There is some evidence that non-nightly use (3–5 times weekly) in patients with primary insomnia might remain safe and effective for longer periods of time (Perlis et al., 2004). Triazolam 0.125 to 0.25 mg (half-life 2–3 h) is also available; however, questions raised about its effect on cognition in the elderly have led to decreased use in this country and withdrawal from the market elsewhere. When a prolonged hypnotic effect is desired, lorazepam (half-life 6–8 h) can be useful in doses ranging from 0.5 to 1 mg.

An alternative to benzodiazepine receptor agonists are small doses of tricyclic antidepressants or trazodone. Psychiatrists often prefer trazodone (half-life 5–9 h) for its low cost and lack of anticholinergic burden. The list of drugs used as hypnotics is long and evidence of efficacy and safety in the elderly institutionalized is not yet available. Hypnotic agents such as ramelteon, which is supposed to bind to melatonin receptors in the suprachaismatic nucleus, mirtazapine or quetiapine in low doses and antihistaminic drugs such as diphenhydramine have been used, although evidence of efficacy, tolerability, and cost effectiveness is not established in this population.

Regardless of which agent is chosen, it is important to avoid long-term use in chronic insomnia, especially when drugs with habituation potential are considered.

Many times patients with advanced dementia have profound deterioration in sleep/wake cycle and limited ability to respond to hypnotics. Some show a reversed pattern being active at night and sleeping profoundly during the day. This can be very frustrating to family members wanting to interact with them or to staff trying to provide care according to a normal diurnal schedule. Such residents are best managed when care is adjusted to their own patterns of sleep and aggressive efforts to restore night sleep are not undertaken.

PHARMACOTHERAPY IN THE NURSING HOME ENVIRONMENT

Regardless of the particular medication chosen or condition treated, several guiding principles should be followed when treating institutionalized frail elderly patients. These principles are informed not only by a body of knowledge accumulated over the years in geriatric medicine but also by nonmedical considerations relating to the unique characteristics of the institutional environment.

1. *Evaluation.* Whenever possible a complete diagnostic inquiry should precede the initiation of treatment with psychotropics even when the presenting symptom implies an obvious direction. A resident with paranoid aggression might need an antibiotic, not an antipsychotic if an intercurrent urinary or respiratory infection is correctly identified as the true cause of her behavior. Sudden anxiety in a previously calm demented elderly person indicates an urgent need to exclude conditions like pulmonary embolism or stroke rather than the assumption of an anxiety disorder and initiation of anxiolytics. A nursing home resident who becomes withdrawn, avoidant of socialization, and seemingly apathetic might not suffer with clinical depression treatable with antidepressants but might simply restrict his activities due to dementia-related executive dysfunction or might suffer with organic apathy, best treated with small doses of stimulants. At times, however, psychotropic drugs have to be given before the clinical evaluation is complete to address acute safety concerns like in an agitated aggressive or imminently suicidal patient or to simply make further examination possible if patient is feared ill with a life-threatening medical condition but does not cooperate.

2. *Nonpharmacological interventions.* Many abnormal behaviors displayed by nursing home residents can subside or be mitigated by nonpharmacological interventions. Research in this area has expanded in the last decade and controlled clinical trials have been conducted showing effectiveness comparable with that shown in drug trials (Cohen-Mansfield, 2001). Individual and group psychotherapy (supportive, interpersonal), informal supportive interactions (validation, life review), interactions involving physical contact or sensory stimulation (massage, aroma therapy, tai chi, etc.), or simple environmental interventions (rocking chairs, pets, or visits by small children) are now being used and have been tested and advocated as an alternative to pharmacological treatment. The ability of a particular institution to insure that such interventions are consistently applied depends on resources like highly motivated and well-trained staff, institutional philosophy of care, staff to resident ratio, etc. It is important to keep in mind, however, that some conditions require immediate somatic treatments. In the presence of severe depression or psychosis for instance, well-intended but ill-informed nursing home providers might delay initiation of needed medication and jeopardize a resident's well-being when the principle of "psychotropics only as a last resort" is applied mechanically.

3. *Target symptoms and quality of clinical observations.* All too often medication is being prescribed for vaguely described conditions like "agitation," "depression," or "nervousness." The more precise the condition treated is being described and documented, the easier it becomes to fully and objectively assess response, both qualitatively and quantitatively. If agitation

were described as "striking out each time care is being delivered during the morning shift" or "calling out loudly and repeatedly at any time of day, most days, and without apparent precipitant" for instance, staff would find it easier to determine the extent to which a psychiatric medication is effective. Ideally, objective psychometric scales should be used but lack of resources or difficulty with standardized administration and interpretation limits their use. Nonetheless, some institutions make good use of the Mini Mental State Exam (Folstein et al., 1975), Geriatric Depression Scale (Yesavage et al., 1983), or similar tools. Sleep logs, serial measurement of weight, counting the number of "prn's" needed, and the number of behavioral observations entered in the chart per week or month are also useful ways to determine to what extent treatment with psychotropics is effective and/or tolerable. Staff education is crucial in recognizing small changes in a resident's condition. A significant decrease in the number of violent outbursts of a demented nursing home resident might be missed as long as the specific behavior still occurs occasionally, if staff is not trained in quantitative behavioral assessment. Many times the psychogeriatric consultant receives conflicting information about the same resident: reports from morning versus evening shift, week day versus weekend, well-established versus temporary staff. This information will need to be reconciled before making a therapeutic decision. Describing specific goals for pharmacological treatment and educating staff in how to measure them can alleviate such inconsistencies.

4. *Defining the proper dose and duration of a medication trial.* With the exception of acute sedation and treatment for some forms of anxiety like panic, psychopharmacological interventions for most problems encountered in nursing homes (agitation, depression, psychosis) take weeks to be effective. Dose titration is rarely guided by objective measures like drug levels but rather requires a "trial and error" approach in determining proper dosage, further prolonging the time one has to wait before therapeutic response can be seen. Oftentimes this slowness in reaching response comes in conflict with the real or perceived needs of institutions, families, or the residents themselves. Unacceptable social behaviors due to frontal lobe syndrome, for example, are even less acceptable during a re-certification state inspection, and administrators expect the problem to be "fixed" faster than pharmacologically possible. The distraught visiting spouse who becomes the target of a demented resident's delusions of jealousy cannot wait for weeks for relief, neither can the depressed, apathetic stroke victim who fails to perform in physical therapy risking to miss the "window of opportunity" when rehabilitation is still clinically possible and insurance coverage in effect. Such unrealistic expectations may lead to premature increments in dose or changing agents altogether with obvious negative

consequences. To compound the challenge of proper dosing, physician visits in nursing homes may be less frequent than necessary for prompt dose titration. Because of this, the psychogeriatric consultant is sometimes required to produce a detailed mapping out of future dose changes with all contingent factors that would influence such changes like side effects, therapeutic response, etc. Most of the time, the well-known tenet of geriatric pharmacology to "start low, go slow" applies: generally nursing home residents will need only small doses of medication because of their increased "neurosensitivity," delayed liver metabolism, and changes in volume of distribution (Abernethy, 1992). For instance, psychosis associated with dementia requires about a third of the risperidone dose used to treat schizophrenia in a younger adult population. Dogmatic "geriatric dose caps" while encouraged by some regulatory "guidelines" are to be avoided though. Oftentimes higher than expected doses of psychotropics are both tolerated and necessary even in the very old. Underdosing when treating severe depression or dangerous aggression can be more dangerous and lethal than overdosing. When high doses are necessary, proper documentation of rationale can protect caregivers from future litigation or regulatory sanctions. Another source of psychiatric problems is when patients already taking unusually high doses of psychotropic medication are first admitted, either from home or other facilities. The admitting physician is tempted to react to the apparent inappropriate drug regimen prescribed, especially if the resident seems calm and content when first examined. The laudable but forced drug reduction leads to reemergence of symptoms. Patients with lifelong history of severe mental illness like Schizophrenia or Bipolar Disorder compensated for years with a particular regimen of antipsychotics or mood stabilizers are deceptively prone to drug discontinuation or reduction when admitted into the nursing home. Once acutely psychotic again, recompensation takes a long time to achieve and sometimes simply restoring the initial treatment regimen is not sufficient. How long a nursing home resident should continue on psychotropic medications can be equally difficult to decide. Probably one of the most justified criticisms of psychotropic prescribing in nursing homes remains the tendency to leave residents on the same regimen even when their condition has been stable for a long time or when further progression in their illness makes the initial target symptoms irrelevant. A resident successfully medicated for physical aggression might still take the same dose of medication 2 years later when she is already bedridden and unable to move, let alone hurt her caregivers.

5. *Monotherapy versus polypharmacy.* Elderly nursing home residents tend to receive a large number of medications due to multiple comorbid medical conditions, some of which become more resistant to treatment, requiring

combination regimens (for instance, hypertension requiring three or even four agents at times). Since psychopharmacological treatment is mostly symptomatic it is not uncommon to see insomnia, delusions, depression, agitation, and anxiety being addressed each with a separate psychotherapeutic agent. Obviously the potential for oversedation and drug interactions in this highly sensitive population increases with each additional medication. Ideally, psychiatric conditions in nursing home residents should be addressed with only one agent. For instance, most antidepressants decrease both depression and anxiety and if the patient also has insomnia and anorexia, the choice of a sedating agent like mirtazapine would conceivably improve all symptoms. There are situations where the synergism between two psychiatric medications is well established: for instance, treating psychotic depression with an antidepressant and an antipsychotic, augmentation of antidepressants with drugs like lithium, thyroid hormone or stimulants, or the use of several agents in florid mania.

6. *Beneficiaries.* For whom treatment with psychotropics is being prescribed should be clearly understood: many times nursing home staff relate better or worse to pharmacological interventions according to their own biases, the philosophy of the institution or the way a particular resident's behavior affects their surroundings. There might be support for medicating an annoying or aggressive resident but not a depressed or delusional one even if in the former nonpharmacological interventions might be more appropriate and the latter might respond only to medication. Family members might request psychotropic medication when the resident shows emotional distress or hostility toward them, or if they have difficulty accepting the resident's rapid mental, functional, and behavioral deterioration. Physicians and nurse practitioners might decide to medicate based on rather brief interactions consistent with the duration and frequency of medical visits in this setting. If the resident is angry and refuses to allow an examination on the day of her appointment, she might be started on an antipsychotic, even if most days this would not be a problem. If a resident is tearful on "doctor day" but not on most other days, her chance increases to have depression added to the long problem list and to be started on an antidepressant. Residents themselves might insist upon receiving psychotropics for subjective reasons like insomnia even if sleep logs contradict their perception. Today, the much vilified "medicating with psychotropics for staff convenience" is no longer a systemic problem in this country's nursing homes (OIG, 2001), Nevertheless, in borderline clinical situations the decision of whether to use psychotherapeutic medications or not can be complicated: first and foremost it should address the well-being of the identified patient, but how this is defined ends up taking into account the values, opinions, and needs of other residents, caretakers, families, and the institution at large.

7. *Disability.* The mere presence of a target symptom or syndrome does not in itself warrant the use of psychotropic medication, especially in this medically and mentally fragile group of patients. A certain level of severity of symptoms and consequent disability are a prerequisite for prescribing medication. For instance, an elderly woman was talking to an imaginary litter of puppies in the corner of her room and asking staff to feed them. She was gratified by her hallucinations, the content of which was consistent with her lifelong love for animals and the clinical context (vascular dementia) was relatively stable. The symptom did not interfere with the woman's ability to function and no medication was prescribed. An elderly man with Parkinson's disease and discrete periods of tearfulness and low mood lasting minutes at a time and occurring several times a week did not receive antidepressant medication as most of the time his prevailing mood was good and he was showing no anhedonia, negativity, or vegetative signs of depression. In deciding to medicate psychopathology, the clinician should try to quantify and document the level of disability involved and weigh it against other factors like adverse effects and expected efficacy of the agent considered.

8. *Iatrogenic illness.* One has to weigh the potential benefit against the adverse effect burden of psychopharmacological treatment. Although generally safe by comparison with other classes of medications, psychotropics can cause a number of *side effects* and complications especially, in frail elderly nursing home residents. For instance "atypical" antipsychotics while better tolerated than the earlier generation "typicals," can still cause restlessness (akathisia), parkinsonism, or dyskinesias, especially in patients with preexistent extrapyramidal pathology like Parkinson's disease. Antidepressants like SSRIs can accentuate apathetic states; anticholinergic drugs (tricyclics, but also paroxetine) can increase confusion (delirium), or cause constipation, urinary hesitancy, blurred vision, and tachycardia. Benzodiazepines can have negative effects on memory and virtually all psychotropics can increase or decrease steadiness in ambulation.

Non-psychotropic drugs widely used in the long-term care setting have well-established negative effects on mental status: for instance, steroids have been associated with organic mania, antiparkinsonians with hallucinosis, antihypertensives with depression, and digoxin, antihistamines, and many others with delirium. Nursing home mental health consultants were used to seeing delirium "epidemics" in nursing homes when amantadine was being prescribed as influenza prophylaxis to all residents. Sometimes agitation, psychosis, or mood symptoms will improve by discontinuing or modifying treatment with such drugs rather than by adding psychotropic medication.

Drug–drug interactions are numerous and an important factor influencing the variability in the efficacy and tolerability to psychotropic medications in nursing home residents. Meperidine and serotonergic antidepressants can cause a life-threatening syndrome consisting of hyperreflexia, rigidity, delirium in patients treated with MAOIs; thiazide diuretics decrease the renal clearance of lithium, the levels of which can rapidly become toxic; nonsteroidal antinflammatory drugs (NSAIDS) can also increase lithium levels while theophylline, verapamil, and diltiazem have the opposite effect. Much has been written about the inhibitors, inducers, and substrates of the hepatic P450 enzyme complex, responsible for the catabolism of many medication and alimentary substances ingested by humans. Carbamazepine for instance is a notorious enzymatic inducer, causing inadvertent decreases in the levels of other medications and even in its own serum level.

The list of psychotropic-induced side effects, unintended psychiatric consequences of nonpsychiatric drugs, and drug-drug interactions seen in the nursing home setting is long and growing. Avoiding iatrogenic consequences in the face of such complexities requires up-to-date knowledge of geriatric pharmacology, and medicine. It is in such circumstances that the value of expert psychogeriatric consultation and a geriatric pharmacist becomes relevant.

9. *Ethical and legal issues.* Decision-making in the practice of nursing home psychopharmacology can be complicated, oftentimes posing difficult dilemmas. For instance, newer, more effective, and better-tolerated medications carry a high price tag and often institutions and individuals are forced to choose based on their ability to afford such treatments. Recent changes in government funding for nursing homes have further accentuated this trend. Starting July 1, 1998, the retrospective cost-based system of payment was phased out, to be replaced with the present prospective-pricing system (PPS). Under the new system, Medicare pays nursing homes an all inclusive per diem rate including drug costs. If the cost of medication and the cost of food and other living comforts in the nursing home are borne by the same total pool of funds, it is easy to imagine situations where a nursing home administrator has to choose between buying fresh rather than canned vegetables or allowing the widespread use of anti-dementia drugs or brand name antidepressants. Inevitably practitioners are forced to consider conflicting priorities. Should an MMSE minimal score be used to qualify residents for cholinesterase inhibitors? Should one subscribe to the practice of switching otherwise stable patients from established brand name antidepressants to similar but not identical generics (e.g., from Lexapro to Citalopram or from Effexor-Extended Release to Venlafaxine-Immediate Release)? Many nursing home residents are passive recipients of care, and their capacity to make informed decisions, including decisions

about psychiatric drugs, is often impaired. Clinical assessments of mental capacity, consent, or "assent," and legal concepts like competency, "health care proxy," "living will," need to be considered. They offer some guidance, but individual presentations can be too complex to eliminate ethical or legal gray areas: should a dying patient who chose comfort care receive antidepressant treatment that can alleviate suffering but conceivably prolong life by restoring appetite? Or should a relative with legal right to make decisions be allowed to prevent treatment of distressing psychosis and agitation in a resident with advanced dementia? Frequently, the theoretical principle of patient autonomy is not applicable to the practice of medicine in the nursing home environment, and providers find themselves forced in paternalistic postures toward patients and families. The litigious environment in which medical practice takes place has not spared long-term care. In many areas written, informed consent for the use of certain drugs is standard practice. The recent "black box" warnings of increased mortality and cerebrovascular events with atypical antipsychotics or of suicide with antidepressants have prompted a range of responses by clinicians and administrators, including total avoidance of such drugs even if the scientific evidence would not support such extremes. The risk/benefit analysis for using psychotropics can be very complicated: Is control of episodic aggression worth the risk of sedation, increased confusion, or increased fall risk? Is electroconvulsant therapy consistent with the concept of comfort care? Should hallucinations and delusions in a Parkinson's disease victim be controlled even if it leads to more neurological disability? Does diabetes or preexistent cerebrovascular disease always preclude the use of some atypical antipsychotics like olanzapine or risperidone even when they are otherwise effective? When institutions and practitioners try to grapple with such complex issues the psychogeriatric consultant can play a constructive role by participating in ethics committees or providing individualized, informed, and balanced opinions to front-line caregivers or administrators.

ACTUAL USE OF PSYCHOTROPICS IN THE NURSING HOME: MYTH, FACT, AND REGULATION

A number of studies in the 1980s confirmed the perception that nursing home residents were being overmedicated to prevent abnormal dementia-related behaviors primarily for staff's convenience rather than in patients' best interest (Avron et al., 1989).

On December 22, 1987, Congress enacted the comprehensive Nursing Home Reform Act (NHRA) attached to that year's Omnibus Budget Reconciliation

Act (OBRA 87 or P.L. 100–203). The legislation took the unprecedented step to regulate in some detail medical and nursing practice in all long-term facilities receiving Medicare or Medicaid funding. It banned "physical or chemical restraints imposed for the purpose of discipline or convenience." It required that restraints be applied only for safety and only upon an explicit physician order. It limited the use of as needed sedatives and it mandated systematic efforts to decrease or discontinue psychotropic medications in residents receiving such medications. The regulations were further refined in 1991, when the focus was broadened from antipsychotics to psychotropics in general. In fact, the very concept of "unnecessary drugs" was defined operationally as medication given (1) in excessive dose, (2) for excessive duration, (3) without monitoring or without adequate indication, (4) in the presence of adverse consequences, and (5) without specific target symptoms.

Initially, OBRA regulations stimulated efforts to minimize psychotropic drug use in nursing homes as shown in a number of studies (Rovner et al., 1992). Prospective drug-reduction studies using provider education as the main intervention showed some promise as well (Avron et al., 1992). However, after 1995, psychotropic drug prescribing in nursing homes started to increase again. The reason for this trend reversal was not clear: Was inappropriate use resurfacing due to inadequate enforcement of existing regulations? Were residents in nursing homes presenting with increased psychopathology? Or, had progress in psychopharmacology led to changes in practice patterns through better-tolerated and more effective drugs? A 2001 study performed by the Office of Evaluations and Inspections (OEI) at the request of an alarmed Senate Special Committee on Aging tried to shed light on these very questions (OIG, 2001). The study was comprehensive and on a large scale. It utilized a variety of sources like drug regimen reviews in 135 nursing homes, on-site visits, detailed reviews of medical records, analysis of survey, and recertification data and interviews with ombudsmen and certification staff. The findings were generally positive: the results indicated that in 85% of residents treated with psychotropics the use was medically appropriate, meaning that drugs were used within regulatory guidelines and had the potential to benefit the recipients. Psychotropics were used inappropriately 8% of the time; "unjustified chronic use," no documented benefit, wrong type of drug for a given diagnosis, or excessive doses were examples of such inappropriate use. In the remaining 7% of cases, insufficient documentation prevented the authors to determine conclusively if the use of psychotropics was or not appropriate. Significantly, the use of psychotropics as "chemical restraints" amounted to only 0.08% of all deficiencies, whereas the "unnecessary psychotropic use" label was attributed in 2% of cases. The authors concluded that in general, psychotropic drug use in nursing home was seemingly appropriate. Obviously both practice and documentation can and should further improve.

In conclusion, nursing home residents as a group have a high prevalence of psychiatric disorders and consequently and frequently have overwhelming needs for proper evaluation and treatment. An increasing number of pharmacological agents have become available to treat conditions like depression, cognitive loss, and agitation. This number is likely to continue to grow. Establishing tolerability and efficacy in this population is not easy and many a times the best evidence available to practitioners consists of extrapolations from studies conducted in younger age groups or in noninstitutionalized elderly. Nevertheless, nursing home residents can benefit from the judicious use of psychotherapeutic medications provided that such use is integrated with good medical and psychiatric evaluation, close monitoring of response and side effects, and application of nonpharmacological interventions.

REFERENCES

Abernethy, D. R. (1992). Psychotropic drugs and the aging process: Pharmacokinetics and pharmacodynamics. In C. Salzman (Ed.), *Clinical geriatric psychopharmacology* (pp. 61–73). Baltimore: Williams & Wilkins.

Alexopoulos, G. S., Jeste, D. V., Chung, H., Carpenter, D., Ross, R., & Docherty, J. P. (2005, January). The Expert Consensus Guidelines Series: Treatment of dementia and its behavioral disturbances. *Postgraduate Medicine, 117*, 45.

Alexopoulos, G. S., Young, R. C., Lieberman, K. W., & Shamoian, C. A. (1987). Platelet Mao activity in geriatric patients with depression and dementia. *American Journal of Psychiatry, 144*, 1480.

Avron, J., Dreyer, P., Connely, K., & Soumerai, S. B. (1989). Use of psychoactive medication and the quality of care in rest homes: Findings and policy implications of a statewide study. *New England Journal of Medicine, 320*, 227.

Avron, J., Soumerai, S. B., Everitt, D. E., et al. (1992). A randomized trial of a program to reduce the use of psychoactive drugs in nursing homes. *New England Journal of Medicine, 327*, 168.

Cohen-Mansfield, J. (2001). Nonpharmacologic interventions for inappropriate behaviors in dementia. *American Journal of Geriatric Psychiatry, 9*, 361.

Cummings, J. L. (2003). Use of cholinesterase inhibitors in clinical practice. *American Journal of Geriatric Psychiatry, 11*, 131.

Cummings, J. L., McRae, T., Zhang, R., et al. (2006). Effects of donepezil on neuropsychiatric symptoms in dementia patients with severe behavioral disorders. *American Journal of Geriatric Psychiatry, 14*, 605.

Folstein, M. F., Folstein, S. E., & McHugh, P. R. (1975). "Mini-mental state": A practical method for grading the mental state of patients for clinicians. *Journal of Psychiatric Research, 12*, 189.

Georgotas, A., McCue, R. E., & Hapworth, W. (1986). Comparative efficacy and safety of MAOIs versus TCAs in treating depression in the elderly. *Biological Psychiatry, 21*, 1155.

Herrman, N., & Eryavec, G. (1993). Buspirone in the management of agitation and aggression associated with dementia. *American Journal of Geriatric Psychiatry, 1*, 249.

Hogan, D. B. (2006). Donepezil for severe Alzheimer's disease [Editorial]. *Lancet, 367,* 1031–1032.

Kallin, K., Gustafson, Y., Sandman, P. O., & Karlsson, S. (2004). Drugs and falls in older people in geriatric care settings. *Aging—Clinical and Experimental Research, 16*(4), 270–276.

Katz, I. R., & Parmelee, P. A. (1994). Depression in the elderly patients in residential care settings. In L. S. Schneider, C. F. Reynolds III, B. D. Lebowiitz, & A. J. Freidhoff (Eds.), *Diagnosis and treatment of depression in late life* (p. 437). Washington, DC: American Psychiatric Press.

Lebert, F., Stekke, W., Hassenbroekx, C., & Pasquier, F. (2004). Frontotemporal dementia: A randomized, controlled trial with trazodone. *Dementia and Geriatric Cognitive Disorders, 17*(4), 355.

Office of Inspector General. (2001, November). *Psychotropic drug use in nursing homes.* Department of Health and Human Services. OEI-02–00.00490.

Oslin, D. W., Streim, J. E., Katz, I. R., et al. (2000, May). Heuristic comparison of sertraline with nortriptyline for the treatment of depression in frail elderly patients. *American Journal of Geriatric Psychiatry, 8,* 141–149.

Perlis, M. L., McCall, W. V., Krystal, A. D., & Walsh, J. K. (2004). Long term non-nightly administration of zolpidem in the treatment of patients with primary insomnia. *Journal of Clinical Psychiatry, 65*(8), 1128.

Reisberg, B., Doody, R., Stoffleer, A., Schmitt, F., Ferris, S., & Mobius, H. J. (2003). Memantine in moderate-to-severe Alzheimer disease. *New England Journal of Medicine, 348,* 1333.

Rovner, B. W., Edelman, B. A., Cox, M. P., & Shmuely, Y. (1992). The impact of antipsychotics drug regulations on psychotropic prescribing practices in nursing homes. *American Journal of Psychiatry, 149,* 1390.

Schneider, L. S., Dagerman, K. S., & Insel, P. (2005). Risk of death with atypical antipsychotic drug treatment for dementia: Meta-analysis of randomized placebo-controlled trials. *JAMA, 294,* 1934.

Schneider, L. S., Dagerman, K., & Insel, P. S. (2006). Efficacy and adverse effects of atypical antipsychotics for dementia: Meta-analysis of randomized, placebo-controlled trials. *American Journal of Geriatric Psychiatry, 14*(3),191.

Sink, K. M., Holden, K. F., & Yaffe, K. (2005). Pharmacological treatment of neuropsychiatric symptoms of dementia: A review of the evidence. *JAMA, 293*(5), 596.

Solai, L. K., Muslant, B. H., & Pollock, B. G. (2001). Selective serotonin reuptake inhibitors for late-life depression: A comparative review. *Drugs and Aging, 18,* 355–368.

Steffens, D. C., Doraiswami, P. M., & McQuoid, D. R. (2001). Bupropion SR in the naturalistic treatment of elderly patients with major depression. *International Journal of Geriatric Psychiatry, 16*(9), 862.

Streim, J. E., Oslin, D. W., Katz, I. R., et al. (2000). Drug treatment of depression in frail elderly nursing home residents. *American Journal of Geriatric Psychiatry, 8,* 150–159.

Tariot, P. N., Fallow, M. R., Grossberg, G. T., Graham, S. M., McDonald, S., & Gargle, I. (2004). Efficacy of SSRI's in geriatric depression. *JAMA, 291*(3), 317.

Tariot, P. N., Podgorski, C. A., Blazina, L., & Leibovici, A. (1993). Mental disorders in the nursing home: Another perspective. *American Journal of Psychiatry, 150,* 1063.

Tariot, P. N., Raman, R., Jakimovich, L., et al. (2005). Divalproex sodium in nursing home residents with possible or probable Alzheimer disease complicated by agitation: A randomized, controlled trial. *American Journal of Geriatric Psychiatry, 13,* 942.

Tariot, P. N., Schneider, L. S., Katz, I. R., et al. (2006). Quetiapine treatment of psychosis associated with dementia: A double-blind randomized, placebo-controlled clinical trial. *American Journal of Geriatric Psychiatry, 14*(9), 767.

Trappler, B., & Cohen, C. (1998, February). Use of SSRI's in the "very old" depressed nursing home residents. *American Journal of Geriatric Psychiatry, 6*, 83–89.

Verdoux, H., Lagnaoui, R., & Begaud, B. (2005). Is benzodiazepine use a risk factor for cognitive decline and dementia? A literature review of epidemiological studies. *Psychological Medicine, 35*(3), 307.

White, E. M., Basinski, J., Fahri, P., et al. (2004, December). Geriatric depression treatment in nonresponders to selective serotonin reuptake inhibitors. *Journal of Clinical Psychiatry, 65*(12), 1634–1641.

Winblad, B., Kilander, L., Eriksson, S., et al. (2006, April). Donepezil in patients with severe Alzheimer's disease: Double-blind, parallel-group, placebo-controlled study. *Lancet, 367*, 1057–1065.

Yesavage, J. A., Brink, T. L., Rose, T. L., et al. (1983). Development and validation of a geriatric depression screening scale: A preliminary report. *Journal of Psychiatric Research, 17*, 37.

14

Insight-Oriented, Interpersonal, and Integrative Psychotherapy

Richard A. Zweig, Patricia Marino,
and *Gregory A. Hinrichsen*

For most older adults, long-term-care placement represents the culmination of a series of traumatic psychological experiences. Their physical integrity has been undermined by chronic illnesses and decline in physical functioning. Their psychological integrity has been severely challenged by an onslaught of stresses, emotional upheaval, and often impairment of the very cognitive abilities that undergird the experience of selfhood. Their social integrity has been fragmented by dislocation from familiar environments, loss of social networks, and the alienating effects of institutionalization. To long-term-care staff, the treatment of these individuals may be overwhelming—all systems appear in decline, yet are complexly interdependent. Interventions to help these patients seem only partially effective and outcomes are rarely certain. Not surprisingly, older long-term-care residents experience higher levels of psychological distress than any other group of elderly (Diagnosis and Treatment of Depression in Late Life, NIH, 1991). Paradoxically, psychological treatment for these residents is rarely commensurate with their distress. Despite documentation of the efficacy of psychological treatments, particularly psychotherapy, for community dwelling elderly (Blazer, 2003; Borson et al., 1989; Gatz et al., 1998; Newton & Lazarus, 1992; Scogin & McElreath, 1994), these treatments remain underutilized in long-term-care settings (Herst & Moulton, 1985; Lichtenberg & Duffy, 2000; Ruckdeschel & Katz, 2004; Shea et al., 1992).

There are signs, however, that psychological and psychiatric treatments are gradually becoming available for psychologically distressed elderly long-term-care residents. Nursing homes are increasingly adopting rehabilitative models of care to maximize residents' functioning. The Omnibus Budget Reconciliation Acts of 1987 and 1989 mandated that nursing homes provide "active treatment" to mentally ill residents, and the acts have improved financial incentives for mental health clinicians serving these elderly residents. Research has documented the potentially deleterious effects of prolonged treatment of institutionalized elderly with chemical and physical restraints (German et al., 1992), and recent legislation has both regulated their use and promoted alternate treatments. Federal guidelines, and recent recommendations of the American Geriatrics Society and the American Association for Geriatric Psychiatry advocate greater use of nonpharmacological interventions to manage depression and other behavioral problems in long-term-care residents (AGS & AAGP, 2003; Ruckdeschel & Katz, 2004). As standards of care have evolved, long-term-care medical personnel have increasingly sought the services of mental health professionals skilled in the use of psychotherapeutic techniques to better manage the aberrant behaviors of elderly residents and reduce their psychological distress. Mental health professionals have responded to the needs of older long-term-care residents by developing psychotherapeutic treatment models (Carpenter et al., 2002; Lichtenberg, 1994; Molinari, 2000) and guidelines for psychotherapeutic treatment (Lichtenberg et al., 1998).

This chapter provides an overview of psychotherapy, a major psychological intervention utilized by mental health clinicians, as a treatment for mentally ill elderly living in the long-term-care setting. Psychotherapeutic interventions are here broadly defined as "planned processes of behavioral change that employ a deliberate application of psychological principles and theory to persons experiencing mental dysfunction or distress" (Smyer et al., 1990). We will emphasize insight-oriented, interpersonal, and integrative psychotherapies and exclude discussions of cognitive-behavioral psychotherapy (which is covered separately in Chapter 15) or of other psychosocial interventions (for an excellent review of these, see Karuza & Katz, 1991). In addition, although we recognize that individuals of varied ages reside in long-term-care settings, our primary focus will be on elderly residents of assisted living or nursing home facilities. To provide an overall framework for understanding the utility of psychotherapy in treating long-term-care residents, this chapter is divided into four main sections: (1) an overview of the theoretical bases for psychotherapy in institutionalized mentally ill older adults, (2) prevalence of mental disorders and the availability of psychotherapeutic treatment in long-term-care facilities, (3) a review of models of psychotherapeutic treatment and their relevance to special problems of elderly long-term-care residents, and (4) an overview of social and environmental factors that effect the utility of psychotherapy in the long-term-care setting.

THEORETICAL BASES FOR PSYCHOTHERAPY

Treatment models for insight-oriented, interpersonal, and integrative psycho-therapies are derived from theoretical and empirical research in psychology, medicine, and sociology. These models share the perspective that late-life psy-chopathology results from the interaction of biopsychosocial stressors (e.g., illness, loss) and risk factors (e.g., interpersonal dynamics, coping styles, social context). Psychotherapy in the long-term-care setting is specifically based on research in three primary areas that will be briefly reviewed: (1) developmental psychology and psychodynamic theory, (2) stress and coping research and health psychology, and (3) social and environmental psychology.

Developmental Psychology and Psychodynamic Theory

Early work in the field of developmental psychology held that cognition and personality develop incrementally until the individual reaches early adulthood or maturity. However, other theorists have argued that personality continues to develop throughout the life-span. Erikson (1950) posited that each era of the life-cycle is characterized by developmentally specific intrapsychic tasks. The task of older adulthood is to develop an integrated sense of self and to stave off despair and meaninglessness. Indeed, maintaining an inner sense of self-continuity despite physical and environmental changes is often seen as a central theme in the lives of older adults (Atchley, 1989; Griffin & Grunes, 1990; Tobin, 1989). The mechanisms through which older individuals maintain a sense of self-continuity are varied and complex. For example, Neugarten (1977) has suggested that most middle-aged and older adults view many typically stressful life changes (e.g., launching of children, physical decline, the loss of a spouse) as expectable and normative. When these stressors occur "on time," individuals have often psychologically rehearsed for them, and typically cope adequately. It is only when stressors are unrehearsed, unpredictable, or "off time" that they pose psychological crises.

The psychological impact of illness for some older individuals may be best understood when viewed within a developmental context. The following case example is illustrative:

Example.   A 55-year-old divorced woman suffered a right middle cerebral artery stroke leaving her with left hemiparesis, confining her to a wheelchair, and ulti-mately prompting a psychotic depression that required hospitalization. Following her stabilization on psychotropic medication and discharge to a nursing home, she was referred for psychotherapy. In the course of her psychological treatment, she said that prior to her stroke and after having launched her children from the home, she had obtained a divorce and had looked forward to establishing her own career. She was in the midst of completing a bachelor's degree when the stroke occurred, which left her disabled, financially destitute, and stripped of the autonomy she had so cherished.

Other developmental changes appear to enhance older adults' management of their social and emotional well-being. One such normative developmental change is socioemotional selectivity, a process whereby older adults tend to selectively engage in close, familiar interpersonal relationships to optimize energy expenditure and maximize positive emotional experiences. A growing body of empirical research (Carstensen, 1992) supports the universality of this adaptive developmental process in older adulthood. A second normative developmental trend, identified in research on emotion and aging, suggests greater emotional resilience in late life. In cross-sectional studies, older adults show greater cognitive complexity and self-regulation of affect and more flexible reasoning when faced with emotion-laden dilemmas when compared with younger adults (Issacowitz et al., 2000; LaBouvie-Vief et al., 1989; Magai & Passman, 1997). A growing body of research finds that older adults "exercise greater control of affective arousal by acting proactively to avoid conflict or the escalation of conflict—show greater affective control, greater avoidance of stressors, engage in less negative start-up with partners, and de-emphasize the negative in interpersonal relations" (Magai & Passman, 1997).

In sum, research in adult development and aging suggests that normative developmental changes such as socioemotional selectivity and improved affective self-regulation may help buffer the impact of late-life stressors for most older adults. The derailment of these developmental trends, the experience of difficulties in resolving phase-specific developmental tasks, the disruptions in self-continuity, or the developmental "timing" of life stressors may be some of the determinants of psychopathology in later life.

Psychodynamic theory and research provide a second perspective through which psychopathology may be understood, and upon which psychotherapeutic techniques with medically ill older adults may be based. Psychodynamic theory holds that how an individual copes with life stresses is strongly influenced by early-life experiences, personality structure, characteristic psychological defenses, and unconscious fears and impulses. Illnesses that diminish ego functioning and produce increased dependency may trigger unresolved inner conflicts and overwhelm defenses (Solomon & Szwabo, 1992). Because of the complex interplay of these factors, the conscious and unconscious meaning to an individual of life stresses is highly idiosyncratic. This subjective meaning may determine how the individual reacts emotionally and perceives others. For example, a medical condition may cause one person to reject others' help because it is perceived as a threat to autonomy. For another individual, the same condition will trigger persistent demands for others' assistance because of fears of being abandoned. A psychodynamic understanding of an individual's modal personality type and characteristic coping styles, defenses, and fears may thus be used as a basis for psychological intervention (Griffin & Grunes, 1990; Groves & Kucharski, 1987; Newton & Jacobowitz, 1999; Nordhus & Nielsen, 1999).

Late-life theorists such as Gutmann (1988) have also argued that a physically-ill older adult's psychological reactions to physical decline often have their roots in the subjective meaning of that decline. The following vignette illustrates this issue:

> A woman in her early eighties was transferred to a medical rehabilitation unit for muscle weakness which was attributed to a late-onset post-polio syndrome. While her functioning was only mildly compromised, she felt markedly distraught and humiliated by her condition and the thought of staying on a rehabilitation unit. During the psychological consultation, she reported that as a child with polio, she could not participate in activities with others and had felt deeply ashamed. Once cured of her childhood polio, she had enjoyed robust health and had never spoken again of that time in her life. Now, the return of a milder form of her childhood illness had shattered her view of herself as fiercely independent, and caused her to re-experience intense feelings of humiliation and anger more appropriate to her childhood illness than to her current one.

Based on developmental and psychodynamic theory and research, integrative and insight-oriented psychotherapies with older physically-ill long-term-care residents can have multiple objectives. First, psychotherapy helps identify the predispositions (i.e., personality structure, developmental context) that the older individual brings to his/her experience of the illness, and clarifies the subjective meaning of the illness to the individual. In fact, clarifying the subjective meaning may in itself have lasting psychotherapeutic benefit to the medically ill (Viederman & Perry, 1980). Second, psychotherapeutic interventions may be utilized to limit maladaptive behaviors and restore an older individual's sense of self-continuity, even in the context of dementia (Frey et al., 1992; Hausman, 1992). Third, as long-term-care staff come to understand the meaning of an individual's behavior, counterproductive interpersonal interactions may be reduced. Finally, as meanings are clarified and adaptive behaviors are fostered, the individual gains a sense of mastery over the traumatizing illness.

Stress, Coping, and Health Psychology

Most residents of long-term-care facilities experience high levels of stress. Therefore, it is vital to recognize the interdependence of physical and psychological health among older adults in long-term care. Most would meet criteria of the *Diagnostic and Statistical Manual of Mental Disorders*, Fourth Edition, Text Revisions

(*DSM-IV-TR*; American Psychiatric Association, 2000), for one or more "extreme psychosocial stressors" by virtue of acute or enduring physical illness. Life in a long-term-care facility confronts residents with an ongoing series of daily stresses—from the interpersonal demands of sharing a room with another person to the physical and medical changes that often precipitate long-term-care admissions. A sizable number of studies have generally documented the deleterious mental and physical health effects of stressful life circumstances (Kaplan, 1983) and specifically the negative emotional impact of physical health problems (Moos, 1984; Symister & Friend, 2003; Watson et al., 1999). The growing fields of health psychology and behavioral medicine testify to interest in better understanding the mind–body interface and in developing ways to help patients to better cope with illness.

Little research has specifically addressed how long-term-care residents cope with these stresses. However, a large body of social and behavioral science literature has documented that different strategies for coping with stressful life circumstances are associated with psychological well-being (Folkman, 1984; Snyder & Ford, 1987). Theory suggests that when life experiences "tax or exceed" an individual's available resources the individual appraises what can be done to cope with them (Lazarus & Folkman, 1984). Coping theory portrays people as active responders to stressful events, who engage in problem-focused efforts to change the stressful event, cognitive efforts to change the meaning of the event so that it is less stressful, or emotion-focused efforts to contend with the dysphoric affects aroused by the event. Coping theory also suggests that people draw upon existing resources to deal with stressful situations including physical health and energy, positive beliefs, problem-solving skills, social skills, social support, and material resources.

Research has examined how people cope with a variety of chronic medical conditions. The psychological, practical, and interpersonal demands of different chronic medical conditions often vary (Antoni, 2003; Biegel et al., 1991). The degree to which an individual successfully copes with the demands of a particular illness may partly depend on aspects of premorbid functioning and psychosocial factors. For example, an individual who has a life-long pattern of conscientiously attending to work- and family-related responsibilities may contend better with the demands of dietary vigilance and daily insulin injections characteristic of severe diabetes than someone with a pattern of neglecting responsibility. An individual with rheumatoid arthritis who highly valued physical attractiveness and independence may adapt less successfully to the potentially crippling effects of arthritis than someone for whom these attributes were less valued. Nonetheless, research has indicated that successful adaptation to chronic illness requires acknowledgment of the medical problem only as one aspect of one's identity, and a flexible use of internal and external resources to deal with the emotional and practical problems engendered by the condition (Burish & Bradley, 1983).

Studies in psychoimmunology suggest that coping ability, emotional distress, and immune system functioning are interrelated. Several psychosocial variables including poor social support and distress have been associated with immune system factors that are relevant to the body's response to illness (Anderson, 1998; Levy et al., 1991; Stowell et al., 2001). Individuals who adapt poorly to chronic medical problems often become depressed. Untreated depression has been associated with impaired immune function (Asnis & Miller, 1989) and poor medical compliance (DiMatteo et al., 2000) thus increasing the patient's risk for further medical problems and possible medical relapse (Watson et al., 1999). The negative impact of depression on close social relationships (Weissman & Paykel, 1974) may also impede the use of social support as a coping strategy and poor support has been tied to impaired immune function (Cohen, 1988), when utilized social support has been found to serve a protective function regardless of the stressor (Cohen & Symes, 1985; Wolkow & Ferguson, 2001). Preliminary studies in psychoimmunology indicate that how individuals cope with chronic medical illness may influence both their future mental and physical health. Research on stress and immunity within a cancer population has found that stressful situations may trigger specific neurological, endocrine, and immunological responses (Antoni, 2003; McEwen, 1998). Psychosocial factors such as one's ability to cope and manage stress have been shown to predict greater survival rate in cancer patients (Fawzy et al., 1997).

From a coping perspective a physically ill individual at a long-term-care facility is confronted with a formidable series of stresses. Serious physical health problems are one of the most serious threats to well-being. The emotional toll taken by these stresses often trigger acute psychological and physiological distress symptoms in individuals who are otherwise well adjusted (Koocher, 1996). Placement in long-term care may underscore the threat and reduce expectations of functional improvement. Coping resources that might be drawn upon to deal with life stresses prior to long-term-care facility entry now may be unavailable or less useful in the new environment: physical health problems often diminish physical energy; society does not engender a set of positive beliefs about long-term-care facilities but rather the opposite; established problem-solving skills that worked well in the community may not work in an institutional setting; social support in the form of friends or family may not be readily available. As a consequence the long-term-care resident may experience diminished resources for developing alternative coping skills and decreased expectations about the utility of engaging in any type of coping thus engendering feelings of helplessness (Seligman, 1975). For residents with cognitive impairments the process of coping is further compounded by the loss of mental processes that are critical to the whole coping enterprise. Clinical reports suggest that there are long-term-care residents who make successful adaptations to the stresses of chronic physical health problems and life in an institutional setting. However, the processes that promote successful coping within the long-term-care setting, for the most part, have not been studied. Much of the research in the area of successful adaptation and an individual's ability to be transformed and even grow after a stressful or traumatic experience has focused primarily on diagnosis of medical illness and bereavement (Folkman & Greer, 2000; Tedeschi & Calhoun, 1996).

When faced with stressful life situations including loss and environmental changes long-term-care residents may find meaning and growth in their experience. Neimeyer (2001) suggests that individuals attribute meaning to their environment through constructing narratives that hold their unique interpretation of events. The process of formulating their personal narratives helps people to understand their emotions and their coping pattern. The new insights gained through constructing a narrative may enable individuals to generate alternatives and more adaptive ways of coping.

Facilitating coping should result in reductions in depression, anxiety, subjective distress, enlarged loss of control, and related psychiatric phenomena. Psychotherapy may facilitate this process by helping the resident to reappraise or reassess the life circumstances that made placement in the long-term-care setting necessary, to take stock of remaining resources and build new resources to facilitate coping, and to learn to utilize existing or new coping strategies to maintain emotional equilibrium. Another goal of psychological intervention may be to help the individual optimize social functioning and management of medical aspect of the disease process (Pollins, 1995).

Social and Environmental Psychology

Efforts by an individual to cope with physical illness and other stresses, including disruptions in social and family relationships, obviously take place within and are affected by the physical and interpersonal environment of the long-term-care setting. Clinical observations of the stressors encountered by the residents in long-term-care settings underscore the importance of the environment as a potent modifier of stressors (Baldwin, 1992). Specific models have been proposed to account for the interface between individual coping and the institutional environment (Moos & Lemke, 1985). Over the past 40 years social and behavioral scientists have examined the influence of institutional settings for the elderly (ranging from "senior citizen housing" to nursing homes) on their residents. Their research has documented that physical and neighborhood characteristics of the setting, social and recreational aspects of the environment, staffing patterns, and other factors directly or indirectly influence the social, physical, and emotional well-being of elderly residents (Moos & Lemke, 1985; Timko & Moos, 1991).

In long-term-care residences in particular, institutions that facilitate environmental stimulation, interaction with other residents, greater choice, and autonomy have residents who function better (Moos & Lemke, 1985; Sotile & Miller, 1998). A basic theme that runs throughout much of this research is the question of autonomy versus security (Parmelee & Lawton, 1990); that is, how an institution balances the resident's need to exercise some measure of control over the environment and the institution's mandate to provide a safe structured setting. Institutional decisions that impose limitations on residents' autonomy may strip them of autonomy and a sense of control over their environment. Concern about the potentially helplessness-engendering aspects of institutions was most forcefully articulated by Goffman (1961) in his treatise on the "total" institution. Researchers such as Langer and Rodin (1975, 1977) have tested interventions designed to increase feelings of control in long-term-care residents. In one study, enlarging long-term-care residents' decision-making responsibilities was associated not only with enhanced emotional and social well-being but also with dramatically reduced death rates compared with controls. Carpenter and colleagues (2002) proposed the use of empowerment to treat depression in long-term-care residents with mild to moderate dementia. Perceptions of personal control were important for the resident's quality of life even when control was specific to daily choices and routines (Carpenter et al., 2002; Perlmuter & Eds, 1998). These findings and those of others suggest that psychotherapeutic interventions that support feelings of autonomy and control in older adults lead to a decrease in morbidity and improve survival (Langer & Rodin, 1975). Others have found, however, (Schulz & Hanusa, 1979) that raising residents' expectations about control without providing substantive opportunities to exert control may actually be harmful.

Several research studies have suggested that the psychological impact of one's environment is determined by the balance between the functional capacity of the individual and what is available in the environment—or "person-environment fit" (Kahana, 1982). Lawton and Nahemow (1973) have proposed that for each person there is a level of demand or "press" from the immediate environment that facilitates maximum performance. They suggest that there are negative consequences for the individual when there is too little or too much demand relative to an individual's capacities. One corollary of this perspective (known as the "environmental docility hypothesis") is that as the mental and physical vigor of an individual diminishes, the well-being of that individual becomes proportionately more dependent on the immediate environment. Thus there is an ongoing transaction between the individual and the environment. Particularly in long-term-care settings, the support offered by care providers and staff may enhance feelings of autonomy and control (Sotile & Miller, 1998).

Efforts to enhance coping and emotional well-being in psychotherapy require a simultaneous accounting for individual capacity and environmental opportunities. A better "fit" between resident and the long-term-care facility may be identified by a clearer understanding of the resident's psychological strengths and vulnerabilities and the constraints and resources within the facility. The therapist can educate the staff about the resident's unique psychology, which then may guide staff in how to optimally interact with the resident. By helping the resident to more fully reckon with the problems that required long-term-care placement, the resident should then be better able to engage in a more realistic discussion of what options exist within the long-term-care setting to make daily life more satisfying and increase perceived autonomy. Such a process should result in enhanced feelings of control for both the patient and staff—with reductions in patient distress and staff frustration.

MENTAL DISORDERS AND THE AVAILABILITY OF PSYCHOTHERAPEUTIC TREATMENT IN LONG-TERM-CARE SETTINGS

Epidemiology

As indicated in other chapters in this volume, the prevalence of potentially treatable mental disorders among long-term-care residents is strikingly high. As many as 80% of elderly individuals residing in nursing homes (German et al., 1992) or assisted-living facilities (Rosenblatt et al., 2004) suffer from a mental disorder; as many as 26% experience noncognitive syndromes such as mood, anxiety, or psychotic disorders (Rosenblatt et al., 2004). Further, 6% to 14% of older residents are estimated to suffer from major depression (Teresi et al., 2001). Of long-term-care residents with dementia, an estimated 40% to 70% have clinically significant psychiatric symptoms (Rosenblatt et al., 2004; Rovner & Katz, 1993).

Other manifestations of potentially treatable mental disorders, while less well studied, are alarmingly high in long-term-care residents. For example, 30% to 50% of elderly residents manifest symptoms of "minor depression" that may predispose to more severe depression (Rovner & Katz, 1993). Findings from the Collaborative Studies of Long-Term-Care report that approximately 25% to 50% of residents exhibit subsyndromal mood or anxiety symptoms or other behavioral disturbances (Morgan et al., 2001) that may be treatable with non-pharmacological approaches such as psychotherapy (AGS & AAGP, 2003; Ruckdeschel & Katz, 2004). The rate of life-threatening behaviors (e.g., refusal of food or medications, or intentional self-harm) has been conservatively estimated at 95/100,000 in nursing home residents or almost five times the suicide rate for this age group (Osgood & Theilman, 1990). An estimated 11% to 23% of nursing home residents suffer from personality disorders (Hing, 1987; Teeter et al., 1976) characterized by emotional distress and disturbed interpersonal interactions and that may predispose to severe mental disorders. Other treatable disorders known to be prevalent in community-dwelling elderly (e.g., anxiety disorders, adjustment disorders, sleep disorders) have been less well researched, but are likely present in high rates among long-term-care residents.

Despite the high prevalence of both major and minor mental disorders among elderly long-term-care residents, evidence suggests that these disorders frequently are undetected or inadequately treated. Teetor et al. (1976) found missed or incorrect psychiatric diagnosis in 68% of nursing home residents with mental disorders. Using data from the Institutional Population Component of the 1987 National Medical Expenditure Survey, Shea et al. (1992) reported that less than 40% of nursing home residents with mental illness uncomplicated by dementia received any mental health treatment. Those residents who are older and physically ill and are thereby at greater risk for depression (Parmelee et al., 1989) are the least likely to be offered treatment. A more recent study of assisted-living-facility residents with noncognitive psychiatric disorders found that only 42% were adequately treated (Rosenblatt et al., 2004). Lack of effective psychotherapeutic or somatic treatment has been associated with increased morbidity and mortality (Rovner & Katz, 1993), medical rehospitalization (Lipzin, 1992), and increased overall health-care utilization (Mumford et al., 1982). The gap between the high prevalence of mental disorders and the inadequate mental health services currently delivered in long-term-care settings warrants further explanation (see Chapter 2 for a more complete discussion of the nursing home as a psychiatric hospital).

Barriers to Accessing Psychotherapeutic Treatment

Gerontological researchers have long argued that few elderly receive mental health services not only because of their own biases against using these services but because of barriers raised by inadequate public and private insurance coverage of mental health services, institutional public policies, and lack of an adequate geriatric mental health work force (Jeste et al., 1999; Smyer et al., 1990). Significant barriers continue to exist; yet, in the past ten years there has been some improvement in access to appropriate services for nursing home residents with mental health problems. Improvement has coincided with increased professional attention to the mental health needs of residents of long-term care (Lichtenberg et al., 1998; Molinari & Hartman-Stein, 2000) and novel models of treatment of depression in medically ill individuals (Unutzer et al., 2002). Despite efforts by the federal government, many long-term-care residences are de facto mental health care settings but often lack the professional resources to address the psychiatric and psychosocial needs of residents (Streim & Katz, 2004). Older mentally ill long-term-care residents may go misdiagnosed and untreated due to the problems inherent in diagnosing mental disorder in the context of physical illness. Biological, psychological, and social factors are interdependent; behavior problems may be secondary to physical illness; physical symptoms may mask a psychological disorder. Distinguishing whether behavioral problems evidenced by a resident reflect the resident's poor adaptation, a staff member's mismanagement of the patient, or both, is difficult to discern (Streim & Katz, 2004).

Some institutional and economic barriers to the delivery of mental health services in long-term-care facilities are declining. By mandating active treatment of mentally ill nursing home residents, improving payment and eliminating caps on mental health services under Medicare/Medicaid, and opening long-term-care facilities to qualified psychologist and social work consultants, the 1987 OBRA legislation improved access to psychotherapy services for mentally ill residents. Most residents of nursing homes are dual eligible (i.e., qualify for both Medicare and Medicaid), yet most states do not elect to reimburse through Medicaid the Medicare co-pay. This situation discourages providers from delivering mental health services in nursing homes (Karlin & Duffy, 2004; Molinari & Hartman-Stein, 2000). Policies of local Medicare carriers for what is considered "medically necessary" services to nursing home residents vary widely and some insurance carriers have held that a diagnosis of dementia or of Alzheimer's disease are grounds for denial of reimbursement of psychotherapy or other mental health services (Karlin & Duffy, 2004). This situation was remedied by vigorous lobbying from aging interest groups. Since psychologists became eligible in 1989 to be reimbursed through the Medicare program for psychotherapeutic services, increasing numbers of them are providing services in nursing homes. The limited number of mental health-care professional trained in geriatrics is another barrier to access to quality mental health services.

Staff attitudes often reveal ageist biases: depression in the nursing home is viewed as inevitable; mental health problems are attributed to "aging"; older individuals are perceived as incapable of change (Levy & Benaji, 2002). Referral for psychotherapy may also be constrained by biological reductionism, or an overemphasis on biological factors and an underemphasis on psychosocial factors that contribute to functioning (Estes & Binney, 1989). Recent studies indicate that psychotherapy is underutilized as a treatment for depression in older adults based on treatment guidelines and it can be reasonably assumed that this is very much the case in long-term-care facilities (Wei et al., 2005).

For example, Cohen (1989) points out that health-care providers often assume that depression in an individual with dementia must have a biological etiology; the role of psychosocial factors, especially in early dementia, are underrecognized. Staff countertransference, or the emotional response of staff to older long-term-care residents, presents another barrier to access for psychotherapeutic services (Genevay & Katz, 1990). Institutional staff often avoid close interaction with residents who are emotionally distressed in order to manage their own discomfort (Duffy, 1999; Gunther, 1987). Thus, for a variety of reasons, long-term-care staff may underrecognize the presence, source, and psychotherapeutic treatability of mental disorders in elderly long-term-care residents.

Indications for Psychotherapy in Long-Term-Care Residents

Some have sought to clarify guidelines for appropriate psychotherapeutic treatment of problems common to elderly long-term-care residents (Cohen, 1990; Goldfarb, 1955; Lewis & Rosenberg, 1990; Lichtenberg & Duffy, 2000; Miller, 1989; Rovner & Katz, 1993; Sadavoy & Robinson, 1989; Smith & Kramer, 1992). "Standards for psychological services in long-term care facilities" published by Psychologists in Long-Term Care (Lichtenberg et al., 1998) include recommendations for psychotherapeutic treatment in long-term-care facilities. Guidelines summarized in Table 14.1 regarding the use of insight-oriented, interpersonal, or integrative psychotherapy. Use of behavior management or psychosocial interventions would likely require less stringent criteria than those in Table 14.1. Our summary of referral guidelines may be grouped into three main criteria.

First, for psychotherapy to be warranted, a mental disorder must be present. Signs of mental disorder may be expressed explicitly (through depressive, anxious, or psychotic symptoms or significant behavior problems) or implicitly (e.g., interpersonal conflict with staff; behavior inconsistent with goal of rehabilitation). Second, the patient must evidence some capacity to engage in the

TABLE 14.1. Proposed Indications for Psychotherapy in the Nursing Home Setting

Presence of mental disorder
    Depressive, anxious, or psychotic symptoms
    Evidence of significant behavior problems
    Demanding, disruptive, or dependent behaviors
    Interpersonal conflict with staff
    Behavior inconsistent with goal of rehabilitation

Capacity to engage in psychotherapy
    Some capacity to communicate with others
    Some awareness that a problem exists, and motivation toward mastery
      of problem
    Some capacity for retention/carry-over

Possible additional factors
    Presence of signs of personality disorder
    Symptoms subclinical in degree
    Somatic treatment only partially effective or contraindicated

Source: Adapted from Goldfarb, 1954; Miller, 1989; Sadavoy & Robinson, 1989; Cohen, 1990; Lewis & Rosenberg, 1990; Smith & Kramer, 1992; Rovner, 1993; Lichtenberg, et al., 1998; Duffy, 1999.

psychotherapeutic process. This capacity requires at least a limited ability to communicate with others, an understanding that a problem exists, a willingness to remedy the problem, and a capacity to retain some of the products of the therapeutic session. Thus, psychotherapy is indicated for some individuals with dementia. Just as long-term-care residents with dementia may retain partial capacity to make decisions about their care, so too may their capacity to engage in psychotherapy be relative rather than absolute. Third, other factors such as the presence of personality disorder, a subclinical presentation of psychiatric symptoms, and a contraindication for or partial response to somatic treatment may indicate that an evaluation for psychotherapy is warranted. We hasten to add, there is a paucity of research on the criteria regarding which long-term-care residents would most profit from psychotherapy. Some argue that criteria for psychotherapy eligibility are wider than those we have outlined. Duffy (1999) believes that even individuals with markedly limited language skills may benefit by supportive psychotherapy and points to the large repertoire of nonverbal means of communication that are available to client as well as therapist. These communications include subvocal communication of affect, kinesic communication (e.g., facial expressions), autonomic communication (e.g., posture, pupil dilation), and tactile communication (e.g., touch). Further, given that mid-brain regions are often spared in dementia, some have suggested that affect-focused psychotherapeutic interventions may remain effective despite loss of communication ability (Duffy, 1999; Lichtenberg & Duffy, 2000).

PSYCHOTHERAPEUTIC TREATMENT MODELS

As noted, a large body of research argues for the utility of a psychotherapeutic approach to the problems of elderly long-term-care residents. However, what is the efficacy of psychotherapeutic treatments for younger as well as older individuals? Efficacy rates of 60% to 70% have been repeatedly demonstrated in meta-analytic studies of psychotherapy as a treatment for individuals of mixed ages (Smith, Glass, & Miller, 1980). More recently, clinical and empirical research has examined the effectiveness of psychotherapy with community-dwelling and institutionalized elderly. This literature may be broadly grouped into five sections: (1) individual psychotherapy, (2) group psychotherapy, (3) specialized techniques for older adults with depression, (4) specialized techniques for older adults with personality disorder, and (5) specialized techniques for older adults with dementia.

Individual Psychotherapy

There is general agreement that community-dwelling elderly with mental disorders can be successfully treated with slightly modified forms of insight-oriented psychodynamic and interpersonal psychotherapy (IPT) (Lebowitz et al., 1997; Niederhe & Schnieder, 1994; Scogin & McElreath, 1994). Similarly, clinical reports have long supported the utility of psychotherapy with institutionalized older adults. Goldfarb (1955, Goldfarb & Sheps, 1954) found that older nursing home residents could overcome feelings of helplessness through their alliance with a therapist. Grunes (1984) and others (Carpenter et al., 2002; Cohen, 1985; Hausman, 1992; Kahana, 1987; Ronch & Maizler, 1977; Sadavoy & Robinson, 1989; Solomon & Szwabo, 1992; Spayd & Smyer, 1988; Unterbach, 1994) have suggested that even brief forms of individual psychotherapy can assist institutionalized older adults to cope adaptively with physical illness, adjust to greater dependency on others, and maintain a sense of self-continuity. Psychotherapeutic efforts may also assist staff and family to better understand and manage a resident's behavior (Molinari, 2000; Tobin, 1989, 1999).

These clinical reports have been supported by a developing evidence base of empirical research. In a study of brief individual psychotherapy for community-based elderly with major depressive disorder, 70% of subjects evidenced substantial improvement and therapeutic gains that were maintained at a 1-year follow-up and those treated with brief dynamic psychotherapy demonstrated comparable gains to those treated with cognitive-behavioral approaches (Gallagher-Thompson & Steffen, 1994; Thompson et al., 1987). Brief insight-oriented individual psychotherapy also reduces symptoms in older adults with mild depression (Lazarus et al., 1987). Early studies of elderly long-term-care residents also demonstrated favorable results. Goldfarb and Turner (1952–1953) found that even infrequent psychotherapeutic contact improved the symptoms of 49% of mentally ill residents. Power and McCarron (1975) reported that a modified psychotherapeutic approach reduced psychiatric symptoms in withdrawn elderly residents. Frey et al. (1992) demonstrated that brief counseling significantly enhanced long-term-care residents' self-esteem and sense of self-continuity. In a preliminary study of an integrative approach that incorporates psychodynamic techniques to treat depression in patients with dementia, Carpenter et al. (2002) found measurable improvement in patients' depressive symptoms. These studies and others (Hyer et al., 2005) suggest the potential for significant benefit from insight-oriented or integrative psychotherapy approaches.

Related psychotherapeutic techniques, such as reminiscence and life review therapy, are also purported to improve mood and enhance self-understanding and self-continuity among long-term-care residents. Recent reviews find some empirical support for these approaches (Finnema et al., 2000; Kasl-Godley & Gatz, 2000; Molinari, 1999), although few controlled trials have been conducted in long-term settings.

In sum, a growing body of clinical and empirical evidence supports the rationale for insight-oriented and integrative individual psychotherapy as a treatment for elderly long-term-care residents with mood disorders. Further research will be needed to replicate and expand the existing research base on psychotherapy for long-term-care residents, examine whether therapeutic gains are maintained over time, and clarify which common factors or psychotherapeutic techniques are effective for designated mental disorders in elderly in long-term care.

Group Psychotherapy

Group psychotherapy is an intervention that is particularly well suited for residents in a long-term-care setting. It is an effective alternative to individual psychotherapy enabling clinicians to treat a greater number of residents using fewer resources (Molinari, 2000). Group psychotherapy has been used with the elderly to reduce aberrant behavior, dependency, and social withdrawal and isolation, as well as to enhance self-esteem, adaptive problem solving, and affiliation with others (Ripeckyj & Lazarus, 1984; Spayd & Smyer, 1988). In institutionalized elderly, it has also been proposed as a means to enhance social skills, communication and memory skills, and emotional self-control (Herst & Moulton, 1985; Molinari, 2000).

Group psychotherapy also may produce a sense of belonging and adjustment to living in a long-term-care setting. Insight-oriented psychodynamic and cognitive-behavioral forms of group therapy have been found to reduce symptoms of depression and anxiety in clinically depressed community-dwelling elders (Steurer et al., 1984). In long-term-care residences, group approaches have been studied primarily through self report of group participants. Empirical research regarding interpersonal or integrative group psychotherapy is less common. Limited research on reminiscence group psychotherapy demonstrates positive effects of the therapy on depression, hopelessness, and life satisfaction (Haight, Michel & Hendrix, 2000). Preliminary studies suggest that group psychotherapy improves residents' psychological well-being, self-reliance, and sense of personal control (Christopher, et. al., 1988; Kasl-Godley & Gatz, 2000; Moran & Gatz, 1987; Rattenbury & Stones, 1989). Long-term-care residents, like others who participate in group therapy, may benefit from a group's ability to allow participants to learn that they were not alone (Bonhote et al., 1999). Given the proven utility of group psychotherapy approaches in institutional settings, further research to evaluate the psychological and psychosocial outcomes and use of this modality are likely.

Specialized Techniques: Older Adults with Depression

Existing models of insight-oriented and supportive psychotherapy have recently been refined in an effort to develop specialized techniques to treat depressive disorders (American Psychiatric Association, 1989). The theoretical basis of these models is that depression has both biological and psychosocial etiologies.

An individual's personality is held to play a pivotal role in determining how the individual reacts to intrapsychic or interpersonal stressors and regulates self-esteem. In addition, an individual's capacity to relate interpersonally is theorized to mediate the ability to successfully contend with loss, transition, and interpersonal conflicts. Thus, maladaptive personality development or poor interpersonal functioning is viewed as a factor contributing to vulnerability to depression. Six major psychotherapeutic modalities have been identified as efficacious in the treatment of depression in older adults: cognitive-behavioral therapy (CBT), psychodynamic psychotherapy, problem-solving therapy (PST), life review therapy, family interventions, and IPT. At least some research evidence supports their efficacy (Karel & Hinrichsen, 2000).

Relevant to the focus of this chapter, we believe that IPT holds promise as a useful treatment for depressed older long-term-care residents. IPT has some elements of psychodynamic psychotherapy and supportive psychotherapy. Unlike psychodynamic psychotherapy, however, IPT does not focus on personality change but rather on change of relevant interpersonal behaviors and reduction of depressive symptoms (Weissman et al., 2000). IPT was originally developed as a time-limited treatment for younger adults (Weissman et al., 2000). Within a psycho-educational and empowerment ethos, the therapeutic focus of IPT is on one or two of four interpersonally relevant problem areas: Role transitions, interpersonal disputes, grief, or interpersonal deficits. These four problem areas encompass many of the problems that are often discussed in the course of psychotherapy with long-term-care residents. IPT has been found to be effective in both acute and maintenance treatment of major depression in mixed aged groups of adults (see Frank and Spanier, 1995 for review). Two pilot studies of IPT in the treatment of acute depression in older adults exist as well as a study of an abbreviated form of IPT (Interpersonal Counseling, IPC) in the treatment of depressive symptoms in older adults with medical problems (Mossey et al., 1996). A larger continuation-maintenance study of older adults with recurrent major depression found that IPT as well as antidepressant medication significantly reduced rates of recurrence of major depression (Reynolds et al., 1999). In routine practice settings IPT has also been reported to be useful for older adults (Hinrichsen & Clougherty, in press).

An overall model of the psychotherapeutic management of depression in elderly long-term-care residents may be derived from an adaptation and integration of models of insight-oriented, supportive, and IPT. This proposed integrated model has three basic goals: (1) identification and clarification of the depressive experience and its internal and external precipitants, (2) limitation of maladaptive behavior and facilitation of effective coping, and (3) restoration of emotional self-regulation, effective social functioning, self-continuity, and mastery.

Various specific techniques are utilized to achieve these goals. Symptoms and interpersonal problems are reviewed; education is provided regarding the nature of depression; emotional states and subjective versus objective perceptions of events are identified; pre-morbid and current strengths and limitations are assessed. The patient-therapist relationship plays a critical role in this form of psychotherapy, both in providing an empathic environment and in enhancing interpersonal learning: Self-defeating interpersonal behaviors are confronted, and more adaptive mechanisms are supported; verbalization and effective communication are practiced and encouraged; testing of subjective perceptions is fostered; when indicated, the therapist may actively advocate on behalf of the resident, or assist staff to understand the interpersonal behavior of the resident. Restoration of effective functioning may require various techniques: Mourning for internal and external losses is facilitated; strengths and limitations are reappraised; strategies to maintain emotional regulation and resolve interpersonal conflicts are promoted; self-mastery and a new sense of identity are highlighted and integrated. The following case vignette is illustrative:

An 83-year-old married woman suffered a right CVA with a dense left hemiplegia, leaving her dependent on others for most ADLs, and prompting her nursing home admission. Earlier in her life she had worked as an English teacher, loved to read and to travel, and had prided herself on her ability to manage an array of household and family affairs. In her later years she served as a caregiver to her ailing husband. Her stroke, while sparing much of her intellect, left her feeling suddenly useless and helpless, "like I'd lost part of myself," with little interest in activities and with steady weight loss. In the course of psychotherapy, as she began to survey her remaining attributes, she recognized that her capacity to be opinionated could now be enlisted to control aspects of her care; her ability to call up visual memories of her travels could be used for entertainment and for solace; her family still valued her advice. She also became reconciled to her limitations, as she realized that she could no longer be a "female Atlas" who takes on the problems of others; she could no longer control many of her life's circumstances; while she yearned for independence and to return home, this was not possible. Despite her stroke, she began to again view herself as capable and whole, with accompanying stabilization of her weight and a lifting of her dysphoria.

Specialized Techniques: Older Adults with Personality Disorder

The diagnosis of personality disorder is used to describe individuals who display patterns of culturally nonnormative inner experiences, traits, and maladaptive behaviors that are associated with impaired social or occupational functioning or subjective distress (*DSM-IV-TR*, APA, 2000). These disorders encompass a variety of behavioral characteristics: some individuals with personality disorder may be self-aggrandizing, hypersensitive to criticism, and unable to empathize with others; others may be aloof, solitary, and indifferent; still others may be submissive, uncomfortable when alone, and excessively dependent. Although previously underrecognized and thought to be rare, late-life personality disorder is now viewed as prevalent and purported to be linked to the onset, course, and treatment outcome of Axis I disorders such as depression among community-dwelling elderly (Rosowsky, Abrams, & Zweig, 1999). Personality disorder in the elderly is associated with a higher prevalence of early-onset depression (Abrams et al., 1994; Ames & Molinari, 1994), recurrent depression, comorbid anxiety disorder, past suicide attempts (Kunik et al., 1993), and negative life events (Vine & Steingart, 1994). Further, while depressed elderly without personality disorder respond well to standardized psychotherapeutic and/or somatic approaches (Niederhe & Schneider, 1998; Scogin & McElreath, 1994), elderly with personality disorder experience increased depressive symptom severity, greater residual symptoms following standardized psychotherapeutic treatment (Gradman et al., 1999; Thompson et al., 1988; Vine & Steingart, 1994), and persisting decreases in functioning and quality of life, even following remission of most depressive symptoms (Abrams et al., 1998, 2001).

In the nursing home population, as mentioned previously, an estimated 11% to 23% of residents have a diagnosable personality disorder (Hing, 1987; Teeter et al., 1976), but this syndrome has only received scant attention in the long-term-care literature (Lichtenberg & Duffy, 2000). Individuals with untreated personality disorder often create havoc for medical personnel by sabotaging treatment efforts, provoking and disturbing other residents, and inciting intra-staff conflict.

Insight-oriented psychodynamic and integrative psychotherapy approaches appear efficacious for adults with personality disorder (Leichsenring & Leibling, 2003; Livesley, 2001) yet there are no empirical studies examining its use in treating long-term-care residents. Clinical reports suggest that these approaches are effective in reducing pathological acting out (e.g., sabotaging of treatment), reducing maladaptive patterns of interaction, and improving the emotional control of personality disordered elderly long-term-care residents (Molinari, 2000; Sadavoy, 1987; Sadavoy & Dorian, 1983; Zweig, 2003; Zweig & Agronin, 2006). The following case vignette is illustrative:

> A 73-year-old widowed woman was admitted to the nursing home following hemicolectomy for metastatic cancer. She had additional medical problems and was quite debilitated and reliant on others for assistance with ADLs. She was estranged from her children and was only rarely in contact with siblings. Her medical prognosis was poor. She alternately denied the seriousness of her condition and tearfully stated that the surgery was unsuccessful and she was "waiting to die." As her medical problems worsened, she became demanding and verbally abusive toward nursing staff whom she perceived as withholding of the care she required. As conflicts with staff escalated, she threatened to suicide and to refuse medications, but withdrew these threats later. Her psychotherapeutic treatment consisted of setting limits on her manipulative threats, reaching agreement regarding appropriate ways to manage feelings of hopelessness and suicidality, clarifying that anger precipitated by her helpless and painful condition was misdirected at staff, and enlisting staff in efforts to understand and better manage her behavior. The threats and conflicts lessened, her family contacted her more often, and shortly thereafter she died rather quietly.

IMPACT OF SOCIAL AND ENVIRONMENTAL FACTORS

The impact of social and environmental factors, most notably the institutional environment and staff behaviors, has been increasingly recognized in discussions of psychotherapy in (Lawton, 1999) long-term-care settings. As noted earlier, numerous studies have documented the importance of social and environmental factors on the general emotional well-being of community and institutionally residing elderly. The older individual's interpersonal environment has also been shown to affect the course of major depression in community-dwelling elderly (Hinrichsen, 1993; Hinrichsen & Emery, 2005; Hinrichsen & Pollack, 1997; Zweig & Hinrichsen, 1993). It therefore seems likely that the effectiveness of psychotherapy for elderly living in long-term-care settings partly depends on aspects of the institutional environment and the interpersonal context provided by primary care staff.

Elderly long-term-care residents whose physical, psychological, and social integrity have been compromised require a facilitating psychological environment to begin the psychotherapeutic process of self-restoration (Duffy, 1999). Yet, certain attributes of the institutional environment militate against this goal. The long-term-care environment is often impersonal; staff upon whom residents depend change frequently and unpredictably; privacy and autonomy are compromised; the nature of one's interpersonal relationships is often dictated by one's care needs; rooms and roommates change; if medically hospitalized, the security of having a bed and a "home" is often only guaranteed for a limited time (Kennedy, 2000; Molinari, 2000). Further, some institutions organize service delivery in a manner that instills dependency in residents and creates a cycle of helplessness, recurrent demands, and increased staff utilization (Gatz et al., 1985).

As noted, the interpersonal environment created by primary care staff is likely critical to the genesis, course, and treatment outcome of mentally ill long-term-care residents. However, caring for community-dwelling depressed elderly patients has in itself been tied to feelings of anger, depression, and anxiety in caregivers (Hinrichsen et al., 1992). While less well studied, similar emotional reactions are likely elicited in long-term-care staff caring for residents with these problems. In particular, nursing aides have the most direct contact with nursing home residents; yet, they usually contend with enormous job stress and are often underappreciated and underpaid despite the fact that they may have valuable insights into optimal psychosocial care of their residents (Kramer & Smith, 2000). Gunther (1987) has observed that "the price a dedicated and effective rehabilitation staff pays for significant therapeutic involvement with seriously damaged patients is periodic subjective distress and impaired professional behavior" (p. 219). More commonly, he noted, institutional staff respond to physically and psychologically traumatized patients by avoiding true empathic contact with the patient, repressing the patient's and their own distress, and failing to attend to behavioral principles in delivering care (Duffy, 1999). Thus, for psychotherapy to be effective, interventions must target the emotional responses and behaviors of primary staff as well as those of the mentally ill resident.

CONCLUSION

Mental disorders are prevalent in elderly long-term-care home residents. Although mental health treatment is still underutilized in this setting, the provision of psychological treatment is on the rise. Psychotherapy, based on a body of well-developed theory and grounded in research, has been shown to be effective in treating mental illness in community-dwelling elderly and in groups of institutionalized elders. Existing models of psychotherapy are being modified to treat the special clinical problems found in residents of long-term-care facilities; barriers to treatment are being identified, and guidelines for psychotherapeutic treatment are being developed; the social and environmental conditions that enable psychotherapy in long-term-care facilities are being clarified.

However, the delivery of mental health services, including psychotherapy, to elderly long-term-care residents is in a nascent stage. Future treatment programs will likely continue to borrow from existing models of psychiatric and rehabilitative care and employ mental health clinicians to further develop methods for the early detection of mental illness, maximize the physical rehabilitation of residents suffering from mental illness, and develop educational programs for primary staff and family members of residents. Therein will the treatment needs of this underserved population be met and the public policy mandate for "active treatment" be realized.

REFERENCES

Abrams, R. C., Alexopoulos, G. S., Spielman, L. A., et al. (2001). Personality disorder symptoms predict declines in global functioning and quality of life in elderly depressed patients. *American Journal of Geriatric Psychiatry, 9:* 67–71.

Abrams, R. C., Rosendahl, E., Card, C., et al. (1994). Personality disorder correlates of late and early onset depression. *Journal of the American Geriatrics Society, 42:* 727–731.

Abrams, R. C., Spielman, L. A., Alexopoulos, G. S., & Klausner, E. (1998). Personality disorder symptoms and functioning in elderly depressed patients. *American Journal of Geriatric Psychiatry, 6:* 24–30, Win 1998.

American Geriatrics Society and American Association for Geriatric Psychiatry (2003). Consensus statement on improving the quality of mental health care in U.S. nursing homes: Management of depression and behavioral symptoms associated with dementia. *Journal of the American Geriatrics Society, 51:* 1287–1298.

American Psychiatric Association (2000). *Diagnostic and statistical manual of mental disorders* (4th ed. rev). Washington DC: American Psychiatric Association.

American Psychiatric Association (1989). *Treatments of psychiatric disorders: A task force report of the American Psychiatric Association.* Washington DC: American Psychiatric Association.

Ames, A., & Molinari, V. (1994). Prevalence of personality disorders in community-living elderly. *Journal of Geriatric Psychiatry and Neurology, 7:* 189–194.

Anderson, B. (1998, August). Stress, immune and endocrine responses following a psychological intervention for women with regional breast cancer. Paper presented at the International Congress of Behavioral Medicine, Copenhagen, Denmark.

Antoni, M. H. (2003). *Stress management intervention for women with breast cancer.* Washington DC: American Psychiatric Association.

Asnis, G. M., & Miller, A. H. (1989). Phenomenology and biology of depression—potential mechanisms for neuromodulation of immunity. In A. H. Miller (Ed.), *Depressive disorders and immunity* (pp. 53–63). Washington DC: American Psychiatric Press.

Atchley, R. C. (1989). A continuity theory of normal aging. *Gerontologist, 29:* 183.

Baldwin, B. (1992) Stress in the elderly: Environments of care. In M. L. Wykle, E. Kahana, & J. Kowal (Eds.), *Stress and health among the elderly* (pp. 197–208). New York: Springer.

Biegel, D. E., Sales, E., & Schulz, R. (Eds.). (1991). *Family caregiving in chronic illness.* Newbury Park, CA: Sage.

Blazer, D. (2003). Depression in late life: Review and commentary. *Journal of Gerontology: Medical Sciences, 58A(3),* 249–265.

Bonhote, K., Romano-Egan, J., & Cornwell, C. (1999). Altruism and creative expression in a long-term older adult psychotherapy group. *Issues in Mental Health Nursing, 20:* 603–617.

Borson, S., Liptzin, B., Nininger, J., & Rabins, P. (1989). *A report of the task force on nursing homes and the mentally ill elderly.* Washington DC: American Psychiatric Association.

Burish, T. G., & Bradley, L. A. (Eds.). (1983). *Coping with chronic illness: Research and applications.* New York, NY: Academic.

Carpenter, B., Ruckdeschel, K., Ruckdeschel, H., & Van Haitsma, K. (2002). R-E-M Psychotherapy: A manualized approach for long-term care residents with depression and dementia. *Clinical Gerontologist, 25:* 25–49.

Carstensen, L. L. (1992). Social and emotional patterns in adulthood: Support for socio-emotional selectivity theory. *Psychology and Aging, 7:* 331–338.

Christopher, F., Loeb, P., Zaretsky, H., & Jassani, A. (1988). A group psychotherapy intervention to promote the functional independence of older adults in a long-term rehabilitation hospital: A preliminary study. *Physical and Occupational Therapy in Geriatrics, 6:* 51.

Cohen, G. (1985). Mental health aspects of nursing home care. In E. L. Schneider, C. J. Wendland, A. W. Zimmer, N. List, & M. Ory (Eds.), *The teaching nursing home* (pp. 157–164). New York: Raven Press.

Cohen, G. (1989). Psychodynamic perspectives in the clinical approach to brain disease in the elderly. In D. E. Conn, A. Grek, & J. Sadavoy (Eds.), *Psychiatric consequences of brain disease in the elderly: A focus on management* (pp. 85–99). New York: Plenum.

Cohen, G. (1990). Psychopathology of mental health in the mature and elderly adult. In J. E. Birren, & K. W. Schaie (Eds.), *Handbook of the psychology of aging* (pp. 359–371). San Diego: Academic.

Cohen, S. (1988). Psychosocial models of the role of social support in the etiology of physical disease. *Health Psychology, 7*: 269.

Cohen, S., & Syme, S. L. (1985). *Social support and health*. Orlando, FL: Academic.

Diagnosis and Treatment of Depression in Late Life. (1991). (Reprinted from NIH Consensus Development Conference Consensus Statement 1991 November 4–6: 9(3)). Bethesda MD: NIH.

DiMatteo, M. R., Lepper, H. S., & Croghan, T. W. (*2000*). Depression is a risk factor for noncompliance with medical treatment: Meta-analysis of the effects of anxiety and depression on patient adherence. *Archives of Internal Medicine, 160(14): 2101–2107.*

Duffy, M. (1999). Reaching the person behind the dementia: Treating comorbid affective disorders through subvocal and nonverbal strategies. In M. Duffy (Ed.), *Handbook of counseling and psychotherapy with older adults* (pp. 577–589). New York: Wiley.

Erikson, E. (1950). *Childhood and society*. New York: W. W. Norton.

Estes, C., & Binney, E. A. (1989). The biomedicalization of aging: Dangers and dilemmas. *The Gerontologist, 29:* 587–596.

Fawzy, F., Fawzy, H., Hyun, C., & Wheeler, J. (1997). Brief, coping-oriented therapy for patients with malignant melanoma. In J. Spira (Ed.), *Group therapy for medically ill patients* (pp. 133–164). New York: Guilford Press.

Finnema, E., Droes, R. M., Ribbe, M., & Van Tilburg, W. (2000). The effects of emotion-oriented approaches in the care of persons suffering from dementia: A review of the literature. *International Journal of Geriatric Psychiatry, 15:* 141–161.

Folkman, S. (1984). Personal control and stress and coping process: A theoretical analysis. *Journal of Personality and Social Psychology, 46:* 839–852.

Folkman S., & Greer S. (*2000*). Promoting psychological well-being in the face of serious illness: When theory, research and practice inform each other. *Psycho-Oncology, 9(1): 11–9.*

Frank, E., & Spanier, C. (1995). Interpersonal psychotherapy for depression: Overview, clinical efficacy, and future directions. *Clinical Psychology: Science and Practice, 2:* 349–369.

Frey, D. E., Kelbley, T. J., Durham, L., & James, J. (1992). Enhancing the self esteem of selected male nursing home residents. *Gerontologist, 32:* 552–557.

Gallagher-Thompson, D., & Steffen, A. M. (1994). Comparative effects of cognitive-behavioral and brief psychodynamic psychotherapies for depressed family caregivers. *Journal of Consulting and Clinical Psychology, 62:* 543–549.

Gatz, M., Fiske, A., Fox, L., Kaskie, B., Kasl-Godley, J., McCallum, T., et al. (1998). Empirically validated psychological treatments for older adults. *Journal of Mental Health & Aging, 4:* 9–46.

Gatz, M., Popkin, S. J., Pino, C. D., & VandenBos, G. R. (1985). Psychological interventions with older adults. In J. E. Birren, & K. W. Schaie, *Handbook of the Psychology of Aging* (2nd ed., pp. 755–785). Van Nostrand Reinhold, New York.

Genevay, B., & Katz, R. S. (1990). *Countertransference and older adults*. Newbury Park: Sage.

German, P. S., Rovner, B. W., Burton, L. L., Braut, L. J., & Clark, R. (1992). The role of mental morbidity in the nursing home experience. *Gerontologist, 32:* 152–158.

Goffman, E.(1961). *Asylums: Essays on the social situation of mental patients and other inmates*. Garden City, NY: Doubleday.

Goldfarb, A. I., & Sheps, J. (1954). Psychotherapy of the aged III: Brief therapy of interrelated psychological and somatic disorders. *Psychosomatic Medicine, 16:* 209.

Goldfarb, A. (1955). Psychotherapy of aged persons IV: One aspect of the psychodynamics of the therapeutic situation with aged persons. *Psychoanalitic Review, 42:* 180–187.

Goldfarb, A. I., & Sheps, J. (1954). Psychotherapy of the aged III: Brief therapy of inter-related psychological and somatic disorders. *Psychosomatic Medicine, 16:* 209.

Goldfarb, A., Turner, H. (1952). Psychotherapy of aged persons II: Utilization and effectiveness of brief therapy. *American Journal of Psychiatry, 109:* 916.

Gradman, T., Thompson, L., Gallagher-Thompson, D. (1999). Personality disorders and treatment outcome. In E. Rosowsky, R. Abrams, & R. Zweig (Eds.), *Personality disorders in older adults: Emerging issues in diagnosis & treatment* (pp. 69–94). Mahwah: Erlbaum.

Griffin, B. P., & Grunes, J. M. (1990). A developmental approach to psychoanalytic psychotherapy with the aged. In R. A. Nemiroff, & C. A. Colarusso (Eds.), *New dimensions in adult Development* (pp. 267–283). New York: Basic Books.

Groves, J. E., & Kucharski, A. (1987). Brief psychotherapy. In T. P. Hackett, & N. H. Cassem (Eds.), *Massachusetts general hospital handbook of general hospital psychiatry* (2nd ed., pp. 309–331). Littleton, MA: PSG Publishing Co.

Grunes, J. M. (1984). Brief psychotherapy with the aged: A clinical approach. In J. P. Abrahams, & V. J. Crooks (Eds.), *Geriatric mental health* (pp. 97–107). Orlando: Grune & Stratton.

Gunther, M. S. (1987). Catastrophic illness and the caregivers: Real burdens and solutions with respect to the behavioral sciences. In B. Caplan (Ed.), *Rehabilitation psychology desk teference* (pp. 219–243). Gaithersburg, MD: Aspen Publications.

Gutmann, D. L. (1988). Late onset pathogenesis: Dynamic models. *Topics in Geriatric Rehabilitation, 3:* 1.

Haight, B. K., Michel, Y., & Hendrix, B. K. (1998). Life review: Preventing despair in newly relocated nursing home residents. *International Journal of Aging and Human Development, 47:* 119–142.

Hausman, C. (1992). Dynamic psychotherapy with elderly demented patients. In G. M. Jones, & B. L. Miesen (Eds.), *Care-giving in dementia: Research and applications* (pp. 181–198). New York: Tavistock/Routledge.

Herst, L., & Moulton, P. (1985). Psychiatry in the nursing home. *Psychiatric Clinics of North America, 8:* 551.

Hing, E. (1987). National Center for Health Statistics: Use of nursing homes by the elderly, preliminary data from the 1985 National Nursing Home Survey. Advance Data from Vital and Health Statistics, No. 135, DHHS Pub. No. ADM 87-1516. US Government Printing Office, Washington, DC.

Hinrichsen, G. A., & Clougherty, K. F. Interpersonal psychotherapy for depressed older adults. Washington, DC: *American Psychological Association* (2006).

Hinrichsen, G. A., & Hernandez, N. (1993). Factors associated with recovery and relapse from major depressive disorder in the elderly. *American Journal of Psychiatry, 150:* 1820.

Hinrichsen, G. A., Hernandez, N., & Pollack, S. (1992). Difficulties and rewards in family care of the depressed older adult. *Gerontologist, 32:* 486.

Hinrichsen, G. A., & Emery, E. E. (2005). Interpersonal factors and late-life depression. *Clinical Psychology: Science and Practice, 12:* 264–275.

Hinrichsen, G. A., & Pollack, S. (1997). Expressed emotion and the course of late-life depression. *Journal of Abnormal Psychology, 106:* 336–340.

Hyer, L., Carpenter, B., Bishmann, D., & Wu, H. (2005). Depression in long term care. *Clinical Psychology: Science and Practice, 12:* 280–299.

Isaacowitz, D. M., Charles, S. T., & Carstensen, L. L. (2000). Emotion and cognition. In F. I. M. Craik, & T. A. Salthouse (Eds.), *Handbook of aging and cognition* (2nd ed., pp. 593–631). Mahwah: Erlbaum.

Jeste, D. V., Alexopoulos, G. S., Bartels, S. J., Cummings, J. L., Gallo, J. J., Gottlieb, G. L., Halpain, M. C., et al. (1999). Consensus statement on the upcoming crisis in geriatric mental health. *Archives of General Psychiatry, 56:* 848–853.

Kahana, E. (1982). A congruence model of person-environment interaction. In P. G. Windley, & T. O. Byert (Eds.), *Aging and the environment: Theoretical approaches* (p. 97). New York: Springer.

Kahana, R. J. (1987). Geriatric psychotherapy: Beyond crisis management. In J. Sadavoy, & M. Leszcz (Eds.), *Treating the elderly with psychotherapy: The scope for change in later life* (pp. 233–263). Madison: International Universities Press.

Kaplan, H. B. (Ed.). (1983). *Psychosocial stress: Trends in theory and research.* New York: Academic.

Karel, M. J., & Hinrichsen, G. (2000). Treatment of depression in late life: Psychotherapeutic interventions. *Clinical Psychology Review, 20:* 707–729.

Karlin, B. E., & Duffy, M. (2004). Geriatric mental health policy: Impact on service delivery and directions for effecting change. *Professional psychology: Research & Practice, 35:* 509–519.

Karuza, J., & Katz, P. R. (1991). Psychosocial interventions in long-term care: A critical overview. In P. Katz, R. Kane, & M. Mezey (Eds.), *Advances in long term care* (Vol. 1, pp. 1–27). New York: Springer.

Kasl-Godley, J., & Gatz, M. (2000). Psychosocial interventions for individuals with dementia: An integration of theory, therapy and a clinical understanding of dementia. *Clinical Psychology Review, 20:* 755–782.

Kennedy, G. (2000). *Geriatric mental health care: A treatment guide for health professionals.* New York: Gilford.

Koocher, G. P. (1996). Pediatric oncology: Medical crisis intervention. In R. J. Resnick, & R. H. Roszensky (Eds.), *Health psychology through the life span, practice and research opportunities* (pp. 213–225). Washington, DC: American Psychological Association.

Kramer, N. A., & Smith, M. C. (2000). Training nursing assistants to care for nursing home resident with dementia. In V. Molinari (Ed.), *Professional psychology in long term care: A comprehensive guide* (pp. 227–256). New York: Hatherleigh Press.

Kunik, M. E., Mulsant, B. H., Rifai, A. H., Sweet, R., Pasternak, R., Rosen, J., & Zubenko, G. S.(1993). Personality disorders in elderly inpatients with major depression. *American Journal of Geriatric Psychiatry, 1:* 38–45.

Labouvief, G. V., DeVoe M., & Bulka, D. (1989). Speaking about feelings: Conceptions of emotion across the life span. *Psychology and Aging 4:* 425–437.

Langer, E. J., & Rodin, J. (1975). The effects of choice and enhanced personal responsibility for the aged: A field experiment in an institutional setting. *Journal of Personality and Social Psychology 34:* 191.

Lawton, M. P. (1999). Environmental design features and the well-being of older persons. In M. Duffy (Ed.), *Handbook of counseling and psychotherapy with older adults* (pp. 350–363). New York: Wiley.

Lawton, M. P., & Nahemow, L. (1973). Ecology and the aging process. In C. Eisdorfer, & M. P. Lawton (Eds.), *The psychology of adult development and aging* (pp. 619–674). Washington, DC: American Psychological Association.

Lazarus, L. W., Groves, L., Gutmann, D., Ripekyj, A., Frankel, R., Newton, N., Grunes, J., et al. (1987). Brief psychotherapy with the elderly: A study of process and outcome. In

J. Sadavoy, & M. Leszcz (Eds.), *Treating the elderly with psychotherapy: The scope for change in later life* (pp. 265–293). Madison: International Universities Press.

Lazarus, R. S., & Folkman, S. (1984). *Stress, Appraisal, and Coping*. New York: Springer.

Lebowitz, B. D., Pearson, J. L., Schneider, L. S., Reynolds, C. F. III, Alexopoulos, G. S., Bruce, M. L., Conwell, Y., et al. (1997). Diagnosis and treatment of depression in late life: Consensus statement update. *Journal of the American Medical Association, 278:* 1186–1190.

Leichsenring, F., & Leibling, E. (2003). The effectiveness of psychodynamic therapy and cognitive behavior therapy in the treatment of personality disorders: A meta-analysis. *American Journal of Psychiatry, 160:* 1223–1232.

Lewis, L., & Rosenberg, S. J. (1990). Psychoanalytic psychotherapy with brain-injured adult psychiatric patients. *The Journal of Nervous and Mental Disease, 178:* 69.

Levy, B. R., & Banaji, M. R. (2002). Implicit ageism. In T. D. Nelson (Ed.), *Ageism: Stereotyping and prejudice against older persons* (pp. 49–75). Cambridge, MA: The MIT Press.

Levy, S., Herberman, R., Lippman, M., D'Angelo, T., & Lee, J. (1991). In M. ten Have-de Labije, & H. Balner (Eds.), *Coping with cancer and beyond: Cancer treatment and mental health* (pp. 67–75). Amsterdam: Swets & Zeitlinger.

Lichtenberg, P. (1994). *A guide to psychological practice in geriatric long term care*. Binghampton, NY: Haworth Press.

Lichtenberg, P. A., & Duffy, M. (2000). Psychological assessment and psychotherapy in long-term care. *Clinical Psychology: Science and Practice, 7:* 317–328.

Lichtenberg, P. A., Smith, M., Frazer, D., Molinari, V., Rosowsky, E., Crose, R., Stillwell, N., et al. (1998). Standards for psychological services in long-term care facilities. *The Gerontologist, 38:* 122–127.

Lipzin, B. (1992). Nursing home care. In J. E. Birren, R. B. Sloane, & G. Cohen (Eds.), *Handbook of mental health and aging* (2nd ed., pp. 833–852). San Diego: Academic.

Livesley, W. J. (2001). *Handbook of personality disorders: Theory, research, and treatment*. New York: Guilford.

Magai, C., & Passman, V. (1997). The interpersonal basis of emotional behavior and emotion regulation in adulthood. In M. P. Lawton, & K. Schaie (Eds.), *Annual review of geriatrics and gerontology* (Vol. 17, pp. 104–137).

McEwen, B. (1998). Protective and damaging effects of stress mediators. *New England Journal of Medicine, 338:* 171–179.

Miller, M. (1989). Opportunities for psychotherapy in the management of dementia. *Journal of Geriatric Psychiatry and Neurology, 2:* 11.

Molinari, V. (1999). Using reminiscence and life review as natural therapeutic strategies in group therapy. In M. Duffy (Ed.), *Handbook of counseling and psychotherapy with older adults* (pp. 154–165). New York: John Wiley & Sons.

Molinari, V. (Ed.). (2000). *Professional psychology in long term care*. New York: Hatherleigh Press.

Molinari, V., & Hartman-Stein, P. (2000). Psychologists in long-term care: Overview of practice and public policy: Introduction to the special series. *Clinical Psychology: Science and Practice, 7:* 312–316.

Moos, R. H. (Ed.). (1984). *Coping with physical illness 2: New perspectives*. New York: Plenum.

Moos, R. H., & Lemke, S. (1985). Specialized living environments for older people. In J. E. Birren, & K. W. Schaie (Eds.), *The handbook of the psychology of aging* (2nd ed., p. 864). New York: Van Nostrand Reinhold.

Moran, T. A., & Gatz, M. (1987). Group therapies for nursing home adults: An evaluation of two treatment approaches. *Gerontologist, 27:* 588.

Morgan, L. A., Gruber-Baldini, & A. L., Magaziner, J. (2001). Resident characteristics. In S. Zimmerman, P. D. Sloane, & J. K. Eckert (Eds.), *Assisted living* (pp. 144–172). Baltimore, MD: Johns Hopkins University Press.

Mossey, J. M., Knott, K. A., Higgins, M., & Talerico, K. (1996). Effectiveness of a psychosocial intervention, interpersonal counseling, for subdysthymic depression in medically ill elderly. *Journal of Gerontology: Medical Sciences, 51A:* 172–178.

Mumford, E., Schlesinger, H. J., & Glass, G. (1982). The effects of psychological intervention on recovery from surgery and heart attacks: An analysis of the literature. *American Journal of Public Health 72:* 141.

National Institutes of Health Consensus Development Panel on Depression in Late Life. (1992). Diagnosis and treatment of depression in late life. *Journal of the American Medical Association, 268:* 1018–1024.

Neimeyer, R. A. *(2001).* Reauthoring life narratives: Grief therapy as meaning reconstruction. *Israel Journal of Psychiatry & Related Sciences. 38(3–4): 171–183.*

Newton, N. A., & Jacobowitz, J. (1999). Transferential and counter-transferential processes in therapy with older adults. In M. Duffy (Ed.), *Handbook of counseling & psychotherapy with older adults* (pp. 21–40). New York: Wiley.

Newton, N., & Lazarus, L. (1992). Behavioral and psychotherapeutic interventions. In J. E. Birren, R. B. Sloane, & G. Cohen (Eds.), *Handbook of mental health and aging* (2nd ed., pp. 699–719). San Diego: Academic.

Neugarten, B. L. (1977). Time, age, and the life cycle. *American Journal of Psychiatry, 136:* 887.

Niederehe, G., & Schneider, L. S. (1998). Treatments for depression and anxiety in the aged. In P. E. Nathan, & J. M. Gorman (Eds.), *A guide to treatments that work* (pp. 270–287). New York: Oxford.

Nordhus, I. H., & Nielsen, G. H. (1999). Brief dynamic psychotherapy with older adults. *Journal of Clinical Psychology, 55:* 935–947.

Osgood, N., & Theilman, S. (1990). Geriatric suicidal behavior. In S. J. Blumenthal, & D. Kupfer (Eds.), *Suicide over the life cycle* (pp. 341–379). Washington DC: American Psychiatric Association Press.

Parmelee, P., Katz. I. R., & Lawton, M. P. (1989). Depression among institutionalized aged: Assessment and prevalence estimation. *Journal of Gerontology, 44:* 22.

Parmelee, P. A., & Lawton, M. P. (1990). The design of special environments for the aged. In J. E. Birren, & K. W. Schaie (Eds.), *Handbook of the psychology of aging* (3rd ed., p. 465). San Diego: Academic.

Perlmuter, L. C., & Eads, A. S. (1998). Control: Cognitive and motivational implications. In J. Lomranz (Ed.), *Handbook of aging and mental health: An integrative approach* (pp. 45–67). New York: Plenum.

Pollins, I. (1995). *Medical crisis counseling: Short-term therapy for long-term illness.* New York: Norton.

Power, C. A., & McCarron, L. T. (1975). Treatment of depression in persons residing in homes for the aged. *Gerontologist, 15:* 132.

Rattenbury, C., & Stones, M. J. (1989). A controlled evaluation of reminiscence and current topics discussion groups in a nursing home context. *Gerontologist, 29:* 768.

Reynolds, C. F., III, Frank, E., Perel, J. M., Imber, S. D., Cornes, C., Miller, M. D., Mazumdar, S., et al. (1999). Nortriptyline and interpersonal psychotherapy as maintenance therapies for recurrent major depression: A randomized controlled trial in patients older than 59 years. *Journal of the American Medical Association, 281:* 39–45.

Ripeckyj, A. J., & Lazarus, L. W. (1984). Management of old age—Psychotherapy: Individual, group, and family. In D. Kay, & G. Burrows (Eds.), *Handbook of studies on psychiatry and old age* (pp. 375–388). Amsterdam: Elsevier Science Publishers B. V.

Rodin, J., & Langer, E. (1977). Long-term effects of a control-relevant intervention. *Journal of Personality and Social Psychology, 35:* 891.

Ronch, J., & Maizler, J. (1977). Individual psychotherapy with the institutionalized aged. *American Journal of Orthopsychiatry 47:* 275–283.

Rosenblatt, A., Samus, Q. M., Steele, C. D., Baker, A. S., Harper, M. G., Brandt, H., Rabins, P. V., et al. (2004). The Maryland assisted living study: Prevalence, recognition, and treatment of dementia and other psychiatric disorders in the assisted living population of central Maryland. *Journal of American Geriatrics Society, 52:* 1618–1625.

Rosowsky, E., Abrams, R. C., & Zweig, R. A. (1999). *Personality disorders in older adults: Emerging issues in diagnosis and treatment.* Mahwah: Erlbaum.

Rovner, B. W., & Katz, I. R. (1993). Psychiatric disorders in the nursing home: A selective review of studies related to clinical care. *International Journal of Geriatric Psychiatry, 8:* 75–87.

Ruckdeschel, K., & Katz, I. R. (2004). Care of dementia and other mental disorders in assisted living facilities: New research and borrowed knowledge. *Journal of the American Geriatrics Society, 52,* 1771–1773.

Sadavoy, J., & Dorian, B. (1983). Treatment of the elderly characterologically disturbed patient in the chronic care institution. *Journal of Geriatric Psychiatry, 16:* 223.

Sadavoy, J. (1987). Character disorders in the elderly. In J. Sadavoy, & M. Leszcz (Eds.), *Treating the elderly with psychotherapy: The scope for change in later life* (pp. 175–229). Madison: International Universities Press.

Sadavoy, J., & Robinson, A. (1989). Psychotherapy and the cognitively impaired elderly. In D. E. Conn, A. Grek, & J. Sadavoy (Eds.), *Psychiatric consequences of brain disease in the elderly: A focus on management* (pp. 101–135). New York: Plenum.

Schulz, R., & Hanusa, B. H. (1979). Environmental influences on the effectiveness of control- and competence-enhancing interventions. In L. C. Perlmuter, & R. A. Monty (Eds.), *Choice and perceived control* (p. 315). Hillsdale, NJ: Erlbaum.

Scogin, F., & McElreath, L. (1994). Efficacy of psychosocial treatments for geriatric depression: A quantitative review. *Journal of Consulting and Clinical Psychology, 62:* 69–74.

Seligman, M. E. P. (1975) *Helplessness.* San Francisco: Freeman.

Shea, D. G., Smyer, M. A., & Streit, A. (1992, November): Receipt of mental health treatment by nursing home residents. Presented at the 45th Annual Meeting of the Gerontological Society of America, Washington DC.

Smith, M. C., & Kramer, N. A. (1992, November). Psychotherapy with persons with dementia. Paper presented at the Annual Meeting of the Gerontological Society of America, Washington DC.

Smith, M. L., Glass, G. V., & Miller, T. I. (1980). *The benefits of psychotherapy.* Baltimore: Johns Hopkins University Press.

Smyer, M. A., Zarit, S. H., & Qualls, S. H. (1990). Psychological intervention in the aging individual. In J. E. Birren, & K. W. Schaie (Eds.), *Handbook of the psychology of aging* (3rd ed., pp. 375–403). San Diego: Academic.

Snyder, C. R., & Ford, C. E. (Ed.). (1987). *Coping with negative life events.* New York: Plenum.

Solomon, K., & Szwabo, P. (1992). Psychotherapy for patients with dementia. In J. E. Morley, R. Coe, R. Strong, & G. T. Grossberg (Eds.), *Memory function and aging-related disorders* (pp. 295–319). New York: Springer.

Sotile, W. M., & Miller, H. S. (1998). Helping older patients to cope with cardiac and pulmonary disease. *Journal of Cardiopulmonary Rehabilitation, 18:* 124–128.

Spayd, C. S., & Smyer, M. A. (1988). Individual interventions for nursing home residents. In M. Smyer, M. Cohn, & D. Brannon (Eds.), *Mental health consultation in the nursing home* (pp. 100–122) New York: New York University Press.

Steurer, J. L., Mintz, J., Hammen, C. L., Hill, M. A., Jarvik, L. F., McCarley, T., Motike, P., et al. (1984). Cognitive behavioral and psychodynamic group psychotherapy in the treatment of geriatric depression. *Journal of Consulting and Clinical Psychology, 52:* 180.

Stowell, J. R., Kiecolt-Glaser, J. K., & Glaser, R. (2001). Perceived stress and cellular immunity: when coping counts. *Journal of Behavioral Medicine, 24:* 323–339.

Streim, J. E., & Katz, I. R. (2004). Clinical psychiatry in the nursing home. In D. G. Blazer, D. C. Steffens, E. W. Busse (Eds.), *Textbook of geriatric psychiatry* (3rd, pp. 139–161). Washington, DC: American Psychiatric Publishing.

Symister, P., & Friend, R. (2003). The influence of social support and problematic support on optimism and depression in chronic illness: A prospective study evaluating self-esteem as a mediator. *Health Psychology, 22:* 123–129.

Tedeschi, R. G., & Calhoun, L. G. (*1996*). The posttraumatic growth inventory: Measuring the positive legacy of trauma. *Journal of Traumatic Stress, 9(3):* 455–471.

Teeter, R. B., Garetz, F. K., Miller, W. R., & Heiland, W. F. (1976). Psychiatric disturbances of aged patients in skilled nursing homes. *American Journal of Psychiatry, 133:* 1430.

Teresi, J., Abrams, R., Holmes, D., et al. (2001). Prevalence of depression and depression recognition in nursing homes. *Social Psychiatry and Psychiatric Epidemiology, 36:* 613–620.

Thompson, L., Gallagher, D., & Breckenridge, J. (1987). Comparative effectiveness of psychotherapies for depressed elders. *Journal of Consulting Clinical Psychology, 52:* 385.

Thompson, L., Gallagher, D., & Czirr, R. (1988). Personality disorder and outcome in the treatment of late-life depression. *Journal of Geriatric Psychiatry, 21:* 133–146.

Timko, C. & Moos, R. H. (1991). A typology of social climates in group residential facilities for older. *Journal of Gerontology, 46:* S160–S169.

Tobin, S. (1989). Issues of care in long term settings. In D. E. Conn, A. Grek, & J. Sadavoy (Eds.), *Psychiatric consequences of brain disease in the elderly: A focus on management* (pp. 163–187). New York: Plenum.

Unterbach, D. (1994). An ego function analysis for working with dementia clients. *Journal of Gerontological Social Work, 22:* 83–94.

Unutzer, J., Katon, W., Callahan, C. M., Williams, J. W., Hunkeler, E., Harpole, L., Hoffing, M., et al. (2002). Collaborative care management of late-life depression in the primary care setting. *Journal of American Medical Association, 288:* 2836–2845.

Viederman, M., & Perry, S. W. (1980). Use of a psychodynamic life narrative in the treatment of depression in the physically ill. *General Hospital Psychiatry, 2:* 177.

Vine, R., & Steingart, A. (1994). Personality disorder in the elderly depressed. *Canadian Journal of Psychiatry, 39:* 392–398.

Watson, M., Haviland, J., Greer, S., Davidson, J., & Bliss, J. (1999). Influence of psychological response on survival in breast cancer: A population-based cohort study. *The Lancet, 35:* 1331–1136.

Wei, W., Sambamoorthi, U., Olfson, M., Walkup, J. T., & Crystal, S. (2005). Use of psychotherapy for depression in older adults. *American Journal of Psychiatry, 162:* 711–717.

Weissman, M. M., Markowitz, J. C., & Klerman, G. L. (2000). *Comprehensive guide to interpersonal psychotherapy.* New York: Basic Books.

Weissman, M., & Paykel, E. (1974). *The depressed woman.* Chicago: University of Chicago Press.

Wolk, R. L., & Goldfarb, A. I. (1967). The response to group psychotherapy of aged recent admissions compared with long term mental hospital patients. *American Journal of Psychiatry, 123:* 1251.

Wolkow, K. E., & Ferguson, H. B. (2001). Community factors in the development of resiliency: Consideration and future direction. *Community Mental Health Journal, 37:* 489–498.

Zweig, R. A. (2003). Personality disorders in older adults: Managing the difficult patient. *Clinical Geriatrics, 11:* 22–25.

Zweig, R. A., & Agronin, M. (2006). Personality disorders. In M. E. Agronin, & G. J. Maletta (Eds.), *Principles and practice of geriatric psychiatry* (pp. 449–469). York, PA: Lippincott, Williams, & Wilkins.

Zweig, R. A., Hinrichsen, G. A.(1993). Factors associated with suicide attempts in depressed older adults: A prospective study. *American Journal of Psychiatry, 150:* 1687–1692.

15

Cognitive and Behavioral Therapy

Jurgis Karuza and *Paul R. Katz*

This chapter provides an overview of cognitive and behavioral interventions primarily in nursing home settings. The first section defines behavioral and cognitive therapies, and discusses their need with frail elderly institutionalized populations. The next section presents a selected review of the empirical literature on behavioral and cognitive interventions in nursing homes. The final section discusses issues in the implementation of these procedures in nursing homes. Although increasing numbers of older adults are residing in assisted-living facilities, and the prevalence of dementia, behavioral problems, and depression are high (e.g., Guber-Baldini, Boustani, Sloane and Zimmerman, 2004), there are few studies examining the effectiveness of cognitive and behavioral-based interventions specifically in assisted-living facilities. A reasonable expectation would be that cognitive and behavioral therapeutic approaches could be implemented effectively in assisted-living settings, but additional empirical work is needed to determine the generalizability of these approaches, especially given the different staffing and organizational structure, and regulatory environment, in assisted-living facilities.

COGNITIVE AND BEHAVIORAL THERAPY—AN OVERVIEW

Behavior Therapy

Behavior Therapy represents a collection of interventions that focus on identifying specific behavioral problems associated with clients' presenting complaints, and teaching clients to change these behaviors. Often defined as the application of learning principles to the treatment of maladaptive behavior (e.g., Krasner, 1971), behavior therapy draws its theoretical roots from operant and classical conditioning (e.g., Pavlov, 1927; Skinner, 1974; Watson, 1925), social learning theory (Bandura, 1977, 1986), and others. These theories have generated a range of behavioral interventions, such as systematic desensitization, biofeedback, social skills training, and lifestyle modification approaches.

There are two key characteristics of a behavioral approach. The first is the reliance on a functional analysis of behavior. Psychological and behavioral dysfunctions are viewed as resulting from learning experiences in which the environment shapes and reinforces maladaptive behavior. In changing the undesired behaviors, behavior therapists and clients attempt to alter these environmental factors, and build in new prompts and reinforcement for desired behaviors. Therapists and clients typically work as partners in this effort, and use the outcomes of these interventions to guide further treatment efforts.

A second defining characteristic of behavioral interventions is the focus on clearly specifying the treatment, assessing the outcome (e.g., Mahoney, 1974) and conducting controlled outcome studies to evaluate the effectiveness of behavioral interventions. Further, when interventions are shown to be effective, a clear protocol for implementation is typically provided so that the procedures can be replicated in other settings.

The fields of Behavioral Gerontology (e.g., Burgio and Burgio, 1986) and Behavioral Geriatrics (Hussian, 1984) have applied these behavioral approaches to older populations. These interventions are used to treat specific response deficits, such as appropriate voiding, good hygiene, self-care, ambulation, and social interaction. Such behaviors are often amenable to specific behavior therapy techniques, and do not require more lengthy and costly psychotherapies that focus on large-scale personality modifications (Hussian, 1984).

Cognitive Therapy

From the perspective of cognitive-based therapeutic approaches, the underlying cognitions of a person influence their mental health problem, such as depression. It is assumed that negative emotions and maladaptive behaviors result from maladaptive thoughts. It follows, then, that treating mental health problems requires modifying the patient's cognitions. A variety of approaches have been developed to directly or indirectly restructure the ways patients think about themselves, their problems, and their lives. One example is Ellis' Rational Emotional Therapy (Ellis, 1962), which views negative emotions and inappropriate behavior as resulting from illogical thinking. Another is Meichenbaum's (1977) Self-instructional Trainings, which changes patients' thoughts about themselves by teaching patients to talk to themselves in more positive and constructive ways. A third example is Beck's Cognitive Behavior Therapy (Beck, 1984), which helps patients to identify, challenge, and reinterpret the illogical and negative thoughts and self-perceptions that underlie depression (Beck and Young, 1985).

A common theme running through these approaches is that patients can be consciously aware of their thought patterns and that there is little need for analytic interpretation by the therapist, as in more classic psychotherapeutic approaches. Although the therapist style varies, from more directive in Rational Emotive Therapy, to more Socratic in Cognitive Behavior Therapy, the relationship between therapist and patient is a collaborative one, with the patient assuming a major role in the therapeutic effort. This is in contrast to more psychoanalytic approaches where the therapist is, in effect, the active therapeutic agent of change. Although behavioral-based approaches and cognitive-based approaches use behavioral change methods, cognitive-based approaches see behavior change as a means to achieve cognitive change rather than an end "in and of" itself.

Rationale for Cognitive and Behavioral Therapies in Nursing Homes

Cognitive and behavioral therapies in nursing homes are types of nonpharamacologic interventions. Several reviews (e.g., Camp, Cohen-Mansfield, and Capezuti, 2002; Cody, Beck, and Svarstad, 2002; Cohen-Mansfield, 2005; 2001; Snowden, Sato, Roy-Byrne, 2003; Verkaik, van Weert, and Francke, 2005) discuss the variety of interventions developed, such as sensory stimulation, social interaction, and environmental interventions, and the range of problems addressed, such as reducing agitated behavior, and improving affect and function. A number of studies have been published, most demonstrating modest positive effects. However, drawing conclusions from this literature can be problematic since the studies are frequently underpowered, rely on weaker, nonrandomized controlled designs, and fall prey to subject selection biases and measurement validity concerns.

The prevalence of psychological and behavioral problems in nursing homes defines a clear need for these nonpharmacological interventions, including behavior and cognitive therapies. Historically, the prevalence rates for depression among nursing home residents have ranged from 11% to 78%, depending on the severity of the disorder (e.g., Jones, Marcantonio, and Lusti, 2002; Parmalee, Katz, and Lawton, 1992; Schnelle, Wood, and Schnelle, 2001; Teresi, et al., 2001). In a recent survey of Ohio nursing home residents, Levin et al. (2007) found 48% of residents with an active depression diagnosis. Compounding the problem is the frequent underdiagnosis and undertreatment of depression in nursing homes (Brown, Lapne, & Lusti, 2002; Burns et al., 1993; Smyer, Shea, & Streit, 1994) and in assisted-living settings (Magsi and Malloy, 2005). Further, a survey of skilled nursing facilities conducted by Zimmer, Watson, and Treat (1984) found that 64% of residents had significant behavior problems, and 23% were described as having serious behavior problems. A similar high frequency of functional problems, such as incontinence, ambulation difficulties, was reported by Burgio and Burgio (1986). Undertreatment of these depressive and behavioral problems creates additional risks for nursing home patients including functional decline, increased hospitalization, decreased quality of life, and mortality (American Geriatrics Society and American Association of Geriatric Psychiatry, 2003).

At the same time, consideration of cognitive and behavioral interventions is reinforced by the Nursing Home Reform Act that was part of the Omnibus Budget Reconciliation Act of 1987 and various professional guidelines, such as the American Geriatric Society's position statement on psychotherapeutic medications in the nursing home (American Geriatrics Society, 1997), which discourages the indiscriminant use of psychotropic drugs and encourages the use of nonpharmacological treatments. Recent studies point out the danger of offsetting adverse effects associated with atypical antipsychotic drugs (Schneider et al., 2006), and suggest that non pharmacological interventions may be more acceptable to nursing home residents (Burgio & Sinnott, 1990). Cognitive and behavioral therapies particularly are useful for dealing with at least two general types of disorders. First, they can address a variety of functional issues and include interventions to enhance autonomy and activities of daily living (ADLs) and decrease disruptive or assaultive behaviors that may be secondary to dementia. Second, they can target the range of mental health and psychiatric disorders such as depression and dementia.

REVIEW OF STUDIES ON BEHAVIORAL AND COGNITIVE THERAPIES IN NURSING HOMES

The sections below provide a selected review of behavioral and cognitive therapies in nursing homes. Although the literature on cognitive and behavioral therapies in nursing home settings is limited, existing research supports the viability of a number of specific approaches (for additional reviews of earlier studies, see Hussian, 1984; Burgio & Burgio, 1986; Karuza & Katz, 1991; for specific intervention protocols, see Lundervold & Lewin, 1992). Additional new work from the Maryland Assisted Living Study (Lyketsos et al., 2007; Rosenblatt et al.,

2007) that demonstrates the impact of dementia and dementia treatment on resident outcomes, suggest promising avenues for research.

Functional Issues

Exercise/ambulation

Physical activity and physical fitness have been related to reduced mortality for the population in general (Blair et al., 1989) and for older adults specifically (Rakowski and Mor, 1992). Exercise may exert its protective effect through its impact on coronary artery disease, blood pressure, glucose metabolism and insulin resistance, bone density, and other factors. Further, exercise can improve muscle strength and function, which is particularly relevant for older populations who are at risk for falls, fractures, and reduction in ADLs related to muscle dysfunction (Fiatarone and Evans, 1993). Finally, exercise has been shown to enhance psychological function in older adults (Powell, 1974). Behavioral interventions to increase exercise among nursing home patients have typically targeted ambulation, muscle strength, and flexibility/endurance (Baum et al., 2003).

Ambulation. Ambulation studies have demonstrated that walking can be increased through simple behavioral procedures. An early study by MacDonald and Butler (1974), using a single-subject design, showed that verbal prompts to walk, and interaction with staff contingent on walking, increased ambulation in two nursing home residents who had been previously transported by wheelchair. Burgio et al. (1986) extended these procedures to eight nursing home residents who were physically capable of walking but were transported to meals by wheelchair. Nursing home staff was trained to prompt subjects to walk from the entrance to the dining area to the table, and to verbally reinforce any walking. Significant increases in walking occurred and were maintained through the 4-month follow-up. Further, as the study progressed, seven of the subjects did not require staff assistance for most sessions.

Muscle strength. The position statement of the American College of Sports Medicine (1990) includes recommendations for both muscle-strengthening as well as endurance exercises for adults of all ages. Several studies have demonstrated that high-intensity resistance training produces dramatic increases in muscle strength in older individuals, including frail elderly up to 100 years of age (Fiatarone & Evans, 1993). Using an 8-week weight-lifting protocol based on standard rehabilitation principles of progressive-resistance training, Fiatarone et al. (1990) showed significant increases in muscle strength, size, and functional mobility among 10 frail nursing home residents averaging 90 years of age. Subjects exercised three times per week, with three sets of eight repetitions per leg at each session. The load was adjusted to provide 50% of a one-repetition maximum in the first week, and 80% at subsequent weeks. Such high-intensity protocols may be necessary, as little or no increase in muscle strength has been shown with low- to moderate-resistance training in older adults. Effective implementation of exercise programs can be enhanced by incorporation of behavioral and cognitive approaches to motivate and reinforce patients' initiating and maintaining weight lifting. Such techniques include provider education and encouragement of patients, using patient-determined daily weight-lifting goals (within provider-set guidelines), and the provision of feedback on patient progress.

Flexibility/endurance. A behavioral procedure to enhance stationary bicycle riding was reported by Perkins et al. (1986). Subjects were eight male residents in a nursing home care unit at the Jackson Mississippi V A Medical Center, who ranged from 46 to 78 years of age. Treatment involved prompting bicycle riding through posting distance goals and providing immediate feedback and gold stars to subjects on whether these goals were met, providing colored buttons for met goals during the first 3 weeks, providing T-shirts for 4 consecutive weeks of met goals, and announcing successful exercisers in an in-house newsletter distributed to staff and residents. Prompts and rewards were gradually eliminated over time to examine maintenance of exercise. Results showed significant increases in bicycle riding during the course of treatment, which was consistently maintained in six of eight subjects. Although health outcomes were not assessed, this study supported the effectiveness of behavioral strategies in promoting exercise in nursing home residents. Improved grip strength, spinal flexion, chair-to-stand time, ADLs, and self-rating of depression were reported for 20 nursing home residents following a 7-month program of twice-weekly 45-minute exercise sessions (McMurdo & Rennie, 1993). Exercise involved repetitive upper- and lower-limb range of motion and muscle strengthening in a seated position. Notable in this study was the 64% to 100% attendance rate (averaging 91%) at sessions and the 75% completion rate for exercise participants at 7 months.

Overall, exercise interventions appear to be both physiologically sound and feasible for even frail nursing home residents. Sample sizes in most studies reviewed were small, and further research is needed to identify strategies to enhance maintenance of exercise in older (as well as younger) populations. Nevertheless, a number of behavioral approaches to implementing programs to enhance activity are currently available for incorporation in nursing home settings.

Incontinence

One of the most serious problems in nursing home residents is incontinence, with prevalence rates pegged at 50% (Mohide, 1986). The economic cost of managing incontinence in 2000 has been estimated at $2.85 billion a year in institutions (Hu et al., 2003). Typically, the problem is assumed to be an inevitable and irreversible consequence of aging and treated by use of long-term indwelling catheters or diapers. With attendant risks of infection and skin ulceration, neither of these approaches is ideal. Behavioral-based approaches offer the promise of being effective management alternatives for at least some residents.

At the outset, it is important to distinguish among the common types of incontinence, since the relevance and effectiveness of behavioral techniques will vary with the type of incontinence. Of the four basic types of persistent urinary incontinence—overflow, stress, urge, and functional incontinence-behavioral interventions are seen as potentially relevant for all but overflow incontinence, which typically requires surgical intervention or catheterization (Ouslander, 1991).

A number of behavioral techniques have been developed that vary in the involvement of the patient and staff members. These have been described extensively elsewhere (e.g., Burgio & Burgio, 1986; National Institutes of Health Consensus Development Conference, 1990; Ouslander, 1991) and include pelvic muscle exercises, biofeedback, bladder training, bladder retraining, and prompted voiding.

Pelvic muscle exercises. This approach provides exercises that strengthen the pelvic floor muscles; it results in greater closing force on the urethra. The efficacy of this treatment has ranged from 30% to 90% in reported studies (Wells, 1990).

Biofeedback techniques. Biofeedback has been used to teach patients to exert greater control over urine storage. Patients are given muscle exercises and are provided with immediate feedback on how well they are controlling sphincter, detrusor, and abdominal muscles. Patients with stress or urge incontinence benefit from these techniques, with complete control achieved by 20% of the patients and improvement in urinary control found in an additional 30% (National Institutes of Health Consensus Development Conference, 1990).

Bladder training. This approach teaches patients to void at regular times during the day. The logic is to "catch the patient" before the incontinence occurs. This is especially relevant to those patients who suffer from urge and functional incontinence. Cure rates of 10% to 15% have been found using these techniques (National Institutes of Health Consensus Development Conference, 1990).

Bladder retraining. This method attempts to restore the normal pattern of urination by teaching the patient to gradually expand the intervals between voiding by techniques such as learning to resist the sensation of urgency or developing a voiding schedule by the clock (Burgio & Burgio, 1986). To be successful, bladder retraining interventions call for a patient who is cooperative and motivated and who has sufficient mental function to participate in the training program. Overall, studies of bladder training efficacy report high cure rates, ranging from 44% to 90%. The outcomes, however, do vary with initial bladder capacity (Burgio & Burgio, 1986). Although this approach is more demanding on the patient, it has the advantage of less direct staff involvement.

Prompted voiding. In this approach, staff members develop a frequent void-ing schedule for residents, periodically check the residents' dryness, prompt the resident to void, and reinforce the resident for voiding. Although the typical schedule for prompted voiding is 1 to 2 hours, it has been suggested that a less intensive 3-hour schedule may be effective for some residents (Burgio et al., 1994).

Prompted voiding has been shown to be most relevant for incontinence that is due to the poor functional level of patients. Up to 75% of all nursing home patients show significant reductions in incontinence with this procedure (Schnelle, 1990; Schnelle et al., 1983). More recent reviews (e.g., Eustice Roe & Paterson, 2000) indicate only limited evidence of prompted voiding effective-ness in the short term, much less in the long term.

Although behavioral techniques have been found to have the greatest potential for success, several caveats should be noted. Most of the studies on the efficacy of behavioral techniques have been tested on younger, community-based, more functional adults (Burgio & Burgio, 1986). The rates of efficacy with nursing home residents are less clear. The cost-effectiveness of behavioral techniques compared to other approaches, such as use of diapers, is also a consideration (Schnelle et al., 1993). A major barrier to the success of behavioral techniques is the cognitive impairment and low level of functioning of residents (Ouslander, 1990, 1991). An important consideration in maximizing the effectiveness of behavioral approaches to the management of incontinence in nursing homes is the appropriate selection of patients who can benefit from behavioral techniques and the development of an effective staff organization to monitor and implement the intervention. Guidelines for the selection process and specific intervention procedures are available (e.g., Schnelle et al., 1993).

Bathing

Downs and colleagues tested two modeling interventions to reduce avoid-ance of whirlpool baths among nursing home residents (Downs et al., 1988). Residents, who had previously demonstrated apprehension and resistance toward the lifting and lowering of their chairs (needed to enter and exit the whirlpool bath), were randomized to one of two modeling conditions, participant mod-eling or filmed modeling, or to no treatment. Participant modeling involved breaking the bath time into small, incremental steps that the therapist demon-strated and the residents then practiced with verbal reinforcement and assistance as needed. Participant modeling was conducted in both group and individual formats. Filmed modeling involved presenting the same information as in par-ticipant modeling but using a film of peers demonstrating these procedures. Consistent with empirical guidelines, filmed models first displayed apprehen-siveness about the bath but then modeled coping skills that enabled them to complete the bathing routine successfully. Both modeling approaches have been shown to be effective for a range of fears and avoidance behaviors (Bandura, 1986). Results showed the greatest improvements with participant modeling, followed by filmed modeling, and no significant change for the no-treatment group. Participant modeling appeared most effective when administered in individual format, as single residents who remained fearful were shown to disrupt the progress of other group members. Further, some family members objected to the group bathing format, even though groups consisted of same-sex residents and residents remained clothed throughout the procedure. The authors suggest means of reducing barriers to group participant modeling, including screening or pretraining the most disruptive residents, and preceding participant modeling with filmed modeling of both individual and group approaches. In a more recent study (Hoeffer et al., 2006), certified nursing assistants who received training in a person-centered approach that could be used when bathing agitated, demented residents were more likely to demonstrate more gentle and verbal support behaviors and experience less distressed behaviors from the resident during bathing, compared to control groups.

Eating

There is some evidence that eating dependency among nursing home residents can be successfully addressed by employing behavioral interventions (Baltes & Zerbe, 1976; Lewin et al., 1989). For example, in a series of single-case design studies by Lewin et al. (1989), behavioral techniques were successful in reducing food dependence in two of three severely cognitively impaired female nursing home residents. A behavioral strategy of prompting coupled with social reinforcement was used with two women who were largely dependent on staff for feeding. The intervention was successful with one woman, who increased her rate of independent feeding behaviors at meals from 25% to 50% during baseline to 75% to 100% following the intervention. The third woman, who fed herself independently but had low food intake at meals, was found to significantly increase her food consumption after an intervention that consisted of serving her preferred foods in small containers and giving her verbal praise for eating. In a related vein, Simmons, Alessi, and Schnelle (2001) found that a behavioral intervention consisting of verbal prompts was effective increasing the fluid intake in cognitively impaired nursing home residents

These case studies show the promise of behavioral interventions as ways to increase the feeding independence of nursing home residents. The pattern of results also highlights the difficulty of implementing behavioral strategies with residents who are severely impaired cognitively. The paucity of recent studies examining behavioral approaches to facilitate feeding independence among nursing home residents is puzzling, given the prevalence of feeding dependence and its associated costs. Further work is clearly needed to develop and evaluate new behavioral techniques.

Psychiatric Disorders

Dementia

Behavioral interventions have targeted several behavioral and cognitive difficulties associated with dementia, including conversational skills, wandering/inappropriate behaviors, and disruptive/assaultive behaviors.

Conversational skills. Memory aids have been one approach used to improve patterns of conversation with demented patients. For example, using a single-subject design, Bourgeois (1993) reported that a "memory book" consisting of simple statements and photographs of familiar people and events resulted in improved quality of conversations between pairs of demented patients. Similarly, providing a card with a listing of relevant names or daily routines, combined with prompting to use the card, increased conversation among residents (Bourgeois, 1990).

Wandering/inappropriate behaviors. Hussian (1988) used environmental cues and verbal prompts with five demented male patients in an attempt to reduce inappropriate voiding, climbing into the beds of other patients, entering the nursing station, and attempting to leave a protective environment; these techniques were also used to increase ability to locate relevant ward items (e.g., patient's own bed). Cues included a bright yellow sign on the door of the rest room, a bright sign with the patient's name over his bed, tape on the floor in front of the exit door, and colored signs near other relevant ward items. During the first phase of study, staff prompted the patients to attend to the cues; in a subsequent phase, cues alone were provided. All patients showed at least an 86% improvement in problem behaviors relative to periods when no interventions were provided; these improvements persisted even when cues alone (without prompts) were provided. Similarly, Hussian and Brown (1987) demonstrated that placing an eight-strip grid of clearly visible, horizontal masking tape stripes 57.2 cm from exit doors significantly reduced exiting from the ward by demented patients. The investigators attribute this effect to the observation that demented patients often see two-dimensional patterns as three dimensional and thus pause or stop at flat grid patterns that nondemented patients would cross over.

These interventions are relatively straightforward and logical. In settings in which hallways and rooms look alike, the environment is handicapping, particularly to cognitively impaired patients. Patients can easily become confused about which is the correct room to enter or exit. Changing the environment by providing clear signs identifying key areas, combined with staff reinforcement of the patients' attending to these signs or, in some cases, providing clear floor grids, produces clear changes in patient behavior. Whether these changes will be maintained over long periods of time using the above protocols or whether additional maintenance efforts are needed remains to be studied.

Disruptive/assaultive behaviors. Behavioral models and approaches for decreasing disruptive and assaultive behaviors among nursing home patients have been described. For example, Cariaga et al. (1991) identified specific impairments among disruptive vocalizers as well as staff-reported utilization and perceived effectiveness of various existing interventions. Using a behavior-analytic perspective and drawing from literature with other populations, the authors suggested behavioral interventions that could be tested for dealing with this clinically meaningful problem. In addition, Lundervold and Lewin (1992) provide specific examples of behavioral programs for decreasing such inappropriate behaviors.

Reducing aggression during bathing was described by Lundervold and Lewin (1992). The resident was an elderly woman with Alzheimer's disease in a foster care setting who would bite, hit, and/or pinch her caregiver during the morning routine of bathing and dressing. These behaviors would occur while she was sitting, with caregivers leaning in front of her to undress, toilet, sponge-bathe, and dress her. To change this routine, the resident was instructed to stand facing away from the caregiver and hold onto the towel bar to prevent herself from falling. If she let go of the bar, the caregiver lowered her to the floor so she would not injure herself and instructed her to stand and grab the bar again. For bathing, the resident was placed in the bath, again facing away from the caregiver and holding onto the bar, and instructed to wash herself with her other hand. This new routine had several features: by having the resident face away from the caregiver, it removed a stimulus for hitting (i.e., having the caregiver bend down in front of the resident), and having the resident hold onto the bar and bathe herself did not leave her hands free to harm the caregiver. Additional evidence for the effectiveness of nursing assistant–based behavioral treatment approach to reduce agitation and behavioral disturbance of residents can be seen in a study of a dementia care units (Lichtenberg, Kemp-Havican, Macneill, & Schafer Johnson, 2005) and a study of staff behaviors during personal care routines (Roth, Sevens, Burgio, & Burgio, 2002).

Depression

Behavioral approaches

Behavioral approaches typically view depression as resulting from a loss of previous reinforcers (Lewinsohn, 1974), a process particularly salient in frail, institutionalized patients. Treatment focuses on helping patients increase the availability of pleasant activities. Goddard and Carstensen (1986) applied this approach to the treatment of an 86-year-old depressed nursing home resident who was confined to a wheelchair and had recently broken her wrist. An applied behavior analysis indicated significant loss of reinforcers, particularly during morning and evening hours. Treatment involved increasing the patient's access to self-initiated pleasant activities (identified by the patient), with special focus on the morning and evening, and verbally reinforcing her positive self-statements and actions. Improvements were found in daily mood ratings, which persisted through a 6-week follow-up. Anecdotally, staff and visitors commented about the positive changes in the patient. It should be noted, however, that her score on the Geriatric Depression Scale (Brink et al., 1982), though improved, was still in the mildly depressed range.

Cognitive therapy for depression

Behavioral therapy targets patients' negative beliefs and maladaptive means of processing information. Depressed patients are viewed as having negative beliefs about themselves as failures, the world as joyless, and the future as hopeless resulting from cognitive errors (Beck, 1967). Therapy focuses on helping patients recognize and test these negative beliefs, and develop more adaptive styles for viewing the world. Beck (1967) identifies six such systematic cognitive errors:

1. *All or none thinking.* The tendency to view things in black and white terms.
2. *Overgeneralizaton.* Tendency toward broad sweeping conclusions.
3. *Arbitrary inference.* Tendency to draw unwarranted negative conclusions from available information—jumping to conclusions.
4. *Personalization.* Taking personal responsibility for negative events that are beyond the person's control.
5. *Magnification and minimization.* Tendency to overestimate the importance of negative events and minimizing the significance of positive events.
6. *Selective abstraction.* Tendency to focus on negative details of situations and take them out of context.

These logical errors are evident in the "automatic thoughts" that are habitual and often go unnoticed in depressed patients. These thoughts come between things that happen to a person and their emotional reaction. A major goal of cognitive therapy is to have patients notice their automatic thinking and not accept it on face value.

The main components of cognitive therapy are to teach patients

- to identify their automatic thought patterns
- to challenge their negative and illogical thoughts
- to interpret events more rationally.

Developing a friendly and mutually respectful therapeutic relationship is important so that the interrelations among the patient's thoughts, feelings, and actions can be explored and changed. These nonspecific therapeutic ingredients help foster the collaborative relationship between patient and therapist (Thompson et al., 1986). The therapist, while expected to be a critical thinker, should not force the patient into accepting the therapist's point of view.

At the start of treatment it is recommended (Newman & Beck, 1990) that a comprehensive diagnostic evaluation be given to make sure that the depression is not secondary to another psychological disorder, or that there is not an underlying organic disorder, such as hypothroidism, that should be considered. The severity of the depression, especially if it is associated with suicidal tendency, should be determined. In more severe cases, medication may be indicated. Cognitive therapy is short term. An average of 12 to 16 sessions is typically reported in outcome studies (e.g., Beck et al., 1985). Patient age (Jarrett et al., 1991; Sotsky et al., 1991), and intelligence (Haaga et al., 1991) have been found to be unrelated to cognitive therapy outcome, although these conclusions are best treated as preliminary (Whisman, 1993).

Cognitive therapy has been done with older people individually and in groups (Thompson, et al., 1986). The first session typically focuses on developing the therapeutic rapport, defining the problem and setting the goals of the treatment and educating the patient about the relationship between thoughts, moods, and behaviors that are part of the cognitive therapy model. Early on, patients are taught self observational skills to help identify automatic thinking. Often patients are given "homework" where they track frequent negative thoughts or record their thoughts in depressive situations in a "Daily Thought Record." In addition to describing upsetting thoughts, patients are asked to write down more objective and adaptive thoughts they may have and to document any improvements in their moods. Although potentially effective, some patients may have qualms about doing homework. In keeping with the collaborative nature of the therapy, the therapist should not "order" the patient to do homework, and make sure that the homework is tied to the content of the sessions.

A major component in cognitive therapy is to teach patients to challenge their automatic thoughts and to generate new more accurate and adaptive ones. Patients are taught to question themselves when they have upsetting thoughts by asking questions such as "What evidence is there to support or refute my thoughts?" "How else could I view this situation?" "Realistically, what is the worst thing that could happen in this situation?," and "Even if there is reason to believe that my depressing viewpoint is warranted, what can I do to help remedy the situation?" (Newman & Beck, 1990). Other techniques used to challenge the thinking of patients include role playing, the therapist playing "devil's advocate" arguing in favor the patient's negative thoughts.

Use of imagery techniques can be helpful in altering negative belief systems. In using imagery, patients are asked to imagine life in the future, solving current problems, or effectively dealing with threatening situations. Also common to cognitive therapy is the use of behavioral techniques, especially at the start of therapy. Techniques such as developing schedules for activities, assertiveness practice, and problem-solving techniques are used to engage the patient in changing his or her behavior in constructive ways and to overcome the negative and hopeless views patients have that come with lethargy and inactivity.

Fears of relapse are not uncommon. Thompson et al. (1986) recommend several ways to deal with relapse including, reinterpreting a mild depressive episode as a chance to practice the skills learned in therapy, or scheduling a few "booster" sessions a month apart before the termination of therapy.

The effectiveness of behavioral and cognitive-behavioral therapies for depression has been clearly demonstrated for the population in general (e.g., Elkin et al., 1989; Sotsky, et al., 1991), as well as for the elderly (e.g., Gallagher & Thompson, 1982, 1983; Thompson, et al., 1987). Most of the research has focused on unipolar depression. Less clear is the effectiveness of cognitive therapies with bipolar disorders and dysthymia, the so-called depressive personality, (Newman & Beck, 1990). Outcome studies that compare cognitive therapy to pharmacotherapy, provide additional evidence for the attractiveness of cognitive therapy with adults (Dobson, 1993) and more specifically in older adults. Jarvik et al. (1982), compared older adult outpatients who were diagnosed as having a major depressive disorder and were treated with tricyclic antidepressants to a placebo group and to patients assigned to psychodynamic or cognitive/behavioral therapy that were conducted in groups. After 26 weeks of treatment, the patients receiving the tricyclics improved compared to the placebo group. About one-third of the patients who received the psychotherapies showed some improvement, but only 12% showed clear remission of their depression as measured by the Hamilton Rating Scale for Depression (Hamilton, 1967). Steuer et al. (1984) found 40% of the patients who went through a 9-month course of cognitive/behavioral or psychodynamic therapy went into remission. Beutler et al. (1987) compared group cognitive therapy with supportive intervention, and a pharmacological treatment using Alprazol, a minor tranquilizer. Improvement in depression was found under all treatments, with the greatest improvement found in the cognitive therapy group.

Other studies have found Cognitive Behavioral Therapeutic approaches to be effective in treatment of generalized anxiety disorders in older adults (Wetherell, Gatz, & Craske, 2003), discontinuation of benzodiazepine among adults with generalized anxiety disorder (Goesselin et al. 2006), and treatment of persistent insomnia in general practice patients (Espie et al., 2007).

Taken together, these results indicate that in older adults, short-term psychotherapeutic interventions, including cognitive therapy, can be effective in treating older adults.

Cognitive therapy in the nursing home

The track record of cognitive therapy would suggest that it would be effective with nursing home resident. Still, there is some question whether the effectiveness of cognitive therapy in treating community-based adults generalizes to treating institutionalized older adults, many with dementia. The irony is that given the prevalence of depression among nursing home residents there has been a paucity of controlled studies of cognitive interventions with nursing home residents.

One exception is the study by Abraham et al., (1992) that examined group-based psychotherapeutic-based interventions in nursing homes. Using a controlled study they tested the effectiveness of nurse-led 24-week cognitive, focused imagery, and discussion group interventions with depressed patients. Subjects were enrolled if they had a score of 11 or higher on the Geriatric Depression Scale (or a score of 10 with clinical evidence of depressive symptomlogy), had sufficient hearing, verbal, and comprehension skill to participate in group session, absence of major cognitive impairment, absence of antidepressant medication, and no history of endogenous depression. Although no significant changes were found in depression, hopelessness or life satisfaction scores for the patients enrolled in the three treatment groups, there were significant increases in cognitive scores after treatment in the cognitive therapy and focused visual imagery groups. In an interesting tangential study Cook (1998) found Cognitive Behavioral Therapy was effective in managing the chronic pain of nursing home residents without serious cognitive impairment.

SOME CONSIDERATIONS FOR BEHAVIORAL AND COGNITIVE THERAPY IN THE NURSING HOME

Clearly, more controlled studies that compare behavioral and cognitive therapies to pharmacological interventions as well as to other psychotherapeutic approaches in nursing homes are called for. Nevertheless, the broader positive results with these therapies for depressed patients in general, and the positive changes noted in nursing home residents, make behavioral and cognitive-behavioral therapies potentially usable as treatment options for depression in nursing home patients.

A major advantage of both behavioral and cognitive therapies for nursing home residents is that they provide an alternative to pharmacological treatment, with its attendant dangers of polypharmacy. (The reader is referred to Chapter 14 for a more complete discussion of depression, and to Chapter 13 for psychopharmacological considerations.) The range of medical conditions, medications, difficult life situations, and psychosocial issues that are particularly prevalent in nursing home residents underscores the importance of incorporating cognitive and behavioral therapies rather than relying on pharmacological management alone.

The importance of assessment and targeting the use of cognitive therapy with patients with the best prognosis is important. Several studies and reviews have pointed out (Newman & Beck, 1990; Thompson et al., 1986; Thompson et al., 1990) that cognitive therapies may not be optimal or sufficient by themselves for severe depression, especially when coupled with suicidal ideation, bipolar disorders, dysthymic disorders, or depression overlayed by dysthymia or dementia. Rather than argue for cognitive therapies being a panacea, cognitive therapy should remain a potential treatment of choice in certain cases.

Some concerns temper an unbridled enthusiasm for cognitive therapies. As Thompson et al. (1986), and others raise (Gatz & Smyer, 1992; Smyer, et al., 1990), there may be special considerations in doing cognitive therapy with older adults especially in institutional long-term-care environments. The prevalence of perceptual problems, mild cognitive impairments, and decreased ability to retain new information, and reduced functional levels in older adults may make it more difficult to teach and practice the skills that are part of cognitive therapy. This problem is compounded in nursing homes, which typically have a more frail and disabled population. Compensatory strategies can offset some of these problems, such as making physical adjustments, e.g., brighter lighting, use of big print, or restructuring the cognitive training by adopting many of the "tricks" that have been found to improve learning and memory, such as building in redundancy and repetition in presentation of material, frequent practice and rehearsal opportunities for patients and frequent reinforcement of the patients (Thompson, et al., 1986). Thompson et al (1986), also recommend leveling with the older adult, offering a balanced presentation to the older adult patient which clearly states that cognitive therapy may be difficult but not beyond the grasp of most older adults.

An added consideration in developing both cognitive and behavioral therapeutic approaches is the tendency for older adults and their family to shift responsibility for the cure of the problem onto the health professional (Karuza, et al., 1992). This tendency, if anything, can be expected to be more pronounced in a nursing home, with its "medical" overtones, and the tendency of staff to reinforce dependent behaviors (Baltes et al., 1983). Given the dynamics of cognitive and behavioral therapy, such a passive stance by older adults may make it difficult to develop collaborative therapeutic relationships between therapists and patients. Setting up the ground rules, assumptions, and expectations of these therapies at the outset becomes very important.

PERSPECTIVES: KEEP IT SIMPLE (KIS) IS OFTEN BEST

A range of physical, mental health, and adjustment problems are responsive to formal interventions, which include behavioral and cognitive as well as more traditional medical and psychiatric/psychological therapies. However, it is important to note that "just because a hammer is available, not every problem is necessarily a nail." These points have been made by several authors in poignant ways. The late B. F. Skinner, a father of behavioral approaches, provided a series of behavioral insights on his own aging (e.g., Skinner, 1983; Skinner and Vaughan, 1983), in which he described a number of minor and practical environmental adjustments to compensate for changing capacities associated with aging. Similarly, Oneal (1986) presented a series of case studies illustrating the sometimes easily overlooked simple solutions. For example, she described a nursing home resident who refused to remain in bed at night. Instead, this resident continuously jumped up, ripped off her nightgown, and walked around the room nude and mumbling. The author ultimately determined that the resident hated the nightgown, which had been a gift from a sister whom she also hated. The social worker asked the patient to pick out a new nightgown from a catalogue and then purchased it for the resident; thereafter, the resident's nighttime problems disappeared. Although a behavioral intervention could have been developed to reinforce staying in bed, this social worker's simple solution was correct, sensitive to the patient's needs, and effective. Finally, Dallam (1987) gave examples of disruptive behaviors that were calmed by the nurse's touch or kind words or by the presence of another resident. In the efforts to provide clinically and cost-effective interventions for complex problems, these examples underscore the need to allow for the possibility that simple, humane solutions sometimes exist. It is when these solutions cannot be found that behavior, cognitive, and traditional psychotherapy and medical interventions become necessary.

ORGANIZATIONAL ISSUES

Staff Training

One question that arises in using both cognitive and behavior therapy in the nursing home is who will be doing the therapy. Studies have used different therapists, ranging from psychologists to nurses, nursing assistants, and other health-care providers. As the list of eligible providers of mental health services in long-term-care settings expands, a question can be raised regarding whether the outcomes are equivalent with different professional providers. In a therapeutic approach, such as cognitive therapy, a special set of skills is necessary to assess patients appropriately and to conduct the therapeutic sessions. How much training and at which level best prepares therapists and produces the best patient outcomes is an important question for future research.

Implementation of behavioral and cognitive interventions may be done individually in the context of typical therapy sessions, in group settings, or through more general implementation by nursing home staff under the supervision of a behavioral/cognitive specialist (e.g., psychologist). Programs to train staff in these interventions have been reported. Ray and colleagues (Ray et al., 1993) conducted a controlled trial of a program to reduce antipsychotic drug use in nursing homes. Direct-care staff (physicians, nurses, nursing assistants, and others) were trained in medication withdrawal/monitoring and concurrent behavioral management approaches. Results showed decreases in antipsychotic medication use and physical restraint and no increase in behavior problem frequency. Mixed results have been reported for nursing assistant training. Cohn et al. (1990) found that a five-session program in behavioral management resulted in increases in both knowledge and self-reported use of these skills among nursing assistants. However, Smyer et al. (1991) reported that this program produced improvements in knowledge but did not improve performance. This last study provides an important caveat that reflects a common behavioral principle that information alone is often insufficient to change behavior. Producing meaningful changes in the behavior of health-care providers may be best accomplished by combining training with appropriate and ongoing prompts and reinforcers to staff for using the new skills.

As pointed out in many reviews (e.g., Cody, Beck, & Svarstad, 2002; Cohen-Mansfield, 2005) any nursing home–based intervention implementation must recognize the manifold internal and external forces that shape the nursing home environment. Organizational factors such as work environment and culture, including presence of quality improvement processes, and commitment to resident and staff empowerment, staffing levels, organizational arrangements such as policy and procedures, social factors, such as quality of interdisciplinary relationships, relationship with families, the actual physical setting and layout, and the available technology and resources can be significant barriers to or facilitators to behavioral and cognitive therapeutic interventions. Enhancing the practice styles of nursing home staff can be daunting and requires a commitment and acceptance of the staff, administrators, and families to education, communication and flexibility. In addition, consideration of external challenges such as regulatory forces and funding levels can help determine the feasibility of implementing these interventions and their long-term sustainability.

REFERENCES

Abraham, I. L., Neundorfer, M. M., & Currie, U. (1992). Effects of group interventions on cognition and depression in nursing home residents. *Nursing Research, 41:* 196–202.

American Geriatrics Society. (1997). Position statement psychotherapeutic medication in the nursing home. Retrieved November 19, 2008, from http://www.americangeriatrics.org/products/positionpapers/psychot.shtml

American College of Sports Medicine. (1990). The recommended quantity and quality of exercise for developing and maintaining cardiorespiratory and muscular fitness in healthy adults. *Medicine and Science in Sports and Exercise, 22:* 265–274.

American Geriatrics Society and American Association of Geriatric Psychiatry. (2003). Consensus statement on improving the quality of mental health care in US nursing home. *Journal of the American Geriatrics Society, 51:* 1287–1298.

Baltes, M. M., Honn, S., Barton, E. M., et al. (1983). On the social ecology of dependence and independence in elderly nursing home residents: A replication and extension. *Journal of Gerontology, 38:* 556–564.

Baltes, M. M., & Zerbe, M. B. (1976). Independence training in nursing home residents. *Gerontologist, 16:* 428–432.

Bandura, A. (1986). *Social foundations of thought and action: a social cognitive theory.* Englewood Cliffs, NJ: Prentice-Hall.

Bandura, A. (1977). *Social learning theory.* Englewood Cliffs, NJ: Prentice-Hall.

Baum, E. E., Jarjoura, D., Polen, A. E., et al. (2003). Effectiveness of a group exercise program in a long-term care facility: A randomized pilot trial. *Journal of the American Medical Association, 4:* 74–80.

Beck, A. T. (1967). *Depression: Clinical, experimental, and theoretical aspects.* New York: Harper & Row.

Beck, A. T., & Young, I. E. (1985). Cognitive therapy of depression. In D. Barlow (Ed.), *Clinical handbook of psychological disorders: A step by step treatment manual* (pp. 206–224). New York: Guilford.

Beutler, L. E., Scogin, F., Kirkish, P., et al. (1987). Group cognitive therapy and alprazolarn in the treatment of depression in older adults. *Journal of Consulting Clinical Psychology, 55:* 550–556.

Blair, S. N., Kohl, H. W. III, Paffenbarger, R. S. Jr., et al. (1989). Physical fitness and all-cause mortality: A prospective study of healthy men and.women. *Journal of the American Medical Association, 262:* 2395–2401.

Bourgeois, M. S. (1993). Effects of memory aids on the dyadic conversations of individuals with dementia. *Journal of Applied Behavior Analysis, 26:* 77–87.

Bourgeois, M. S. (1990). Enhancing conversation skills in patients with Alzheimer's disease using a prosthetic memory aid. *Journal of Applied Behavior Analysis, 23:* 29–42.

Brink, T. L., Yeasavage, L. A., Lum, O. et al. (1982). Screening tests for geriatric depression. *Clinical Gerontology, 1:* 37–43.

Brown, M. N., Lapne, K. L., & Lusti, A. F. (2002). The management of depression in older nursing home residents. *Journal of the American Geriatrics Society, 50:* 69–76.

Burgio, L. D., Burgio, K. L., Engel, B. T., & Tice, L. M. (1986). Increasing distance and independence of ambulation in elderly nursing home residents. *Journal of Applied Behavior Analysis, 19:* 357–366.

Burgio, L. D., & Burgio, K. L. (1986). Behavioral gerontology: Application of behavioral methods to the problems of older adults. *Journal of Applied Behavior Analysis, 19*(4): 321–328.

Burgio, L. D., McCormick, K. A., Scheve, A. S., et al. (1994). The effects of changing prompted voiding schedules in the treatment of incontinence in nursing home residents. *Journal of the American Geriatrics Society, 42:* 315–320.

Burgio, L. D., & Sinnott, J. (1990). Behavioral treatments and pharmacotherapy: Acceptability ratings by elderly individuals in residential settings. *Gerontologist, 30:* 811–816.

Burns, B. J., Wagner, H. R., Taube, J. E., Magazner, J., Permutt, T., & Landerman, L. R. (1993). Mental health service use by the elderly in nursing homes. *American Journal of Public Health, 83:* 331–337.

Camp, C. J., Cohen-Mansfield, J., & Capezuit, E. (2002). Mental health services in nursing homes: Use of nonpharmacologic interventions among nursing home residents with dementia. *Psychiatry Services, 53:* 1397–1404.

Cariaga, J., Burgio, L., Flynn, W., & Martin, D. (1991). A controlled study of disruptive vocalizations among geriatric residents in nursing homes. *Journal of the American Geriatrics Society, 39:* 501–507.

Cody, M., Beck, C., & Svarstad, B. L. (2002). Mental health services in nursing homes: Challenges to the use of nonpharmacologic interventions in nursing homes. *Psychiatry Services, 53:* 1402–1406.

Cohen-Mansfield, J. (2001). Nonpharmacologic interventions for inappropriate behaviors in dementia. *American Journal of Geriatric Psychiatry, 9:* 361–381.

Cohen-Mansfield, J. (2005). Nonpharmacological interventions for persons with dementia. *Alzheimer's Care Quarterly, 6:* 120–145.

Cohen-Mansfield, J., & Mintzer, J. E. (2005). Time for change: The role of nonpharmacological interventions in treating behavior problems in nursing home residents with dementia. *Alzheimer Disease and Associated Disorders, 19:* 37.

Cohn, M. D., Horgas, A. L., & Marsiske, M. (1990). Behavior management training for nurse aides: Is it effective? *Journal of Gerontological Nursing, 16:* 21–25.

Cook, A. J. (1998). Cognitive-behavioral pain management for elderly nursing home residents. *Journals of Gerontology Series B: Psychological Sciences and Social Sciences, 53:* 51–59.

Downs, A. F. D., Rosenthal, T. L., & Lichstein, K. L. (1988). Modeling therapies reduce avoidance on bathtime by the institutionalized elderly. *Behavior Therapy, 19:* 359–368.

Elkin, I., Shea, M. T., Watkins, J. T., et al. (1989). NIMH treatment of depression collaborative research program: General effectiveness of treatments. *Archives of General Psychiatry, 46:* 971–982.

Ellis, A. (1962). *Reason and emotion in psychotherapy.* New York: Lyle Stuart.

Espie, C. A., MacMahon, K. M., Kelly, H. L., et al. (2007). Randomized clinical effectiveness trial of nurse administered small-group cognitive behavior therapy for persistent insomnia in general practice. *Sleep, 30:* 574–584.

Eustic, S., Roe, B., & Paterson, J. (2000). Prompted voiding for the management of urinary incontinence in adults. *Cochrane Database Systematic Reviews* CD002113.

Fiatarone, M. A., & Evans, W. J. (1993). The etiology and reversibility of muscle dysfunction in the aged. *Journal of Gerontology, 48*(special issue), 77–83.

Fiatarone, M. A., Marks, E. C., Ryan, N. D., et al. (1990). High-intensity strength training in nonagenarians-Effects on skeletal muscle. *Journal of the American Medical Association, 263:* 3029–3034.

Gallagher, D., & Thompson, L. (1982). Treatment of major depressive disorder in older adult outpatients with brief psychotherapies. *Psychotherapy Theory Research Practice, 19*: 482–490.

Gallagher, D. E., & Thompson, L. W. (1983). Effectiveness of psychotherapy for both endogenous and nonendogenous depression in older adult outpatients. *Journal of Gerontology, 38:* 707–712.

Goddard, P., & Carstensen, L. L. (1986). Behavioral treatment of chronic depression in an elderly nursing home resident. *Clinical Gerontology, 4:* 13–20.

Goesselin, P., Ladouceur, R., Morin, C. M., et al. (2006). Benzoiazepine discontinuation among adults with GAD: A randomized trial of cognitive behavioral therapy. *Journal of Consulting and Clinical Psychology, 74:* 908–918.

Gruber-Baldini, A. L., Boustani, M., Sloane, P. D., & Zimmerman, S. (2004). Behavioral symptoms in residential care/assisted living facilities: prevalence, risk factors, and medication management. *Journal of the American Geriatrics Society, 52:* 1610–1617.

Haaga, D. A. F., DeRubeis, R. J., Stewart, B. L., & Beck, A. T. (1991). Relationship of intelligence with cognitive therapy outcome. *Behavior Research and Therapy, 29:* 277–281.

Hoeffer, B., Talerico, K. A., Rasin, J. et al. (2006). Assisting cognitively impaired nursing home residents with bathing: Effects of two bathing interventions on caregiving. *Gerontologist, 46:* 524–532.

Hu, T. W., Wagner, T. H., Bentkover, J. D., et al. (2003). Estimated economic costs of overactive bladder in the United States. *Urology, 61:* 1123–1128.

Hussian, R. A., & Brown, D. C. (1987). Use of two-dimensional grid patterns to limit hazardous ambulation in demented patients. *Journal of Gerontology, 42,* 558–560.

Hussian, R. A. (1984). Behavioral geriatrics. *Behavior Modification Program, 16:* 159–183.

Hussian, R. A. (1988). Modification of behaviors in dementia via stimulus manipulation. *Clinical Gerontology, 8:* 37–43.

Jarrett, R. B., Eaves, G. G., Grannemann, B. D., et al. (1991). Clinical, cognitive and demographic predictors of response to cognitive therapy for depression: A preliminary report. *Psychiatry Research, 37:* 245–260.

Jones, R. N., Marcantonio, E. R., & Lusti, A. F. (2003). Prevalence and correlates of recognized depression in US nursing homes. *Journal of the American Geriatrics Society, 51:* 1404–1409.

Karuza, J., & Katz, P. R. (1991). Psychosocial interventions in long-term care: A critical overview. In P. R. Katz, R. L. Kane, & M. D. Mezey (Eds.), *Advances in long-term care* (Vol 1). NewYork: Springer.

Karuza, J., Zevon, M. A., Gleason, T., et al. (1992). Models of helping and coping, responsibility attributions and well being in community elderly and their helpers. *Psychology and Aging, 5:* 194–208.

Krasner, L. (1971). Behavior therapy. *Annual Review of Psychology, 22:* 483–582.

Levin, C. A., Levin Wie, W., Akincigil, A., et al. (2007). Prevalance and treatment of diagnosed depression among elderly nursing home residents in Ohio. *Journal of the American Medical Directors Association, 8:* 585–594.

Lewin, L. M., Lundervold, D., Saslow, M., & Thompson, S. (1989). Reducing eating dependency in nursing home patients: The effects of prompting, reinforcement, food preference and environmental design. *Journal of Clinical and Experimental Gerontology, 11:* 47–63.

Lewinsohn, P. M. (1974). Clinical and theoretical aspects of depression. In K. S. Calhoun, H. E. Adams, K. Mitchell (Eds.), *Innovative treatment methods in psychopathology.* New York: Wiley.

Lichtenberg, P. A., Kemp-Havican, J., Macneill, S. E., & Schafer Johnson, A. (2005). Pilot study of behavioral treatment in dementia care units. *Gerontologist, 45:* 406–410.

Lundervold, D. A., & Lewin, I. M. (1992). *Behavior analysis and therapy in nursing homes.* Springfield, IL: Charles C. Thomas.

Lyketsos, C. G., Samus, Q. M., Baker, A., et al. (2007). Effect of dementia and treatment of dementia on time to discharge from assisted living facilities: The Maryland Assisted Living Study. *Journal of the American Geriatrics Society, 55:* 1031–1037.

MacDonald, M. L., & Butler, A. K. (1974). Reversal of helplessness: Producing walking behavior in nursing home wheelchair residents using behavior modification procedures. *Journal of Gerontology, 29:* 97–101.

Magsi, H., & Malloy, T. (2005). Underrecognition of cognitive impairment in assisted living facilities. *Journal of the American Geriatrics Society, 53:* 295–298.

Mahoney, M. J. (1974). *Cognition and behavior modification.* Cambridge, MA: Ballinger.

McMurdo, M. E. T., & Rennie, L. (1993). A controlled trial of exercise by residents of old people's homes. *Age and Ageing, 22:* 11–15.

Meichenbaum, D. (1977). *Cognitive behavioral modification.* Morristown, NJ: General Learning Press.

Mohide, E. A. (1986). The prevalence and scope of urinary incontinence. *Clinics in Geriatric Medicine, 2:* 639–655.

National Institutes of Health Consensus Development Conference. (1990). Proceedings of Consensus Development Conference on Urinary Incontinence in Adults. Bethesda, MD, October 3–5, 1988. *Journal of the American Geriatrics Society, 38:* 265–272.

Newman, C. F., & Beck, A. T. (1990). Cognitive therapy of affective disorders. In B. Wolman, & G. Stricker (Eds.), *Depressive disorders* (pp. 343–367). New York: Wiley.

Oneal, E. (1986). A simple way to modify behavior. *Geriatric Nursing, 7:* 45.

Ouslander, J. G. (1991). New approaches to the diagnosis and treatment of incontinence in the nursing home. In P. R. Katz, R. L. Kane, & M. D. Mezey (Eds.), *Advances in long-term care.* (Vol 1., pp. 61–80). New York: Springer.

Ouslander, J. G. (1990). Urinary incontinence in nursing homes. *Journal of the American Geriatrics Society, 38:* 289–291.

Parmalee, P., Katz, I. R., & Lawton, M. P. (1992). Indices of depression in long-term care settings. *Journal of Gerontology, 47:* 189–196.

Pavlov, I. P. (1927). *Conditioned reflexes.* (G. V. Aurep, Trans.). London: Oxford.

Perkins, K. A., Rapp, S. R., Carlson, C. R., & Wallace, C. E. (1986). A behavioral intervention to increase exercise among nursing home residents. *Gerontologist, 26:* 479–481.

Powell, R. R. (1974). Psychological effects of exercise therapy upon institutionalized geriatric mental patients. *Journal of Gerontology, 29:* 157–161.

Rakowski, W., & Mor, V. (1992). The association of physical activity with mortality among older adults in the Longitudinal Study of Aging. *Journal of Gerontology: Medical Science, 47:* 122–129.

Ray, W. A., Taylor, J. A., Meador, K. G., et al. (1993). Reducing antipsychotic drug use in nursing homes—A controlled trial of provider education. *Archives of Internal Medicine, 153:* 713–721.

Roth, D. L., Stevens, A. B., Burgio, L. D., & Burgio, K. L. (2002). Timed event sequential analysis of agitation in nursing home residents during personal care interactions with nursing assistants. *Journals of Gerontology Series B: Psychological Science and Social Science, 57:* 461–468.

Schneider, L. S., Tariot, P. N., Dagerman, K. S., et al. (2006). Effectiveness of atypical antipsychotic drugs in patients with Alzheimer's disease. *New England Journal of Medicine, 355:* 1525–1538.

Schnelle. J. F., Ouslander, J. G., Osterweil, D., & Blumenthal, S. (1993). Total quality management: Administrative and clinical applications in nursing homes. *Journal of the American Geriatrics Society, 41:* 1259–1266.

Schnelle, J. F., Traughber, B., Morgan, D. B., et al. (1983). Management of geriatric incontinence in nursing homes. *Journal of Applied Behavior Analysis, 6:* 235–241.

Schnelle, J. F. (1990). Treatment of urinary incontinence in nursing home patients by prompted voiding. *Journal of the American Geriatrics Society, 38:* 356–360.

Schnelle, J. F., Wood, S., Schnelle, E. R., & Simmons, S. F. (2001). Measurement sensitivity and the Minimum Data Set depression quality indicator. *Gerontologist, 41:* 401–405.

Simmons, S. F., Alessi, C., & Schnelle, J. F. (2001). An intervention to increase fluid intake in nursing home residents: Prompting and preference compliance. *Journal of the American Geriatrics Society, 49:* 926–933.

Skinner, B. F., & Vaughan, M. (1983). *Enjoy old age: A program of self-management.* New York: Norton.

Skinner, B. F. (1974). *About behaviorism.* New York: Knopf.

Skinner, B. F. (1983). Intellectual self-management in old age. *American Psychologist, 38:* 239–244.

Smyer, M., Brannon, D., & Cohn, M. (1991). Improving nursing home care through training and job redesign. *Gerontologist, 32:* 327–333.

Smyer, M. A., Shea, D. G., & Streit, A. (1994). The provision and use of mental health services in nursing homes: Results from the National Medical Expenditure Survey. *American Journal of Public Health, 84:* 284–287.

Snowden, M., Sato, K., & Roy-Byrne, P. (2003). Assessment and treatment of nursing home residents with depression or behavioral symptoms associated with dementia: A review of the literature. *Journal of the American Geriatrics Society, 51(9):* 1305–1317.

Sotsky, S. M., Glass, D. R., Shea, M. R., et al. (1991). Patient predictors of response to psychotherapy and pharmacotherapy: Findings in the NIMH Treatment of Depression Collaborative Research Program. *American Journal of Psychiatry, 148:* 997–1008.

Teresi, J., Abrams, R., Holms, D., et al. (2001). Prevalence of depression and depression recognition in nursing homes. *Social Psychiatry and Psychiatric Epidemiology, 36:* 613–620.

Thompson, L. W., Gallagher, D., & Breckenridge, J. S. (1987). Comparative effectiveness of psychotherapies for depressed elders. *Journal of Consulting and Clinical Psychology, 55:* 385–390.

Thompson, L. W., Davies, R., Gallagher, D., & Krantz, S. E. (1986). Cognitive therapy with older adults. *Clinical Gerontology, 5:* 245–279.

Verkaik, R., van Veert, J. C., & Francke, A. L. (2005). The effects of psychosocial methods on depressed, aggressive and apathetic behaviors of people with dementia: A systematic review. *International Journal of Geriatric Psychiatry, 20:* 301–314.

Watson, J. B. (1925). *Behaviorism.* New York: Norton.

Wells, T. (1990). Pelvic (floor) muscle exercise. *Journal of the American Geriatrics Society, 38:* 333–337.

Wetherell, J. L., Gatz, M., & Craske, M. G. (2003). Treatment of generalized anxiety disorder in older adults. *Journal of Consulting and Clinical Psychology, 71:* 31–40.

Whisman, M. (1993). Mediators and moderators of change in cognitive therapy of depression. *Psychological Bulletin, 114:* 248–265.

Zimmer, J. G., Watson, N., & Treat, A. (1984). Behavioral problems among patients in skilled nursing facilities. *American Journal of Public Health, 74:* 1118–1121.

16

Family Interventions

Lee Hyer, Shailaja Shah, and *Amanda Sacks*

Annually within the United States, almost 2 million adults are admitted to one of 16,800 NHs (Hyer & Intrieri, 2006). The recent growth of assisted-living facilities, now estimated at over 36,000 facilities serving about 1 million residents (see Hyer & Intrieri, 2006) complements these nursing homes (NHs) within the spectrum of long-term-care (LTC) facilities. The decision to relocate to an LTC facility, such as an NH or assisted-living facility (ALF), is a major transition point in an older adult's life and the family.

The decision to place a loved one in an LTC facility may be a long and agonizing one for family carers (Dellasega & Mastrian, 1995). It evokes various emotions. "Nursing homes" are not "hospitals" from the perspective of the residents and most family members. Most people in our culture will spend some portion of their final phase of life in such settings (Hyer & Intrieri, 2006). In addition, there is a sense of role loss because of placement. There is also evidence that staff frequently underutilize the expertise of family caregivers in implementing a treatment plan for the elderly individual (Naleppa, 1996). Placement in LTC does not relieve the attendant emotional depression. In effect, the caregivers need to be prepared for this new stage of care.

In this chapter, we discuss the predictors of institutionalization. Further, the need to intervene with families to ease this phase of caregiving is addressed. After placement, the importance of continuing to work with family caregivers and various family interventions is emphasized to help acclimatize the patient and family to the new environment. There is little research to indicate the type of support that will effectively smooth the transition during this difficult phase (Bowers 1988; Dellasega & Mastrian 1995). We also address taxonomy of families in LTC and provide an assessment protocol for assistance with families.

ADMISSION ISSUES

The decision to place an older adult is multifactorial and often involves patient demographics, caregiver characteristics, and patient health status (Buhr, 2006). At a personal level, the decision to relocate to an LTC facility is a major transition point in the life cycle of the family. For the identified patient, institutionalization is a tangible response to an imbalance between an individual's functional ability and the resources available for their care. This imbalance can result from limitations of their environment, caregivers, and resources available in their home settings and is often compounded by demands related to an accumulation of both medical and mental health issues. For the family, stress does not abate; indeed it most often increases.

Patient factors, such as living alone (Gaugler, Kane, & Clay, 2003), being white (Gaugler et al., 2003), and being older (Gaugler et al., 2000), are associated with higher rates of institutionalization. Studies that include dementia characteristics have all revealed that higher levels of cognitive and functional impairment, as well as the presence of difficult behaviors are associated with an increased likelihood of placement (Gaugher et al., 2000; Yaffe et al., 2002). In general, factors related to caregiving, including perceived stress or burden (Gaugler et al., 2003; Yaffe et al., 2002), feeling trapped in the caregiving role (Gaugler et al., 2000), health problems (Hebert et al., 2001), and poor self-rated health (Gaugler et al., 2003) have all been implicated as causal factors in predicting institutionalization. Buhr et al. (2006) conducted a longitudinal caregiver study (n = 2200 caregivers) over a 4-year period. They found that caregivers' reasons for placement included the need for more skilled care (65%), caregiver's health (49%), patients' dementia-related behavioral disturbance (46%), and the need for more assistance (23%). The authors further emphasized that the caregiver's reasons were valid and placement occurred due to caregiver and patient factors evident in the year prior to placement. Importantly, Buhr and colleagues recommend routine screening of caregivers for accounts of low life satisfaction, dementia problem behaviors, or high task demand in routine office visits.

Among the top 20 disease diagnoses reported in the MDS Active Resident Information Report (Centers for Medicare and Medicaid Studies, 2002, 2004) are mental health problems. The prevalence of mental and cognitive disorders, including depressive disorders, anxiety disorders, and organic brain damage, is striking

(Jones, 2002). In a comparison of the 1985 and 1997 surveys, almost all residents had more than one condition present at admission and more than half had three or more admitting diagnoses (Sahyoun, Pratt, Lentzner, Dey, & Robinson, 2001). An inability to function independently has become a theme that underlies the many different diseases found in LTC settings (see Hyer & Intrieri, 2006). In effect, residents are becoming sicker and have more mental health problems.

Heath and coworkers (2006) classified residents in LTC as actively rehabilitating, dying, and surviving. Although any taxonomy of LTC residents is wanting, it is clear that the largest proportion of LTC residents comprise those which can be classified as "surviving." This term is intended primarily to reflect the fact that such residents are not undergoing actively rehabilitative efforts, due to the static nature of their impairments or the chronicity of the conditions; however, their prognosis has not been formally determined to be immediately limited. The most typical of these residents are those with various stages of dementias such as Alzheimer's disease. Such slowly progressive dementias often have caused functional impairment that requires institutional care but has not yet led to immediate threats to continued survival. Such dementing illnesses may either be explicitly identified as the primary diagnosis for the individual or be listed among a variety of chronic conditions that have accumulated to an extent that institutional placement was required (Table 16.1).

TABLE 16.1. Typology of Long-Term-Care Residents

NATURE OF RESIDENT	TYPICAL MEDICAL DIAGNOSES	CHARACTERISTIC MENTAL HEALTH ISSUES	COMMON "RED FLAG" PRESENTATIONS
Actively rehabilitating	Acute stroke; Joint fracture/ replacement; Major surgery; Limb amputation; Deconditioning after prolonged medical hospitalization	Self-care challenges; Conflicts over body image; Pain management	Slowed progress in rehabilitation; Accelerating somatic complaints; Anorexia
Actively dying	Metastatic cancers; End-stages of progressive chronic diseases	Pain; Depression; Anxiety; Psychiatric features of brain lesions	Isolation and withdrawal; Hallucinations; Delirium
Surviving	Dementias; Heart disease; Stroke; Advanced parkinsonism; Emphysema	Learned helplessness; Adjustment reactions; Restlessness	Dementia-related behaviors; Weight loss; Resistance to care; Excessive call bell use

Physical problems and psychiatric diagnoses augment adjustment problems in LTC. The 1999 National Center for Health Statistics National Nursing Home Survey (see Hyer & Ragan,2003) found that nearly 75% of nursing home residents received help with three or more activities of daily living (ADLs). As many as 80% of nursing home residents have dementia or another diagnosable psychiatric disorder (Rovner et al., 1990). Furthermore, anywhere between 6% and 24% have a major depressive disorder diagnosis, 30% to 50% have minor depression or dysthymia and as many as 35% to 45% manifest depressive symptoms. MDS reports 14.6% of long-term-care patients have been diagnosed with anxiety disorder, though this rate may be deceptively low when given the limitations in reporting anxiety symptoms within the MDS (Centers for Medicare and Medicaid Studies, 2004). The Centers for Medicare and Medicaid Services (2004) report a 97% increase in antidepressant medications for all residents from 12.6% to 24.9% over the past five years. Weintraub, Datto, Streim, and Karz (2002) suggest that currently 35% to 60% of nursing home residents receive antidepressant medication.

THE TRANSITION

Information that family caregivers receive does not prepare them for the LTC experience. Often it includes a list of facilities with only one visit before admission. Families have not had a chance to discuss the move with nurses or other health-care professionals and feel anxious and isolated (Reed & Morgan, 1999). Health-care providers do not have as a priority to support families in the decision-making process for LTC placement. Problematic too is the fact that many health-care providers who treat acute problems are largely uneducated about LTC and are ill prepared to assist families. The timing of educating and informing families about placement is also unclear. Most of the time professionals may not bring up this issue until later in the course of the illness. At that point, it may be a crisis situation and caregivers may feel pressured and make a "last resort" decision. This may lead to feelings of guilt. The families' difficulties during transition, resulting in emotions such as sadness, loneliness, anger, and resentment have been described in a study by Dellasega and Mastrian (1995). In some families placement may be viewed as a means of coping, due to lack of time, money and motivation (Townsend, 1990). In other cases, placement was considered as a stressor, as it posed new and different challenges (emotions of grief and guilt, doubts about quality of care after placement) (Matthieson, 1989).

Educating families about the type of various facilities and levels of care provided is of utmost importance. Importantly, families need to be advised on issues such as what questions to ask and what to look for when visiting facilities. Hopefully, this information process will involve input from the identified patient.

The different levels of care available in a facility need to be addressed, as well as whether a continuum of care is available (independent living, assisted living, skilled nursing care). The staff interactions with residents need to be observed as it will give fairly good insight into the type of facility. The financial aspects of living in a long-term-care facility need to be addressed; who pays for care, what happens when private funds run out, and what happens when Medicaid benefits are the only resource of payment. Issues such as how does the facility handle progression of illness when caring for someone in an assisted living; do they "age in place" or are they moved to a nursing home. In addition, it is now evident that LTC facilities that provide a psychosocial model of care with psychiatry and psychology optimize quality of life (Hyer & Intrieri, 2006). Families should be apprised of existence of this in the LTC facility also.

IMPORTANCE OF FAMILIES

Families play an important role in the quality of care and quality of life in LTC. Among LTC residents family involvement has been associated with better psychological care (Greene & Monahan, 1982; McCallion, Toseland, & Freeman, 1999) and higher provision of certain types of treatment (Anderson, Lyons, & West, 2001). Higher life satisfaction has been reported for ALF residents who receive at least monthly visits from family members (Mitchell & Kemp, 2000), and quality of the social environment is important to resident satisfaction and feeling "at home" (Sikorska, 1999). Port et al. (2005) found few differences between the family caregivers of ALFs and NHs across several health and sociodemographic characteristics. In addition, caregivers seem to tailor their involvement to the specific abilities of the resident—ALF caregivers sent more letters, used the telephone for assistance, and provided help with IADLs than nursing home caregivers.

It is widely accepted that as we age marital relationships add emotional support and act as a source of positive affect. Cartensen's (1992) socioemotional selectivity theory (SST) asserts that an important goal of later life is to enhance emotional closeness. As individuals age, they become less concerned with gaining new information and forming new friendships, and more interested in nurturing close family ties (Carstensen, Isaacowitz, & Charles, 1999). Older people apparently desire to nurture stable and consistent relationships. In a path analysis Whisman, Uebelacker, and Weinstock (2004) found that depressive symptoms were significantly related to marital dissatisfaction with greater depressive severity associated with greater marital dissatisfaction. It appears further that marital dissatisfaction at later life is associated with unfairness of role allocation, higher levels of disagreement, keeping opinions to self, avoiding calm discussions, and having heated arguments (Bookwala & Jacobs, 2004).

Research suggests that it is important to keep family members involved in the care of residents (Port et al., 2005). This is especially important at the beginning of the transition into LTC. There is also a special need for families of dementia residents, as there is a demand for the social and emotional connection regarding historical background, care decisions, social and personal care, and advocacy. "Caregiving" then is multifaceted and beyond basic resident needs. Whatever tasks are involved, caregiving remains critical to the treatment of the new resident. What the tasks for caregiving were at home are not less but different, occurring in a social context. In truth, little is known of the reciprocal impact that patients and caregivers have on one another in LTC. At this transition moment into an LTC, clarity and improvement in the new caregiving role will no doubt impact positively on the overall health of the family as well as the patient. We discuss this below.

Burden

There is considerable burden of caring for an elder with dementia (Schultz, & Martire, 2004). At some point in the course of the illness about 40% of families must place the affected person in an LTC facility. As noted, this process is neither smooth nor does it lead to less distress (Lieberman & Fisher, 1999). In general, both cross-sectional and longitudinal data suggest that instrumental burdens decrease, but other burdens increase—caregiver health, well-being, depression, and life satisfaction show little change following LTC placement. Placement in LTC does not relieve the attendant emotional dysphoria. In effect, the caregivers need to be prepared for this new stage of care. Problems with the severity of the patient's functional deficits and a reduction of caregiver burden do not trump the quality of the family relationships and the efficiency of the decision-making.

Conventional wisdom that a caregiver will be relieved of a great burden when a family member is moved to a nursing home has been challenged (see Schulz et al., 2004). Moving a family member to an LTC facility can challenge the strengths of the healthiest family system and can magnify occult problems. For example, a daughter who no longer has to bathe, dress, and feed her mother, now has to negotiate for her parent's care at the facility, worry that she is being well-cared for, and deal with her own guilt over "putting mother away."

The real-world balance tasks of what families should assist with and what to back off from remain unknown. On the one hand, families and staff in NH report problems when families interfere too much in the care of the resident—fostering excess disability. The number one problem with many residents in LTC involves their interaction with their loved one in the LTC facility or the staff in that facility. On the other hand, family members are neither aware of nor can they answer specific questions regarding the specifics of care. Simmons and Ouslander (2005), for example, found that resident and family satisfaction differed with incontinence and mobility care, as many caregivers could not answer basic questions about incontinence and mobility care and their reports are insensitive to care management.

Interventions with the Family

There is a simple and logical thing to do: Staff need to include the family carers in most aspects of care and do so over time. During the initial assessment of residents on admission to a facility and at regular intervals thereafter, this process should unfold. This will enable staff to find out more about their resident's likes and dislikes, routines, recreational activities, and hobbies. This type of ongoing interaction will also cultivate an environment of collaboration and will help the family members feel part of the treatment/care at the home. Staff members on the team including nurses, social workers, and nurse's aides must take this opportunity also to educate families that the environment of the patient's room can be made to resemble that at home. They can educate families to bring in personal care items, family photos, furniture, and plants to help individuals acclimatize smoothly to the new environment. Staff also need to support families and inquire into their needs and clarify what their expectations from the LTC might be. Some families may still want to be part of daily care routines and such wishes may need to be respected. In addition, families need to be educated that they continue to have a role in showing affection by touching, and hugging, as residents, including those who have dementia, still have needs for intimacy and feeling loved. When dementia-related behavior problems do arise, families need to be informed. Interventions such as behavior modification and/or medication can be discussed as needed. Fortunately, these formulations are discussed and accounted for in the MDS care plans. The family should be involved.

That said, we highlight three areas of intervention based on three separate literatures. We discuss caregiver models of intervention, staff training, and family systems theory.

Caregiving models of family involvement

The construct of caregiving as it applies to families loses little of its importance in LTC. Several extant models of caregiving have applicability to LTC. In a meta-analysis of caregiving Sorensen, Pinquart, and Duberstein (2002) indicate that the effect size for extant interventions is low-moderate (14–41) In effect, the strength of the intervention for caregivers of dementia patients is consistent but anemic. When a resident lives in an LTC facility, the actual burden of the objective amount of care provided by the caregiver is reduced. Now the focus of caregiving shifts from objective burden to psychoeducation, family involvement, and coping. Interestingly, these are the areas of most benefit for caregiving in general (Sorensen et al., 2002).

There is considerable variability in the success of caregiver intervention programs (Roth, Mittelman, Clay, Madan, & Haley, 2005). They run the gamut from counseling-focused interventions to very clear objective support in the form of goods and services. Across all programs, individual programs mildly outperform group interventions (Sorensen et al., 2002) and comprehensive programs show more success than narrow ones (Schulz et al., 2002). In addition, as the efficacy of these programs is more understood, the mediating effects of social support, lower stressful appraisals, and adaptive coping become more evident (Haley, Levine, Brown, & Bartolucci, 1987).

There are however several models of outpatient caregiver programs that have proven effective. For several years Mittelman and colleagues (Mittelman, Epstein, & Pierzchala, 2003) provided a caregiver intervention in a community setting and addressed the social support network of spouses of dementia patients. This intervention consisted of individual and family sessions, as well as groups, and ad hoc telephone counseling. Results showed that over a 9.5-year period the counseling and support intervention outperformed usual care in delaying nursing home placement for the resident (Mittelman, Ferris, Shulman, Steinberg, & Levin, 1996), significantly reduced appraisals of memory problems and disruptive behaviors (Mittelman, Roth, Haley, & Zarit, 2004), and resulted in reduced depressive symptoms over time for the caregivers (Mittelman, Roth, Coon, & Haley, 2004). In another study on this data set, structural equation modeling revealed that the number of support persons and satisfaction with the support network increased as a function of the intervention; this in turn mediated a significant proportion of the intervention's impact on caregiver depression and caregiver stress appraisals (Roth et al., 2005). While these studies have not been carried out in LTC, the translation of the caregiving behaviors to this setting is both logical and appealing.

Other caregiver treatment models, involving structured psychoeducation programs (Hepburn, et al. 2006), cognitive training (ACTIVE; Ball et al., 2002), programs that tailor interventions to the caregiver-care receiver dyad (Resources for Enhancing Alzheimer's Health project (REACH); Gallagher-Thompson et al., 2003), have also been applied to dementia. These models have addressed the caregiver directly using a problem-solving process, either preventively or via treatment. A cooperative communication Intervention (Partners in Caregiving; Pillemer et al., 2003) was also designed as an intervention to increase cooperation and effective communication between family members and nursing home staff. In all, the role of the caregiver is critical in the adjustment of the resident's life. Again, these models, while well studied, have not been used in LTC.

Implied in these models is the importance of coping. In 2006, the Family Caregiver Alliance (2006a, 2006b) endorsed the importance of knowledge of primary (objective) and secondary (role strains and intrapsychic coping) stressors in the family adjustment whether in or out of LTC. Coping was a key measure in this taxonomy. One coping model applicable for caregiving in LTC is the Stress/ Health model (Pearlin et al., 1990). This model holds that the primary stressors placed on the caregiver include the level of the resident's cognitive impairment, the frequency of patient problem behaviors, number of hours per week spent providing physical assistance with instrumental or personal ADLs, and helping the patient negotiate the health-care system. A second set of stressors resulting from the primary ones include conflict in the family or at least a decrease in relationship quality, as well as role-related problems such as missing work. It is this secondary set of stressors that impact on caregivers of LTC residents. In general, if the demands exceed the resources, there are problems—increased burden and depression (Schultz & Martire, 2004).

In sum, these models have considerable appeal and promise. Caregiving is certainly a complex process. It changes in structured ways only when residence in LTC occurs; objective burden goes down. The models noted above have not been directly applied to LTC. Their strength involves individually tailored interventions that address problems of the care receiver and the stress of the caregiver. Ultimately the caregivers in LTC must

- acknowledge the disease
- make the cognitive/emotional shift about the disease
- develop emotional tolerance
- negotiate control issues with resident and staff
- establish realistic expectations
- gauge the resident's capacities
- work with staff
- design opportunities for satisfying moments in LTC
- be objective (acquire Power of Attorney, help with finances, etc.).

Staff training

Staff training is a strategy for improving the care and quality of life of NH residents. Staff training provides staff members with knowledge and skills to identify and address the unmet needs of residents. Staff training interventions, however, seldom result in meaningful changes in staff behavior or skill use after the designated training period. Staff members can learn skills that will improve care, but they are not likely to continue to use those skills after training (Burgio & Stevens, 1998; Hyer & Intrieri, 2006).

There are reasons for this. Characteristics of the NH culture strongly contribute to staff performance and to the sustainability of new skills after initial training. NH culture is affected by staffing levels and staff turnover, management and supervisory practices, opportunities for professional growth, incentives and recognition, regulatory demands, and the interprofessional and interpersonal relationships among staff members (see Stevens & Hochhalter, 2006). In general, CNAs report feeling underappreciated and poorly supervised. Often the culture of their work environment is one in which too few people are available to provide the quality of care that they would like to provide. Very high turnover among staff members in all NH positions means that supervisors and coworkers come and go regularly (see Hyer & Intrieri, 2006). Therefore, both the content of staff training and the culture into which new knowledge and skills are introduced are critical determinants of the impact that a staff development program has on staff behavior and resident care.

What is most relevant here is that, when CNA competences and environmental press are not well balanced in an NH, quality of care, staff performance, and workforce stability are threatened. There is evidence that skills training can increase staff members' knowledge (Gilbert & McMahon, 2004; Martin, Rozon, McDowell, Cetinski, & Kemp, 2004), but changes in knowledge and skill use after staff training dissipate over time, if steps are not taken to maintain and continue to develop new competencies (Burgio et al., 2002). For example, McCallion et al. (1999) provided staff training on communication skills for use with residents who have dementia coupled with consultation-type monthly follow-ups. Resident depression and agitation improved after training. Staff members were more knowledgeable about strategies for managing problem behaviors 3 months after training, but the increase in knowledge did not persist 3 months after follow-up consultations ceased.

Hyer and Intrieri (2006) offer several models for staff training that impact on both resident and family. One model is provided by Stevens and Hochhalter (2006), the Informed Teams model (Boettcher, Kemeny, DeShon, & Stevens, 2004; Burgio et al., 2002; Stevens et al., 1998). First, training is mandatory and time is allotted for new skills to develop. Enforcement of mandatory attendance policies is an indicator of an organization's commitment to a staff development program. If an NH administrator and director of nursing are not willing or able to require staff participation in training, then the organization is probably not ready for change. Second, skill acquisition is not likely with didactic sessions alone. A combination of short interactive in-services, exercises and one-the-job training is more likely to be effective than any of the three alone. These skills involve combinations of empathy responses, problem-solving tasks, motivational enhancement interventions, and behavior modification. Third, effective teaching in a staff development program uses activities that demonstrate respect for staff members in all positions and for the designated duties of each position. NH leaders and trainers must model respect for all staff members. Fourth, supervisors in NHs require separate training on how to be a good supervisor. RNs and LPNs rarely have experience or training as a supervisor, and often feel unprepared to serve as a manager/supervisor. Although these skills come naturally to some, one should not assume that all supervisors have the skills needed to fill that role. Finally, incentives motivate staff members to try new skills initially. Continued motivation requires that staff members find new skills useful and that the culture of the work environment supports skill use with constructive feedback and recognition.

The importance of staff training cannot be underestimated. In effect, the residents' quality of life is largely dependent on their family. Family in LTC now involves both blood linage and staff, the new family. The extent to which staff respond empathically and clinically to residents depends on training and on commitment of the facility.

Family system

The family is the most influential interpersonal context throughout life. It has been suggested that several family members may be involved in caregiving and that the health decline of an elder with dementia involves multiple generations (Mellins & Blum, 1993). A report from the House Select Committee on Aging (U.S. House of Representatives, 1987) suggests that the average American woman can expect to spend 18 years of her life helping a family member who has health impairments. Odds were 1 out of 6 that a parent or spouse aged 65 or older would require some form of assistance. When this occurs, the family system is affected, even when the residence is now in an LTC facility (Mellins & Blum, 1993). Perhaps then it is prudent to have a sense about the family and its rules of operation (family systems).

Mitriani et al. (2006) provides a structural family approach as an explanatory model for the influence of family functioning on dementia caregivers. Family structural functioning is a major contributor to the caregiver stress process, specifically the way in which such structure impacts on the transition of an elder with dementia to a long-term-care facility. A conceptualization of family system then becomes essential in providing care in disease management and in enhancing quality of life for the elder with dementia (Lieberman & Fisher, 1999). An elder with dementia decline (cognitive loss and dependence in ADLs and behavioral disturbances) and their demands represent important stressors to the family resulting in family conflicts, high rates of psychological (anxiety, depression, insomnia), economic, and physical (arterial hypertension, propensity to infections) health problems (Engelhardt, Dourado, & Laks, 2005).

FAMILY SYSTEM THEORY

Family systems theory emphasizes the stability of patterns throughout the lifetime. A family system is composed of the individuals within the family who serve to maintain the homeostasis. This is due to the roles that each member fulfills. Individuals in the family system become dependent on each member to fulfill their roles that consist of psychological and behavioral aspects (Minuchin, 1974).

Cohesion and stability are the bases for this function of the family system (Steinglass, 1980). Members are able to function in the family in ways that are consistent with their own strengths and their weaknesses, while helping the family function as a whole. Such patterns of relating are consistent and predictable and therefore serve as a safe haven. Roles, communication patterns, and subsequent family structure have been reinforced over many years.

Any intervention, including one involving treatment of the elder with dementia in LTC, needs to integrate the family system (Hyer & Intrieri, 2006). Due to the longevity in stability of the family system and how it affects individuals throughout their lives, it becomes important to understand the type of system from which the elder with dementia has emerged and developed in order to better understand how the family may react to, process, and interact with issues related to a dementia diagnosis in the family (Mitrani et al., 2005). These systems are generally stable across situations and will impact the processing of a dementia diagnosis and transition of the elder into a living facility.

As discussed above, disclosure of a dementia diagnosis and the decision to relocate the elder with dementia to an LTC facility is disruptive to the family system, including both spouse and adult children. According to the ABCX model of family stress, such an event creates change in the family organization, the resources of the whole family must address this event, and the family defines this event in the context of the family's goals, values and overall organization (Hill, 1958). The family unit may even change in order to regain organization. Monitoring and assessing family dynamics then become important clinical tools for promoting the utilization of optimal care (Brubaker, 1990). In effect, family functioning is both a source of stress when dealing with transition to long-term care and a resource. This idea is consistent with the stress-process model conceptualized by Pearlin, Mullan, Semple, and Skaff (1990) in which stress will disorganize the family, however can also be protective from this stressor.

The dementing individual loses a fundamental role in the family, either discretely or gradually. Inevitably there is a role reversal and role ambiguity, wherein the family member with a dementia is now the recipient of care. The decision-making is now allocated to a family member(s) who formerly conceptualized the recipient as an autonomous individual. Such role reversal results in alienation and confusion. A role transition unfolds, whereby family members become engaged in activities to preserve functioning of the family. Often this results in a deviation from their standard role.

Family Taxonomy

We extend a taxonomy of family types previously provided by Goldstein (1996). The following description provides an overview of different family styles and possible methods of handling issues related to the care of an LTC resident with a dementia diagnosis. In this system some of the families demonstrate being enmeshed or disengaged only; some have the additional features of being impulsive, at odds, or overstressed. In addition, as with any therapy dynamic, the involved clinician will experience reactions to each type of family, and an awareness of these patterns assists in the provision of optimal care.

At the start, we want to emphasize this: all families are impacted by the admission of their relative to LTC and many handle this well. We address here the families that do not address this well.

Enmeshed family

Definition.   This family is one in which members are inextricably tied to one another for a sense of identity. Boundaries, as far as roles within the family, are unclear in these types of families (Hoffman, 1981). A defining quality of this family is lack of appreciation of members as being separate individuals with their own thoughts and feelings. Often in such families there are cross-generational alliances in which a parent is allied with a child, excluding a third member of the family, in order to deflect conflict between two parental figures (Hoffman, 1981). Family members tend to relinquish a sense of being autonomous due to a heightened sense of belonging to the family unit and, as such, independent exploration may be discouraged (Minuchin, 1974).

Modes of Relating.   Family members engage in modes of relating that incorporate projection and projective identification. Projection is a process in which members of the family, perhaps without full awareness, take difficult or unacceptable feelings and perceive such feelings as coming from a family member rather than from within. In projective identification, the member of the family that has such feelings projected onto him/her identifies with the feelings that are being projected onto them. Enmeshed families avoid discussing genuine feelings and thoughts about one another by repetitively arguing (Nichols & Schwartz, 2003). Feelings of guilt and shame may be pervasive in this family type. In this context communication patterns are characterized by assumptions about what others are thinking. The result is that, due to communications not truly capturing needs and feelings of family members, individuals within the enmeshed family feel misunderstood and not validated.

Problems with Family.   In an enmeshed family system the prospect of dealing with an individual with dementia is most often overwhelming for the family system. Due to the lack of clear roles throughout the family history, the members of the family are in turmoil and confused as to role assignments of the various responsibilities involved in the dementia diagnosis and sequelae. Such families may be inefficient in making decisions regarding the diagnosis and may attempt avoiding issues related to the dementia diagnosis, in part due to the rigid conceptualization of the role of the elder with dementia in the family. The adjustment for both the family and elder with dementia that follows the decision to enter an LTC facility is riddled with feelings of guilt. For example, as the dementing patient expresses statements of wanting to be at home, an enmeshed family becomes emotionally confused and guilty, resulting in excessive visiting and emotional reasoning, disturbing LTC personnel in their care (Goldstein, 1996). Often there exists a feeling of indebtedness whereby a family member believes they must atone for perceived negative treatment throughout the lifetime of dementing relative (Ory, Yee, Tennstedt, & Schulz, 2000). This feeling may have been perpetuated through an enmeshed family dynamic in which feelings of guilt tend to unite family members. This enmeshed family interaction, whereby the elder with dementia elicits guilt in the family members for the decision to institutionalize can contribute to caregiver distress (Mitrani et al., 2005). Feelings of guilt and high avoidance of conflict, therefore, contribute to anxiety and depression in family members (Fisher & Lieberman 1996). Staff may have frequent communication with family members due to family members' internal feelings of wrong doing and a need to alleviate such negative feelings.

At times an enmeshed family can be cohesive and maintain functioning (Schwartz, 1995). Strengths within this family variation include a sense of loyalty and attachment that can be utilized to foster cooperation (Mitrani et al., 2005). But, even here, when confronted with a dementia diagnosis or a need to transition to an LTC facility, disorganization is present. There may be chaotic arguments within the family and subsequent projection of affect onto the clinician, whereby the clinician may be made to feel incompetent (usually due to demands for a second opinion) or blameworthy. It is important for the clinician to be consistent and concise in his/her approach to this type of family.

CASE VIGNETTE

Ms. V is a 93-year-old retired nurse, who had been living independently up until a diagnosis of dementia. She had one very involved daughter, who checked up on mother for medication administration and financial needs. Ms. V began to have increasing difficulty with ADLs, ultimately needing a home care aide. Unfortunately, the aide was not "good enough" as per Ms. V and was fired by the daughter. This happened on four separate occasions and over the next 6 months. Her level of dementia had progressed to where she needed 24-hour care, including assistance with ADL care. The treatment team recommended that Ms. V be placed in an LTC facility. Ms. V refused.

The daughter chose a facility close to her home and placed her mother. Immediately Ms V had problems. She repeatedly asked to "go home."

(continued)

The daughter visited daily in the first week. Staff at the facility spoke with the daughter and explained that decreasing the frequency of visits may help patient acclimatize to the facility. The daughter then visited once per week in the next 3 weeks and Ms. V did seem to adjust. However, the daughter could not stay away as "mother may not be cared for well." On several occasions she accused staff of minor care slights reflective of neglect. She also called other siblings to assist with the LTC facility that did "not understand" their mother. In addition, she continued to ask to "go home" when she saw her daughter. Upon consultation, the facility care providers met with Ms. V and the daughter set limits and reflected the problems in care. They also discussed the mother's routine at home. Ms. V missed interacting with friends and going out. A care plan was put together whereby she was able to have regular visits from friends. The daughter also started to take mother out to restaurants and to visit family. The daughter was also asked to assist in care and later to lessen her visits. There was a drastic improvement in Ms. V's demeanor. Over the next 2 years, Ms. V seemed to adjust well in the LTC, occasionally asking to go home

Disengaged family

Definition.   Individuals within this family type function in an absence of strong connections and relationship ties, as if there is no sense of belonging to family (Hoffman, 1981).

Modes of Relating.   In a disengaged family, there may be rigid cross-generational boundaries. Specifically, the spouses may have a relationship that is not shared with the younger generation, resulting in lack of sharing care and affection with all members. This mode of relating may result in family members feeling deprived of basic emotional needs. Disengaged families tend to avoid conflict by distancing from one another. Avoiding contact can also be physical distance, such as not being at home as a family unit, or emotional distance, such as discussion that occurs on a superficial level that does not disclose feelings. Lack of reciprocity may be a factor in these families such that, when feelings are disclosed, there is a lack of awareness of this disclosure or attempt at communication and therefore may be perceived as lack of reciprocal interaction.

Feelings generally are not communicated and therefore individuals within the family feel isolated and on their own when processing events from the environment. Individuals typically communicate on an intellectual level. Due to the relative lack of feelings of loyalty in this family, there is a diminished sense of interdependence and subsequent request for support when needed (Minuchin, 1974).

Problems with Family. This family has been relatively uninvolved in the activities of one another's lives throughout their history. In dealing with a family member with dementia then this family might initially withdraw from one another. Feelings may be processed privately and therefore the ambiguity of each member's experience may lead to anxiety. Caregiver stress is the result. Typically, the dementing relative who enters an LTC facility lacks full awareness of the rationale for such a move, is reluctant, or is uninvolved in the decision-making. In turn, the family struggles to deal with this dynamic, usually by avoiding or feeling guilty. Interestingly, given the emotional turmoil and confusion often involved in such a decision, the disengaged family may respond in an uninvolved manner, thereby avoiding conflict.

Impulsive families

Definition. This type of family has weak control over impulses. In fact, there exists a narrow range of communicating affect. These families experience events in a concrete action-oriented manner—interruptions (Camp, 2000)

Modes of Relating. There is a sense of impatience which manifests as task-oriented behavior such that members engage in action before thought about potential consequences and ways decisions may affect the family unit.

Problems with Families. Impulsive families may tend to listen to and act immediately on what is told to them in a professional setting. Typically these families react by reducing dissonance quickly and do not allow discomfort or ambiguity to be tolerated. As such, the health-care provider may choose to slow the process of health-care decisions and allow for better decision-making. Having them partake in the activities of the NH is especially important.

Overstressed families

Definition. An overstressed family may fall on the spectrum of either a disengaged or enmeshed family type. Typically this family is high on expressed emotion (EE), a harbinger of relapse, increased psychiatric problems and health-care utilization, and morbidity. This family seems to evolve due to diminished family resources. Financial strains or other preexisting stressors may render the family vulnerable to stress. This is most manifest during the transition to LTC. The disorganized manner of dealing with fundamental matters of living that involve sustainability (e.g., finances), or being proactive are faulty and result in problems. These problems in turn become stressors for more problems.

Modes of Relating. Overstressed families tend to become overwhelmed by emotionality that may compromise communicating effectively and being task oriented. An overstressed family may act out in an irritated or aggressive manner toward one another due to the stresses induced by the external factors. In addition, there may be a tendency to diminish expression of emotion due to family members not wanting to burden the family with additional stressors.

Problems with Families.   The transition of an elder with dementia to LTC in an overstressed family may be an overwhelming prospect. Problems can range from high EE and poor decision-making to being shut down with little input regarding the decision. Unfortunately, like most of these problem family styles, this pattern also does not allow for careful consideration of the issues.

CASE VIGNETTE

Ms. H is a 78-year-old woman with a past psychiatric history of bipolar disorder and now diagnosed with a dementia. She lives with the younger daughter L, who has a family of her own and is stressed. She also has another daughter, who lives an hour away who is very devoted. She is always accompanied by both daughters for appointments. Ms. H has been maintained by an outpatient multidisciplinary team (consisting of a geriatric psychiatrist and a geriatric social work case manager). Over the past 6 months, Ms. H has started to have increasing sleep disturbance and pacing. None of the medication trials have helped. L is overwhelmed having to take care of mother and her own 5-year-old son, and calls the treatment team frequently in "crisis" stating mother needs help, and that she "cannot keep caring for her." On one visit, the treatment team explained the various options for LTC, giving the daughters and the patient suggestions to visit LTC facilities. They visit several facilities and, with some expressed emotion decide on one. The other daughter has been "concerned" about the possible move but realizes that she cannot help as much and agrees to placement. After the move, daughter L feels guilty and wants to take mother back home. The mother, on the other hand, has some problems in the home but has adjusted relatively well. LTC staff meet with the patient and daughters and explain how she (L) can still continue to be active in mother's care by visiting regularly, and assisting staff with bathing and dressing routines (as Ms. H is resistant at times). The staff also asks L to come and spend time with mother. In addition, provision is made for L to see the social worker and discuss issues related to guilt as well as how to deal her sister and with her family.

Families at odds

Definition.   A family at odds with one another may lay on the spectrum of enmeshed to disengaged with regards to pattern of relating. However, the current state of the family is one in which the members are currently at odds with one another, most likely brought on by multiple stressors inherent in the transition to long-term care. LTC transition elicits decisions that need to be made such that values and beliefs come to the forefront of how families engage in with the elements of long-term care. Differing values and beliefs among family members, specifically in the context of perspectives on the transition to long-term care, may result in a family at odds. An imbalanced family system arises when members are given more resources or responsibilities throughout the family history (Schwartz, 1995). This may result in a dynamic of polarization such that members of the family may take on roles that are either in competition or opposed to one another, additionally creating a family at odds with one another.

Modes of Relating.   A family at odds with one another may relate in a way that promotes competition with one another as well as encouraging opposition, through framing issues in a manner that results in members choosing sides.

Problems with Families.   Logistical issues such as location of placement, type of placement, power of attorney, and other types of legal issues such as judging level of competency may become contentious. A clinician may serve as a mediator in this context, hearing each perspective and attempt to find points where agreement is reached (Table 16.2).

Assessment

It is important to involve families in treatment of residents of LTC. This is so for several reasons, but most especially because the family can assist in the care of the resident across time. Assessment is part of this process, as it provides a plan of action for the resident, an understanding by the family of what is being done, and a request for cooperation and assistance in the plan. The intent is not to change the family. It is to provide information regarding what is being done and why this is important. The extent to which the family becomes involved then is less important than an understanding of the care plan. This assessment-as-treatment plan involves four parts; assessment and validation, psychoeducation, problem solving, and a crisis plan.

Assessment of family and validate position

This involves an understanding of the type of family system (see above) and how the family may assist in care or can best be informed about treatment. In effect, to enhance quality of life for both the family and the elder (with dementia) understanding the dynamics of the family, may aid in acknowledging the patterns present and what can be expected. Recognizing the underlying tendencies within the family can be useful in conceptualizing how a given family may react and how the elder in LTC may adjust. The aforementioned levels of dysfunction

TABLE 16.2. Family Types

	MODES OF COMMUNICATION	TRANSITION TO LONG-TERM CARE	STRENGTHS	TREATMENT
Enmeshed family (Minuchin, 1974)	Avoiding direct communication about needs External focus on the cause of the problem	Conflict and guilt (i.e. aware that placement is appropriate but stagnant in the idea that the elder with dementia should be in the home) Feelings of guilt are exacerbated by guilt inducing statements of the elder Feelings of obligation are pervasive and behavior by family members is motivated by obligation	Supportive and cohesive Family closeness such that there may be useful knowledge and insight about one another Express Affect which is conducive to developing enhanced communication	Psychoeducation Encourage and help establish the use of concrete roles for each member in the transition to long-term care through assessing the strength of each member (i.e. one member may organize the move while another may deal with the facility). In addition, members may feel connected to the family member if they can do some hands on tasks such as picking out clothes Suggestions for autonomous communication patterns (i.e. expressing what one feels rather than how another may feel or behave) Help the family to predict what circumstances may lead to a conflict and have suggestions for conflict resolution that promote listening skills and autonomous communication of feelings and perceptions of the situation at hand Promote acknowledgment and appreciation of the individual contribution each member has in the transition
Disengaged family (Minuchin, 1974)	Avoidance of conflict Alienation from one another Denial or diminishment of the dementing condition in the elder due to the need of avoidance of emotional sequelae (i.e. loss, guilt) Emphasis on independence and autonomy	Suppressed guilt and sadness such that there are psychosomatic complaints Elder is expected or encouraged to be independent in their emotional transition to long-term care	Placement to long term care is overtly and rationally understood May establish structure such as logistics and scheduling of long-term-care placement efficiently due to repressed emotion	Clinician can help establish roles and schedules for members Clinician can encourage overt expression of feelings in both the elder and the family members about the transition in order to foster affection and understanding Develop a sense of loyalty to the transition to long term care by appealing to their intellectual sense through psychoeducation about the process of a dementing illness and the necessity of long term care

Continued

TABLE 16.2. Continued

	MODES OF COMMUNICATION	TRANSITION TO LONG-TERM CARE	STRENGTHS	TREATMENT
Impulsive families	Aspects of impatience in dealing with external factors as well as with one another Decisions, in general are made abruptly and may have a variety of consequences that are not prepared for	Facility placement may occur abruptly without deliberation about type of facility and such logistics	Task oriented Desire to engage in action sooner rather than later	Emphasize the importance of careful consideration and what issues should be taken into consideration (i.e. distance of the facility form family) Give different options for long-term placement as well as presenting other issues as options
Overstressed families (Goldstein, 1996)	Displacement of aggression and frustration of the situation on one another		This may be a temporary state of the family brought on be the circumstance of transition to long term care There is acknowledgment of needing help and appreciation of the opportunity for resources that may reduce the stress of the family	Each individual to take responsibility of their own feelings Small and doable modifications of activities to reduce stress (may not have to do with the elder with dementia) Emphasis of caring for oneself outside of the context of the elder with dementia
Families at odds (Goldstein, 1996)	Polarization—Individuals are on one side of an issue or another	Contention and disagreement about many factors Legal involvement	Potential to reach agreements about the elder and their placement such that the family is collectively supported	Helping each side to be heard Frame issues in a speculative or conceptual way such that discussion is encouraged

in communication and roles in the family, regardless of their relationship to the patient (i.e., spouse or child), can contribute to caregivers with high levels of burden (Tremont, David, & Bishop, 2006). Families develop coping strategies based on previous exposure to stressful situations (Brubaker, 1990). Knowledge of the family system then can assist in what strategies to use in the current stress situation (Mitriani et al., 2005).

There are formal assessment scales. Mitriani et al. (2005) adapted the Structural Family Systems Ratings (SFSR-DC), an observational measure of family interaction, for dementia caregivers, in order to determine the impact of familial interaction on caregiver emotional functioning. Subscales derived from the adaptation of the scale include those highly related to family problems and systems issues (see case vignettes). The SFSR-DC provides theoretically sound dimensions for conceptualizing family dynamics and, implicitly, how such dynamics impact on the families' adjustment to placing the elder with dementia into long-term care. In addition, each dimension represents a point at which there can be intervention by the clinician (Table 16.3).

To this we have added several marker questions that flesh out the types of problem families we have been discussing (Table 16.4).

TABLE 16.3. Structural Family Systems Ratings (SFSR-DC) Domains

Caregiver leadership—caregiver not fulfilling leadership role or deriving validation from other members of their leadership

Enmeshment vs. disengagement—high degree of closeness or intrusion by family members vs. absence of engagement and rigid boundaries

Family maladjustment to the dementia diagnosis—conceptualization of the abilities of the care recipient (i.e., assigning roles that are consistent or inconsistent with cognitive abilities)

Focus on the identified patient—the extent to which the family focuses or expresses negativity about elder with dementia

Conflict resolution—the approach the family takes to managing tasks or conflict

Supportive functioning—family support or negativity toward central caregiver

TABLE 16.4. Marker Questions for Family System

How will each type of family experience the stress?

How does the family define the stressful event and its impact on the family structure?

What are the resources that they see as available to them?

What types of resources would they be inclined to utilize?

Will the family be active or passive in their involvement?

What is the level of expressed emotion in the family?

How controlling is the family?

How are family duties shared?

How do families handle conflict?

How do families talk to one another?

Psychoeducation

This is a no nonsense representation of problems. It is a formulation of the physical and mental health issues that require care and work in LTC. In regards to depression, for example, the health-care provider represents that the commonness of the problem, the chronic state of its features, the lowered functioning that results, and the problems that result in relationships. In a sense it is an expectation setter, a problem manifesto, and treatment guide. How the family may want to partake in the LTC plan is encouraged but optional. The objective is to that they are aware of the plan and can assist and not be a problem.

Problem solving

This involves two features of the family: where problems develop and where help can be initiated. Problems are present due to several identified areas, including level of involvement with resident, poor family coping (e.g., high expressed emotion), and loss of the active role of a family member. Again, the health-care provider is not there as a family therapist but as an informant and coach finessing possible transparent problems. The family can help on many fronts, including basic support (visits), taking care of necessary business, and eliciting other family members for defined issues.

Crisis plan

This is a plan that can be implemented with the family if a problem evolves. This includes a change in health status of the resident or other family member. This plan should address end of life issues, the occurrence of a negative event in the LTC facility, or some high probability issue within the family that can occur (e.g., competency, POA issues).

CONCLUSION

Families maintain their influence throughout the lifespan. The family affects the life of the resident and, therefore, requires attention by the health-care provider in LTC. This chapter discussed the importance of understanding the family, its history, dynamics, communication patterns, and strengths. The goal is to appreciate this influence in the LTC treatment of the resident. Optimal treatment then involves an assessment and engagement of the family. We provided several ideas on how to involve and care for the family, a taxonomy of family systems, and an assessment plan. Through such an understanding, the clinician working with the family has the ability to aid in developing balance and harmony to the family system, facilitate personal growth of family members, and affect the care of the resident.

REFERENCES

Anderson, R., Lyons, J., & West, C. (2001). The prediction of mental health use in residential care. *Journal of Gerontological Nursing, 37:* 313–322.

Ball, K., Berch, D., Helmers, K., Jobe, J., Leveck, M., Marsiske, M., et al. (2002). Effects of cognitive training interventions with older adults: A randomized controlled trial. *Journal of American Medical Association, 288:* 2271–2281.

Boettcher, I. F., Kemeny, B., DeShon, R. P., & Stevens, A. B. (2004). A system to develop staff behaviors for person-centered care. *Alzheimer's Care Quarterly, 5*(3): 188–196.

Bookwala, J., & Jacobs, J. (2004). Age, marital processes, and depressed affect. *The Gerontologist, 44*(3): 328–338. Gerontological Society of America.

Bowers, B. (1988). Family perceptions of care in a nursing home. *The Gerontologist, 28:* 361–367.

Brubaker, T. H. (1990). A contextual approach to the development of stress associated with caregiving in later-life families. In M. A. Stephens, J. H. Crowther, S. E. Hobfoll, & D. L. Tennenbaum (Eds.), *Stress and coping in later-life families.* Washington: Hemisphere Publishing Corporation.

Buhr, G., Kuchibhatla, M., & Clipp, E. (2006). Caregivers' reasons for nursing home Placement: Clues for improving discussions with families prior to the transition. *The Gerontologist, 46*(1): 52–61.

Burgio, L. D., Stevens, A. S., Burgio, K. L., Roth, D. L., Paul, P., & Gerstile, J. (2002). Teaching and maintaining behavior management skills in the nursing home. *The Gerontologist, 42:* 487–496.

Camp, C. J. (2000). Clinical research in long term care: What the future holds? In V. Molinari (Ed.). *Professional psychology in long term care: A comprehensive guide* (pp. 401–423). New York: Hatherleigh Press.

Carstensen, L. L. (1992). Social and emotional patterns in adulthood: Support for socioemotional selectivity theory. *Psychology and Aging, 7*(3): 331–338.

Carstensen, L. L., Isaacowitz, D. M., & Charles, S. T. (1999). Taking time seriously: A theory of socioemotional selectivity. *American Psychologist, 54*(3), 165–181.

Centers for Medicare and Medicaid Services. (2002). Revised long term care resident assessment instrument. User's manual for the minimum data set (MDS), version 2. Atlanta, GA: Center for Medicare and Medicaid Services.

Centers for Medicare and Medicaid Services (2004). MDS active resident information Report: Fourth quarter 2004. Retrieved March 8, 2005 fromhttp://www3.cms.hhs.gov/states/mdsreports/res2.asp.

Dellasega, C., & Mastrian, K. (1995). The process and consequences of institutionalizing an elder. *Western Journal of Nursing Research, 17:* 123–140.

Engelhardt, Dourado & Laks, J. (2005). Alzheimers disease and the impact on caregivers. *Revista Brasileira de Neurologia, 41*(2): 5–11.

Family Caregiver Alliance (2006a). *Caregiver assessment: Principles, guidelines, and strategies for change.* Report from the national consensus conference (Vol I). San Francisco: Author.

Family Caregiver Alliance (2006b). *Caregiver assessment: Principles, guidelines, and strategies for change.* Report from the national consensus conference (Vol II). San Francisco: Author.

Gallagher-Thompson, D., Coon, D., Solano, N., Ambler, C., Rabinowitz, Y., & Thompson, L. (2003). Changes in indices of distress among Latino and Anglo female caregivers of elderly relatives with dementia: Site specific results from the REACH National Collaborative Study. *The Gerontologist, 45*: 580–591.

Gaugler, J., Edwards, A., Femia, E., Zarit, S., Stephens, M., & Townsend, A. (2000). Predictors of institutionalization of cognitively impaired elders: Family help and the timing of placement. *Journal of Gerontology: Psychological Sciences, 55B*, 247–255.

Gaugler, J., Kane, R., Clay, T., & Newcomer, R. (2003). Caregiving and institutionalization of cognitively impaired older people: Utilizing dynamic predictors of change. *The Gerontologist, 43*: 219–229.

Gilbert, M. E., & McMahon, J. K. (2004). Nursing-oriented in-services: Providing meaningful education to direct nursing care providers. *Journal of Gerontological Nursing, 30*: 54–56.

Greene, V., & Monahan, D. (1982). The impact on visitation on patient well-being in nursing homes. *The Gerontologist, 7*: 57–67.

Goldstein, M. (1996). Working with families. In W. E. Reichman, & P. R. Katz (Eds.), *Psychiatric care in the nursing home.* New York: Oxford University Press.

Haley, W., Levine, E., Brown, S., & Bartolucci, A. (1987). Stress, appraisal, coping, and social support as predictors of adaptational outcome among dementia caregivers. *Psychology and Aging, 2*: 323–330.

Heath, J. Gartenberg, M., & Beagin, E. (2006). Blending mental health services into the geriatric medical care of long term care facility residents. In L. Hyer, & R. Intrieri (Eds.), *Treatment in long-term care: Geropsychological interventions.* New York, Springer .

Hepburn, K., Lewis, M., Natayan, S., Center, B., Tirnatore, J., Bremer, K., & Nelson, L. (2006). Partners in caregiving: A psychoeducational program affecting dementia family caregivers' distress and caregiving outlook. *Clinical Gerontologist, 29*: 53–70.

Hebert, R., Dubois, M., Wolfson, C., Chambers, L., & Cohen, C. (2001). Factors associated with long-term institutionalization of older people with dementia: Data from the Canadian study of health and aging. *Journal of Gerontology: Medical Sciences, 56A*, 693–699.

Hill, R. (1958). Generic features of families under stress. *Social Casework, 48*: 139–150.

Hoffman, L. (1981). *Foundations of family therapy.* New York: Basic Books.

Hyer, L., & Intrieri, R. (2006). *Treatment in long-term care: Geropsychological interventions.* New York: Springer.

Hyer, L., & Ragan, A. (2003). Training in long-term care facilities: Critical issues. *Clinical Gerontologist, 25*: 197–239.

Jones A. (2002). The national nursing home Survey: 1999 Summary. *National center for health statistics. Vital health stat 13*(152). Retrieved March 8, 2005 from http://www.cdc.gov/nchs/data/series/sr_13/srl3_152.pdf.

Lieberman, M., & Fisher, L. (1999). The effects of family conflict resolution and decision making on provisions of help for elders with Alzheimer's disease. *The Gerontologist, 39* (2), 156–166.

Martin, L. S., Rozon, L., McDowell, S., Cetinski, G., & Kemp, K. (2004). Evaluation of a training program for long-term care staff on bathing techniques for persons with dementia. *Alzheimer's Care Quarterly, 5*(3): 217–229.

Mathieson, V. (1989). Guilt and grief: when daughters place mothers in nursing homes. *Journal of gerontological nursing, 15*: 11–21.

McCallion, P., Toseland, R. W., Lacey, D., & Bandks, S. (1999). Educating nursing assistants to communicate more effectively with nursing home residents with dementia. *The Gerontologist, 5*, 546–558.

Mellins, C., & Blum, M. (1993). Family network perspectives on caregiving. *Generations*, *17* (1): 21–27.

Minuchin, S. (1974). *Families and family therapy*. Cambridge, MA: Harvard University Press.

Mitchell, J., & Kemp, B. (2000). Quality of life in assisted living homes: A multidimensional analysis. *Journal of Gerontology: Psychological Sciences*, *55B*: 117–127.

Mittelman, M. (2005). Taking care of the caregivers. *Current Opinion in Psychiatry*, *18*(6), 633–639.

Mittelman, M., Epstein, C., & Pierzchala, A. (2003). *Counseling the Alzheimer's caregiver: A resource for healthcare providers*. Washington, DC: American Medical Association.

Mittelman, M., Ferris, S., Shulman, E., Steinberg, G., & Levin, B. (1996). A family intervention to delay nursing home placement of patients with Alzheimer's disease: A randomized controlled trial. *Journal of American Medical Association*, *276*: 1725–1731.

Mittelman, M., Roth, D., Coon, D., & Haley, W. (2004). Sustained benefit of supportive intervention for depressive symptoms in Alzheimer's caregivers. *American Journal of Psychiatry*, *661*: 850–856.

Mittelman, M., Roth, D., Haley, W., & Zarit, S. (2004). Effects of a caregiver intervention on negative caregiver appraisals of behavior problems in patients with Alzheimer's disease: Results of a randomized trial. *Journal of Gerontology*, *59B*: 27–34.

Mitriani, V., Feaster, D., McCabe, B., Czaja, S., & Szapocznik, J. (2005). Adapting the structural family systems rating to assess the patterns of interaction in families of dementia caregivers. *The Gerontologist*, *45*(4): 445–455.

Naleppa, M. (1996). Families and the institutionalized elderly: A review. *Journal of Clinical Nursing*, *8*(6): 723–730.

Nichols, M. D., & Schwartz, R. C. (2003). *Family therapy: Concepts and methods* (6th ed.). New Work: Allyn and Bacon.

Ory, M. C., Yee, J. L., Tennstedt, S. L., & Schulz, R. (2000). The extent and impact of dementia care: Unique challenges experienced by family caregivers. In R. Schulz (Ed.), *Handbook on dementia caregiving: Evidence-based interventions for family caregivers* (pp. 1–33). New York: Springer..

Pearlin, L., Mullan, J., Semple, S., & Skaff, M. (1990). Caregiving and the stress process: An overview of concepts and their measurements. *The Gerontologist*, *30:* 583–594.

Pillemer, K., Suitor, J., Henderson, Jr., M., Meador, R., Schultz, L., Robison, J., & Hegeman, M. (2003). A cooperative communication intervention for nursing home staff and family members of residents. *The Gerontologist*, *43:* 96–106.

Port, C., Zimmerman, S., Williams, S., Dobbs, D., Williams, C., & Preisser, J. (2005). Families filling the gap: Comparing family involvement for assisted living and nursing home residents with dementia. *The Gerontologist*, *45*, 88–96.

Reed, J., & Morgan, D. (1999). Discharging older people from hospital to care homes: Implications for nursing. *Journal of advanced nursing*, *29:* 819–825.

Roth, D., Mittelman, M., Clay, O., Madan, A., & Haley, W. (2005). Changes in social support as mediators of the impact of a psychosocial intervention for spouse caregivers of persons with Alzheimer's disease. *Psychology and Aging*, *20:* 634–644.

Rovner B. W., German, P. S., Broadhead, J., Morriss, R. K., Brant, L. J., Blaustein, J., & Folstein, M. F. (1990) The prevalence and management of dementia and other psychiatric disorders in nursing homes. *International Psychogeriatrics*, *2*(1): 13–24.

Sahyoun, N. R., Pratt, L. A., Lentzner, H., Dey, A., & Robinson, K. N. (2001). The changing profile of nursing home residents: 1985–1997. *Aging Trends*, *4:* 1–8.

Schulz, R., Belle, S. H., Czaja, S. J., McGinnis, K. A., Stevens, A., & Zhang, S. (2004). Long-term care placement of dementia patients and caregiver health and well-being. *Journal of American Medical Association*, *292*(8): 961–967.

Schultz, R., & Martire, L. (2004). Family caregivers of persons with dementia: Prevalence, health effects, and support strategies. *American Journal of Geriatric Psychiatry, 12:* 240–249.

Schulz, R., O'Brien, Czaja, S., Ory, M., Norris, R., Matire, L., et al. (2002). Dementia caregiver intervention research: In search of clinical significance. *The Gerontologist, 42:* 589–602.

Schwartz, R. C. (1995). *Internal family systems therapy.* New York: The Guiliford Press.

Sikorska, E. (1999). Organizational determinants of resident satisfaction with assisted living. *The Gerontologist, 39:* 450–456.

Simmons, S., & Ouslander, J. (2005). Resident and family satisfaction with incontinence and mobility care: Sensitivity to intervention effects. *The Gerontologist, 45:* 318–326.

Steinglass, P. (1980). Assessing families in their own home. *American Journal of Psychiatry, 137:* 1523–1529.

Sorensen, S., Pinquart, M., & Duberstein, P. (2002). How effective are interventions with caregivers? An updated meta-analysis. *The Gerontologist, 42:* 356–372.

Stevens, A., & Hochhalter, (2006). Meeting the needs of nursing home residents and staff: The informed teams model of staff development. In L. Hyer, & R. Intrieri (Eds), *Treatment in long-term care: Geropsychological interventions.* New York: Springer.

Stevens, A. B., Burgio, L. D., Bailey, E., Burgio, K. L., Paul, P., Capilouto, E., Nicovich, P., et al. (1998). Teaching and maintaining behavior management skills with nursing assistants in a nursing home. *The Gerontologist, 38:* 379–384.

Townsend, A. (1990). Nursing home care and family caregivers' stress. In M. A. Stephens, J. Crowther, S. Hobfal, & D. Tannebaum (Eds.), *Stress and coping in later life families* (pp. 267–286). New York: Hemisphere.

Tremont, G., David, D., & Bishop, D. (2006). Unique contribution of family functioning in caregivers of patients with mild to moderate dementia. *Dementia and Geriatric Cognitive Disorders, 21*(3), 170–174.

Weintraub, D., Datto, C., Streim, J., & Katz, I. (2002). Second-generation issues in the management of depression in nursing homes. *Journal of the American Geriatrics Society, 50(12):* 2100–2101.

Whisman, M., Uebelacker, L., & Weinstock, L. M. (2004). Psychopathology and marital satisfaction: The importance of evaluating both partners. *Journal of Consulting and Clinical Psychology, 72(5):* 830–838. American Psychological Association.

Yaffe, K., Fox, P., Newcomer, R., Sands, L., Lindquist, K., Dane, K., & Covinsky, K. (2002). Patient and caregiver characteristics and nursing home placement in patients with dementia. *Journal of American Medical Association, 287*(16): 2090–2097.

17

Environmental and Milieu Interventions

Jiska Cohen-Mansfield and *Rene P. Laje*

The majority of nursing home residents suffer from dementia (Rovner et al., 1990). The cognitive decline that occurs with the natural course of dementia is always associated with memory problems, and at times with other difficulties including depressed affect or apathy, and often involves the emergence of disturbed affect or behaviors that are bothersome to others or indicative of the resident's discomfort. These dementia-related symptoms and behaviors were, for many years, either ignored or treated with physical restraints or psychotropic medication. In the past 2 decades, new research has advanced the understanding of affect, function, and behavior in dementia so that many problems can be treated, and often prevented, through modification of the social and physical environment. These interventions thus help to enhance the quality of life for people with dementia and give relief to staff and families. In this chapter, we will review the rationale for such interventions and the evidence for their use. We use the terms "environmental and milieu interventions" in their wide definition to include both the physical environment as well as the social environment, including the way staff members treat residents and the tools they use to improve care.

PURPOSE OF INTERVENTIONS

The living situation of an individual with cognitive impairment can have a considerable effect on overall well-being. As cognition declines and familiarity with surroundings lessens, people with dementia rely more and more on their environment to address their needs. A setting that accommodates the bio-psycho-social needs of the individual may be effective in slowing cognitive decline, improving affect, and decreasing undesirable behaviors. The social and physical environment needs to be designed to address the affective needs, cognitive abilities and behavioral symptoms of the specific resident. The chapter begins with a discussion of behavior problems and their conceptualization. We then proceed to describe treatment through milieu and environmental interventions to improve behavior, affect, and cognition.

Description of Problem Behaviors/Agitated Behaviors

Research shows that dementia-related behaviors (labeled interchangeably as problem behaviors, agitated behaviors, or behavioral disturbances) in the nursing home fall into three categories: verbally agitated behaviors, physically non-aggressive behaviors, and physically aggressive behaviors (Cohen-Mansfield et al., 1989). Verbally agitated behaviors include screaming, cursing, overly frequent calls for attention, verbal bossiness or pushiness, complaining or whining, negativism, temper outbursts, or making strange or menacing noises. Physically nonaggressive behaviors include general restlessness, performing repetitious mannerisms, pacing, trying to get to a different place without apparent cause, inappropriate handling of objects, aimless walking, and inappropriate dressing or undressing. Physically aggressive behaviors include hitting, pushing, scratching, kicking, and grabbing things or people.

GENERAL THEORETICAL FRAMEWORK

The relationship between dementia and problem behaviors raises the question of why people with dementia so often develop undesirable behaviors. There are several theories that point to factors in the environment that may ultimately contribute to problem behaviors and affect: behavioral theory, the environmental vulnerability model, the unmet needs model, and models of depressed affect.

Behavioral Model

According to the behavioral model, a problem behavior is controlled by its antecedents and consequences (Figure 17.1). Antecedents include triggers that

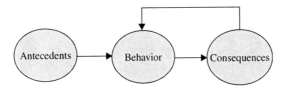

FIGURE 17.1. Behavioral model. © Cohen-Mansfield, 1998. All rights reserved.

initiate the behavior, such as the view of the exit door eliciting an attempt to exit the institution; consequences refer to the reaction to the behavior, such as when screaming is followed by attention from staff members, a response that reinforces the screaming behavior. Interventions based on a behavioral model aim to change these relationships in the environment. For example, changing the antecedents through camouflaging of the exit door may reduce exit-seeking behavior. Changing the contingencies for attention may reinforce appropriate rather than inappropriate behavior.

The Environment Vulnerability Model

The environmental vulnerability model (Figure 17.2) asserts that the process of cognitive decline causes a vulnerability to the environment, which leads to a lower threshold at which stimuli affect behavior. A stimulus that may elicit an appropriate response in a person without cognitive impairment may generate problem behaviors in a person with cognitive impairment. This model is based on the concepts of person–environment congruence (French et al., 1974; Kahana, 1982) and the environment-behavioral model (Lawton, 1990), which suggest that for optimal functioning, a match is needed between the person's needs and abilities and the demands of the environment, as they relate to those needs and abilities. For any level of competence, there is a range of environmental demands that is favorable. The environmental docility hypothesis (Lawton & Simon, 1968) states that as personal competence decreases, the environment becomes a more potent determinant of behavioral outcome. The idea that the environment has a potent role in affecting behavior does not, however, clarify the way in which a mismatch between the person and the environment results in behavior problems. Two opposing explanations are that the environment provides overstimulation relative to the abilities of persons with dementia (exemplified by the progressively lowered stress threshold theory described below) or that the environment is understimulating and may cause sensory deprivation (as described in the unmet need theory below). Although there are studies supporting both notions, and either may apply under certain circumstances, more often research results support the understimulation notion, i.e., the idea that lack of

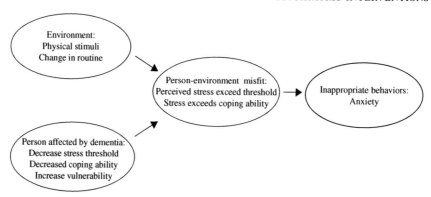

FIGURE 17.2. Environmental vulnerability/progressively lowered stress threshold. © Cohen-Mansfield, 1998. All rights reserved.

sufficient and appropriate stimulation is at the heart of certain types of problem behaviors and the environment needs to be modified to match the individual's stimulation needs and capabilities.

A related concept is that dementia results in a progressively lowered stress threshold (Hall, 1994; Hall & Buckwalter, 1987). Essentially, this theory asserts that persons with dementia progressively lose their coping abilities and their comprehension of their environment, and therefore perceive their environment as more stressful, thereby having a lower threshold for encountering stress. Anxiety and inappropriate behavior can result as environmental stimuli exceed the person's stress threshold. Excess levels of stress can be caused either by environmental stimuli that would otherwise be considered normal but cannot be processed by the person with dementia because of the lowered threshold for stress, or by inappropriate environmental stimulus levels as well as physical stressors, such as pain. Interventions based on the environmental vulnerability model often focus on the need for a quiet and untaxing environment, such as shutting off the intercom or providing a quiet unit (Cleary et al., 1988; Meyer et al., 1992).

Unmet Needs Model

The unmet needs model (Figure 17.3) describes a ripple effect of the cognitive decline. Because of the disease process, the person with dementia has difficulty in meeting his/her needs because of a decreased ability to communicate needs and provide for oneself. This encompasses all aspects of one's being: physical, emotional, mental (e.g., cognitive need for intellectual stimulation, need for meaningful activity), and social. The nursing home environment provides for basic needs, such as need for food and shelter. However,

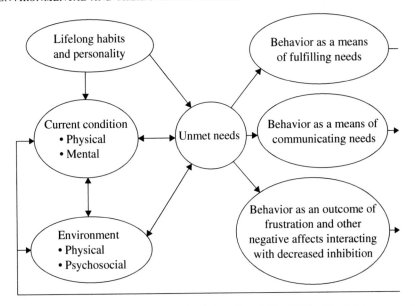

FIGURE 17.3. Unmet needs model. © Cohen-Mansfield, 1998. All rights reserved. Reprinted with permission from Cohen-Mansfield and Taylor (1998).

most often it does not fit the lifelong habits and personality, preferences, and specific needs of the individual. The loss in the ability to communicate and to perform tasks, combined with the environment's lack of understanding of the person and deficiencies in individualizing care, results in unmet needs (Algase et al., 1996; Cohen-Mansfield & Deutsch, 1996; Cohen-Mansfield & Werner, 1995). Problem behaviors emerge as an attempt to meet or to communicate those needs. Research has shown some of the general needs that people with dementia are trying to communicate or diminish through agitated behavior; these are described below.

Pain/health/physical discomfort

Studies have demonstrated the relationship of pain and health with verbal agitation (Cohen-Mansfield et al., 1990). In fact, one study reported an increase in negativity in people who had fevers (Hurley et al., 1992), and another showed a relationship between level of agitation and the presence of infection (Cohen-Mansfield et al., 1994). Individuals who are cognitively intact may yell out when they are experiencing pain. For people with dementia, the same reaction to pain may occur. Vocally disruptive behavior may also be an attempt to communicate the discomfort under circumstances in which a cognitively impaired individual is no longer able to communicate more directly. At times, it may be exacerbated by the frustration of not experiencing understanding or relief despite communicating the pain. The relationship between agitation and pain is supported by a small study (Douzjian et al., 1998) in which five of eight residents receiving analgesic medication showed significant improvement in their behavior and could therefore be taken off psychoactive medication.

The association between pain or health and physically aggressive or physically nonaggressive behaviors is less clear, although Ryden et al. (1991) did find a relationship between physical aggression and urinary tract infections. In contrast, people who engage in physically nonaggressive behavior (e.g., pacing) have been reported to have fewer medical diagnoses than other nursing home residents and to have better appetites. However, Mutch (1992) found that people who demonstrate physically nonaggressive behaviors, such as pacing, might be suffering from akathesia, an inner sense of restlessness, caused by a reaction to antipsychotic drugs.

Sleep disturbance or fatigue is another aspect of health that has been linked to problem behaviors (Cohen-Mansfield et al., 1990, 1995). The impairment of circadian rhythms that is characteristic of Alzheimer's disease (Friedman et al., 1993) may also be related to behavioral problems. In particular, an increase in behavioral problems in elderly individuals with dementia that occurs in the evening hours, beginning at a time near sunset, has been termed sundowning (Bliwise, 1994).

Uncomfortable environmental conditions present another possible trigger of problem behaviors. In an observational study of the nursing home environment, problem behaviors tended to increase when it was cold at night, and requests for attention increased when it was hot during the day (Cohen-Mansfield & Werner, 1995). These findings suggest that uncomfortable temperatures may cause or contribute to some behavioral problems.

Mental discomfort evident in affective states: Depression, anxiety, and frustration

These affective processes may result from the individual's confrontation with decreasing abilities or other unmet needs, such as loneliness and boredom. Research revealed a relationship between verbal/vocal problem behaviors and depressed affect (Cohen-Mansfield & Marx, 1988; Cohen-Mansfield & Werner, 1999). This finding may in part be explained by the fact that the same group also had more physical pain, which is known to relate to depressed affect, or that this group was more cognitively intact and therefore better able to communicate their moods (via complaints or other negative comments) to caregivers than those manifesting other types of behavioral problems. The relationship between depressed affect and physically nonaggressive behaviors or aggressive behaviors is less clear, with some studies showing a relationship and others showing none (Cohen-Mansfield & Marx, 1988; Cohen-Mansfield & Werner, 1998b, 1999; Leonard et al., 2006; McShane et al., 2000).

Need for social contacts/social isolation

Verbal/vocal problem behaviors, as well as some physically nonaggressive behaviors other than pacing and wandering, tended to increase in frequency when nursing home residents were alone and tended to decrease when they were with others. Similarly, such behaviors decreased when staffing levels increased (Cohen-Mansfield & Werner, 1995). These findings suggest that loneliness or the need for social contact may be at the root of these behaviors. This idea is supported by an intervention study (Cohen-Mansfield & Werner, 1997), in which social interaction was more beneficial in decreasing verbal and vocal problem behaviors than was the mere provision of pleasant stimuli, such as music.

In addition, loneliness is highly correlated with depressed affect, and social interaction and contact interventions are therefore also appropriate for improving affect. The most effective intervention for loneliness seems to be a positive interaction with a person who is meaningful to the elderly person (Cohen-Mansfield & Werner, 1997).

Inadequate level of stimulation (too low, too high, inappropriate)/sensory deprivation

Problem behaviors have been attributed to overstimulation that cannot be processed because of the dementia (Cleary et al., 1988; Johnson, 1989; Meyer et al., 1992). However, an observational study of the nursing home (Cohen-Mansfield et al., 1992) did not support this hypothesis. In fact, observations from this study found that the nursing home was a relatively monotonous place. Routine is the rule, and activities and stimulation are infrequent (Cohen-Mansfield et al., 1992). Most problem behaviors increased when the older person was inactive and decreased when structured activities were offered (Cohen-Mansfield & Werner, 1995).

The opposite view, that problem behaviors result from sensory deprivation and understimulation, has also been proposed. According to this view, the person with dementia has a reduced ability to obtain stimulation and process it. In addition, many of those suffering from dementia also have vision and hearing deficits that further decrease their ability to process stimuli. Finally, many of the nursing homes in which persons with dementia reside offer few activities or other positive stimulation. All of these factors result in a state of sensory deprivation to which the person responds with either self-stimulation or behaviors that manifest discontent because of this unmet need for stimulation. Moreover, studies on social deprivation in younger populations have shown that sensory deprivation can result in hallucinations and perceptual distortions, which may in turn cause problem behaviors. Even without hallucinations or perceptual changes, the sensory deprivation may evoke feelings of fear, loneliness and boredom, all resulting in the manifestation of problem behaviors. Several studies showed that providing sensory stimulation to nursing home residents decreased behavioral disturbances in general and vocally disruptive behaviors in particular (Birchmore & Clague, 1983; Mayers & Griffin, 1990; Zachow, 1984).

Theoretical Frameworks for Affect

Depressed affect has been conceptualized as resulting from lack of control and a sense of helplessness (Seligman, 1974, 1975) or to insufficient reinforcing activities (Lewinsohn & Youngren, 1976); it has also been linked to loneliness (Cohen-Mansfield & Parpura-Gill, 2007). All of these models can be used to address depressed affect in persons with dementia. For example, according to the lack of control/increased helplessness model, in order to decrease depressed affect, one needs to increase a sense of control and/or decrease helplessness. Providing opportunities for persons with dementia to exercise control, such as making decisions about meals or clothes or caring for a plant, may also be used to target depression in this population (Langer & Rodin, 1976). Another method that has helped to alleviate depression in this population involves affirmation of self. This has been successfully achieved through identifying previous and current roles of individuals with dementia and developing interventions that utilize aspects of these roles to alleviate agitation or distress (Cohen-Mansfield et al., 2000, 2006).

TYPES, USE, AND EFFICACY OF ENVIRONMENTAL AND MILIEU INTERVENTIONS

Sensory Enhancement/Relaxation Interventions

Sensory interventions provide stimulation and can thereby ease agitation through the senses. These interventions include massage (touch), music/white noise (auditory), aromatherapy (olfactory), and sensory stimulation, which may be a combination of these approaches.

Massage has been tested alone and in combination with other interventions. A study of 14 community-dwelling elderly by Rowe and Alfred (1999) reported that using slow-stroke massage alone was beneficial in decreasing nonphysical agitation, but there was no change in verbal agitation. Another study on nursing home residents with dementia found that when using massage alone, participants' anxiety scores declined, but this study did not measure agitation (Sansone & Schmitt, 2000). Moreover, Snyder et al. (1995) revealed that hand massage alone did not lower agitation scores but did produce a relaxation response.

Studies show that when *massage* is used in combination *with other interventions,* treatment is more effective. Ballard et al. (2002) found that when applying Melissa officinalis (lemon balm) to residents' faces and arms twice a day, residents were significantly less agitated than residents who had massage with placebo (sunflower oil). Moreover, Smallwood et al. (2001) found that when comparing aromatherapy and massage (AM), aromatherapy and conversation, and massage only, AM showed the greatest benefits in reducing motor agitation in people with severe dementia. Another study tested the effects of expressive physical touch with verbalization on anxiety and difficult behaviors and found that this intervention does lower anxiety and reduces the number of episodes of problem behaviors (Kim & Buschmann, 1999). In combining calm music with hand massage, one study did not find a cumulative effect; however, the author did find that using the interventions together or alone significantly reduced agitation in residents up to 1 h after the intervention (Remington, 2002).

Music intervention is used for two general purposes: for relaxation during meals or bathing or to provide sensory stimulation. Music interventions ranged from listening to a music tape (in some studies, with headphones) to a music therapy session, which included musical games, dancing, movement, and singing. In using music for relaxation during bathing, two studies found that music was effective in reducing aggressive behaviors and demonstrated a trend for decreasing other problem behaviors (Clark et al., 1998; Thomas et al., 1997). Of the four studies that examined the relaxing impact of quiet music during mealtimes, two reported a significant decline in agitation during lunchtime (Denney, 1997; Goddaer & Abraham, 1994) and one found a significant decline during the evening meal (Hicks-Moore, 2005); however, the fourth did not demonstrate an effect during dinner (Ragneskog et al., 1996). Several studies reported a reduction in verbal agitation or agitation in general while patients listened to music on a tape or DVD player (Cohen-Mansfield & Werner, 1997; Gerdner, 2000; Gerdner & Swanson, 1993; Tabloski, 1995). In about half of these studies, the music was individualized to match the person's preferences, whereas other studies used soft or classical music. The effect of music was reported to occur primarily during the listening sessions and to be reduced after the conclusion of the session. Two other studies found that using music therapy, which included singing, playing instruments, and dancing, resulted in a significant decrease in agitation (Brotons & Pickett-Cooper, 1996; Svansdottir & Snaedal, 2006). Finally, a study of 30 Alzheimer's-unit residents who wandered found that music therapy activities (listening, playing percussion instruments, singing, and movement or dance) promoted more seating behavior than did reading aloud to residents. This was conducted in one-to-one sessions with the therapist, and whenever possible, the content of the session was individualized to match the resident's past preferences (Groene, 1993).

White noise may induce relaxation and sleep and thereby decrease nocturnal restlessness. Positive results have been reported in some, but not all, cases (Burgio et al., 1996; Young et al., 1988).

There are three studies on *aromatherapy* intervention used alone for agitation, and all three included lavender as one type of scent. Holmes et al. (2002) found that 60% of the participants showed a reduction in agitation when a lavender stream was presented compared with a stream of water, for which there was no change. The other two studies (Gray & Clair, 2002; Snow et al., 2004) did not see a change in agitation with the introduction of the intervention. As mentioned above, the use of lemon balm via massage was found to be effective in reducing agitation when compared with a placebo aroma (Ballard et al., 2002).

Social Contact—Real or Simulated

Social contact involves interacting with humans, pets, or technologies that simulate such contact. There have been very few studies on *one-to-one interaction* despite the positive effects it appears to have with people who have dementia and are agitated. Cohen-Mansfield and Werner (1997) found that one-to-one interaction provided to 41 nursing home residents for half an hour per day for 10 days was effective in decreasing verbally disruptive behaviors by 54%, a reduction that was significantly larger than the control condition of the same duration. The importance of social interaction was also displayed in the findings by Runci et al. (1999). They demonstrated that interaction in Italian was superior to interaction in English when each was combined with music therapy in reducing vocal agitation in an 81-year-old Italian woman suffering from dementia.

There are five studies that suggest a beneficial effect of *animal-assisted therapy* for people with dementia who are agitated. An intervention consisting of 1-h daily visits with a dog for 5 days showed a trend toward improvement ($p < .07$) for 33 hospital patients on a geriatric psychiatry unit (some of the patients suffered from dementia) on the Irritable Behavior scale of the Multidimensional Observation Scale rated for the week of treatment (Rovner et al., 1996). These results may underestimate the impact of the intervention in that a greater effect might have been seen with ratings taken immediately after treatment. One-half hour sessions with a dog resulted in significantly lower levels of agitation than half an hour sessions with only the researcher present in 28 special care unit residents (Churchill et al., 1999). Moreover, the presence of a pet at home was related to a lower prevalence of verbal aggression in a study of 65 people suffering from dementia (Fritz et al., 1995). Finally, seven participants who had six sessions of animal-assisted therapy biweekly for about 3 months measured lower on scores on the Behave-AD posttreatment compared with a control group (Kanamori et al., 2001).

One study on *simulated animal-assisted therapy* (Libin & Cohen-Mansfield, 2004) found that when presented with either a plush cat or a robotic cat, the nine participants with dementia manifested a reduction in agitation. Simulated animal-assisted therapy is an innovative intervention technique, which may offer an alternative to pet therapy for people who suffer from allergies or for facilities that cannot provide staff time to care for a pet.

Simulated interaction is an intervention that involves either audiotapes or videotapes of family members that are presented to the resident in an attempt to alleviate agitation. Three studies reported a significant positive impact of Simulated Presence Therapy or Audio Presence Intervention, an audiotape that contains a relative's portion of a telephone conversation, with pauses that allow the older person to respond to the relative's questions (Camberg et al., 1999; Miller et al., 2001; Woods & Ashley, 1995). A different type of simulated social contact, videotapes of family members talking to nursing home residents, was reported to result in an average decrease of 46% in verbally disruptive behavior during exposure to the videotape (Werner et al., 2000). In contrast, a generic videotape of reminiscence and relaxation did not result in reduction in agitation (Hall & Hare, 1997).

Two studies used mirrors as prompts to simulate or enhance interaction with the person with dementia. One study used a mirror at the exit door to simulate the presence of another person and decrease the nonaggressive agitation behavior of wandering (Mayer & Darby, 1991). With this intervention, contacts with the door decreased from 76.2% to 35.7%. This technique may be useful for facilities that lack funding for technological interventions or for those that do not have family members available to make audio or videotapes. Another study of 100 residents with dementia (Tabak et al., 1996) used mirrors as prompts while administering care to examine changes in resident behavior. The authors reported that using mirrors increased residents' awareness of self-care and improved communication between nurses and residents.

Structured Activities

Structured activities range from trivia games to puzzles. Surprisingly, there has been little research measuring the impact of structured activities in reducing agitation in people with dementia. A positive impact of activities is reported by Aronstein et al. (1996), who presented 15 nursing home residents with recreational interventions including manipulative (e.g., bead maze), nurturing (e.g., doll), sorting (e.g., puzzles), tactile (e.g., fabric book), sewing (e.g., lacing cards), and sound/music (e.g., melody bells). Fourteen episodes of agitation were observed in five residents, and the interventions were judged as helpful in alleviating agitation in 57% of these episodes. In addition, Kolanowski et al. (2005) examined the difference among the following activities: (1) activities matched to skill level only; (2) activities matched to style of interest only; and (3) combinations of the activities. The authors found that all activities helped reduce agitation in people with dementia. Moreover, Rovner et al. (1996) used a combination of Activities, Guidelines for psychotropic medications, and Educational rounds (A.G.E.) to test the effect on behavior, psychotropic drug use, and restraint use. They found that compared with the control group, the intervention group demonstrated fewer behavior disorders, lower antipsychotic drug use, and reduced use of restraints. Another study of group activities that were provided to three patients (Sival et al., 1997) yielded inconclusive results.

There have been recent studies on the use of *self-identity* tools to help in the design of structured activities. Cohen-Mansfield and colleagues (2000, 2006) found that some sense of personal self continues to exist even in advanced stages of dementia, especially the familial role. The use of activities based on persons' most important self-identity roles resulted in a decrease in agitation (Cohen-Mansfield et al., 2006). In addition, individualizing activities based on knowledge of what experiences are pleasant for persons with dementia has been used to treat depressed affect in this population (Teri & Logsdon, 1991; Teri et al., 1997).

Self-affirming interventions also target the improvement of affect. These include *reminiscence therapy,* which encourages persons with dementia to talk about their pasts and may utilize audiovisual aids such as old family photos and objects. Reminiscence can enhance individuals' sense of identity, sense of worth, or general well-being (Brooker & Duce, 2000), and it may also stimulate memory processes. *Validation therapy,* in which a therapist accepts the disorientation of a person with dementia and validates his or her feelings, was developed by Naomi Feil (1982). This self-affirming intervention is based on the assumption that persons return to unfinished conflicts in their pasts, providing a background for meaningful conversations addressing their emotions.

Two studies used *outdoor walks* for wanderers and found that this intervention led to decreases in inappropriate behavior and an increase in pleasure (Cohen-Mansfield & Werner, 1998b; Holmberg, 1997). Both studies involved interpersonal contact during the walk, though that was more pronounced in Holmberg's (1997) study, which also included singing and holding hands.

In addition, one study found that the use of a *therapeutic bike* significantly reduced depression scores in older adults with dementia who resided in long-term care facilities (Buettner & Fitzsimmons, 2002). The study included 70 residents with dementia who scored four or greater on the Geriatric Depression Scale. The participant rode in a wheelchair device attached to the back portion of a bicycle, which was driven by a staff member. After 2 weeks of riding with the staff member daily and discussing the experience with other participants in a group format, participants were significantly less depressed.

Memory books are booklets that contain autobiographical, daily schedule, and problem resolution information (Bourgeois et al., 2001). When nursing assistants were trained to use memory books, nursing home residents showed improvement in conversation and affect.

Environmental Interventions

Like social and activity interventions, environmental interventions can provide multiple benefits to residents in long-term care institutions by improving function and affect and decreasing agitated behaviors.

Modifications to the physical environment are crucial for optimizing performance of activities of daily living (ADL) in that they adjust the surroundings (including physical access, temperature, color, furniture, or wall design) to facilitate the activity for both older person and caregiver. The extent of environmental adaptation varies from decreasing clutter to providing grab bars or handrails. For decreasing the risk of falling, lowering bed height, placing mattresses on the floor, using hip protectors, improving light on the way to the bathroom, and improving call systems have been used. Enhanced visibility of toilets increased their utilization (Namazi & Johnson, 1991), and eating behavior improved with better light and increased contrast between plates and the table (Koss & Gilmore, 1998). In order to optimize ADL care, it is also crucial to pay attention to demands on the caregiver. Some tasks require more than one caregiver, whereas others require technology or modifications in environmental design to spare caregivers discomfort or injuries (Cohen-Mansfield & Parpura-Gill, 2007), which can be common (Cohen-Mansfield et al., 1996).

Environmental cues, such as placing frequently needed items in a specified location, using labels and signs (Brawley, 1997), wearing large wristwatches, or placing a card with important information in a pocket, have been used to simplify orientation. Signs require large font and high contrast to increase orientation. Nursing homes have also used color-coding or structural changes (Gibson et al., 2004) or placed pictures of residents or meaningful memorabilia in display cases outside their rooms to improve orientation (Namazi et al., 1991; Nolan et al., 2001). Clear labels on public toilets are useful for decreasing incontinence (Day & Calkins, 2002).

Two studies showed that free *access to an outdoor area* can result in decreased agitation (McMinn & Hinton, 2000; Namazi & Johnson, 1992). When the person has control over the ability to go outdoors, that control is expected to be of additional therapeutic benefit beyond that of the outdoor walk experience.

A *natural environment*, consisting of recorded songs of birds, babbling brooks, or small animals, together with large, bright pictures matching the audiotapes, and offering foods such as pudding, was presented during shower time. This resulted in significant reductions in agitation in the treatment group of 15 nursing home residents, in comparison with a control group of 16 residents who received usual care (Whall et al., 1997). A simulated home environment and a nature environment, each composed of visual, auditory, and olfactory stimuli, were compared in a study of nursing home residents who wander. Results showed a trend toward less trespassing, exit seeking, and other agitated behaviors in the altered environments, as compared with the unit's usual décor (Cohen-Mansfield & Werner, 1998a).

Bright light therapy (BLT) has been used to improve sleep and reduce agitation, which can result from fatigue or circadian rhythm disturbances. The time of day and the duration of the treatment may have an effect on whether or not it is beneficial to the participant. Consistently, research has shown that when BLT is offered in the morning, it significantly helps participants sleep better (Ancoli-Israel et al., 2002; Fetveit & Bjorvatn, 2005; Fetveit et al., 2003, 2005; Lyketsos et al., 1999). Ancoli-Israel et al. (2002) reported that when comparing groups who either received 2 h of BLT in the morning, daytime, or evening or dim red light in the evening, only participants who received BLT in the morning had sleep benefits. Another study found that with only 30 min a day of BLT, participants exhibited significantly reduced motor restless behavior (Haffmans et al., 2001). One study reported that BLT works only in certain situations, that is, BLT was beneficial to people who had intact vision, but it did not make a difference in sleep for people who were visually impaired (Van Someren et al., 1997). Two studies, however, found that BLT did not affect sleep. Dowling et al. (2005) offered BLT for 1 h every morning Monday through Friday and found no change in sleep duration. Another study provided 45 min of BLT every morning for 4 weeks and reported that there was no change in sleep; however, there was a significant reduction in behavior problems and agitation (Skjerve et al., 2004).

Low vision accommodation, in the form of *light intensity* and enhanced *visual contrast* (achieved by the colors of tablecloths, napkins, etc.), during evening meals resulted in a significant decrease in agitation during the interventions, compared with pre- and post-intervention (Koss & Gilmore, 1998).

Two articles describe a reduction in agitation after the initiation of a *reduced-stimulation environment*. The first study involved camouflaged doors; small tables for eating; small-group activities; neutral colors on pictures and walls; no televisions, radios, or telephones (except one for emergencies); a consistent daily routine; and an educational program for staff and visitors concerning the use of touch, eye contact, slow and soft speech, and allowing residents to make choices (Cleary et al., 1988). As a result, both agitation and use of restraints declined (no statistical test for agitation was presented). The second study (Meyer et al., 1992) included elimination of television, radio, stereo, or piano playing; use of quiet voices by staff at all times; relocation of the public entrance to an area that was out of sight of the residents; and reduced telephone use. Observation of 11 residents before and after the changes showed a statistically significant decrease in agitated behavior.

An *enhanced-stimulation environment* refers to a combination of stimuli delivered to different sensory modalities, including sight, hearing, touch, and smell. Multisensory rooms are referred to as "Snoezelen" rooms. The term derives from two Dutch words that mean "sniffing and dozing" (McKenzie, 1995). The purpose of a Snoezelen room is to create a sense of relaxation by stimulating the senses, thus decreasing agitation and/or depression. A key component in determining the success of the multisensory interventions is the presence of a nurse or recreation therapist to ensure proper use of the room. Sensory stimuli presented in a Snoezelen room include (1) auditory: soft music, beach sounds, water sounds, or birds singing; (2) visual: mirror ball, cloud scene, bubble column, or fiber optic spray; (3) tactile: massage chair, box of sand, fuzzy toy, or vibrating pillow; (4) olfactory: aromatherapy with essential oils such as Melissa or lavender oil (Ball & Haight, 2005).

Several studies examined the benefits of a multisensory room for older adults. Holtkamp and colleagues (1997) found that during the intervention phase of the study, behavioral problems decreased. Another study reported that compared with sitting in a living room or garden, when people sat in a Snoezelen room, they experienced less sadness (Cox et al., 2004). Finally, a study that tested the difference between reminiscence therapy and sitting in a Snoezelen room discovered that both interventions were effective in reducing agitated behaviors in older adults with dementia (Baillon et al., 2004).

Combination Therapies

Combination therapies often combine pharmacological and nonpharmacological techniques, which may include structured activities and nursing interventions. Studies that examined an individualized approach where treatment plans were adapted to the needs of the participant showed a significant decrease in problem behaviors or agitation (Matthews et al., 1996; Hinchliffe et al., 1995; Holm et al., 1999). For example, Holm and collaborators (1999) found that by creating an individualized treatment plan for each patient that involved pharmacological and nonpharmacological interventions on admission and again upon discharge, they were able to significantly reduce problem behaviors and preserve cognitive and functional abilities. Others used a group approach. As mentioned above, Rovner and coworkers (1996) found that providing an activity program (with music, exercise, relaxation, reminiscence, and word games), reevaluation of psychotropic drugs, and educational rounds resulted in significant reduction in agitation. Another study, however, reported worsening of behaviors with a group intervention approach (Wimo et al., 1993).

Many of the interventions that are presented as single interventions are, in fact, combination interventions, and therefore, it is not possible to determine which component is the active ingredient. For example, a Snoezelen room is supposed to help because of the provision of sensory stimulation. Yet, it usually involves a one-on-one interaction with a therapist, which may be the more potent intervention.

FUTURE DIRECTIONS

There has been considerable research in the past 20 years on interventions that benefit older adults with dementia in long-term care. Studies show that by applying environmental/milieu interventions through sensory enhancement, social contact, structured activities, or environmental modifications, agitation can be reduced or even eliminated. Although the bulk of this evidence is positive, it is mostly based on small studies with considerable methodological limitations. There is a need to enhance this body of research both in terms of the range of approaches taken and in terms of the quality and size of the studies. For this research agenda to materialize, a funding body that focuses on environmental and milieu interventions in dementia is required. As the body of evidence grows on which interventions benefit which individuals, future research is needed in identifying how to help facilities implement these findings. Long-term care facilities continue to struggle with how to help alleviate the suffering associated with agitation in dementia and need more assistance in order to implement the findings from research.

In addition, this evidence needs to be presented on the federal level to demonstrate the importance of enacting legislation that would require long-term care facilities to employ these interventions and provide them with the resources to do so. Funding sources need to be allocated to reimburse facilities for the supplies and personnel needed to ensure that environmental and milieu interventions are not the exception, but the rule.

Acknowledgment This research for this chapter was funded by grant AG010172 from the National Institute on Aging.

REFERENCES

Algase, D. L., Beck, C., Kolanowski, A., et al. (1996, November/December). Need-driven dementia-compromised behavior: An alternative view of disruptive behavior. *American Journal of Alzheimer's Disease, 11*(6), 10–19.

Ancoli-Israel, S., Martin, J. L., Kripke, D. F., Marler, M., & Klauber, M. R. (2002). Effect of light treatment on sleep and circadian rhythms in demented nursing home patients. *Journal of the American Geriatrics Society, 50*(2), 282–289.

Aronstein, Z., Olsen, R., & Schulman, E. (1996). The nursing assistants' use of recreational interventions for behavioral management of residents with Alzheimer's disease. *American Journal of Alzheimer's Disease, 11*(3), 26–31.

Baillon, S., Van Diepen, E., Prettyman, R., Redman, J., Rooke, N., & Campbell, R. (2004). A comparison of the effects of Snoezelen and reminiscence therapy on the agitated behaviour of patients with dementia. *International Journal of Geriatric Psychiatry, 19*(11), 1047–1052.

Ball, J., & Haight, B. (2005, October). Creating a multisensory environment for dementia: The goals of a Snoezelen room. *Journal of Gerontological Nursing, 31*(10), 4–10.

Ballard, C. G., O'Brien, J. T., Reichelt, K., & Perry, E. K. (2002). Aromatherapy as a safe and effective treatment for the management of agitation in severe dementia: The results of a double-blind, placebo-controlled trial with Melissa. *Journal of Clinical Psychiatry, 63*(7), 553–558.

Birchmore, T., & Clague, S. (1983). A behavioral approach to reduce shouting. *Nursing Times, 79*(16), 37–39.

Bliwise, D. L. (1994). What is sundowning? *JAGS, 42*(9), 1009–1011.

Bourgeois, M., Dijkstra, K., Burgio, L., & Allen-Burge, R. (2001). Memory aids as an augmentative and alternative communication strategy for nursing home residents with dementia. *Augmentative and Alternative Communication, 17,* 196–210.

Brawley, E. C. (1997). *Designing for Alzheimer's disease: Strategies for creating better care environments.* New York: John Wiley.

Brooker, D., & Duce, L. (2000). Wellbeing and activity in dementia: A comparison of group reminiscence therapy, structured goal-directed group activity and unstructured time. *Aging and Mental Health, 4*(4), 354–358.

Brotons, M., & Pickett-Cooper, P. K. (1996). The effects of music therapy intervention on agitation behaviors of Alzheimer's disease patients. *Journal of Music Therapy, 33*(1), 3–18.

Buettner, L. L., & Fitzsimmons, S. (2002). AD-venture program: Therapeutic biking for the treatment of depression in long-term care residents with dementia. *American Journal of Alzheimer's Disease and Other Dementias, 17*(2), 121–127.

Burgio, L., Scilley, K., Hardin, J. M., Hsu, C., & Yancey, J. (1996). Environmental "white noise": An intervention for verbally agitated nursing home residents. *Journal of Gerontology: Psychological Sciences and Social Sciences, 51B*(6), 364–373.

Camberg, L., Woods, P., Ooi, W. L., et al. (1999). Evaluation of simulated presence: A personalized approach to enhance well-being in persons with Alzheimer's disease [see comments]. *Journal of the American Geriatrics Society, 47*(4), 446–452.

Churchill, M., Safaoui, J., McCabe, B., & Baun, M. (1999). Using a therapy dog to alleviate the agitation and desocialization of people with Alzheimer's disease. *Journal of Psychosocial Nursing, 37*(4), 16–24.

Clark, M. E., Lipe, A. W., & Bilbrey, M. (1998). Use of music to decrease aggressive behaviors in people with Dementia. *Journal of Gerontological Nursing, 24*(7), 10–17.

Cleary, T. A., Clamon, C., Price, M., & Shullaw, G. (1988). A reduced stimulation unit: Effects on patients with Alzheimer's disease and related disorders. *The Gerontologist, 28*(4), 511–514.

Cohen-Mansfield, J., Culpepper, W. J. I., & Carter, P. (1996). Nursing staff back injuries, prevalence and costs in long-term care facilities. *American Association of Occupational Health Nurses, 44*(1), 9–17.

Cohen-Mansfield, J., & Deutsch, L. (1996). Agitation: Subtypes and their mechanisms. *Seminars in Clinical Neuropsychiatry, 1*(4), 325–339.

Cohen-Mansfield, J., Golander, H., & Arnheim, G. (2000). Self-identity in older persons suffering from dementia: Preliminary results. *Social Science and Medicine, 51,* 381–394.

Cohen-Mansfield, J., & Marx, M. (1988). Relationship between depression and agitation in nursing home residents. *Comprehensive Gerontological Behavior, 2,* 141–146.

Cohen-Mansfield, J., Marx, M. S., & Rosenthal, A. S. (1989). A description of agitation in a nursing home. *Journals of Gerontology, 44*(3), M77–M84.

Cohen-Mansfield, J., Marx, M. S., & Werner, P. (1992). Observational data on time use and behavior problems in the nursing home. *Journal of Applied Gerontology, 11*(1), 111–121.

Cohen-Mansfield, J., & Parpura-Gill, A. (2007a). Bathing: A framework for intervention focusing on psychosocial, architectural and human factors considerations. *Archives of Gerontology and Geriatrics, 45*(2), 121–135.

Cohen-Mansfield, J., & Parpura-Gill, A. (2007b) Loneliness in elderly persons: a theoretical model and empirical findings. *International Psychogeriatrics, 19*(2), 279–294.

Cohen-Mansfield, J., Parpura-Gill, A., & Golander, H. (2006) Utilization of self-identity roles for designing interventions for persons with dementia. *Journals of Gerontology: Psychological Sciences, 61B,* 202–212.

Cohen-Mansfield, J., & Taylor, L. (1998). Assessing and understanding agitated behaviors in older adults. In M. Kaplan & S. B. Hoffman (Eds.), *Behaviors in dementia: Best practices for successful management.* (pp. 25–44). Baltimore, MD: Health Professions Press.

Cohen-Mansfield, J., & Werner, P. (1995). Environmental influences on agitation: An integrative summary of an observational study. *American Journal of Alzheimer's Care and Related Disorders and Research, 10*(1), 32–37.

Cohen-Mansfield, J., & Werner, P. (1997). Management of verbally disruptive behaviors in nursing home residents. *Journal of Gerontology: Medical Sciences, 52A*(6), 369–377.

Cohen-Mansfield, J., & Werner, P. (1998a). The effects of an enhanced environment on nursing home residents who pace. *The Gerontologist, 38*(2), 199–208.

Cohen-Mansfield, J., & Werner, P. (1998b). Visits to an outdoor garden: Impact on behavior and mood of nursing home residents who pace. In B. Vellas, J. Fitten, & G. Frisoni (Eds.), *Research and practice in Alzheimer's disease* (pp. 419–436). Paris, France: Serdi.

Cohen-Mansfield, J., & Werner, P. (1999). Outdoor wandering parks for persons with dementia: A survey of characteristics and use [in process citation]. *Alzheimer Disease and Associated Disorders, 13*(2), 109–17.

Cohen-Mansfield, J., Werner, P., & Freedman, L. (1995). Sleep and agitation in agitated nursing home residents: An observational study. *Sleep, 18*(8), 674–680.

Cohen-Mansfield, J., Werner, P., & Marx, M. S. (1990). Screaming in nursing home residents. *Journal of the American Geriatrics Society, 38*(7), 785–792.

Cohen-Mansfield, J., Werner, P., & Marx, M. S. (1992). The social environment of the agitated nursing home resident. *International Journal of Geriatric Psychiatry, 7*(11), 789–798.

Cohen-Mansfield, J., Werner, P., & Marx, M. S. (1994). The impact of infection on agitation: Three case studies in the nursing home. *American Journal of Alzheimer's Care and Related Disorders and Research, 9*(4), 30–34.

Cox, H., Burns, I., & Savage, S. (2004, February). Multisensory environments for leisure: Promoting well-being in nursing home residents with dementia. *Journal of Gerontological Nursing, 30,* 37–45.

Day, K., & Calkins, M. P. (2002). Design and dementia. In R. B. Betchel & A. E. Churchman (Eds.), *Handbook of environmental psychology* (pp. 374–393). Indianapolis, IN: Wiley.

Denney, A. (1997, July). Quiet music: An intervention for mealtime agitation. *Journal of Gerontological Nursing, 23,* 16–23.

Douzjian, M., Wilson, C., Shultz, M., et al. (1998). A program to use pain control medication to reduce psychotropic drug use in residents with difficult behavior. *Annals of Long-Term Care, 6*(5), 174–179.

Dowling, G. A., Hubbard, E. M., Mastick, J., Luxenberg, J. S., Burr, R. L., & Van Someren, E. J. (2005). Effect of morning bright light treatment for rest-activity disruption in institutionalized patients with severe Alzheimer's disease. *International Psychogeriatrics, 17*(2), 221–236.

Feil, N. (1982). *Validation: The Feil method.* Cleveland, OH: Feil.

Fetveit, A., & Bjorvatn, B. (2005). Bright-light treatment reduces actigraphic-measured daytime sleep in nursing home patients with dementia. *American Journal of Geriatric Psychiatry, 13*(5), 420–423.

Fetveit, A., Skjerve, A., & Bjorvatn, B. (2003). Bright light treatment improves sleep in institutionalized elderly—an open trial. *International Journal of Geriatric Psychiatry, 18*, 520–526.

French, J., Rodgers, W., & Cobbs, S. (1974). Adjustment as person-environment fit. In G. V. Coelho, D. A. Hamburg, & J. E. Adams (Eds.), *Coping and adaptation* (pp. 316–333). New York: Basic Books.

Friedman, L., Brooks, J. O. I., Bliwise, D. L., & Yesavage, J. A. (1993). Insomnia in older adults. *American Journal of Geriatric Psychology, 1*(2), 153–159.

Fritz, C., Farver, T., Kass, P., & Hart. L. (1995). Association with companion animals and the expression of noncognitive symptoms in Alzheimer's patients. *Journal of Nervous and Mental Disease, 183*(7), 459–463.

Gerdner, L. A. (2000). Effects of individualized versus classical "relaxation" music on the frequency of agitation in elderly persons with Alzheimer's disease and related disorders. *International Psychogeriatrics, 12*(1), 49–65.

Gerdner, L. A., & Swanson, E. A. (1993). Effects of individualized music on confused and agitated elderly patients. *Archives of Psychiatric Nursing, 7*(5), 284–291.

Gibson, M. C., MacLean, J., Borrie, M., & Geiger, J. (2004). Orientation behaviors in residents relocated to a redesigned dementia care unit. *American Journal of Alzheimer's Disease and Other Dementias, 19*(1), 45–49.

Goddaer, J., & Abraham, I. L. (1994). Effects of relaxing music on agitation during meals among nursing home residents with severe cognitive impairment. *Archives of Psychiatric Nursing, 8*(3), 150–158.

Gray, S. G., & Clair, A. A. (2002). Influence of aromatherapy on medication administration to residential-care residents with dementia and behavioral challenges. *American Journal of Alzheimer's Disease and Other Dementias, 17*(3), 169–174.

Groene, R. W. (1993). Effectiveness of music therapy 1:1 intervention with individuals having senile dementia of the Alzheimer's type. *Journal of Music Therapy, 30*(3), 138–157.

Haffmans, P. M. J., Sival, R. C., Lucius, S. A. P., Cats, Q., & Van Gelder, L. (2001). Bright light therapy and melatonin in motor restless behaviour in dementia: A placebo-controlled study. *International Journal of Geriatric Psychiatry, 16*, 106–110.

Hall, G. R. (1994). Caring for people with Alzheimer's disease using the conceptual model of progressively lowered stress threshold in the clinical setting (Vol. 29, Chap. 1, pp. 129–141). Nursing Clinics of North America.

Hall, G. R., & Buckwalter, K. C. (1987). Progressively lowered stress threshold: A conceptual model for care of adults with Alzheimer's disease. *Archives of Psychiatric Nursing, 1*(6), 399–406.

Hall, L., & Hare, J. (1997). Video respite for cognitively impaired persons in nursing homes. *American Journal of Alzheimer's Disease, 12*(2), 117–121.

Hicks-Moore, S. L. (2005). Relaxing music at mealtime in nursing homes: Effects on agitated patients with dementia. *Journal of Gerontological Nursing, 31*(12), 26–32.

Hinchliffe, A. C., Hyman, I. L., Blizard, B., & Livingston, G. (1995). Behavioural complications of dementia—Can they be treated? *International Journal of Geriatric Psychiatry, 10*, 839–847.

Holm, A., Michel, M., Stern, G. A., et al. (1999). The outcomes of an inpatient treatment program for geriatric patients with dementia and dysfunctional behaviors. *The Gerontologist, 39*(6), 668–676.

Holmberg, S. K. (1997). Evaluation of a clinical intervention for wanderers on a geriatric nursing unit. *Archives of Psychiatric Nursing, 11*(1), 21–28.

Holmes, C., Hopkins, V., Hensford, C., MacLaughlin, V., Wilkinson, D., & Rosenvinge, H. (2002). Lavender oil as a treatment for agitated behaviour in severe dementia: A placebo controlled study. *International Journal of Geriatric Psychiatry, 17*(4), 305–308.

Holtkamp, C. C., Kragt, K., van Dongen, M. C., van Rossum, E., & Salentijn, C. (1997). Effect of snoezelen on the behavior of demented elderly. *Tijdschrift voor Gerontologie en Geriatrie, 28*(3), 124–128.

Hurley, A. C., Volicer, B. J., Hanrahan, P. A., Houde, S., & Volicer, L. (1992). Assessment of discomfort in advanced Alzheimer patients. *Research in Nursing and Health, 15*, 369–377.

Johnson, C. J. (1989). Sociological intervention through developing low stimulus Alzheimer's wings in nursing homes. *American Journal of Alzheimer's Care and Related Disorders and Research, 4*(2), 33–41.

Kahana, E. (1982). A congruence model of person–environment interaction. In M. P. Lawton, P. G. Windley, & T. O. Byerts (Eds.), *Aging and the environment: Theoretical approaches* (pp. 97–121). New York: Springer.

Kanamori, M., Suzuki, M., Yamamoto, K., et al. (2001). A day care program and evaluation of animal-assisted therapy (AAT) for the elderly with senile dementia. *American Journal of Alzheimer's Disease and Other Dementias, 16*(4), 234–239.

Kim, E. J., & Buschmann, M. T. (1999). The effect of expressive physical touch on patients with dementia. *International Journal of Nursing Studies, 36*, 235–243.

Kolanowski, A. M., Litaker, M., & Buettner, L. (2005). Efficacy of theory-based activities for behavioral symptoms of dementia. *Nursing Research, 54*(4), 219–228.

Koss, E., & Gilmore, G. C. (1998). Environmental interventions and functional ability of AD patients. In B. Vellas, J. Fritten, & G. Frisoni (Eds.), *Research and practice in Alzheimer's disease* (pp. 185–192). Paris, France: Serdi.

Langer, E. J., & Rodin, J. (1976). Effects of choice and enhanced personal responsibility for the aged: A field experiment in an institutional setting. *Journal of Personality and Social Psychology, 34*(2), 191–198.

Lawton, M. P. (1990). Adjustment. Environmental adjustment. *Abstracts in Social Gerontology, 33*(1), 33–34.

Lawton, M. P., & Simon, B. (1968). The ecology of social relationships in housing for the elderly. *The Gerontologist, 8*(2), 108–115.

Leonard, R., Tinetti, M. E., Allore, H. G., & Drickamer, M. A. (2006). Potentially modifiable resident characteristics that are associated with physical and verbal aggression among nursing home residents with dementia. *Archives of Internal Medicine, 166*, 1295–1300.

Lewinsohn, P. M., & Youngren, M. A. (1976). The symptoms of depression. *Comprehensive Therapy, 2*(8), 62–69.

Libin, A., & Cohen-Mansfield, J. (2004). Therapeutic robocat for nursing home residents with dementia: Preliminary inquiry. *American Journal of Alzheimer's Disease and Other Dementias, 19*(2), 111–116.

Lyketsos, C., Veiel, L., Baker, A., & Steele, C. (1999). A randomized, controlled trial of bright light therapy for agitated behaviors in dementia patients residing in long-term care. *International Journal of Geriatric Psychiatry, 14*(14), 520–525.

Matthews, E. A., Farrell, G. A., & Blackmore, A. M. (1996). Effects of an environmental manipulation emphasizing client-centred care on agitation and sleep in dementia sufferers in a nursing home. *Journal of Advanced Nursing, 24*, 439–447.

Mayer, R., & Darby, S. J. (1991). Does a mirror deter wandering in demented older people? *International Journal of Geriatric Psychiatry, 6*, 607–609.

Mayers, K., & Griffin, M. (1990). The play project—Use of stimulus objects with demented patients. *Journal of Gerontological Nursing, 16*(1), 32–36.

McKenzie, C. (1995). Brightening the lives of elderly through Snoezelen. *Elderly Care, 7*(5), 1.

McMinn, B. G., & Hinton, L. (2000). Confined to barracks: The effects of indoor confinement on aggressive behavior among inpatients of an acute psychogeriatric unit. *American Journal of Alzheimer's Disease, 15*(1), 36–41.

McShane, R., Cohen-Mansfield, J., & Werner, P. (2000). Predictors of aggressive behaviors. *Research and Practice in Alzheimer's Disease, 3*, 183–188.

Meyer, D. L., Dorbacker, B., O'Rourke, J., Dowling, J., Jacques, J., & Nicholas, M. (1992). Effects of a "quiet week" intervention on behavior in an Alzheimer boarding home. *American Journal of Alzheimer's Care and Research, 7*(4), 2–6.

Miller, S., Vermeersch, P. E. H., Bohan, K., Renbarger, K., Kruep, A., & Sacre, S. (2001). Audio presence intervention for decreasing agitation in people with dementia. *Geriatric Nursing, 22*(2), 66–70.

Mutch, W. J. (1992). Parkinsonism and other movement disorders. In J. C. Brocklehurst, R. C. Tallis, & H. M. Fillit (Eds.), *Textbook of geriatric medicine and gerontology* (p. 423). Edinburgh: Churchill Livingstone.

Namazi, K. H., & Johnson, B. D. (1991). Environmental effects on incontinence problems in Alzheimer's disease patients. *American Journal of Alzheimer's Care and Related Disorders and Research, 6*, 16–21.

Namazi, K. H., & Johnson, B. D. (1992). Pertinent autonomy for residents with dementias: Modification of the physical environment to enhance independence. *American Journal of Alzheimer's Care and Related Disorders & Research, 7*(1), 16–21.

Namazi, K. H., Rosner, T. T., & Rechlin, L. (1991, November/December). Long-term memory cuing to reduce visuo-spatial disorientation in Alzheimer's disease patients in a special care unit. *American Journal of Alzheimer's Care and Related Disorders and Research, 6*(6), 10–15.

Nolan, B. A. D., Mathews, R. M., & Harrison, M. (2001). Using external memory aids to increase room finding by older adults with dementia. *Activities Directors' Quarterly for Alzheimer's and Other Dementia Patients, 2*(4), 13–18.

Ragneskog, H., Brane, G., Karlson, I., & Kihlgren, M. (1996). Influence of dinner music on food intake and symptoms common in dementia. *Scandinavian Journal of Caring Science, 10*, 11–17.

Remington, R. (2002). Calming music and hand massage with agitated elderly. *Nursing Research, 51*(5), 317–323.

Rovner, B. W., German, P. S., Broadhead, J., et al. (1990). The prevalence and management of dementia and other psychiatric disorders in nursing homes. *International Psychogeriatrics, 2*(1), 13–24.

Rovner, B. W., Steele, C. D., Shmuely, Y., & Folstein, M. F. (1996). A randomized trial of dementia care in nursing homes. *Journal of the American Geriatrics Society, 44*(1), 7–13.

Rovner, B. W., Zisselman, P. M., & Shmuely-Dulitzki, Y. (1996). Depression and disability in older people with impaired vision: A follow-up study. *Journal of the American Geriatrics Society, 44*(2), 181–184.

Rowe, M., & Alfred, D. (1999). The effectiveness of slow-stroke massage in diffusing agitated behaviors in individuals with Alzheimer's disease. *Journal of Gerontological Nursing, 25*(6), 22–34.

Runci, S., Doyle, C., & Redman, J. (1999). An empirical test of language-relevant interventions for dementia. *International Psychogeriatrics, 11*(3), 301–311.

Ryden, M. B., Bossenmaier, M., & McLachlan, C. (1991). Aggressive behavior in cognitively impaired nursing home residents. *Research in Nursing and Health, 14*(2), 87–95.

Sansone, P., & Schmitt, L. (2000). Providing tender touch massage to elderly nursing home resident: A demonstration project. *Geriatric Nursing, 21*(6) 303–308.

Seligman, M. E. P. (1974). Depression and learned helplessness. *The psychology of depression: Contemporary theory and research* (pp. 83–113). Washington, DC: Winston-Wiley.

Seligman, M. E. P. (1975). *Helplessness: On depression, development, and death.* San Francisco, CA: W.H. Freeman.

Sival, R. C., Vingerhoets, R. W., Haffmans, P. M., Jansen, P. A., & Ton Hazelhoff, J. N. (1997). Effect of a program of diverse activities on disturbed behavior in three severely demented patients. *International Psychogeriatrics, 9*(4), 423–430.

Skjerve, A., Holsten, F., Aarsland, D., Bjorvatn, B., Nygaard, H. A., & Johansen, I. M. (2004). Improvement in behavioral symptoms and advance of activity acrophase after short-term bright light treatment in severe dementia. *Psychiatry and Clinical Neurosciences, 58,* 343–347.

Smallwood, J., Brown, R., Coulter, F., Irvine, E., & Copland, C. (2001). Aromatherapy and behaviour disturbances in dementia: A randomized controlled trial. *International Journal of Geriatric Psychiatry, 16,* 1010–1013.

Snow, A. L., Hovanec, L., & Brandt, J. (2004). A controlled trial of aromatherapy for agitation in nursing home patients with dementia. *Journal of Alternative and Complementary Medicine, 10*(3), 431–437.

Snyder, M., Egan, E. C., & Burns, K. R. (1995, March/April). Efficacy of hand massage in decreasing agitation behaviors associated with care activities in persons with Dementia. *Geriatric Nursing, 16*(2), 60.

Svansdottir, H. B., & Snaedal, J. (2006). Music therapy in moderate and severe dementia of Alzheimer's type: A case-controlled study. *International Psychogeriatrics, 18*(4), 1–9.

Tabak, N., Bar-Tal, Y., & Cohen-Mansfield, J. (1996). Clinical decision making of experienced and novice nurses. *Western Journal of Nursing Research, 18*(5), 534–547.

Tabloski, P. A. (1995). The use of music to calm agitated nursing home residents. *The Gerontological Society of America, 35*(1), 210–211.

Teri, L., & Logsdon, R. G. (1991). Identifying pleasant activities for Alzheimer's disease patients: The pleasant events schedule-AD. *The Gerontologist, 31*(1), 124–127.

Teri, L., Logsdon, R. G., Uomoto, J., & McCurry, S. M. (1997). Behavioral treatment of depression in dementia patients: A controlled clinical trial. *Journals of Gerontology: Psychological Sciences, 52B*(4), 159–166.

Thomas, D. W., Heitman, R. J., & Alexander, T. (1997). The effects of music on bathing cooperation for residents with dementia. *Journal of Music Therapy, 34*(4), 246–259.

Van Someren, E. J., Kessler, A., Mirmiran, M., & Swaab, D. F. (1997). Indirect bright light improves circadian rest-activity rhythm disturbances in demented patients. *Biological Psychiatry, 41*(9), 955–963.

Werner, P., Cohen-Mansfield, J., Fischer, J., & Segal, G. (2000). Characterization of family-generated videotapes for the management of verbally disruptive behaviors. *Journal of Applied Gerontology, 19*(1), 42–57.

Whall, A., Black, M., Groh, C., Yankou, D., Kupferschmid, B., & Foster, N. (1997). The effect of natural environments upon agitation and aggression in late stage dementia patients. *American Journal of Alzheimer's Disease, 12*(5), 216–220.

Wimo, A., Nelvig, A., Nelvig, J., et al. (1993). Can changes in ward routines affect the severity of dementia? A controlled prospective study. *International Psychogeriatrics, 5*(2), 160–180.

Woods, P., & Ashley, J. (1995). Simulated presence therapy: Using selected memories to manage problem behaviors in Alzheimer's disease patients. *Geriatric Nursing, 16*(1), 9–14.

Young, S. H., Muir-Nash, J., & Ninos, M. (1988). Managing nocturnal wandering behavior. *Journal of Gerontological Nursing, 14*(5), 6–12.

Zachow, K. M. (1984). Helen, can you hear me? *Journal of Gerontological Nursing, 18*(8), 18–22.

18

Staff Education in Long-Term Care Facilities

David K. Conn and *Joy Richards*

Fifteen years ago Rovner and Katz (1993) declared that nursing homes "are the modern mental institutions for the elderly, but the training of staff and physicians, processes of care, and the recognition and treatment of mental disorders lag behind the current state of scientific knowledge." Indeed, lack of trained staff continues to be frequently cited as one of the key problems in the care of nursing home residents. Recent guidelines recommend that long-term care homes "should have an education and training program for staff related to the needs of residents with depression and/or behavioral concerns" (Canadian Coalition for Seniors' Mental Health, 2006). There is evidence that poor education and training can compromise resident care and safety (Anderson et al., 2005). This chapter will explore some of the key issues related to the education of staff in the long-term care setting. In exploring this issue it is important to bear in mind that although education is necessary, it is often not sufficient to improve clinical practice. Enabling care providers to make the transition from "knowing" to "doing" is complex and multifaceted, and the process of successful knowledge transfer and knowledge utilization will vary among different practice settings.

A recent study from Australia (Jones et al., 2007) highlighted the exodus of registered nurses from residential care facilities, reporting that they have been increasingly replaced by carers with little or no expertise in psychiatric illness or disorders of cognitive decline. They emphasize that this "de-professionalizing" of care has important implications for the well-being of all nursing home residents, particularly those with complex mental health problems. The study also highlighted the lack of training in the areas of mental health and dementia (Jones et al., 2007). Other studies have highlighted the training needs of social workers in nursing homes, emphasizing the importance of skills in assessing the resident's social and emotional needs (Brown, 1999). Primary care physicians working in long-term care are also seen as a priority target audience for psychiatric educational programs (Conn & Silver, 1998).

EDUCATIONAL PRINCIPLES

The World Health Organization published a consensus statement on education in psychiatry of the elderly in 1998 (WHO, 1998). The document focused on basic principles and needs. It was emphasized that education in this field should follow modern principles of adult education. Educational programs should

(a) provide clear learning objectives centered on the learner's needs,
(b) ensure that learners are actively involved in the process,
(c) address attitudes and skills as well as knowledge,
(d) be appropriate for the context and culture of the learner,
(e) be systematically evaluated, and
(f) be ready to challenge assumptions and acknowledge controversy where it exists.

The document provided an outline of key areas in geriatric mental health that should be considered in any educational course. A core curriculum primarily derived from the learning needs of health professionals is outlined. There were a number of important recommendations with regard to teaching methods. Formal education should fit with different learning styles and the best way of accomplishing this is to make a variety of teaching formats available for learners. These may include large and small group teaching, tutorials, and seminars. Education for multidisciplinary groups can facilitate teamwork and dispel interprofessional misperceptions. It is noted that many who work with the elderly do so under pressure and may feel they have no time to teach; however, every activity of a clinical service is a potentially fruitful educational opportunity. The use of innovations and information technology such as distance-based education, videoconferencing, and the use of the Internet and computer teaching modules are highlighted. Finally, it is noted that teaching thrives in association with research and encourages critical thinking in learners.

EDUCATION IN THE NURSING HOME

The nursing home is a unique environment in which to develop educational programs. As noted above, there are small numbers of staff with professional qualifications and a large number of staff with limited educational backgrounds. Maas et al. (1996) reported that 90% of all resident care is carried out by health-care aides who have high school education or less, receive little more than minimum wage, obtain limited training; and receive minimal long-term benefits, recognition, or support for their physically and emotionally difficult work. It is also worth noting that there are likely to be culturally sensitive issues to address. Particularly in urban areas, many of the long-term care staff members are foreign born. It has also been noted that a culture of long-term care is different from acute care in that there is generally less emphasis and value on training and few incentives to encourage staff change or motivation. Physicians working in nursing homes are often there on a part-time basis while maintaining outside practices. Funding tends to limit the number of allied health professionals such as psychologists, occupational therapists, and physiotherapists.

Lieff and Silver (2007) point out that it is important to understand the structure and administration of an institution in order for an educational program to be successful. They also note that any new educational endeavor must take into account issues such as shifts occurring over a 24-h period, level of administrative support, efficient use of available time, accessibility to staff within the nursing home, funding, and the motivation and incentives for attendees.

It is critical to emphasize the need for support from administration in the development and facilitation of educational programs. Indeed, the degree of support offered by administration has been shown to have a direct effect on the success rate of mental health training programs in nursing homes (Chartok et al., 1988). Active encouragement, releasing staff from other duties, rewards, and recognition can all enhance participation and attendance at educational events.

A number of different models have been utilized in the development of mental health educational programs. In facilities that have active mental health consultants such as visiting psychiatrists or a psychogeriatric consultation service, these providers can be actively involved in both formal and informal teaching. A great deal of teaching can take place at the bedside or at the nursing station in conjunction with case discussions. The term "teachable moment" nicely captures such important opportunities. In other models, in-house experts are utilized. Kaye and Robinson (2007) have described the role of the psychogeriatric nurse consultant in long-term care facilities. They emphasize that the nursing staff make up the vast majority of professional caregivers and their work is often physically and mentally arduous. Unlike other health-care professionals, nurses remain with their residents throughout their shift and are unable to escape the unrelenting nature of behaviorally disordered residents. This leads to increased stress levels and a need for support. Stolz Howard (1978) links the role of nurse clinician and mental health consultant in defining the functions of the psycho-geriatric nurse consultant. These functions include

(a) Responding to staff requests for assistance with specific nursing interventions in the provision of care.

(b) Assisting staff to extract and coordinate information from their nursing assessments to further understand a problem.

(c) Assisting them to integrate their knowledge of the resident's behavior with the theory that behavior has meaning.

(d) Providing support for the staff around difficult clinical issues through care-planning conferences, educational programming, and remaining involved with the staff/client for the duration of the problem.

(e) Identifying aspects of a problem that may be systems related and may be impacting on the clinical situation. Facilitating problem-solving sessions to reduce the effect of these issues on the staff/residents is an important component of this role.

(f) Providing weekly supportive counseling to residents which then assists staff to care for the residents in their own milieu.

(g) Providing didactic teaching sessions to aides, registered nursing assistants, registered nurses and other multidisciplinary team members in accordance with the biopsychosocial model.

(h) Helping staff to consider and identify possible underlying psychiatric syndromes.

(i) Facilitating staff and families to work as collaborative partners in difficult situations.

(j) Helping staff to determine which residents may need referral to a psychiatrist or a psychologist.

Kaye and Robinson (2007) also point out that nurses in long-term care are in a unique position in that their tasks are clearly defined, but the satisfactions are often nebulous. They note that positive feelings related to care can be severely diminished when a nurse is confronted with racial slurs, aggression, accusations, sexual disinhibition, or screaming. In addition, the nursing staff must interact with many family members and deal with their varying coping styles. Staff must be prepared to deal effectively with a barrage of complaints, anger, and accusations that they "aren't doing enough." They note that ethical, moral, legal, professional, and personal issues often blend to produce a picture of great complexity. Nurses, therefore, need a highly developed sense of tolerance to be able to deal simultaneously with the varied physical and emotional demands, expectations, and ambiguities. It is clear that staff need both comprehensive training and also support. In discussing the development of a behavior management program, Rewilak (2007) highlights the need to reduce the level of staff stress and describes a "stress inoculation paradigm." In this paradigm, stressful situations are redefined as problems that require solutions and one of the solutions is to break down a stressful event into a series of stages and to use internal dialogue or self talk to cope with the stress.

NEEDS ASSESSMENT

The development of any teaching program should begin with a needs assessment. It is important to make a distinction between perceived, unperceived, and misperceived needs. Surveys and focus groups are useful in documenting perceived needs. On the other hand, the care provider may be unaware of certain needs that might be identified only by an educator or an administrator. These may be identified through the clinical experience of the consultant, literature on the topic, or chart audits.

As well, there is a concern that discussions of nursing within the long-term care sector tend to sentimentalize and decomplexify the skill and knowledge involved in nurses' interpersonal or relational work with older patients and their families. It is therefore important, when assessing nursing's educational needs, to understand the kind of language used by nurses at every level of the nursing hierarchy—the language of relationships—particularly when asked to identify individual learning needs, present evidence, or justify decisions regarding clinical practice. For example, a study by Weinberg (2003) revealed that despite carefully nurtured professionalism among nursing staff in a large urban academic teaching hospital, most nurses failed to connect explicitly how time to do the "little things" enabled them to do the big things—assess patients, monitor their progress, plan care, and carry out medical interventions. Therefore, in the routinized environment of long-term care settings, this requires not only special attention but can also provide unique insights into learning opportunities. By leveraging what nurses mean by "knowing patients," educational assessment and activities can be intertwined with the fact that getting to know patients is an integral part of nurses' daily activities. However, this "knowing" does not involve some superficial friendliness or attempt to develop personal intimacy; rather, knowing patients means knowing about a patient's medical needs and progress, not just their personal stories and dreams. Knowing a patient involves learning about the physical and emotional dimensions of a patient's illness, finding out how the patient responds to treatment, managing complex medication regimes, and discerning what resources the patient and their families will need to cope with the gradual or sudden cognitive and physical declines in their health status over time. Thus, knowing the patient is a professional, not a personal, activity and should be imbedded into ongoing learning assessment and educational activities.

A number of studies have focused on needs assessments concerning mental health in the long-term care setting (Canar & Johnson, 1986; Glass & Todd-Atkinson, 1999). In the latter study, the self-perceived learning needs of 319 nurses in 14 nursing facilities were evaluated. Many continuing education needs were highlighted with particular emphasis on behavioral problems, management skills, and drug therapy/interactions. Canar and Johnson developed a tool resulting in identified mental health need statements, which were sorted into 18 categories for the development of in-service education programs. An Australian study of nurses assessed the geriatric mental health knowledge of registered nurses employed in long-term care through use of a standardized examination. The participants were found to be unprepared for the reality of caring for the mental health needs of an older population and to have knowledge deficits related specifically to suicide, the prevalence of mental illness, mental health, and ethnicity and a number of issues regarding dementia (Hsu et al., 2005).

BARRIERS

Numerous barriers that prevent nurses from undertaking training have been described. Eley et al. (2006) surveyed 1000 nurses working in residential care facilities in Queensland, Australia. Despite educational opportunities, the nurses indicated that there were numerous barriers to their participation. These included lack of time, registration fees, distance to training, availability of relief staff, and issues related to leave.

A study of approaches and barriers to continuing education for staff in long-term care facilities was also carried out in Ottawa, Ontario (Ross et al., 2001). The study was based on in-depth interviews with key informants at the administrative level. The authors noted that a major emphasis is placed on individual responsibility for learning and that efficiency and cost-effectiveness constituted major underpinnings of corporate responsibility for continuing education. Continuing education is viewed as a vehicle to quality care for residents and personal and professional growth for staff. The barriers listed included fiscal restraints, understaffing, and a general lack of financial and human resources. The respondents also viewed limited and unequal access of staff to learning opportunities as a barrier. Programs for night staff were viewed as particularly problematic as there are so few staff members on at night. Other barriers included difficulty in tailoring educational programs for staff with diverse needs and backgrounds, the fact that English was not always the prevalent language of some members of staff and overall staff motivation. Some responders felt that staff members did not always recognize their learning needs and, therefore, did not value the offerings of continuing education programs, and for others confidence in their ability to learn was problematic.

Less evident or discussed in the literature is an interesting paradox that is neither accidental nor natural but comes in great part from the logical consequence of the fact that nurses and their organizations place such a heavy emphasis on nursing's and nurses' *virtues* rather than on their *knowledge* and *concrete contributions*. Because of the real and perceived nature of long-term care nursing work, there is an unspoken myth within the nursing profession, which suggests that registered nurses (i.e., RNs, Registered Practical Nurses, Licenced Practical Nurses) who work within this sector do so because they could "not quite cut it" within the acute care sector. This myth is further perpetuated by the power of what Gordon and Nelson (2006) refer to as the "virtue script" in nursing. When asked to describe or justify their work, nurses all too often rely on traditional caring discourse that presents the nurse as the good, trusting, passionate figure, failing to recognize the knowledge and skill that nurses must have in order to care for patients, particularly those in long-term care. Gordon and Nelson (2006) raise concerns that with its images of hearts, hands, and angels, this virtue script sentimentalizes and trivializes what is in fact complex and highly skilled knowledge work in all sectors of health care. It makes the caring that nurses give appear to be *feeling* as opposed to *cognitive work* and thus it paves the way for nice—rather than educated—women, or men, to replace the educated, experienced nurses who are critical to patient care, particularly in long-term care.

Finally, inadequacies in nursing education in general also contribute to the problem of learning and education, which is often exacerbated within the long-term care sector. Historically, nursing education is based on a punitive model of learning that originated in the church and the military. Although moving nursing education into the university has helped its discourse, the fact remains that few nurse educators or nursing home administrators for that matter can tolerate nursing students or staff nurses who challenge their positions and teachings. The profession and organizations representing practice environments for health-care professionals should be encouraging and rewarding respectful disagreement. Instead, students fear that speaking out may result in a poor grade or even failure, particularly in clinical courses, where the evaluation of performance is much more subjective than in the classroom. Where and how do nurses learn how to have reasoned debate? Where do they discuss how to challenge prevailing thought in respectful, objective ways? Rarely do they find this in nursing education, and they certainly do not find it in the workplace, where even unionized nurses often fear retaliation for speaking out about important issues such as conditions that jeopardize patient safety (Manson, 2006).

DESIGN AND IMPLEMENTATION OF
EDUCATIONAL PROGRAMS

Having obtained a needs assessment, it is then important to plan and implement a specific education program. The target audience needs to be determined and the curriculum defined with appropriate learning objectives. It is then necessary to determine who will teach the program and the logistics of how it will be delivered.

The practical aspects of where and when the program will take place are critical. In order to avoid frustration, it is necessary to obtain the clear support of administrators and to make it possible for staff to attend educational sessions. This can be very difficult in a busy facility with limited levels of staff. It should be noted that a single educational intervention is unlikely to result in long-term change in the behavior of staff. Longitudinal programs are much more likely to meet with success. Programs that utilize CD-ROMs or the Internet may be more practical as they allow the participant to work when they have available time and allow for much more flexibility.

In order to increase effectiveness, the teacher should actively involve the learner and maximize interactions between teacher and student. It is often helpful to utilize a variety of different teaching methods (e.g., workshops, role playing, individual assignments). It is important to create a positive atmosphere in which the student feels comfortable and engaged and to use material that is highly relevant (e.g., clinical case vignettes). A number of small group methods that encourage participation have been developed (e.g., the use of games).

Ross et al. (2001) describe a number of suggestions for overcoming barriers to education as related by long-term care administrators. These included the use of more informal and self-directed learning resources, maximizing the use of internal expertise and sharing of resources with other long-term care facilities. The respondents identified a variety of ways to increase staff attendance, which included increased supervisory support; the involvement of staff in the planning, preparation, and presentation of educational sessions; and the provision of relevant, informative, practical, and interesting content. Other suggestions included improved marketing strategies, disseminating new information in newsletters, on bulletin boards, and in pay envelopes. Finally, it was noted that having students from various schools and colleges within the facility demonstrated the importance of learning to staff.

MEASURING EFFECTIVENESS

Evaluation is a critical component of any educational program. Outcome measures can include: (a) the participants' satisfaction with or perception of the program; (b) changes in the participants' degree of knowledge, skill, or attitude;

(c) changes in the participants' actual performance or behavior in the clinical setting; (d) changes in the mental health status of individuals receiving care from the participants; and (e) the cost/benefit ratio associated with the program (Lieff & Silver, 2007).

Aylward et al. (2003) reviewed the literature on the effectiveness of continuing education in long-term care settings. Forty-eight studies met the selection criteria with the majority of them taking place in the United States. Nineteen of the studies were focused on residents with mental health issues and 10 evaluated "chemical or physical restraint reduction." New knowledge was generally provided in a training program format. The length of training ranged from a 10-min educational session to 56 h or seminars with the average length of training being approximately 4 h often in a series of one-half or 1-h seminars, on a weekly basis. The training methods were relatively similar, comprising combinations of handouts, audio/visual material, lectures, seminars, experiential learning, role play activities, and group discussion. The authors pointed out that only 13 of the 48 studies utilized enabling or reinforcing factors in the form of organizational or system support or change to facilitate the transfer of the new knowledge or behavior to the workplace. Seven of the studies used a randomized control trial design, 19 used a quasi-experimental design without randomization, and 22 used a descriptive case-study design. Participant satisfaction was evaluated in two studies; staff knowledge, beliefs, or attitudes in 23 studies; staff behavior in 25 studies; and resident outcomes in 14 studies. In almost two-thirds of the studies there was no follow-up evaluation. Of the 17 studies that conducted a follow-up evaluation, 11 studies concluded that changes or improvement in outcomes were sustained at follow-up, four concluded that the changes were not sustained, and two studies found no changes at posttest and also at follow-up. The authors concluded that there is minimal evidence that knowledge gained from training programs is sustained in the long-term and that most studies do not consider organizational and system factors when planning and implementing training initiatives, which may account for difficulties encountered in the sustained transfer of knowledge to practice.

A few recent studies have demonstrated that training programs can improve the residents' outcome. For example, Teri et al. (2005) describe a dementia-specific training program for staff in assisted living residences. The program provided two 4-h workshops augmented by four individualized on-site consultations and three leadership sessions. Following training, residents displayed significantly reduced levels of affective and behavioral distress compared with residents in a control group. In addition, staff who received the training reported less adverse impact and reaction to residents' problems and more job satisfaction compared with control staff. In addition, Proctor et al. (1999) reported that a combination of on-site teaching and consultation by a nurse specialist was associated with lower depression scores in nursing home residents over a 6-month period. There is also evidence that educational programs aimed at physicians, nurses, and other staff can lead to improved prescribing of psychotropic medications (Avorn et al., 1992; Ray et al., 1993).

Stolee et al. (2005) studied factors associated with the effectiveness of continuing education in long-term care. They utilized focus groups to identify staff perceptions of factors that effect transfer of learning into practice and a Delphi technique to refine the list of factors. A list of key factors is provided in Table 18.1. Interestingly, support from management was identified as the most important factor impacting the effectiveness of continuing education. Other

TABLE 18.1. Workplace Factors Affecting the Effectiveness of Continuing Education

Workforce issues

Changing resident population—worker and facility response to these changes
    More complicated care needs creating new staff responsibilities
    Need for new knowledge and skills
    Need for different models of care
Staff resistance to change
    Influenced by tenure (age), desire to maintain "routine," attitudes toward the
        elderly population that reinforce a custodial model of care
    Physician resistance to implement new treatments with which they are not
        familiar
Workforce education
    Nonregulated staff
    Low education requirements
    Continuing education not a priority

Management support

Prioritization of new initiatives (provision of funding, scheduling, staff coverage)
Need for a "whole-team approach," including physician and administration
    involvement in continuing education to facilitate group effort

Resources

Lack of funding for education in long-term care
Lack of physical space (training rooms, space to implement new care approaches) and
    equipment (audiovisual, photocopiers)

Continuing education—learning strategies

Long-term care staff can be overwhelmed by amount of new information
Continuing education often does not take into account varying levels of staff education
    (resulting in material being either too basic or too complex)
Targeting registered staff excludes the majority of frontline workers
Need for expert resources, follow-up support, and networking opportunities

Source: Adapted from Stolee et al. (2005).

factors included staff funding and space resources and the need for ongoing expert support. They concluded that organizational support is necessary for continuing education programs to be effective and that ongoing expert support is needed to enable and reinforce learning. A study of nurses in long-term care indicated that those nurses who participated in more continuing education activities scored higher on a job satisfaction scale (Robertson et al., 1999). Satisfaction with one's job affects self-esteem, stress level, and professional growth (Cavanaugh, 1992).

Berta et al. (2005) discuss factors that contribute to the learning capacity of an organization. Learning capacity is a term used to describe an organization's ability to recognize the value of new knowledge and information, assimilate it, and then apply it to make high-quality decisions. Performance variations can be explained on differences in the rate at which organizations learn, the ease with which they innovate, and differences in the effectiveness of the processes and mechanisms by which new knowledge is applied to decision-making. They outline a series of propositions that highlight factors that are likely to differentiate high capacity "good" organizational learners from low-capacity "poor" learners, operating in the long-term care field. They relate that although evidence-based clinical practice guidelines can lead to improved patient outcomes, they have often not fulfilled their promise in long-term care settings. There are as many examples in the literature of guideline noncompliance as there are implementation success stories. A number of their propositions are of particular interest, for example, "causal ambiguity" is a significant predictor of the ease of knowledge transfer. If there is uncertainty around the utility of the new knowledge, any related new routines or practices may be abandoned for more familiar prior practices. In addition, one study shows that the speed of adoption of a healthcare innovation had more to do with the fit of the innovation to the interests of the parties involved than to the strength of the scientific evidence concerning its benefits. The authors also suggest that the likelihood of guideline adoption increases with the proportion of registered professional nursing staff, but ultimately they suggest that guidelines will be most widely adopted across long-term care facilities when they are reinforced by regulation.

Clearly, adequate funding and support are required for optimal nursing home education programs. The teaching nursing home program in the United States has linked nursing homes with schools of nursing in colleges and universities and is a useful model. It has been suggested that this approach, which attempts to change the nursing home into a more academic environment, has had a direct effect on enhancing the quality of care (Mezey et al., 1997). An overarching goal, which requires collaboration between long-term care facilities and other institutions, is to truly integrate clinical care with education and research. Ultimately, enhancing the quality of care in our long-term care facilities will rely on the success of this integrated approach.

REFERENCES

Anderson, R. A., Bailey, D. E., Corazzini, K., & Piven, M. L. (2005). The power of relationship for high-quality long-term care. *Journal of Nursing Care Quality, 20*(2), 103–106.

Avorn, J., Soumerai, S. B., Everitt, D. E., et al. (1992). A randomized trial of a program to reduce the use of psychoactive drugs in nursing homes. *New England Journal of Medicine, 327*(3), 168–173.

Aylward, S., Stolee, P., et al. (2003). Practice concepts. Effectiveness of continuing education in long-term care: A literature review. *The Gerontologist, 43*(2), 259–271.

Berta, W., Teare, G. F., Gilbart, E., et al. (2005). The contingencies of organizational learning in long-term care: Factors that affect innovation adoption. *Health Care Management Review, 30*(4), 282–292.

Brown, M. (1999, January–February). Psychosocial functions and training needs of social workers in nursing homes: A survey. *Continuum, 19*, 7–13.

Canadian Coalition for Seniors' Mental Health (CCSMH). (2006). National guidelines for seniors' mental health: The assessment and treatment of mental health issues in long term care homes. Toronto: Author. Available at www.ccsmh.ca

Canar, M. J., & Johnson II, J. C. (1986). An employee learning needs assessment concerning mental health needs of residents in a long-term care setting. *Journal of Continuing Education in Nursing, 17*(1), 5–11.

Chartok, P., Nevins, A., Rzetelny, H., & Gilberto, P. (1988). A mental health training program in nursing homes. *The Gerontologist, 28*, 503–507.

Conn, D. K., & Silver, I. L. (1998). The psychiatrist's role in long-term care. *Canadian Nursing Home, 9*, 22–24.

Eley, R., Hegney, D., Buikstra, E., Fallon, T., Plank, A., & Parker, V. (2007). Aged care nursing in Queensland—the nurses' view. *Journal of Clinical Nursing, 16*(5), 860–872.

Glass, Jr., J. C., & Todd-Atkinson, S. (1999). Continuing education needs of nurses employed in nursing facilities. *Journal of Continuing Education in Nursing, 30*(5), 219–228.

Hsu, M. C., Moyle, W., Creedy, D., & Venturato, L. (2005). An investigation of aged care mental health knowledge of Queensland aged care nurses. *International Journal of Mental Health Nursing, 14*, 16–23.

Jones, T. S., Matias, M., Powell, J., Jones, E. G., Fishburn, J., & Looi, J. C. L. (2007). Who cares for older people with mental illness? A survey of residential aged care facilities in the Australian capital territory: Implications for mental health nursing. *International Journal of Mental Health Nursing, 16*, 327–337.

Kaye, A., & Robinson, A. (2007). Helping the nursing staff: The role of the psychogeriatric nurse consultant. In D. K. Conn et al. (Eds.), *Practical psychiatry in the long-term care home: A handbook for staff* (3rd rev. and exp. ed., pp. 289–297). Seattle, WA: Hogrefe and Huber.

Lieff, S., & Silver, I. (2007). Planning mental health education programs. In D. K. Conn et al. (Eds.), *Practical psychiatry in the long-term care home: A handbook for staff* (3rd rev. and exp. ed., pp. 279–287). Seattle, WA: Hogrefe and Huber.

Maas, M., Buckwalter, K., & Specht, J. (1996). Nursing staff and quality of care in nursing homes. In G. S. Wunderlich, F. A. Sloan, & C. K. Davis (Eds.), *Nursing staff in hospitals and nursing homes. Is it adequate?* (pp. 361–425). Washington, DC: National Academy.

Manson, D. J. (2006). Pride and prejudice: Nurses' struggle with reasoned debate. In S. Nelson & S. Gordon (Eds.), *The complexities of care: Nursing reconsidered* (pp. 44–49). Ithaca, NY: Cornell University Press.

Mezey, M. D., Mitty, E. L., & Bottrell, M. (1977). The teaching nursing home programme: Enhancing educational outcomes. *Nursing Outlook, 45,* 133–140.

Nelson, S., & Gordon, S. (Eds.). (2006). *The complexities of care: Nursing reconsidered.* Ithaca, NY: Cornell University Press.

Proctor, R., Burns, A., Stratton Powell, H., et al. (1999). Behavioural management in nursing and residential homes: A randomized controlled trial. *The Lancet, 354,* 26–29.

Ray, W. A., Taylor, J. A., Meador, K. G., et al. (1993). Reducing antipsychotic drug use in nursing homes. A controlled trial of provider education. *Archives of Internal Medicine, 153*(6), 713–721.

Rewilak, D. (2007). Behavior management strategies. In D. K. Conn et al. (Eds), *Practical psychiatry in the long-term care home: A handbook for staff* (3rd rev. and exp. ed., pp. 217–237). Seattle, WA: Hogrefe and Huber.

Robertson, E. M., Higgins, L., Rozmus, C., & Robinson, J. P. (1999). Association between continuing education and job satisfaction of nurses employed in long-term care facilities. *Journal of Continuing Education in Nursing, 30*(3), 108–113.

Ross, M. M., Carswell, A., Dalziel, W. B., & Aminzadeh, F. (2001). Continuing education for staff in long-term care facilities: Corporate philosophies and approaches. *Journal of Continuing Education in Nursing, 32*(2), 68–76.

Rovner, B. W., & Katz, I. R. (1993). Psychiatric disorders in the nursing home: A selective review of studies related to clinical care. *International Journal of Geriatric Psychiatry, 8*(1), 75–87.

Stolee, P., Esbaugh, J. Aylwar, S. et al. (2005). Factors associated with the effectiveness of continuing education in long-term care. *The Gerontologist, 45*(3), 399–409.

Stolz Howard, H. (1978). Liaison nursing. *Journal of Psychosocial Nursing and Mental Health Services, 4,* 35–37.

Teri, L., Huda, P., Gibbons, L. et al. (2005). STAR: A dementia-specific training program for staff in assisted living residences. *The Gerontologist, 45*(5), 686–693.

Weinberg, D. B. (2003). Code Green: Money-driven hospitals and the dismantling of nursing. Ithaca, NY: Cornell University Press.

World Health Organization. (1998). *Education in psychiatry of the elderly: A technical consensus statement.* Geneva: Author.

19

Psychiatric Consultation and Liaison

Gary S. Moak

As has been made abundantly clear elsewhere in this volume, the prevalence of psychopathology among residents of nursing facilities is high and the need for psychiatric services great. Dementia, depression, and delirium, with their high rates of mood symptoms, psychosis, and behavioral disturbance, represent the most pressing needs of many residents. Contemporary nursing homes are de facto geriatric psychiatry facilities (Reichman et al., 1998). Yet nursing homes are primarily designed for the care of residents' medical and surgical problems. Despite two decades of regulatory pressure on facilities to address mental health issues and ensure that effective psychiatric treatment is provided to those residents who need it, there has been no redesign of nursing homes to facilitate the internal provision of mental health care. Thus, a mismatch exists between needs of residents and types of services available.

Most psychiatric services in nursing homes are provided by outside mental health consultants who provide various clinical services. Shortages of geriatric mental health professionals of all disciplines leave some nursing homes without access to psychiatric consultation services. Those mental health consultants available to go to nursing homes find them to be challenging settings. A paucity of psychiatric intervention and services research in the nursing home means that consultants must base their work on consensus rather than evidence-based best practices models. Mental health perspectives are alien to the nursing home culture (MacDonald, 1983). Because of this, psychiatric liaison activities are considered to be especially important. Such services, however, usually are not reimbursed. Reimbursement structures typically constrain psychiatrists into a medical model of consultation despite the need for more comprehensive intervention. Thus, psychiatrists and other mental health professionals who attempt to provide consultation in nursing homes will confront a great, unmet need for services under nonconducive circumstances. Effective psychiatric consultation in nursing homes thus requires great clinical efficiency and flexibility and tight practice management.

   This chapter will review what is known about mental health services in nursing homes and discuss the role and function of psychiatric consultants in these facilities.

WHAT IS KNOWN ABOUT NURSING HOME
PSYCHIATRIC CONSULTATION?

Little is known about the types, availability, or adequacy of mental health services provided in nursing homes. A survey of nursing home directors of nursing in six states revealed that in about one-half of the facilities, the frequency of consultation was considered inadequate (Reichman et al., 1998). Among facilities that have access to consultation services, little is known about the function, the range of interventions, or the effectiveness of the consultants (Bartels et al., 2002; Reichman et al., 1998).

   Prior to the implementation of the nursing home reform provisions of the Omnibus Budget Reconciliation Act of 1987 (OBRA-87), very few nursing residents with mental disorders received explicit psychiatric services (Borson et al., 1987; Streim et al., 2002). Mandates to address the mental health needs of residents triggered an increase in the volume of psychiatric services in regions where such services were available. The swift upturn in Medicare claims for mental health services in nursing homes brought about intense federal government scrutiny of those services and doubts about their appropriateness. This left a perplexing inconsistency: many nursing home patients needing psychiatric treatment were not receiving it, whereas others were receiving unnecessary services, some of which were presumed to be fraudulent or abusive (Streim et al., 2002). Resulting mandates for Medicare compliance and threats of sanctions for noncompliance have made nursing home consulting more complex and stressful.

   Unfortunately, there is no clear consensus about the types of psychiatric services that should be provided in nursing homes, what types of disciplines should provide them, or what expertise they should have (American Geriatrics Society & American Association for Geriatric Psychiatry 2003; Moak & Borson 2000).

Nursing home regulations governing psychiatric treatments are more proscriptive than prescriptive (Ryan et al., 2002). Clinical trials with most classes of psychoactive medication are of limited scope and leave a gap between evidence and practice for clinicians to bridge (Ryan et al., 2002). Recent safety warnings about atypical antipsychotic medications, a mainstay of nursing home psychiatric practice, impose additional risk management challenges for consultants. It is widely accepted that nonpharmacologic interventions ought to be provided, but the evidence for their effectiveness is also limited and many are impractical outside of funded research protocols. Best practice models defining which treatments are appropriate and medically necessary are lacking (Moak & Borson, 2000). Mental health service delivery research is difficult to do in nursing homes, and demonstrating effectiveness is challenging (Brodaty et al., 2003). In sum, the nursing home consulting psychiatrist practices in a complicated, contradictory climate in which need for services is high, many residents are still not receiving the mental health care they need (American Geriatrics Society & American Association for Geriatric Psychiatry, 2003), best practices are not clear, and scrutiny by payers abounds.

Given the lack of clear evidence-based best practices for nursing home psychiatric consultation, what can we say about what good consultation should consist of? The literature is somewhat helpful in this regard and permits some general conclusions. First, nursing home nursing directors (Reichman et al., 1998) are most satisfied when consultation is provided during regularly scheduled visits. Sporadic services in which the consultant comes as needed, only when called, with no regular follow-up is not viewed as satisfactory. Nursing home staff clearly prefer a regular presence in the facility, and most reports in the literature about psychiatric consultation services recommend this.

Beyond this, what else does the literature tell us? The literature on psychiatric consultation in nursing homes is mostly descriptive. Some of these reports include data. Fewer contain outcomes data and only a few of those involve randomized, controlled trials (Bartels et al., 2002). Much of the literature on nursing home psychiatric consultation services comprises descriptions of academic-based programs. The feasibility of delivering many of the recommended programs by community-based agencies or private practitioners is not addressed in the literature.

An opinion survey (Moak et al., 2000) and a descriptive (Samter et al., 1994) study suggest that common patterns of practice may rely very heavily on psychopharmacologic intervention, recommendations for further general medical testing, changes in nonpsychiatric drug regimen, and staff interventions and depend much less upon behavioral intervention, environmental manipulation, individual psychotherapy, and family therapy. Such patterns do not necessarily reflect best practices and may instead reflect therapeutic pragmatism in typical long-term care settings. Even though the emphasis is on biomedical intervention, it seems clear that an eclectic range of psychiatric services requiring broad expertise is likely to be necessary.

Models of Nursing Home Psychiatric Consultation Described in the Literature

Three prevailing models for delivering services have been described. These are psychiatrist-centered, multidisciplinary team, and nurse-centered models. In the psychiatrist-centered model, the primary consultant is a psychiatrist who often works alone. This is the traditional model of consultation, following the standard medical specialty model, and may be the most common model (Moak et al., 2000). In this model, it is not unusual for the psychiatrist to come only in response to being called and to provide no follow-up visit unless called back. As stated above, this model is usually unsatisfactory for effective nursing home mental health services.

A preferable form of the psychiatrist-centered model involves regularly scheduled visits to the home. The consultant "carries" a panel of patients who are followed as clinically indicated. During these visits, new consultations will be performed and established patients may be seen for follow-up when medically necessary. In this model, the psychiatrist may work with other clinicians, but they clearly are ancillary to the psychiatrists with a primary focus on extending the number of patients that can be seen rather than expanding the range of interventions provided.

Psychiatrists who self-identify as geriatric subspecialists are more likely to provide consultation working within the multidisciplinary team model (Conn & Silver, 1998; Moak et al., 2000). Various compositions have been described for such teams. They typically consist of two to five clinicians, including social workers, psychologists, and psychiatric nurses, each with distinct roles and responsibilities. Many provide organized psychiatric liaison activities that are likely to include training and education of staff. In the team model, psychiatrists may provide direct treatment, supervise other clinicians, or both. Supervision may also be provided to the facility staff, such as the social worker, nursing staff, or nurse practitioner, if the facility employs one (Conn & Silver, 1998).

The third model is the nurse-centered model. There are only a few published descriptions of this model (Bartels et al., 2002; Santmyer, 1991). In this model, a nurse clinician comes to the nursing home to provide patient-centered and staff-centered consultation. The nurse clinician may be supervised off-site by a psychiatrist. When a psychiatrist is available to come to the home, the nurse may refer cases to the psychiatrist cases that the nurse deems appropriate for pharmacotherapy. It is important to bear in mind that fee-for-service reimbursement does not cover supervisory services provided by psychiatrists or nurse clinicians.

Since there is no clear evidence-based best practices model, is there an accepted "gold standard" for nursing home consultation services? The literature suggests that mental health services should consist of a multidisciplinary team providing ongoing diagnostic assessments and ongoing treatment (Lichtenberg et al., 1998). Visits to the facility should be regularly scheduled. Services must be medically necessary based on clinical need. Patients should not be seen solely based on the consultants visiting schedule. At each scheduled visit to the facility, only those patients who need to be seen should be seen. Active treatment should be of sufficient intensity to address patients' problems effectively. This might mean weekly visits during the acute phase of treatment and less often in the continuation and maintenance phases. Stable patients should be seen at a frequency (e.g., quarterly) dictated by community standards of care for maintenance management. Services should provide a range of interventions indicated by patients' problems and should include appropriate staff liaison activities.

It is important to view this gold standard as an ideal. In the vast majority of facilities, implementation of the full model is not likely to be practical. Financing mechanisms in the United States generally do not support this vision of comprehensive services outside of funded demonstration projects or research protocols, or absent another source of financial support. In the broader universe of nursing facilities, the intensity and comprehensiveness of psychiatric consultation services are likely to be determined by local manpower availability, fee-for-service reimbursement rates, and other market factors. A psychiatrist in rural practice who must divide his or her time among several outlying facilities, spending an afternoon per month at each will provide a very different range of services than one working as part of a community mental health center geriatric outreach team or in an urban private practice with an office across the street from the nursing home. Each may provide excellent quality service, albeit with different goals and scope of treatment.

GOALS OF NURSING HOME PSYCHIATRIC CONSULTATION

Stated most simply and profoundly, the job of the nursing home consulting psychiatrist should be to attempt to improve the mental health of individual residents whom he or she is asked to see while acting to improve the facility's mental health culture. In endeavoring to achieve this, the consultant should provide the most comprehensive services possible under the circumstances. The scope of interventions should be pragmatic, based upon realistic appraisal of the strengths and weaknesses of each nursing home and the professional resources available to the consultant. Goals must be realistic and achievable and should represent the best compromise possible under the circumstances. Basic goals of consultation might be limited to ensuring that patients have a correct psychiatric diagnosis and that psychopharmacologic agents are used correctly. In contrast, advanced goals might include regular use of behavioral interventions and individual psychotherapy, active monitoring of treatment outcomes and side effects, frequent contact with families, informal liaison with staff, and participation in staff development programs.

TECHNIQUE AND PRACTICE OF NURSING HOME CONSULTATION

Absent data to support an evidence-based consensus about best practices for nursing home psychiatric consultation, what services should the nursing home psychiatric consultant provide and how should he or she attempt to deliver them? An elegant conceptual framework for mental health consultation has been described (Caplan, 1970). The reader interested in nuances of mental health consultative technique for patient-centered consultation in human service organization is referred to this work. The remainder of this chapter will attempt to assist the practitioner in crafting a specific approach to nursing home consultation.

Diagnostic Formulation

Establishing a neuropsychiatric diagnosis is a necessary but not sufficient outcome of the diagnostic assessment process. To be sure, making categorical diagnoses for nursing home patients represents a formidable challenge in its own right. The commotion and lack of privacy characteristic of many nursing homes present a barrier to traditional psychiatric interviewing. The conduct of psychiatric examination may need to be adapted due to this or patients' pathology. Severely demented patients or those who are agitated or delirious may not be able to participate in the standard psychiatric diagnostic interview. In many cases, examining gait, mobility, motor functioning, functional skills, social skills, and perception of the environment may be as useful in diagnosis and management. Information about these neurobehavioral domains and attention, mood, and behavior often can be gleaned more effectively from observing patients feed themselves, interact socially in the milieu, ambulate, or participate in activities than from a structured interview.

Patients' availability to be seen should not be presumed to be automatic. It is not uncommon for a patient to be in physical therapy, attending an activity group, getting a bath, or to be out of the building at the time the psychiatric consultant comes. Consultants should consider whether working with the staff to schedule patient encounters in advance would be helpful. If the psychiatrist has many patients to see, scheduling may not be necessary and flexibility may be more efficient.

It is important to appreciate that the diagnosis has regulatory compliance importance in addition to its clinical role. In fact, obtaining a formal diagnosis often is the sole reason consultation is requested. This occurs, for example, when the nursing home staff wish to establish a diagnosis that supports the use of a psychiatric medication.

Arriving at the appropriate diagnosis, however, may not represent the most useful aspect of the consultative evaluation. A narrative, descriptive formulation of the problem is likely to help others, including attending physicians, staff, quality of care surveyors, and insurance reviewers to appreciate the rationale for treatment. Because of the dearth of mental health experience among most involved parties, use of diagnostic terms commonly used in general medicine may be more suitable than less familiar psychiatric nosology. Distinctions between terms such as "major depressive disorder," "dysthymia," "adjustment disorder with depressed mood" have little meaning to many health-care providers outside of psychiatric programs. Defaulting simply to "depression" is less specific but likely to be better appreciated. On the other hand, a term such as "post-stroke depression," though not part of the official nomenclature, may help link the occurrence of a psychiatric problem to a physical disorder the nursing home team understands better. Multiaxial psychiatric diagnoses rarely are meaningful or useful, but relevant issues should be discussed in the narrative formulation.

Improved diagnostic understanding obviously is an important goal that may improve care (Conn & Silver, 1998; Sakauye & Camp, 1992). For example, recognition that depression is the cause for a common problem such as "agitation" hopefully results in more specific therapy. Problems such as physical aggression, eloping, screaming, refusing to eat, resisting needed care, wandering, and sexually inappropriate behavior distress the staff and often lead to interventions. Usual care often includes sedative medications or behavioral interventions that are counter-therapeutic. Psychiatric consultation may identify more specific syndromal or behavioral features of the problem that lead to more targeted pharmacotherapy or more specific and effective behavioral interventions. Another diagnostic goal of consultation is recognition of the contributions of medical comorbidity and adverse drug effects.

One challenge in performing a nursing home consultation is that ascertaining the reason for the consultation may be difficult. Such information may not be apparent or readily available at the time of consultation, or the stated or manifested reason may be different from the true or latent reason. Staff members present at the time the consultant visits may not know the reason for the consultation. The staff who know the patient best and/or who were involved in originating the consultation request may be unavailable. Those present may be *per diem* personnel or "floats" from other floors. Even those regularly assigned to the same floor may know little about patients with whom they do not work consistently. Further, the lack of mental health orientation often translates into a dearth of documentation in the record about the presenting problem or the patient's mental state or behavior. Thus, it is desirable to identify a reliable informant among the staff and to arrange to meet that person to obtain history at the beginning of the consultation visit.

Once the explicit reason for consultation is identified, the context must be appreciated. Who identified the need? Was it the attending physician, family, or staff? Most often the need for psychiatric intervention is identified by the nursing staff (Samter et al., 1994). Staff perception of the problem, however, often differs considerably from that of the consultant (Lobel et al., 1991) or the family. This dissonance must be addressed as part of the consultation process. If the nursing home staff do not believe that the consultant is responding to their concerns, the consultation will be ineffective. When the staff has a latent agenda, the consultant must identify this and address it.

What about family involvement in the diagnostic process? Family members may not agree with staff over the nature of the problem or the need for psychiatric consultation. There may be disagreement between family members. They may be shocked to learn that the facility has had their relative seen by a psychiatrist. This may reflect ignorance about the patient's condition, misunderstanding about mental illness and modern psychiatry, rationalization, or denial. An essential component of the diagnostic assessment involves determining the extent to which such issues must be addressed. Successful consultation requires negotiating a framework for the consultation with the family.

A number of additional administrative concerns may prompt a request for consultation. Deficiencies cited in recent state survey, safety concerns about classes of medications (i.e., boxed warnings), and biases of the administration or consultant pharmacist about appropriate remedies may motivate requests for consultation. These motivations may not be explicit in the request. Thus, consultants should be aware of the regulatory milieu and how the facility has fared within it recently as well as policies and procedures the facility has adopted to facilitate compliance.

For example, after being cited for preventable patient-to-patient altercations, a facility exhibited a lower threshold for requesting consultation with an underlying agenda of more immediate psychiatric hospitalization of threatening patients. Another example has to do with antipsychotic medication use. Many facilities establish quotas for the use of these medications. When pharmacy data reveal that the quota has been exceeded, there may be an increase in requests to evaluate stable patients in advance of scheduled maintenance visits in order to encourage discontinuation of medication.

Other administratively driven reasons consultations are requested include regulatory requirements to document an extrapyramidal examination for monitoring of antipsychotic medication use, assessment of drug regimen for formulary alternatives to nonformulary medications, determination of competence, and evaluation of suitability for transfer to a dementia unit.

Diagnosis of the Strengths and Weaknesses of the Facility and Its Staff

Successful psychiatric case formulation in nursing homes depends upon good knowledge of the strengths and weaknesses of each facility and its staff. Effective consultants pay attention to these considerations and take time to understand them (Caplan, 1970). Various staff attributes are of particular relevance to the psychiatric consultant. These include understanding of psychiatric problems, communication and behavioral skills, familiarity with the residents, job satisfaction and morale, motivation to work with difficult residents, threshold for tolerating residents' abusive behavior, and ability to work as team members.

The consultant also must recognize the extent to which staff expectations of psychiatric treatment are appropriate and realistic. Nursing home staff can be ill informed about clinical psychiatry and poorly understand psychiatric treatments. They may be naive about treatment and harbor magical thinking about pharmacotherapy and psychotherapy. Thus, they may have inappropriate expectations about pharmacotherapy or request psychotherapy when it clearly is not indicated (MacDonald, 1983). Inappropriate expectations for psychotherapy commonly originate with guilt over not having more time for their patients and a wish for them to have someone to talk to.

Nursing home consultants must rely upon staff report for knowledge of patients' symptoms, behavior, and progress. Patients are often poor historians and staff may be the only available source of information about patients. Staff report may be of poor quality as well, adversely affecting the accuracy of the consultant's initial and ongoing assessment. The reliability and validity of information reported by the staff must be determined.

Why are even the best long-term care nurses sometimes poor informants about mental status and behavior? Once again, the basic culprit is inadequate formal training in psychiatry. Medically and surgically savvy nurses' professional objectivity seems to break down in the realm of mental health problems. Formal knowledge of psychopathology, phenomenology, and psychiatric disorders often is deficient. They may misinterpret the significance of a symptom and then jump to a conclusion using psychiatric vocabulary incorrectly in a way that can be misleading (Leo et al., 2002). For example, they may use the term "mania" to describe hyperactivity and refer to confabulation as delusions.

Another factor that affects the quality of "objective" reporting by nursing home staff is the tendency to underappreciate the extent of patients' cognitive impairment. They may expect patients to function at a higher level than they are capable and interpret helplessness, disorganization, or anxiety as manipulation for attention. Staff can be shockingly unaware of the presence of depression in their patients, especially among those who are cooperative with care and not agitated. They may view such patients as doing well and not in need of further intervention.

Nursing home staff often seems to lack a longitudinal sense of progress. Their impressions of patients seem limited to one shift at a time, often the current or last shift worked or a bygone shift with no perception of progress in the interim. The persistence of residual symptoms may cause them to report that a treatment has been ineffective and to clamor for a change of therapy.

Finally, ageist attitudes and psychiatric stigma may bias the judgment of some staff. Believing that frail elderly patients cannot get better and that psychiatric treatment is futile for them, they may lobby against consultation or subtly undermine treatment. For example, they may report that a very depressed patient who has not responded to a low starting dose of an antidepressant is "doing fine," implying that the patient is better. In some cases, they may overtly or unconsciously undermine treatment initiatives (MacDonald, 1983). The composite effect of these limitations is that consultants may obtain as many different opinions about the condition of a patient as there are staff members to query.

Poor communication patterns also reflect lack of experience working successfully within an interdisciplinary team. Professional and personal boundaries may be weak. Individual agendas may be pursued at the expense of the interdisciplinary treatment plan or nursing care plan. Poorly developed team skills may thwart consensus about the care plan that all staff can accept and carry out. There may be subtle undermining of the consultant's recommendations or frank sabotage of treatment. Nursing home psychiatric consultants must recognize such patterns and handle them as therapeutically as possible.

Ongoing Treatment and Its Monitoring

As stated above, nursing homes prefer ongoing involvement in residents' care as opposed to onetime consultation visits. At one level, they appear to appreciate that successful treatment of psychiatric problems in nursing homes requires active management and that if the consulting psychiatrist does not provide it, no one else will. At a more administrative level, documentation of the outcomes of acute and maintenance therapy, including efficacy and tolerability of interventions, goes a long way toward satisfying regulatory requirements for monitoring of medication use. Many requests for psychiatric consultation will be motivated by regulatory compliance. Regardless of the motivation, continuing involvement in the care of patients with mental health problems ought to be considered a gold standard for nursing home psychiatric consultation.

The consultant must realize that to achieve good outcomes he or she must assume de facto responsibility for directing the psychiatric treatment

(Sakauye & Camp, 1992), both pharmacologic and psychosocial. This should include monitoring of pharmacologic trials, managing side effects, assessing interactions with other health problems and nonpsychiatric medications, and communicating with families. During an acute phase of treatment, the psychiatrist may see a patient much more frequently than the attending physician.

Sophisticated and highly motivated floor nurses may provide some modicum of case management, but more often the staff and attendent reflexively carry out consultants' recommendations. Ambiguity or vagueness should be avoided in making recommendations. Avoid contingencies that require interpretation or discretion. The nursing staff are more likely to feel confident with concrete recommendations written in the style of orders.

Should nursing home consulting psychiatrists actually write orders for the interventions they recommend? There is no absolutely correct answer to this. If the attending physicians have confidence in the consultant, they may authorize the staff to accept any of the consultant's recommendations as attending physician telephone orders, or request that the consultant write the orders directly. In some cases, this may reflect a desire of the nursing home attending physician not to be bothered.

The policies and procedures of many facilities do not allow consultants to write orders. If consultants are permitted to write orders, the nursing home psychiatrist must nevertheless decide whether this practice is appropriate. Requiring the attending physician to order, even by telephone, a treatment recommended by the consultant ensures that he/she is at least aware of changes in treatment. When consultants write orders, attending physicians may abdicate the psychiatric management entirely to the consultant. Consultant psychiatrists then must be prepared to assume full responsibility for all issues that arise around ordered treatments.

Consulting psychiatrists also should carefully consider the need to obtain informed consent for interventions they recommend. If the consultant recommends treatment, then he/she should attempt to engage patients who are capable in an informed consent discussion. If the consultant writes orders for treatment, then the consultant should have an informed consent discussion with the patient or their health-care agent.

Some nursing homes have introduced separate consent forms specifically for psychoactive medications. Such forms are signed by patients or their families at the behest of a facility staff member, a process that rarely involves an adequate informed consent discussion. Consultants should not rely on this process for informed consent, but instead assess the clinical issues and liability risks of each case to decide what more may be needed. Ideally, each consultation should include a documentation of contact with family members or other health-care agents that include notation of an informed consent discussion. In reality, this is not always possible. In some consultation settings it may be necessary to prioritize the level of family contact and involvement in the consent process.

As mentioned previously, prevailing reimbursement systems conduce toward biomedical intervention. While inappropriate psychotherapy may be requested in some cases, in many nursing facilities, the institutional culture promotes over reliance on medication in spite of regulatory pressures to the contrary. The consultant must be vigilant to prevent such forces from biasing residents' care away from needed nonpharmacologic interventions.

In order to prevent this from occurring, the consulting psychiatrist must be facile in making behavioral recommendations (Conn & Silver, 1998) and coaching the staff in their implementation. Such interventions are described elsewhere in this book. Intensive psychotherapy is less often indicated, due to patients' limitations, and may not be feasible due to time and reimbursement constraints (Class & Hendrie, 1995). The techniques of individual psychotherapy can be adapted, however, for the needs of selected nursing home patients. Thus, while psychotherapy may be a less frequently prescribed treatment, in the nursing home, it is no less important (Conn & Silver, 1998). When another clinician provides the psychotherapy, the consulting psychiatrist should monitor the effectiveness of the therapy and document its ongoing medical necessity.

Another way in which nursing home consultation services conform to a "medical model" is that they are predominantly patient focused rather than program (staff) focused. Again, the institutional culture and reimbursement limitations militate against a broader consultative approach. In many cases, however, the need for consultation may have less to do with patients' psychopathology and more to do with family or staff reaction to it or counter-therapeutic facility policies and procedures. When indicated, the consulting psychiatrist should attempt to refocus attention from the identified patient onto the broader system.

After each visit, some form of feedback to the staff should be provided. Well-documented progress notes may provide this, to an extent, and are an otherwise essential aspect of good nursing home psychiatric consultation. If practical, it is useful to maintain copies of consultations and progress notes in the consultant's office where they can be referenced in addressing questions that are posed by telephone between visits. Some nursing homes have a separate mental health section in their patient records in which they require psychiatric notes to be filed. Attending physicians may not remember to look for psychiatric notes there, however, and it may lead to better integration of medical and psychiatric care to write notes in the medical progress note section chronologically in the flow of the attending physician notes, where they will not be missed.

Written notes should be supplemented with informal, verbal feedback to the staff to ensure that the goals of treatment and recommended therapies are properly understood. Beyond this, such contact with the staff provides an opportunity to educate and teach, anticipate pitfalls, identify unrealistic expectations, and assess skepticism about the recommendations and resistance to carrying them out. Such contact most often occurs "curbside." It provides an important means to facilitate rudimentary multidisciplinary team process and staff liaison (see below), whether explicitly or implicitly.

How often should patients be seen in follow up? Obviously, clinical judgment determines this. The frequency should be as often as is medically necessary to ensure safe, effective treatment. Caregiver factors, such as staff reliability, comfort with the plan, and family and staff anxiety, are important to gauge in determining how soon to see the patient again. Nursing facilities are considered outpatient places of service by the Medicare Program. Thus, a good rule of thumb is to see patients with an intensity of services mirroring a standard of care for office-based treatment of similarly ill patients. It is incumbent upon all providers to be familiar with the coverage policies of their local Medicare carrier.

Staff Liaison

In an ideal model of care, liaison is a cornerstone of nursing home psychiatric consultation (Sakauye & Camp, 1992). Medical model consultation, narrowly construed, focuses on diagnosing and treating the identified patient. In contrast, psychiatric liaison attempts to impact the facility and its staff (Streim et al., 2002). This focus has a twofold benefit. First, staff members are better able to understand and implement the consultants' recommendations, improving treatment outcomes for individual patients. Second, through ongoing liaison activity, the staff generalizes principles from individual cases which they then begin to apply more broadly. Many of the staff and facility weaknesses discussed above can be addressed to some extent through longitudinal psychiatric liaison.

Psychiatric liaison occurs in a number of ways, explicit and implicit. Formal activities may include case conferences, behavioral rounds, staff support groups, and in-service education programs. In-service programs are most likely to be supported by facility administration, because continuing education for the staff is a regulatory requirement. Budgetary constraints make facility administrators prone to view other liaison activities as cost ineffective. They tend to be unwilling to spare staff members from direct patient care responsibilities (Bienenfeld & Wheeler, 1989).

Even when administration strongly supports formal liaison activities, the most effective liaison with staff is likely to occur informally and implicitly. One reason for this is that staff themselves may resist attending. They may complain that attending a meeting, no matter how brief, will keep them from completing their patient care assignments. Staff members may feel intimidated to meet with a psychiatrist. They may resist talking about behavioral issues fearing personal disclosure. The consultant should make every effort to create a nonthreatening and informal atmosphere in which the staff feels more open to participate. It is useful for staff support groups to be case centered for this reason. Ironically, if the consultant succeeds in creating a safe environment, discussions may lead to work-related stress and from there to inappropriate revelation of personal problems. Consultants must take care to prevent this from occurring.

Helping staff cope with difficult patients is a foremost goal of liaison work. A main task for the consultant is to make such patients human for the staff (Sakauye & Camp, 1992). Sharing details of patients' biographies and developmental histories may provide a context that helps staff to be more empathic and therapeutic. Consultants may have opportunities to role model therapeutic communication with difficult residents. (Class & Hendrie, 1995; Sakauye & Camp, 1992). They may be able to assist staff members to accept more realistic expectations of themselves, and to set effective limits with demanding patients and families.

Liaison with attending physicians and the facility medical director is also important. While all care in nursing homes requires physician orders, attending physicians are not present frequently. The need to obtain orders by telephone can be a source of tension between physicians and staff that may affect the psychiatric consultation process. Calls from the staff for permission to obtain a consultation or implement consultants' recommendations may be resisted by physicians who do not feel sufficiently in control of their patients' care. Those who harbor frank beliefs that psychiatric intervention in frail nursing home patients is futile will react to such requests with annoyance and outright obstruction. To what extent psychiatric recommendations are ordered and carried out thus depends upon the relationships between the attending physician, staff, family, and consulting psychiatrist. Nurturing these relationships is fundamental to the successful psychiatric consultation-liaison in nursing homes.

Family Intervention

Theoretical and technical aspects of family intervention in nursing home psychiatry are beyond the scope of this chapter. The reader is directed to Chapter Sixteen, *Family Interventions*, in which this essential dimension of nursing home consultation practice is well covered. The family influences whether psychiatric consultation and liaison occur, what services are provided, and how smoothly it works, however. Nuances of the relationship of families to nursing homes that affect psychiatric consultation liaison will be discussed in this section.

The advocacy and health-care surrogate decision-making roles of family members in the care of frail patients are magnified in the nursing home. This usually serves the well-being of patients by helping to ensure that facilities adhere to their clinical missions. The reality, however, is that nursing homes are businesses, and sometimes they behave as if family members are the customers for the product they sell. In many cases, this is apropos, since it is often the family that picks the facility and attending physician, provides consent for admission, points out deficiencies, registers complaints, files grievances when dissatisfied, and decides to transfer the patient elsewhere when irreparably displeased. In responding to family complaints and demands, nursing homes may apply a "customer-is-always-right" ethos.

Unfortunately, when there are empty beds or a patient is private paying, nursing homes may be willing to mollify families whose insistence on services or refusal of treatment may be contrary to the team's assessment of what is in the patient's best interest. Facilities too readily accept refusal of treatment as an expression of "resident's rights" without question. Nursing homes lack a psychiatric culture in which inappropriate refusal of recommended services by patients or family may be seen as resistance to be worked through. The nursing home, in its customer service *modus operandi,* may thwart the efforts of the psychiatrist in its rush to accede to families' demands. It can be stunning to watch a nursing home allow a family member to refuse consent for necessary services in a way that clinically compromises the patient and the facility. This commonly affects psychiatric consultation. Angry families who blame the facility for a patient's behavioral problems often react unenthusiastically to recommendations for psychiatric consultation.

When performing a consultation to which a skeptical family has agreed only reluctantly, the nursing home consulting psychiatrist should recognize such "realpolitik" in considering the best approach. A pragmatic compromise may be unavoidable. The facility administration may prefer that the psychiatrist not "make too many waves." Moreover, the consulting psychiatrist depends upon the good faith of the family to pay bills for consultation services not covered by insurance.

Although taking on family work can be arduous and fraught with peril for the consulting psychiatrist, it is clinically important and a highly rewarding aspect of nursing home practice. Astute nursing home administrators appreciate this. They know that when done well, the involvement of the consulting psychiatrist with patients' family results in improved family satisfaction with the facility.

What are the options for structuring family work? Often it is done informally and sometimes ad hoc. It may take place "curbside" in the facility or over the telephone. Such family contact often can be bundled into patient-centered visits for Medicare and Medicaid billing purposes. When a formal face-to-face meeting with family requiring a significant amount of time is indicated, it is helpful to decide whether this can be considered family therapy, and billed to the patient as such, and whether it is best conducted at the facility or at the consultant's office. It is critical for consultants who hope to spend significant amounts of time meeting with families, to understand the insurance coverage policies for family therapy, both with and without the patient present.

Administrative Work

Nursing home administrations may recognize the valuable contribution consulting psychiatrists can make to their facilities' quality of care through program consultation services. Such functions and their importance have been described. While financial support rarely exists for nondirect-patient-care services, enlightened administrators may be able to find funds in their budgets for a limited amount of program consultation. This work can include quality improvement projects, committee work, staff education and/or supervision, community education programs, and milieu development (Sakauye & Camp, 1992).

WHAT IS THE KNOWLEDGE BASE NEEDED FOR NURSING HOME PSYCHIATRIC CONSULTATION?

Psychiatric consultation in the nursing home is a subspecialized area of practice that requires unique expertise. Knowledge of the diagnosis and treatment of mental disorders in nursing home patients is necessary but not sufficient. To be truly effective, consultants must command the professional authority that accrues from demonstrating intimate familiarity with barriers and obstacles nursing home staff members face in providing care to patients with mental disorders. The consultant also must demonstrate facility in developing practical and implementable interventions. Consultants must be prepared to respond to problems in frail patients that may not be readily diagnosed using interventions that may not be evidence-based and they must do this with limited resources on hand while juggling competing regulatory, reimbursement, and caregiver agendas. The knowledge base nursing home consulting psychiatrists need to accomplish this is summarized in Table 19.1.

MANAGING A SUCCESSFUL NURSING HOME PSYCHIATRIC CONSULTATION PRACTICE

Being able to deliver high quality health care in the twenty first century depends upon scrupulous attention to reimbursement. Nowhere is this more necessary than in nursing home consultation-liaison. Typical fee-for-service reimbursement barely covers direct services to patients and does not include explicitly dedicated payment for liaison activities. Consultants should set realistic expectations so that services are sustainable in contemporary fee-for-service and managed care markets.

Outside of funded research or demonstration projects, liaison work may need to be informal and provided selectively, based on urgency, feasibility, and impact. When possible, a supplementary stipend that pays for liaison services should be negotiated. The likelihood of being able to command such a stipend

TABLE 19.1. Core Competencies for Nursing Home Psychiatric Consultation

Neuropsychiatric diagnosis	Dementia, delirium, and depression, and behavioral syndromes such as agitation, wandering, food refusal, screaming, and self injurious behavior.
Geriatric syndromes	Incontinence, falling, sensory impairment, pain, anorexia, weight loss, failure to thrive, frailty. Nursing home psychiatrists should be familiar with geriatric medicine and psychiatry.
Geriatric pharmacology	Pharmacokinetics and pharmacodynamics in the elderly. Safety and tolerability of psychiatric medications in frail patients including drug-drug and drug-illness interactions. Regulations governing drug prescribing and monitoring requirements. Role and function of consultant pharmacists in nursing homes.
Psychosocial aspects of aging	Especially individual, family, and institutional dynamics related to life in long term care facilities. Death and dying. Role of psychiatric consultation in hospice care.
Nonpharmacologic interventions	Consultants should be familiar with the range of nonpharmacologic interventions that may be used in nursing homes, including individual psychotherapy, behavioral interventions, environmental manipulations, reminiscence, validation therapy, and activities-based therapies (Snowden et al., 2003). Familiarity with the rehabilitation therapies including their utilities and limitations in frail patients with mental disorders, is helpful. The clinician should be able to provide indicated interventions or recommend them and monitor or supervise their provision by other clinicians.
Regulations	Nursing home reform provisions of the Omnibus Budget Reconciliation Act (OBRA) of 1987 and subsequent amendments—definition of unnecessary medication, guidelines for use of hypnotics, antianxiety medications, and antipsychotic medications, use of restraints, the Beers criteria, and quality indicators relevant to psychiatry. Consultants should be familiar with the state survey process.
Medical-legal aspects of nursing home care	Sources of liability in the nursing home. Competence assessment and decision-making capacity to consent to or to refuse treatment. Health care proxy or other surrogate provisions.
Reimbursement issues	Medicare Part A nursing home benefits, Medicaid, Medicare Part B physician payment policy, Nursing home managed care products, Medicare prescription drug plan formulary limitations. Medicare, Medicaid, and commercial insurance plan coverage policies for nursing home mental health services, respective claims coding options, and associated documentation requirements.

depends more on regional market forces and nursing home financial health than the clinical skill of the consultant.

To a certain extent, liaison work can be built into patient-centered services. Medicare recognizes psychiatrists' use of the medical evaluation and management codes (American Medical Association, 2005), which include codes for nursing home services. These codes include allowances for coordination of care with other providers and caregivers and counseling patients or their families about their condition in the various levels of service intensity. Formal family meetings to prepare the family better to care for the patient may be covered as family therapy without the patient present. Medicare coverage policies regarding this service vary from carrier to carrier, however, so providers should understand their carrier's policies.

Is a formal contract with a nursing home necessary in order to provide consultation services? Some data suggests that nursing homes prefer contractual relationships with mental health providers, although the presence of contracts does not seem actually to improve facilities' satisfaction with the services (Reichman et al., 1998). Contracts may serve to reassure nursing homes that expectations of the consultant are explicit. Nursing homes may use the existence of contracts as evidence in surveys that they are providing for the mental health care of their residents. There is no legal requirement for a contract in order for providers to provide services or to receive reimbursement for such services.

CONCLUSION

The needs for mental health services in nursing homes are great, and challenges to delivering them formidable, yet the professional rewards are many. To achieve the important goals of nursing home psychiatry and liaison, the practitioner must command a range of skills beyond diagnosis and treatment of late-life mental disorders. Nursing home consulting psychiatrists must understand the nursing home as an institution with a range of clinical, regulatory, administrative, reimbursement, and organizational cultural issues that affect provision of care within its walls. Consultants must be able to overcome a range of facility foibles. This must be done employing specific knowledge of the nursing homes and skills unique to organizational mental health consultation.

REFERENCES

American Geriatrics Society & American Association for Geriatric Psychiatry. (2003). Consensus statement on improving the quality of mental health care in U.S. nursing homes: Management of depression and behavioral symptoms associated with dementia. *Journal of the American Geriatrics Society, 51,* 1287–1298.
American Medical Association. (2005). *CPT 2006.* Chicago: AMA.

Bartels, S. J., Gary, S. M., & Dums, A. R. (2002). Models of mental health services in nursing homes: A review of the literature. *Psychiatric Services, 53,* 1390–1396.

Bienenfeld, D., & Wheeler, B. (1989). Psychiatric services to nursing homes: A liaison model. *Hospital and Community Psychiatry, 40,* 793–794.

Borson, S., Benjamin L., Nininger, J., et al. (1987). Psychiatry and the nursing home. *The American Journal of Psychiatry, 144,* 1412–1418.

Brodaty, H., Brian M. D., Millar, J., et al. (2003). Randomized controlled trial of different models of care for nursing home residents with dementia complicated by depression or psychosis. *The Journal of Clinical Psychiatry, 64,* 63–72.

Caplan, G. (1970). *The theory and practice of mental health consultation.* New York: Basic Books, Inc.

Class, C. A., & Hendrie, H. C. (1995). The role of the psychiatrist in nursing home settings. *Psychiatric Annals, 25,* 449–452.

Conn, D., & Silver, I. (1998). The psychiatrist's role in long-term care. *Canadian Nursing Home, 9,* 22–24.

Leo, R. J., Sherry, C., DiMartino, S., et al. (2002). Psychiatric consultation in the nursing home: Referral patterns and recognition of depression. *Journal of Psychiatric Research, 53,* 783–787.

Lichtenberg, P. A., Smith, M., Frazer, D., et al. (1998). Standards for psychological services in long-term care facilities. *The Gerontologist, 38,* 122–127.

Lobel, J. P., Borson, S., Hyde, T., et al. (1991). Relationships between requests for psychiatric consultations and psychiatric diagnoses in long-term care. *American Journal of Psychiatry, 148,* 898–903.

MacDonald, M. L. (1983). Behavioral consultation in geriatric settings. *The Behavior Therapist, 6,* 172–174.

Moak, G. S., & Borson, S. (2000). Mental health services in long-term care. Still an unmet need. *The American Journal of Geriatric Psychiatry, 8,* 96–100.

Moak, G. S., Borson, S., & Jackson, J. (2000). *The AAGP long term care survey.* Paper presented at the long-term care consensus conference of the American Association for Geriatric Psychiatry in Washington, DC.

Reichman, W. E., Andrew, C. C., Borson, S., et al. (1998). Psychiatric consultation in the nursing home. A survey of six states. *American Journal of Geriatric Psychiatry, 6,* 320–327.

Ryan, J. M., Samuel, W. K., Daiello, L. A., et al. (2002). Psychopharmacologic interventions in nursing homes: What do we know and where should we go? *Psychiatric Services, 53,* 1407–1413.

Sakauye, K. M., & Camp, C. J. (1992). Introducing psychiatric care into nursing homes. *The Gerontologist, 32,* 849–852.

Samter, J., Braun, J. V., Culpepper II, W. J., et al. (1994). Description of a program for psychiatric consultations in the nursing home. *American Journal of Geriatric Psychiatry, 2,* 144–156.

Santmyer, K. (1991). Geropsychiatry in long-term care: A nurse-centered approach. *Journal of the American Geriatrics Society, 39,* 156–159.

Snowden, M., Kersten, S., & Roy-Byrne, P. (2003). Assessment and treatment of nursing home residents with depression or behavioral symptoms associated with dementia: A review of the literature. *Journal of the American Geriatrics Society, 51,* 1305–1317.

Streim, J. E., Elizabeth, W. B., Arapakos, D., et al. (2002). Regulatory oversight, payment policy, and quality improvement in mental health care in nursing homes. *Psychiatric Services, 53,* 1414–1418.

PART III

SOCIETAL INFLUENCES

20

An Overview of Residents, Care Providers, and Regulation of Medical Practice in the Long-Term-Care Continuum

Suzanne M. Gillespie and *Paul R. Katz*

The complexity of care within the long-term-care (LTC) continuum has increased dramatically over the past several years. This reflects not only increased acuity in the context of exceedingly frail LTC residents but also a demanding regulatory environment. Insight into these factors is vital to optimizing the care rendered by practitioners in LTC settings. In addition, a basic understanding of how general medical care is provided in LTC is a necessary foundation to providing complementary psychiatric care. In this vein, this chapter will provide an overview of nursing homes, their residents, and care providers. Current financing of LTC and legislative influences to care will also be described. Finally, recognizing the recent expansion in assisted living facilities providing LTC, this chapter briefly discusses trends in assisted living, their regulations and financing.

AN OVERVIEW OF LONG-TERM-CARE FACILITIES

In the United States, there are currently approximately 1.43 million residents receiving care in 15,850 nursing homes. These nursing homes provide 1.7 million licensed beds and annually complete 2.5 million discharges. Current nursing home occupancy rate is 86%, reflecting a decline over the past decade. Between

1977 and 2004, the number of residents receiving care increased, whereas the total number of nursing facilities declined. This reflected an overall increase in facility size from an average of 79 beds per facility in 1977 to 107 beds per facility (Centers for Disease Control and Prevention/National Center for Health Statistics, 2004).

On any given day, short-stay residents, whose length of stay is less than 30 days following admission, comprise approximately 10% of the nursing home population. Nine and a half percent of elderly nursing home residents have a length of stay between 30 and 90 days. Long-stay residents (those with length of stay of 90 days or more following admission) account for 80% of the nursing home population over the age of 65 years (Kasper & O'Malley, 2007). Among all nursing home residents, 10% have a length of stay that is more than 3 years. Historically, the rate of discharge of residents with length of stay less than 3 months has doubled, increasing from 46 per 100 beds in 1977 to 92 per 100 beds in 1994. In contrast, the rate of discharge of those with lengths of stay greater than 3 months has not changed significantly. This increase in the number of residents with short length of stay coincides with increased Medicare funding of postacute care in nursing homes (Decker, 2005).

Of nursing homes, roughly 65% operate on a for-profit basis; 25% are voluntary not-for-profit and 10% are government-operated facilities. More than half of nursing homes are part of a larger chain of homes (American Health Care Association, 2007). Eighty percent of nursing homes have between 50 and 199 licensed beds, and only 6.2% of homes offer more than 200 beds (Centers for Disease Control and Prevention/National Center for Health Statistics, 2006). Whereas size and proprietary status have been linked to quality of care, the associations have been inconsistent. The majority of admissions to nursing facilities come from acute hospitals (62%), followed by private residence (23%) and other nursing homes (5%). Not surprisingly, assisted living facilities are becoming a rich source of older adults admitted to nursing facilities, accounting for 8.6% of total admissions (Kasper & O'Malley, 2007).

The number of assisted living facilities in the United States has increased dramatically. In the 1990s, it was the most rapidly growing segment of senior housing. Today, an estimated 1 million older adults live in over 32,000 assisted living facilities and nearly a third of older adults identify assisted living as their preferred option for LTC (Assisted Living Federation of America, 2001; Hawes et al., 2005; Nelson & Binette, 2006). In the next 20 years, assisted living is anticipated to grow by as much as 40% (Adler, 1998). The majority of these facilities are corporately owned and operated. In contrast to nursing homes, there is no federal oversight of assisted living facilities; most oversight occurs at the state level. Further, there is significant state-to-state variability in the laws and regulations for assisted living. This lack of standardization makes comparison to nursing homes at a national level problematic. Further, the evidence-based guiding clinical care in assisted living facilities is less developed than in nursing homes. For these reasons, the remainder of this chapter will focus primarily on nursing home issues. Epidemiology and mental health care in assisted living is discussed in-depth in Chapter 22.

AN OVERVIEW OF NURSING HOME RESIDENTS

As the baby-boomer generation ages, many expect the population of older adults with functional and cognitive impairments to rise proportionately translating into an increased need for care in LTC facilities (Katz, 2004). Current estimates are that once a person reaches 65 years of age, their risk of nursing home admission exceeds 40% (Spillman & Lubitz, 2002). Many facilities have been increasing the amount of postacute hospitalization care they provide, often referred to as transitional care or subacute care.

A decline in length of stay in acute hospitals has greatly influenced this trend. Subacute care is comprehensive care designed for someone who has had an acute illness, injury, or exacerbation of a disease process. It is goal-oriented treatment, generally rendered immediately after acute hospitalization, designed to treat active complex medical conditions and provide therapeutic treatments like complex wound care, postsurgical care, and intensive rehabilitation therapies. The goal of most subacute residents is increased functional independence to allow return to community residences. Subacute care is generally more intensive than traditional nursing facility care but less intensive than acute hospital care. Subacute care residents generally have lengths of stay between several days to a few months. Their care requires frequent patient assessment and review of treatments and progress. Patients discharged from subacute care in skilled nursing facilities tend to be older and sicker than those discharged from hospitals (AHCA, 1996). Similarly, subacute residents in the nursing home tend to have higher levels of medical acuity and require more oversight from the interdisciplinary team than long-stay LTC residents. Many such residents enter the nursing home with various stages of delirium and may thus warrant psychiatric intervention. Further, chronic psychiatric illness prevents many residents from successfully transitioning back to the community.

Factors generally influencing admission to a skilled nursing facility are increasing age, low income, poor social supports, and low social activity. Cognitive impairment and functional impairment, especially incontinence, increase the chances of nursing home placement (Katz & Karuza, 2006).

The typical nursing home resident is a white, unmarried woman over the age of 85 with limited social supports and usually widowed (60%; American Association of Homes and Services for the Aging, 2007; Kasper & O'Malley, 2007). Most people admitted to nursing homes are older adults, with average age at admission of 79 years. Only 9% of nursing home residents are under the age of 65 years. Pediatric residents under the age of 15 years account for only 0.02% of the total nursing home population but are the most functionally impaired of nursing home residents. They frequently have mental retardation/developmental disorders with seizures with and without quadriplegia. Coma is prevalent and care commonly includes tube feedings, oxygen therapy, and physical and occupational therapy (Fries et al., 2005). Nonelderly adult persons in nursing homes have a mean age of 50 years at admission and an average length of stay of less than 2 years. Most of these residents are in the final stages of chronic illnesses like cancer or recovering from traumatic injuries. However, many individuals admitted to nursing homes at younger ages have longer lengths of stay. These individuals tend to have diagnoses like cerebral palsy without mental retardation, quadriplegia from trauma, or other rare syndromes or multiple sclerosis. Similarly, those with mental retardation tend to enter at earlier age and stay an average of 11 years (Spector et al., 2000).

Women are nearly three times more likely to reside in nursing homes than men (AAHSA, 2007). Minority groups, like Native Americans, Asian Americans, and Hispanic Americans, are underrepresented in LTC. There has, however, been a recent trend of more African Americans being admitted to skilled nursing facilities. Similarly, those with developmental disabilities are becoming more common in LTC (see Henderson, Chapter 10; Katz & Karuza, 2006).

Today's population of older adults in the nursing home is sicker than the nursing home population of even 5 years ago. Disease prevalence in nursing home residents is high. Over two-thirds of older adults residing long-term in a skilled nursing facility have multiple medical conditions (Kasper & O'Malley, 2007). At admission, 3.9% of nursing facility residents have pressure sores (AHCA, 2007). Nearly 40% of older adults in the nursing home are diagnosed with congestive heart failure and/or ischemic heart disease. Diabetes and stroke are reported in 22% and 26% of new nursing home admissions, respectively (Kasper & O'Malley, 2007). Chronic obstructive pulmonary disease, hypertension, arthritis, and hip fractures are also prevalent health conditions of nursing home residents (Katz & Karuza, 2006; Kasper & O'Malley, 2007).

Though approximately 25% of older adults residing in nursing homes are diagnosed with dementia, experts postulate that over 50% of nursing home residents meet the diagnostic criteria for dementia (Kasper & O'Malley, 2007; see Gruber-Baldini, et al., Chapter 1). Depression is diagnosed in 20% to 25% of residents (Ryan et al., 2002). Thirty-nine percent of nursing home residents over the age of 65 years are diagnosed with both medical and psychiatric conditions, reflecting a 60% increase in prevalence of comorbid physical and mental diagnoses in this population, when compared with 1999 data (Kasper & O'Malley, 2007). In addition, behavioral issues, such as verbal and social inappropriateness, wandering, and resistance to care, are observed in one-third of nursing home residents (Ryan et al., 2002).

Functional disability is also prevalent in today's nursing home residents. More than half of long-stay LTC nursing home residents require supervision or hand-on assistance from another person in five activities of daily living (eating, dressing, bathing, transferring, and using the toilet room; Kasper & O'Malley, 2007). Cumulative disability is high, with about 75% of nursing home residents requiring assistance in three or more activities of daily living (Katz & Karuza, 2006). Assistance with bathing and dressing is needed by three-fourths of residents. Many residents require a mechanically altered diet consistency and 52% of residents are totally dependent for eating (AHCA, 2007). Difficulty with bladder and or bowel control is reported in nearly 60% of newly admitted and 40% of long-stay nursing home residents over the age of 65 years. Only 59% of elderly long-stay residents are ambulatory, and few (18%) walk independently of assistance or supervision (Kasper & O'Malley, 2007).

AN OVERVIEW OF NURSING HOME CARE PROVIDERS

Physician responsibilities in nursing home care are presented in Table 20.1 (Katz & Karuza, 2006). Medical care in nursing homes is provided in both open

TABLE 20.1. The Physician's Responsibilities in the Nursing Home

Comprehensive admission assessment, including history and physical examination, and review of available medical records

Development of a plan of care in concert with interdisciplinary team members, the resident, and the family that is consistent with the resident's needs and goals

Periodic monitoring of chronic health problems at an appropriate interval, using diagnostic testing, consultation, and pharmacologic and nonpharmacologic interventions as warranted

Prompt and thorough assessment of acute medical problems or change in function, instituting change in the medical treatment plan as indicated

Communication with interdisciplinary team members, the resident, and the family concerning new diagnoses and treatment plans

Periodic review, in concert with the consultant pharmacist, of all medication with regard to ongoing need, adverse effects, and appropriate laboratory monitoring and potential interactions

Optimization of quality of life and function, with special attention to cognition, mobility, falls, skin integrity, nutrition, and continence

Determination of each resident's decision-making capacity and assistance in establishing advance directives

Physical attendance to each resident, with documentation in the medical record in accordance with all state and federal guidelines

Source: Adapted from Katz and Karuza (2006).

and closed models. In the closed model, a facility has medical staff who assume care of residents when they are admitted to the facility. Although closed staffing models are thought to better integrate physicians into the interdisciplinary team and thereby improve the quality of care, further research is needed in this area. The typical nursing home physician is an internist or family medicine physician. Although contemporary data is lacking, older surveys noted that physicians average only 2 h per week in nursing home practice. This would translate into fewer than 20 min per nursing home resident per month. In fact, it appears to be a small minority of physicians that dedicate a significant part of their work time to nursing home care (Katz et al., 1997). Some physicians whose practices are based in skilled nursing facilities are academically trained in geriatric medicine. However, an ongoing workforce shortage of fellowship-trained geriatricians and geriatric psychiatrists has meant that many physicians who practice in skilled nursing facilities have little formal training in LTC. Experts have estimated that the American health-care system will need approximately 36,000 geriatricians by the year 2030. With a current workforce of 7128 certified geriatricians and 1596 certified geriatric psychiatrists and annual graduation rates from fellowship training of approximately 300 and 85 geriatricians and geriatric psychiatrists, respectively, it is unlikely that this goal will be met (Association of Directors of Geriatric Academic Programs, 2007). Thus, the majority of care provided in LTC settings will be through primary care internists and family physicians. Significant shortage of geriatrics specialty-trained nurses has also been reported (Kovner et al., 2002).

Physician assistants and nurse practitioners commonly provide care in nursing homes. These midlevel providers, working with physicians, have been shown to improve resident satisfaction with care and decrease hospitalization rates. Additional research into the advantages and disadvantages of different collaborative patterns of care between physicians and nurse practitioners or physician's assistants is needed.

Patient care and evaluation in the nursing home is largely dependent on nurses and nurse assistants. Nursing facilities are required to provide nurse staffing sufficient to provide the care outlined in its care plans. According to federal guidelines, every nursing home must staff a licensed nurse that acts as charge nurse on each shift, a registered nurse who is on duty at least eight consecutive hours, 7 days a week, and a registered nurse who is designated as the director of nursing. Though recommendations for minimum and optimal staffing at nursing facilities have been made by the Centers for Medicare and Medicaid Services (CMS) based on links to quality of care, current federal regulations do not mandate specific nurse to resident staffing ratios (Harrington & Millman, 2001; Omnibus Budget Reconciliation Act [OBRA] of 1987). However, states may set staffing requirements for nursing facilities, which are often set higher than federal recommendations. Federal guidelines set minimum educational training for nurse aides at 75 h (Harrington & Millman, 2001).

The American Health Care Association (AHCA) reports that 2007 total direct care staffing averages 3.4 h per resident day (HPRD) or roughly 204 min per resident per day. Nurse assistants contribute most direct staff time, at 2.3 HPRD. Licensed nurses and registered nurses contribute 0.8 and 0.3 HPRD, respectively. Despite increasing medical acuity and care needs of nursing home residents, staffs ratios have been relatively stable (AHCA, 2007). It has been estimated that 9 out of 10 nursing homes are inadequately staffed and nearly 8 billion dollars would be needed to bring staffing to adequate levels (ILC-USA Anti-Ageism Task Force, 2006). Staffing issues are critical in that almost all treatment decisions are operationalized through nursing. Timely and accurate assessment of patient needs, efficient communication with physicians, and the translation of physician orders into treatment at the bedside are all very much dependent on nursing availability and acumen. Thus, declines in the quantity and/or quality of nursing staff have direct impacts on physician performance and ultimately on patient care (Katz, 2004).

Turnover of staff nurses represents a significant challenge to nursing home care. A recent national study revealed turnover rates of over 70% for nurse assistants and over 50% each for directors of nursing, staff registered nurses, and licensed practical nurses (Decker et al., 2003). Staff turnover and job vacancies have been associated with resident hospitalization. Organizational culture of a facility may be influential to retaining staff (Katz & Karuza, 2006). Finally, since job vacancies are often filled by short-term staff unfamiliar with residents, variability in care is commonplace.

As alluded to above, medical and nurse staffing in nursing facilities has numerous impacts on psychiatric care. Staffing ratios in skilled nursing facilities are at significantly lower levels than those of acute hospitals. One-to-one caregivers to resident ratios are generally only feasible in emergent or time-limited situations. As primary medical providers are often only physically present in facilities a few hours a week, communication regarding psychiatric and behavioral issues generally occurs through telephone and written means. Therefore, staff skill, experience, and education in psychiatric assessment are invaluable. Moreover, routine medical visits occur on a schedule of every 30 days for the first 90 days following admission and then every 60 days thereafter. Practitioners often rely upon nursing and ancillary staff to identify significant changes in resident condition during the intervals between medical visits and inform them accordingly. This can present a significant challenge, given the frailty of nursing home residents and workforce constraints.

AN OVERVIEW OF NURSING HOME FINANCING

In 2007, the average cost of a private room in a nursing home was $213 per day or $77,745 annually (MetLife Mature Market Institute, 2007). Overall,

Americans spend more than 90 billion dollars per year on nursing home care. Public health programs primarily finance this cost; Medicaid and Medicare account for 65% and 14% of nursing home care payments, respectively. With the high annual costs, those paying for nursing home care out of pocket often deplete their personal funds and turn to public funding. Although purchase of LTC insurance has become increasingly common, at present these policies pay for only a small fraction of nursing home care (Harrington & Millman, 2001). In comparison, assisted living facility base rate averages $2969 per month or $35,628 yearly. Additional care in assisted living settings, like specialized dementia care, generally has additional fees. Nationally, supplemental costs for dementia care services in assisted living average an additional $1110 per month (MetLife Market Research Institute, 2007). Although Medicaid funding has been increasing, most assisted living facility residents pay privately for their care; however, with only approximately 10% of assisted living residents receiving Medicaid support for services, Medicaid financing of assisted living remains minimal relative to its financing of nursing home care (United States Administration on Aging, 2003).

Medicare funding for nursing home costs occurs for certain limited conditions for beneficiaries who require skilled nursing or rehabilitation services. In general, to be covered, beneficiaries must receive services from a Medicare-certified skilled nursing home following a qualifying hospital stay. A qualifying hospital stay is usually a hospital stay of at least 3 days prior to entering a nursing home. Medicare covers only those skilled nursing facility services rendered to help a beneficiary recover from an acute illness or injury. Medicare pays for skilled care in full for the first 20 days in a skilled nursing facility. For days 21 to 100, a co-payment from the resident may be required for skilled nursing facility services. Beyond 100 days, Medicare does not cover skilled nursing facility care (Centers for Medicare and Medicaid Services, 2007). As part of the Balanced Budget Act of 1997, Medicare payments to nursing homes are based on an individual's functional needs and potential for rehabilitation. This prospective payment system, also called PPS, requires careful documentation of functional gains, particularly by rehabilitation therapists. Supplemental increases in reimbursement are made to offset costs of caring for those with HIV/AIDS. Despite the high cost of nursing home care, resources remain constrained. In general, psychiatric conditions are undervalued with respect to reimbursement in LTC. Residents with active psychiatric illness often require increased care and staff time, but mechanisms do not exist for increased reimbursement for those efforts. Shortage of psychiatric specialists trained in nursing home care, combined with relatively low reimbursement rates for care in nursing homes, adds to the challenge of providing optimal mental health care in this setting.

OVERVIEW OF LEGISLATION INFLUENCING CARE
IN THE NURSING HOME

In 1983, the Institute of Medicine published a report documenting significant deficiencies in the care of nursing home residents. The findings of that report influenced the passage of the OBRA in 1987. As the first major revision of nursing home legislation in over 20 years and the first detailed source of clinical expectations for nursing home care, OBRA has had significant impacts on medical care in nursing homes. OBRA set new, higher standards for quality of care provided in nursing facilities certified for reimbursement under Medicare and Medicaid (which includes most skilled nursing facilities) by the CMS. CMS is an agency of the Department of Health and Human Services and is responsible for managing federal health-care programs like Medicare. CMS pays Medicare claims and interprets legislation into written regulations for skilled nursing facilities. Medicaid is a joint federal and state program. CMS interprets federal statues and also writes regulations for Medicaid that are administered by each state's Medicaid program. Federal regulations, including those pertaining to LTC, are compiled in the *Code of Federal Regulations*. Each federal regulation is given a tag number; often called "F-tags." In order to qualify for federal reimbursement under Medicare and Medicaid, facilities must comply with these CMS regulations. OBRA regulations targeted many residents' rights issues, including setting limits on restraint use and regulating the use of psychoactive medications. As noted earlier, assisted living facilities do not operate under such all-inclusive mandates, which some observers believe contributes to significant variability of care practices and quality of care (Zimmerman et al., 2005).

OBRA also mandates comprehensive periodic assessments of all nursing home residents. This is accomplished by the Minimum Data Set (MDS), which surveys a host of clinical issues that are felt to directly relate to the quality of resident care and thus pertinent to effective care planning. A resident's medical regimen must be consistent with the assessment compiled in the MDS. CMS also uses the MDS datasets for individual facilities to compile nursing facility quality measures data, which it reports publicly on its Web site. Measures include outcomes data like prevalence of pain, pressure ulcers, weight loss, and depression as well as rates of vaccination, restraint use, and urinary tract infection. Although publication of these measures is intended to offer a route by which to compare facilities, it has been criticized for lack of standardization of data to account for the substantial variability in disability and medical acuity between different facilities. Quality measures for nursing homes that are publicly reported by CMS are presented in Table 20.2.

Adherence to regulations is assessed by mandatory site-visit surveys. These surveys are mandated every 15 months but occur on average every 12 months.

TABLE 20.2. Quality Measures for Nursing Homes Based on the Minimum Data Set and Publicly Reported by Center for Medicare and Medicaid Services

QUALITY MEASURES	TIME FRAME FOR MDS OBSERVATION*
For long-stay residents	
Percent of long-stay residents given influenza vaccination during the flu season	October 1–March 31
Percent of long-stay residents who were assessed and given pneumococcal vaccination	5 years
Percent of long-stay residents whose need for help with daily activities has increased	7 days
Percent of long-stay residents who have moderate-to-severe pain	7 days
Percent of high-risk long-stay residents who have pressure sores	7 days
Percent of low-risk long-stay residents who have pressure sores	7 days
Percent of long-stay residents who were physically restrained	7 days
Percent of long-stay residents who are more depressed or anxious	30 days
Percent of low-risk long-stay residents who lose control of their bowels or bladder	14 days
Percent of long-stay residents who have/had a catheter inserted and left in their bladder	14 days
Percent of long-stay residents who spent most of their time in bed or in a chair	7 days
Percent of long-stay residents whose ability to move about in and around their room got worse	7 days
Percent of long-stay residents with a urinary tract infection	30 days
Percent of long-stay residents who lose too much weight	30 days
For short-stay residents	
Percent of short-stay residents given influenza vaccination during the flu season	October 1–March 31
Percent of short-stay residents who were assessed and given pneumococcal vaccination	5 years
Percent of short-stay residents with delirium	7 days
Percent of short-stay residents who had moderate-to-severe pain	7 days
Percent of short-stay residents with pressure sores	7 days

Source: Adapted from Department of Health and Human Services, Medicare (2008)
*If multiple MDS items, with different time frames of observation, are used to calculate the quality measure, the longest observation period is presented.

During survey, facility procedures and records are reviewed and quality of care and of life for residents is observed. Failure to meet regulatory standard for care is cited in "a deficiency." Penalties imposed for deficiencies are dependent on the nature and severity of the deficiency and can range from implementation of a corrective action plan to monetary fines, limits on facility admissions, or even facility closure. Inspections may also occur at any time in between mandated surveys as a result of a complaint received by the state. In the years since OBRA was instituted, restraint use in nursing homes decreased significantly, registered nurse staffing increased, and training requirements for certified nursing assistants were established (Wiener et al., 2007).

OBRA mandates that each individual in a nursing facility receive and be provided the necessary care and services to achieve and maintain "the highest practicable physical, medical and psychological well-being" that is obtainable. The facility must ensure that the resident optimally improves or deteriorates only within the limits of that resident's right to refuse treatments and the influence of their illnesses and normal aging. When a resident declines (or fails to improve), a survey team may investigate whether the decline was avoidable. A decline may be determined unavoidable if the resident has been given a careful and thorough assessment and that assessment informs the creation of the resident's care plan. The interventions included in the care plan should be evaluated and revised as necessary.

OBRA requires that a state agency must screen and preapprove the admission of individuals with mental retardation or serious mental illness prior to a nursing facility (F285). This screening is done to ensure that the facility can provide appropriate programs and services to meet the individual's needs. Residents readmitted to a nursing facility from a hospital, or those admitted from a hospital with an anticipated stay of less than 30 days who require treatment at the nursing facility for the same problem for which they were hospitalized, are exempt from screening.

Facilities are required to designate a medical director (F501). Medical directors take on responsibility for implementation of resident care policies and coordination of medical care within a facility. Resident care policies include admission policies, infection control policies, physician practice, and privileges. They oversee the implementation of clinical policies and procedures from the interdisciplinary team. Medical directors oversee ongoing quality improvement initiatives, generally targeting improvements in quality of care. They also oversee attending physicians' adherence to regulations and policies. Record review and rounds allows the medical directors to oversee quality of care provided by monitoring irregularities in care and prescribing practice. Many medical directors have received certification as medical directors and designation as a "CMD" by participation in training programs of the American Medical Director's Association.

Additional regulations require medication review at regular intervals and that each resident's medication regimen includes no unnecessary drugs. Clinical documentation must demonstrate the indication for all drugs, especially psychoactive medications. Unnecessary drugs are those given without indication, at excessive doses, for excessive duration, without adequate monitoring or in setting of significant adverse reaction. Residents without a history of antipsychotic drug use should not be given them unless the medication(s) is/are required to treat a specific diagnosed condition that is documented in the medical record. Those residents receiving psychoactive medications are mandated to receive gradual dose reductions and behavioral interventions, unless a clinical contraindication exists and is documented in the medical record. To date, the impact on quality of care from these guidelines has not been well described in the clinical research literature.

A monthly medication regimen review, comprising a thorough evaluation of medication regimens by a pharmacist, is also required. This review is intended to minimize adverse consequences and unnecessary medication use and ensure proper medication monitoring. A facility must ensure that the medication error rate is less than 5% and that no significant medication errors occur. No errors should occur that cause a resident discomfort or jeopardizes their health and safety.

Again, absent regulations like those that guide care in nursing homes, care in assisted living facilities often resembles care given in other outpatient venues, including traditional primary care practices. A brief summary of selected regulations influencing medical and psychiatric care in the skilled nursing facility is presented in Table 20.3.

TABLE 20.3. Brief Summary of Selected Medicare and Medicaid Requirements for Long-Term-Care Facilities

TAG NUMBER	SUBJECT	REGULATION	GUIDELINE
F285	Preadmission screening for mental illness or retardation	CFR483.20 (m)	A state agency must screen and approve the admission to a nursing facility of anyone with mental retardation or serious mental illness and ensure that a facility can provide the appropriate programs and services to meet the individual's needs.

Continued

TABLE 20.3. Continued

TAG NUMBER	SUBJECT	REGULATION	GUIDELINE
F309	Quality of care	CFR483.25	Each resident must receive and the facility must provide the necessary care and services to attain or maintain the highest practicable physical, mental, and psychological well-being, in accordance with the comprehensive assessment and plan of care. "Highest practicable" is defined as the highest level of functioning and well-being possible, limited only by the individual's presenting functional status and potential for improvement or reduced rate of functional decline.
F319–320	Quality of care: mental and psychosocial functioning	CFR483.25(f)	Based on the comprehensive assessment of a resident, a facility must ensure that a resident who displays mental of psychosocial adjustment difficulty receives appropriate treatment and services to correct the assessed problem and a resident whose assessment did not display a pattern of decreased social interaction and/ or withdrawn, angry, or depressive behaviors, unless that residents' clinical condition demonstrates that such a pattern is unavoidable.
F329–331	Medications, appropriate and unnecessary	CFR483.25(I)(1)	Residents' drug regimens must be free from unnecessary drugs. These are defined as "those given without indication, at excessive doses, for excessive duration, without adequate monitoring or in setting of significant adverse reaction."
F385–386	Physician services	CFR483.40	It is the attending physician's responsibility to participate in the resident's assessment and care planning, monitoring changes in the resident's medical status and providing consultation or treatment when called by the facility. At scheduled visits, physician must review the total plan of care, write sign and date a progress note, and sign and date all orders.

Continued

TABLE 20.3. Continued

TAG NUMBER	SUBJECT	REGULATION	GUIDELINE
F428–430	Medications, drug regimen review	CFR483.60(c)	The drug regimen of each resident must be reviewed at least once a month by a pharmacist. The pharmacist must report irregularities to the attending physician and director of nursing, and reports must be acted upon.
F501	Medical director, required duties	CFR483.75(i)	Each facility must designate a physician to serve as medical director. The medical director is responsible for implementation of resident care policies and the coordination of care in the facility.

Source: Adapted with permission from the American Medical Director's Association (2005).

SUMMARY

Nursing homes and assisted living facilities provide much needed care to an increasingly frail and functionally dependent population. Shortages of nurses and physicians with an expertise in LTC exist. Assuring quality in such settings demands not only a competent and committed workforce but also a knowledge of and sensitivity to the regulatory environment that influences care planning. Diagnosing and treating residents with psychiatric illness in today's nursing homes is challenging, but the potential benefits are immeasurable.

REFERENCES

Adler, S. (1998, August). Get ready for consolidation: Today's product in the pipeline will build tomorrow's big players. *Contemporary Long Term Care, 21*(8), 39–45.

American Association of Homes and Services for the Aging. (2007). *Aging services: The facts.* Retrieved December 22, 2007, Retrieved December 22, 2007, from http://www.aahsa.org/aging_services/default.asp

American Health Care Association. (2007, June). *CMS OSCAR data current surveys, June 2007.* Retrieved December 22, 2007, Retrieved December 22, 2007, from http://www.ahcancal.org/research_data/Pages/default.aspx

American Health Care Association. (1996). *Nursing facility sub-acute care: The quality and cost-effective alternative to hospital care, 1996.* Retrieved January 25, 2008, from http://www.rai.to/subacute.htm

American Medical Director's Association. (2005, November). *Physician responsibilities and guidelines under OBRA '87.* Retrieved December 28, 2007, from http://www.amda.com

Assisted Living Federation of America. (2001). *ALFA's overview of the assisted living industry*. Fairfax, VA: Author.

Association of Directors of Geriatric Academic Programs. (2007, October). *The status of Geriatrics Workforce Study: Training and practice update*. 5(2). Retrieved January 2, 2008, from http://www.americangeriatrics.org/adgap.

Centers for Disease Control and Prevention/National Center for Health Statistics. (2006). *The National Nursing Home Survey: Trends in nursing homes: Trends, from 1973–2004*. Retrieved January 9, 2008, http://www.cdc.gov/nchs/data/nnhsd/nursinghomes1973–2004.pdf

Centers for Disease Control and Prevention/National Center for Health Statistics. *The National Nursing Home Survey (2006, December). 2004 Facility tables: Characteristics staffing & management, table 1*. Retrieved November 5, 2008, from http://www.cdc.gov/nchs/data/nnhsd/nursinghome2006.pdf#01

Centers for Medicare and Medicaid Services. (2007). Medicare coverage of skilled nursing facility care. (CMS Publication No. 10153). Baltimore, MD.

Decker, F. H. (2005) Nursing homes, 1977–1999: What has changed, what has not? Hyattsville, MD: U.S. Department of Health and Human Services, National Center for Health Statistics, Centers for Disease Control. Retrieved January 2, 2008, http://www.cdc.gov/nchs/data/nnhsd/nursinghomes1977_99.pdf

Decker, F. H., Gruhn, P., Matthews Martin, L., et al. (2003). *Results of the 2002 AHCA survey of nursing home staff vacancy and turnover in nursing homes. Health services research and evaluation: American Health Care Association*. Retrieved January 2, 2008, from www.ahcancal.org/research_data/staffing documents/vacancy_turnover_survey2002.pdf (pp. 133–150).

Fries, B. E., Wodchis, W. P., Blaum, C., et al. (2005). A national study showed that diagnoses varied by age group in nursing home residents under age 65. *Journal of Clinical Epidemiology, 58*, 198–205.

Harrington, C., & Millman, M. (2001). *Nursing home staffing standards in state statutes and regulations*. Report prepared for the Henry J. Kaiser Family Foundation, San Francisco. San Francisco, CA: University of California. Retrieved December 28, 2007, from http://www.kff.org

Hawes, C., Phillips, C. D., Holan, S., et al. (2005). Assisted living in rural America: Results from a national survey. *Journal of Rural Health, 21*(2), 131–139.

ILC-USA Anti-Ageism Task Force; Butler R. N., Kim, K., Curran, M. et al. (2006). *Ageism in America*. International Longevity Center—U.S.A. Ltd. New York. Retrieved January 2, 2008, from http://www.ilcusa.org

Katz, P. R. (2004) Chapter 8: Physician practice in long-term care: Workforce shortages and implications for the future. In P. R. Katz, M. D. Mezey, & M. B. Kapp (Eds.), *Vulnerable populations in the long term care continuum*, (pp. 133–150) New York: Springer.

Katz, P. R., & Karuza, J. (2006) Chapter 16: Nursing-home care. In P. Pompei & J. B. Murphy (Eds.), *Geriatric review syllabus: A core curriculum in geriatric medicine* (6th ed pp. 119–125). New York: American Geriatrics Society.

Katz, P. R., Karuza, J., Kolassa, J., et al. (1997). Medical practice with nursing home residents: Results from the National Physician Professional Practice Activities Census. *Journal of the American Geriatrics Society, 45*, 911–917.

Kasper, J., & O'Malley, M. (2007). *Changes in characteristics, needs and payment for care of elderly nursing home residents: 1999 to 2004*. Report prepared for the Henry J. Kaiser Family Foundation, Washington, DC. Retrieved December 28, 2007, from http://www.kff.org

Kovner, C. T., Mezey, M., & Harrington, C. (2002). Who cares for older adults? Workforce implications of an aging society. *Health Affairs, 21*(3), 78–89.

MetLife Mature Market Institute. (2007) The MetLife market survey of nursing home and assisted living costs. Westport, CT: Author. Retrieved December 28, 2007, http://www.MatureMarketInstitute.com

Nelson, B. M., & Binette, J. (2006). *2005 Missouri member survey on long-term care, assisted living, and Medicaid.* Washington, DC: AARP.

Omnibus Budget Reconciliation Act of 1987, Pub. L. No. 100–203, Subtitle C: Nursing home reform (1987).

Ryan, J. M., Kidder, S. W., Dainello, L. A., & Tariot, P. N. (2002). Mental health services in nursing homes: Psychopharmacologic interventions in nursing homes: What do we know and where should we go? *Psychiatric Services, 53,* 1407–1413.

Spector, W., Fleishman, J., Pezzin, L., et al. (2000). The characteristics of long-term care users. Agency for Healthcare Research and Quality, US DHHS Publication no. 00–0049.

Spillman, B. C., & Lubitz, J. (2002). New estimates of lifetime nursing home use: Have patterns of use changed? *Medical Care, 40,* 965–975.

United States Administration on Aging. (2003, November) *Aging internet information notes: Assisted living.* Retrieved January 6, 2008, http://www.aoa.gov/prof/notes/notes_assisted_living.asp

Wiener, J. M., Freiman, M. P., & Brown, D. (2007). *Nursing home care quality: Twenty years after the Omnibus Budget Reconciliation Act of 1987.* Report prepared for the Henry J. Kaiser Family Foundation, Menlo Park, CA. Retrieved January 18, 2008, from http://www.kff.org

Zimmerman, S., Sloane, P. D., Eckert, J. K., et al. (2005, July). How good is assisted living? Findings and implications from an outcomes study. *Journals of Gerontology Series B-Psychological Sciences & Social Sciences, 60*(4), 195–204.

21

Ethical and Medicolegal Issues

Marshall B. Kapp

MENTAL HEALTH NEEDS OF THE NURSING HOME POPULATION

A substantial proportion of the current nursing home residents in the United States need mental health services for cognitive and emotional problems. Late-stage dementia, clinical depression, and other serious, chronic psychiatric illnesses are prevalent in the nursing home population (Yaffe et al., 2002), especially as all but the most severely disabled individuals of all ages (U.S. Department of Health and Human Services, 2001a) increasingly enjoy the availability of a growing array of home- and community-based long-term-care alternatives. In addition, states are under legal and political pressure to move and keep people out of nursing homes for as long as possible (Kapp, 2005). Under both the Americans with Disabilities Act (ADA), 42 U.S.C. §§ 12101–12213, and the Rehabilitation Act, 29 U.S.C. § 794, a nursing home may not deny admission or services to any individual on account of that person's mental disability unless the facility can prove it is unable to properly accommodate that person (Wagner v. Fair Acres Geriatric Center, 1995). The majority of dementia-related deaths still occur in nursing homes (Mitchell et al., 2005), and this is likely to continue (Spillman & Lubitz, 2002) as many clinicians believe nursing homes are the most appropriate setting for older adults with severe mental illness (Bartels

465

et al., 2003). Increasingly, assisted living facilities today also care for many individuals with advanced dementia (Gaddy, 2000).

ASSESSMENT AND TREATMENT REQUIREMENTS

The Regulatory Environment

In recognition of the extensive mental health needs of nursing home residents, Congress included special provisions addressing this concern as part of its massive overhaul of nursing home regulation, the Nursing Home Quality Reform Act, embedded in the Omnibus Budget Reconciliation Act (OBRA) of 1987, Public Law No. 100–203, codified at 42 U.S.C. §§ 1395i-3(a)-(h) and 1396r(a)-(h). The Nursing Home Quality Reform Act contains many of the legislative recommendations made in a 1986 Institute of Medicine report (Institute of Medicine, 1986) that Congress had directed the Department of Health and Human Services (DHHS) to commission. Relevant statutory amendments have been added in several subsequent OBRAs.

Assessment Requirements

OBRA 1987, as implemented by regulations promulgated by DHHS, requires at 42 C.F.R. § 483.20 the following:

(1) The facility must develop a comprehensive care plan for each resident that includes measurable objectives and timetables to meet a resident's medical, nursing, and mental and psychosocial needs that are identified in the comprehensive assessment [that must be created for each resident at the time of admission and reviewed at least quarterly thereafter]. The care plan must describe the following—
   (i) The services that are to be furnished to attain or maintain the resident's highest practicable physical, mental, and psychosocial well-being ...
(1) A nursing facility must not admit, on or after January 1, 1989, any new resident with—
   (i) mental illness, unless the state mental health authority has determined, based on an independent physical and mental evaluation performed by a person or entity other than the state mental health authority, prior to admission,
      (A) that, because of the physical and mental condition of the individual, the individual requires the level of services provided by a nursing facility; and
      (B) if the individual requires such level of services, whether the individual requires specialized services; or
   (ii) mental retardation, unless the state mental retardation or developmental disability authority has determined prior to admission—
      (A) that, because of the physical and mental condition of the individual, the individual requires the level of services provided by a nursing facility; and
      (B) if the individual requires such level of services, whether the individual requires specialized services for mental retardation.

As originally enacted, OBRA 1987's mental illness preadmission screening provision also required annual resident reviews, and consequently this provision was popularly known as PASARR. The obligatory annual review component was repealed by Congress in OBRA 1996, Public Law No. 104–315, and replaced with a requirement to screen when "there is a significant change in physical or mental condition"; hence, the acronym PASRR is the one commonly used currently. The OBRA 1987 legislation was intended to prevent inappropriate placement and warehousing of persons with mental disabilities in Medicaid (Title 19)-certified nursing facilities. The definition of mental illness used in this context is contained in 42 C.F.R. § 483.102 and is displayed in Table 21.1.

An applicant who is found in a Level I screening not to need nursing facility services—i.e., health-related services above the level of room and board that can only be provided in an institutional setting—may not be admitted to a Medicaid

---

TABLE 21.1. Regulatory Definition of Mental Illness

(a) This subpart applies to the screening or reviewing of all individuals with mental illness or mental retardation who apply to or reside in Medicaid-certified NFs regardless of the source of payment for the NF services, and regardless of the individual's or resident's known diagnoses.

(b) Definitions. As used in this subpart—

  (1) An individual is considered to have a serious mental illness (MI) if the individual meets the following requirements on diagnosis, level of impairment and duration of illness:

    (i) Diagnosis. The individual has a major mental disorder diagnosable under the Diagnostic and Statistical Manual of Mental Disorders, 3rd edition, revised in 1987.

      This mental disorder is—

      (A) A schizophrenic, mood, paranoid, panic or other severe anxiety disorder; somatoform disorder; personality disorder; other psychotic disorder; or another mental disorder that may lead to a chronic disability; but

      (B) Not a primary diagnosis of dementia, including Alzheimer's disease or a related disorder, or a non-primary diagnosis of dementia unless the primary diagnosis is a major mental disorder...

    (ii) Level of impairment. The disorder results in functional limitations in major life activities within the past 3 to 6 months that would be appropriate for the individual's developmental stage. An individual typically has at least one of the following characteristics on a continuing or intermittent basis:

      (A) Interpersonal functioning. The individual has serious difficulty interacting appropriately and communicating effectively with other persons, has a possible history of altercations, evictions, firing, fear of strangers, avoidance of interpersonal relations and social isolation;

Continued

TABLE 21.1. Continued

(B) Concentration, persistence and pace. The individual has serious difficulty in sustaining focused attention for a long enough period to permit the completion of tasks commonly found in work settings or in work-like structured activities occurring in school or home settings, manifests difficulties in concentration, inability to complete simple tasks within an established time period, makes frequent errors, or requires assistance in the completion of these tasks, and

(C) Adaptation to change. The individual has serious difficulty in adapting to typical changes in circumstances associated with work, school, family, or social interaction, manifests agitation, exacerbated signs and symptoms associated with the illness, or withdrawal from the situation, or requires intervention by the mental health or judicial system.

(iii) Recent treatment. The treatment history indicates that the individual has experienced at least one of the following:

(A) Psychiatric treatment more intensive than outresident care more than once in the past 2 years (e.g., partial hospitalization or inresident hospitalization) or

(B) Within the last 2 years, due to the mental disorder, experienced an episode of significant disruption to the normal living situation, for which supportive services were required to maintain functioning at home, or in a residential treatment environment, or which resulted in intervention by housing or law enforcement officials.

Source: 42 C.F.R. § 483.102

certified nursing home under any conditions. Applicants needing nursing facility services who additionally need specialized services, as determined in a Level II screening, may be admitted, but the state must then ensure that the specialized services are provided (Linkins et al., 2001). Level I screening concerns the person's need for nursing home services. If the answer to that question is yes, then Level II looks at whether that person needing nursing home services also needs specialized mental health or retardation services.

Treatment Requirements

In large part because of pressure on nursing homes to admit residents quickly from acute care hospitals, the screening process often is truncated, most notably usually dispensing with psychiatric consultation even when it is clinically indicated for seriously demented and depressed individuals (Borson et al., 1997). In addition, shortages in available community mental health expertise plus the costliness of providing mental health services frequently mean that, instead of the legally required specialized services, difficult behavioral problems in the nursing home are treated, by default, by underprepared primary care physicians (Banazak & Glettler, 2000; Snowden et al., 1998).

Compliance with the mental illness assessment requirements imposed by federal law is the responsibility of the public agency designated by each state as its mental health authority, as is providing any specialized services needed by admitted residents, 42 C.F.R. §§ 483.112, 483.130(n). The state's duties apply regardless of the nursing home resident's age (U.S. Department of Health and Human Services, 2001b). Under 42 C.F.R. § 483.120

(a) Definition—
  1. For mental illness, specialized services means the services specified by the state which, combined with services provided by the NF, results (sic) in the continuous and aggressive implementation of an individualized plan of care that—
     (i) Is developed and supervised by an interdisciplinary team, which includes a physician, qualified mental health professionals and, as appropriate, other professionals.
     (ii) Prescribes specific therapies and activities for the treatment of persons experiencing an acute episode of serious mental illness, which necessitates supervision by trained mental health personnel; and
     (iii) Is directed toward diagnosing and reducing the resident's behavioral symptoms that necessitated institutionalization, improving his or her level of independent functioning, and achieving a functioning level that permits reduction in the intensity of mental health services to below the level of specialized services at the earliest possible time.

The state may directly provide, or arrange for the delivery of, appropriate specialized services anywhere within or outside of the nursing facility, in another institution, or in a community setting.

Moreover, 42 C.F.R. § 483.120(c) provides, "The NF must provide mental health or mental retardation services which are of lesser intensity than specialized services to all residents who need such services." These services are less intensive and frequent than those the state must provide and may include, e.g., group or individual counseling, family therapy, and regular companionship. "The treatment of mental illness in the nursing home often falls by default to the primary care physician" (Banazak & Glettler, 2000), although much of the hands on, everyday care is provided by other personnel within the facility (Beck et al., 2002).

Besides federal statutes and regulations that nursing facilities are obliged to comply with as a condition of participation in the Medicaid program, nursing facilities also are covered (as alluded to earlier) by the ADA and the Rehabilitation Act. In addition, the services delivered to nursing home residents are governed by state professional and institutional licensure statutes and regulations, standards of private accrediting bodies such as the Joint Commission on Accreditation of Healthcare Organizations (JCAHO), state elder abuse and neglect laws, and the threat of private civil litigation initiated by or on behalf of individual residents claiming professional malpractice.

CLINICAL PRACTICE GUIDELINES

Besides being aware of their regulatory obligations regarding the mental health assessment and treatment of residents, nursing facility providers also should be guided in this arena by knowledge of pertinent clinical practice guidelines or parameters. For instance, the American Medical Directors Association has published clinical practice guidelines regarding the assessment and treatment of depression (2003), dementia (2005), and altered mental states (1998) in nursing facilities. The Alzheimer's Association Campaign for Quality Residential Care has published recommendations for dementia care practice in nursing homes (Alzheimer's Association Campaign for Quality Residential Care, 2005). In addition to guidelines or parameters developed by professional organizations, the literature is replete with recommended best practices published by knowledgeable individual practitioners (Bright-Long, 2006).

Careful consideration of solid, evidence-based clinical practice guidelines or parameters may help long-term-care providers to improve the quality of their mental health assessment and treatment efforts. Moreover, such consideration has legal risk management considerations too, because many courts are allowing parties in litigation to introduce into evidence-relevant clinical practice guidelines to help prove to the fact finder what the applicable standard of acceptable care is under a particular set of circumstances.

Informed Consent and Compromised Capacity

Federal and state resident rights statutes and regulations, as well as common law precedents and statements of principles of professional organizations, empower nursing home residents to participate in decisions concerning their own lives, including choices about psychiatric and other medical care. These choices may involve specific treatments to be provided within the facility as well as questions concerning discharge from the facility or transfer to another treatment setting. The doctrine of informed choice, popularly but incompletely referred to as the right of informed consent, is the legal embodiment of the fundamental ethical principle of autonomy or self-determination (Faden & Beauchamp, 1986).

For a medical choice to be considered legally and ethically valid, the choice must be made voluntarily, without coercion or undue influence exerted on the decision-maker. In addition, the health-care provider who will be performing a particular medical intervention (e.g., doing a diagnostic procedure or prescribing a medication) has an obligation to assure that the resident's decision is properly informed. Required informational items include a description, in understandable lay language, of at least: the nature of the problem for which the medical intervention is recommended, the prognosis with and without the proposed intervention, reasonably foreseeable risks associated with the proposed intervention, and reasonable alternatives (including nonintervention) and their anticipated risks and benefits.

The third essential element of legally valid medical decision-making is sufficient cognitive and emotional capacity on the part of the decision-maker to engage in a rational process resulting in an autonomous, informed, voluntary choice. As a general rule, the law starts with the presumption that every adult possesses that minimum required level of decisional capacity. This is a rebuttable presumption, however, meaning that it may be overcome by the presentation of sufficient evidence to the contrary.

For many nursing facility residents, compromised cognitive or emotional capacity makes it difficult, if not impossible, for them to provide legally effective and ethically valid informed consent to or refusal of particular medical interventions or placements. This situation presents challenges for clinicians who endeavor to manage the care of those individuals (Grisso & Appelbaum, 1998).

Assessing Decisional Capacity

As a practical matter, the attending physician functions as a gatekeeper for the resident's autonomy. Although only a court may legally adjudicate a person decisionally incompetent and appoint a substitute decision-maker with official authority (i.e., a guardian or conservator), ordinarily the clinician's working assessment regarding the resident's decisional capacity will trigger reliance on the surrogate for acceptance or refusal of medical intervention (Kapp, 2002a). Such reliance, in turn, triggers questions concerning confidentiality and the sharing of information with others absent the resident's express permission; this concern about medical privacy is especially pronounced in light of the protections of personally identifiable health information contained in the federal Health Insurance Portability and Accountability Act and implementing regulations, 45 C.F.R. Part 160 and Subparts A and E of Part 164.

Accurately assessing decisional capacity in particular older individuals can be a complex and difficult assignment (Kapp, 2004a). No simple, reliable instrument or tool exists to make the task quick and easy (Kapp & Mossman, 1996), although continuing attempts to develop measurement instruments to assist in this task persist. Many of these various standardized instruments are useful for measuring mental status for purposes of assisting in making a diagnosis or structuring a therapeutic research plan for the individual, but the instruments are not specifically designed to take the place of clinical judgment in assessing cognitive levels for the legal and ethical purposes of judging decision-making capacity.

Nevertheless, there are some general guidelines, some of which have been published in the medical and legal literature as clinical practice parameters developed by pertinent professional organizations, that the clinician should keep in mind when conducting this type of assessment. The primary point is that decisional capacity should not be evaluated on the basis of the patient's diagnostic label or category, such as dementia, nor solely predicated on the physician's view of the wisdom of the patient's particular choice. Instead, the focus should be placed on the patient's functional ability—i.e., on the thought processes used in arriving at the "good" or "bad" decision. This approach would take into account a patient's clinical diagnosis of dementia or other mental illness but recognize that a diagnosis, by itself, tells us little about the current severity of the patient's condition or the ways in which that diagnosis actually affects the current cognitive and emotional capacity of the individual.

In conducting a functional inquiry, the following sort of basic questions should be explored: (1) Can the resident make and communicate any decisions at all? (2) Does the resident have the ability to present any reasons for the choices made that illustrate at least some degree of personal reflection and serious consideration about the choices? (3) Are the reasons presented by the resident in support of the choices made based on factually accurate suppositions that are logically applied? For instance, in one case an older woman who refused to consent to amputation of her gangrenous leg because she denied the presence of any medical problem other than dirt on her leg that could easily be washed off was properly deemed by the court to be decisionally incapacitated (State Department of Human Services v. Northern, 1978). (4) Is the resident able to comprehend the implications (the likely risks and benefits) of the available alternatives and the choices expressed, as well as the fact that these ramifications apply to that specific resident? (5) Does the resident actually appreciate the ramifications of the choices made for himself or herself?

Capacity needs to be examined on a decision-specific basis; put differently, an individual with dementia may be able to rationally make some kinds of decisions (e.g., whether or not to follow a low salt diet) but not others, such as whether to take powerful psychotropic medications. Therefore, capacity should not necessarily be envisioned as a global matter pertaining to all decisions, although some residents (particularly those in advanced stages of dementia) in fact may be globally incapacitated. For others, though, partial capacity (the ability to make some kinds, but not all kinds, of decisions) is possible. The inquiry should be whether the resident is capable "enough" to make the particular decision in question.

Moreover, capacity may fluctuate for a particular resident according to such variables as time of day, day of the week, physical location of the assessment, comorbidities (especially acute and transient medical problems), other persons available to interact with the resident and support or coerce his choice (Woods & Pratt, 2005), and reactions to medications. Some of these factors may be sufficiently susceptible to manipulation by the physician that discussions with the resident about the care plan can take place in reasonably lucid circumstances. Whenever possible, physicians should try to maximize the resident's ability to participate in medical decisions before they look to a surrogate to act on behalf of the resident.

In most situations, a working assessment of a resident's decisional capacity may be performed adequately by a primary care physician, without the need to consult with a mental health professional. In fact, the resident's attending physician ordinarily knows the resident much better than would a consultant psychiatrist or psychologist who was meeting the resident for the first time. Nevertheless, following initial assessment by the primary care physician, a separate psychiatric consultation is often requested (although this is almost always limited to situations where the resident has disagreed with the physician's treatment recommendations). The consultation request is sometimes motivated by the physician's anxiety about potential legal liability and the desire for a documented second opinion by someone whose expertise a court is likely to respect. Invoking a psychiatric consultation may be especially advisable for residents who have been determined by the PASRR process (outlined above) to suffer from some mental disorder but who appear at least marginally capable of making and expressing their own preferences about medical care. (See Chapter 19 for a thorough discussion of the role of the consultant psychiatrist.)

Clinicians are used to conducting assessments of decisional capacity based on "real-time"—i.e., assessments that evaluate an individual's ability to make medical decisions around the same time the assessment is being conducted. However, for persons who are admitted to a Medicare or Medicaid-participating nursing facility subject to the federal Resident Self-Determination Act, Public Law No. 101–508, §§ 4206 and 4751 (Ulrich, 1999), clinicians may be called upon to conduct retrospective and prospective, rather than just concurrent, assessments under two kinds of circumstances.

For people who enter a facility with a previously executed advance instruction (i.e., living will) or proxy (i.e., durable power of attorney) directive regarding future medical decisions (Moody et al., 2002), questions may be posed about the validity of that advance directive in light of uncertainty concerning the decisional capacity of the resident at the earlier time that execution of the directive took place. For the new resident who desires at the time of admission to execute an advance directive for the first time or to revise an existing one, decisional capacity may be questionable and in need of formal assessment. In both of these situations, a psychiatrist may be requested to conduct a capacity assessment, ordinarily at some time after the resident's admission, aimed at advising the attending physician or a court about the resident's earlier mental ability.

In addition, when a person of questionable capacity indicates a wish to execute or revise a medical directive at the point of admission to a nursing facility, the clinician will have to conduct an evaluation of that individual's ability to make medical choices today that will not become effective until some future time. Further, since advance directives (including the resident's agreement with a physician's "do not resuscitate" or "do not hospitalize" [Lamberg et al. 2005] order) ordinarily are executed by decisionally capable people with the understanding that they will spring into effectiveness only upon the individual's subsequent incapacity, a clinician will be called upon to determine at what moment an advance directive should become operative.

Nursing facilities should consult with their medical staffs and nursing and social service departments, as well as institutional legal counsel, to utilize any relevant professional literature, judicial precedent, statutes, and regulations in the particular jurisdiction to formulate and formally adopt written policies and procedures concerning decisional capacity assessment for facility residents. Institutional protocols should address, at a minimum, (1) when a psychiatric consultation must or should be ordered; (2) under what circumstances the facility's institutional ethics committee should be involved in decision-making for a cognitively impaired resident; (3) in what situations judicial involvement to definitively resolve questions about a resident's decisional capacity ought to be invoked; and (4) the decision-making process for actual (de facto; Karlawish et al., 2002), but not judicially declared (de jure), incapacitated residents with and without formal advance directives. These institutional protocols should be woven into the facility's overall risk management program.

Surrogate Decision-Making

When a resident lacks sufficient cognitive and emotional capacity to make decisions personally, nursing facility staff may not dispense with the requirement that informed consent be obtained prior to initiating a medical intervention. Instead, in that situation, the clinician must deal with a family member (Beeler et al., 1999) or someone else who acts as a surrogate or proxy on the resident's behalf. Surrogate decision-making for a decisionally incapacitated person may occur either through a planned process, such as the resident's prior execution of a durable power of attorney instrument, or an unplanned process resulting in court appointment of a guardian or conservator or facility reliance on the jurisdiction's default family consent statute.

Informed Decision-Making for Research Participation

The generic legal aspects of conducting biomedical or behavioral research involving human participants are governed by extensive federal, 42 C.F.R.

Part 46, and state (Kapp, 2004b) regulations, and they and related ethical considerations have been described at length elsewhere (Coleman et al., 2005; DeRenzo & Moss, 2006). However, given the disproportionate prevalence of mental illness among the nursing facility population, the legal and ethical catch-22 of conducting biomedical and behavioral research using as participants nursing home residents who are too cognitively compromised to make their own decisions presents a particular dilemma (Kapp, 2002b).

On the one hand, progress in developing new interventions that can eventually become part of standard clinical practice in diagnosing and treating medical and psychological problems in nursing home residents or for keeping potential residents in community settings requires that research projects be done in which individuals suffering from the precise problems of interest be the basic units of study (American Geriatrics Society Ethics Committee, 1998). At the same time, though, those very conditions that qualify a person for eligibility as a participant in such a research project frequently make it impossible for that person to take part in a rational, autonomous decision-making process about his or her own participation as a research subject (Dresser, 2001). This paradox is exacerbated by the fact that research participants ordinarily are more vulnerable to possible exploitation, and therefore need more protection, than residents in therapeutic circumstances because of, among other factors, the researchers' potential conflicts of interest (Gatter, 2003).

Thus, research protocols that anticipate the enrollment of participants with severe cognitive impairment, or that want to avoid enrolling those persons, must contain procedures for assessing the decision-making capacity of potential subjects. Specific assessment methods should be expressly built into the initial enrollment phase of the protocol, and therefore subject to the Institutional Review Board's review so that individuals lacking sufficient decision-making capacity can either be excluded at the outset or else have appropriate surrogates identified for them. Moreover, periodic reassessment may be necessary over the course of a long-term research project to be certain that a participant having adequate cognitive capacity when enrolled at the beginning of the protocol still maintains enough capacity throughout the protocol, such that he or she could exercise the right to withdraw if that option were desired (Loue, 2004). Several formal screening devices have been developed to aid but not displace the vital role of professional judgment exercised by researchers in the capacity assessment process (Palmer et al., 2005).

Federal regulations covering biomedical and behavioral research mandate that informed consent for participation be obtained from the "subject or the subject's legally authorized representative," 45 C.F.R. § 46.116 and 21 C.F.R. § 50.20. A problem is that a subject's legally authorized representative is defined in a circular way to mean an "individual or judicial or other body authorized under applicable [presumably state] law to consent on behalf of a prospective subject," 45 C.F.R. § 46.102(d) and 21 C.F.R. § 50.3(m). Hence, state law, even when unclear, controls in this sphere. Technically, family members have no legal authority in this sphere unless there is (1) a guardianship order expressly granting them authority, (2) a durable power of attorney previously executed by the subject giving a specified family member authorization, or (3) a state statute expressly giving a family member authorization to make these kinds of decisions. It is unusual for any of these conditions to be met. Consequently, ordinarily family members lack legal authority. However, ordinarily health-care providers and researchers act as though the family members have legal authority even when those family members really do not have formal authority.

The National Bioethics Advisory Commission proposed that DHHS promulgate regulations and states adopt legislation specifically targeted at biomedical and behavioral research involving participants with serious cognitive impairments (National Bioethics Advisory Commission, 1998). Thus far, however, such specifically targeted regulations have not been promulgated nor, in most states, legislation enacted. Severely cognitively impaired potential research participants, therefore, must continue to rely on the legal protections provided in generic federal and state laws pertaining to human subjects research.

RESTRAINTS IN THE NURSING FACILITY

The use of both physical or mechanical restraints and psychotropic drugs in nursing facilities is a subject addressed extensively in the OBRA 1987 legislation and implementing regulations. Current legal provisions quite clearly convey congressional and executive branch intentions to reduce markedly the unnecessary and inappropriate utilization of these behavior control modalities. These legal provisions carry substantial implications for professionals concerned with the care of mentally compromised nursing facility residents.

Physical or Mechanical Restraints

Defined intentionally broadly by DHHS's Centers for Medicare and Medicaid Services (CMS) as "any manual method or physical or mechanical device, material, or equipment attached or adjacent to the resident's body that the individual cannot remove easily which restricts freedom of movement or normal access to one's body," physical restraints have been a routine part of the institutional long-term-care scene in the United States for hundreds of years. It took a long time before a professional and public perception that the use of physical restraints in nursing facilities in many instances is unnecessary, improper, and even abusive culminated in detailed federal and state regulations.

Federal law provides that "the resident has the right to be free from any physical restraints imposed or psychoactive drug administered for purposes of discipline or convenience, and not required to treat the resident's medical symptoms" as documented in the resident's chart and incorporated into the resident's assessment and care plan, 42 U.S.C. §§ 1396r(c)(1)(A)(ii) and 1395i-3(c)(1)(A)(ii) and 42 C.F.R. § 483.13(a). CMS encourages state surveyors to take an aggressive stance in enforcing these regulatory constraints on nursing facility action. This stance is consciously intended to be consistent with the resident outcome orientation characterizing the nursing home survey process in place since the enactment of OBRA 1987. In addition to federal regulation by CMS tied to a nursing facility's participation in Medicare and Medicaid, providers should also be aware of potential civil liability connected to regulation by the federal Food and Drug Administration of physical restraints as medical "devices."

Moreover, every state guarantees nursing home residents the right to be free from excessive physical restraints as part of each state's resident bill of rights. These state provisions are in accord with both the spirit and letter of the federal requirements.

These governmental provisions limiting the permissible use of physical restraints do not unduly increase the potential negligence or malpractice liability exposure of nursing facilities based on resident falls or wandering. In fact, the opposite is true (Kapp, 1999). Cases holding providers liable for the absence of restraints are far eclipsed in number and size of damages by legal judgments awarded and settlements made on the basis of inappropriate ordering of restraints, failure to monitor and correct their adverse effects on the residents, or errors in the mechanical application of the restraint (Braun & Capezuti, 2000).

Although the question of physical restraint reduction in nursing facilities is no longer a matter for debate but only for implementation, improvements in actual practice have varied considerably among specific facilities and have fluctuated over time. Constant efforts are necessary to keep up positive momentum and prevent backsliding. Nursing homes must develop and carry out policies and procedures to comply with all applicable legal requirements in this regard. Less restrictive alternatives to the use of restraints, including both environmental and administrative changes in the facility, must be explored fully and explained to staff, residents, and families (Kapp, 1998). In recognition of the continual challenge to wean nursing facilities away from their historical dependence on the use of physical restraints, the Nursing Home Quality Initiative launched in November, 2002, by CMS to assist facilities to improve the quality of care and quality of life for all residents (Nedza, 2005) includes a large component aimed at enabling the federally funded Quality Improvement Organizations to work closely with individual facilities on restraint reduction.

Psychotropic Drugs

Prior to the enactment of OBRA 1987, psychotropic drugs were prescribed profusely, and frequently improperly, in American nursing homes. Prescriptions for them commonly were issued in the absence of any specific psychiatric diagnosis for the resident, let alone a comprehensive treatment plan justifying a scientific rationale for the drugs prescribed. Instead of being prescribed on the basis of legitimate medical indications, psychotropics were used routinely for environmental control (e.g., to keep residents from shouting out or running around) or to appease the strenuous demands of family or staff for constraints on resident behavior.

The OBRA 1987 legislation and its implementing regulations, as well as corresponding resident rights laws in every state, aim at inducing major changes from the previously prevailing situation wherein psychotropic drugs often were used for nonpsychiatric treatment purposes (Ryan et al., 2002). 42 C.F.R. § 483.13(a) assures each nursing facility resident "the right to be free from any...psychoactive drug administered for the purposes of discipline or convenience, and not required to treat the resident's medical symptoms." In addition, 42 C.F.R. § 483.25 states that each resident's drug regimen must be free from unnecessary drugs and requires that a resident for whom antipsychotics have not been used previously be given them only to treat a specific condition. Most residents getting antipsychotic drugs must receive gradual dose reductions or drug holidays. The CMS *Interpretive Guidelines for Surveyors*, available at www.cms.hhs.gov/guidanceforlawsandregulations/12_NHs.asp, should be consulted for guidance concerning criteria for unnecessary drugs, specific indications for permissible psychotropic drug prescriptions, behaviors that should not be considered an indication for psychotropic drug use, and drug discontinuation methodologies.

The OBRA statute and regulations, plus voluntary JCAHO standards, recognize the professional consensus that there may be valid therapeutic indications for the prescription of psychotropics for some nursing home residents (American Geriatrics Society & American Association for Geriatric Psychiatry, 2003a). These indications are the documented, persistent, unpreventable existence of one or more of the following specific conditions: schizophrenia, schizoaffective disorder, delusional disorder, psychotic mood disorders (including mania and depression with psychotic features), acute psychotic episodes, brief reactive psychosis, schizophreniform disorder, atypical psychosis, Tourette's disorder, Huntington's disease, and organic mental syndromes (delirium, dementia, and amnestic and other cognitive disorders) with associated psychotic and/or agitated behaviors. Antipsychotics should not be used if the only indication is one or more of the following: wandering, poor self care, restlessness, impaired memory, anxiety, depression (without psychotic features), insomnia, unsociability, indifference to surroundings, fidgeting, nervousness, uncooperativeness, or agitated behaviors that do not represent a danger to the resident or others. Legal standards to which providers are held obviously assume that prescribers will keep abreast of the current professional literature in this sphere and be aware of the various nonpharmacologic interventions (Camp et al., 2002) available to treat nursing home residents with mental health problems.

Even when prescribed for the correct reasons, however, possible drug toxicities and dangerous interactions may be underestimated. Therefore, it is important for facility staff to carefully monitor residents on psychotropics for timely indications of negative side effects. Liability may be imposed for negligence in monitoring and inadequate response even when the resident assessment and initial prescription itself were defensible. Further, when a particular medication is discontinued, adequate monitoring to detect any adverse reactions is a reasonably expected part of the standard of care.

Federal regulations require within each nursing facility a regular pharmacist-conducted drug regimen review. This activity should be incorporated into the facility's more comprehensive drug utilization review program, with which medical and nursing staff should cooperate completely and in an ongoing manner.

Implementation of OBRA 1987's dictates in this arena has met with some resistence and barriers of various sorts, such as ingrained institutional culture (Cody et al., 2002; Svarstad et al., 2001) and inadequate nursing staff (Svarstad & Mount, 2001). However, there is conclusive evidence that, over all, OBRA 1987 and implementing regulations have effectively influenced practice within nursing facilities so as to cause a reduction in the use of psychotropic drugs. The evidence is still inconclusive, though, regarding the ultimate issue of the actual effect of a reduction in the use of psychotropic drugs on the quality of care and quality of life for the intended beneficiaries, namely, nursing facility residents who would otherwise be at risk of receiving those drugs (Hughes et al., 2000; Van Haaren et al., 2001).

CONCLUSION

Substantial gains have been made over the course of the past 2 decades, often with legal prodding, in the quality of mental health assessment and treatment in American nursing homes. Nevertheless, there remains much room for improvement in this domain as many residents do not yet receive the mental health services they need or still receive only inappropriate or insufficient services (U.S. Department of Health and Human Services, 2003). The law is not adequate by itself (Kapp, 2003). To supplement the present regulatory environment, clinically effective and ethically humane treatment of our most vulnerable citizens compels (among other things) advocacy of public policy changes (American Geriatrics Society & American Association for Geriatric Psychiatry, 2003b) that will embody refinements in the assessment process, the use of outcomes-based quality measures, and payment policies geared to improve access to and quality of mental health services (Streim et al., 2002).

REFERENCES

Alzheimer's Association Campaign for Quality Residential Care. (2005). *Dementia care practice: Recommendations for assisted living residences and nursing homes.* Chicago: Author.

American Geriatrics Society Ethics Committee. (1998). *Position statement: Informed consent for research on human subjects with dementia.* New York: Author.

American Geriatrics Society & American Association for Geriatric Psychiatry. (2003a, September). Consensus statement on improving the quality of mental health care in U.S. nursing homes: Management of depression and behavioral symptoms associated with dementia. *Journal of the American Geriatrics Society, 51,* 1287–1298.

American Geriatrics Society & American Association for Geriatric Psychiatry. (2003b, September). Recommendations for policies in support of quality mental health care in U.S. nursing homes. *Journal of the American Geriatrics Society, 51,* 1299–1304.

American Medical Directors Association. (1998). *Clinical practice guideline: Altered mental states.* Columbia, MD: Author.

American Medical Directors Association. (2003). *Clinical practice guideline: Depression.* Columbia, MD: Author.

American Medical Directors Association. (2005). *Clinical practice guideline: Dementia.* Columbia, MD: Author.

Banazak, D. A., & Glettler, E. (2000). From policy to practice: Physicians' views on OBRA and mental health resources in long-term care. *Journal of the American Medical Directors Association, 1,*14–20.

Bartels, S J., Miles, K. M., Dums, A. R., & Levine, K. J. (2003, November). Are nursing homes appropriate for older adults with severe mental illness? Conflicting consumer and clinician views and implications for the Olmstead decision. *Journal of the American Geriatrics Society, 51,* 1571–1579.

Beck, C., Doan, R., & Cody, M. (2002, Spring). Nursing assistants as providers of mental health care in nursing homes. *Generations, 26,* 66–71.

Beeler, J., Rosenthal, A., & Cohler, B. (1999, September). Patterns of family caregiving and support provided to older psychiatric residents in long-term care. *Psychiatric Services, 50,* 1222–1224.

Borson, S., Leobel, J. P., Kitchell, M., Domoto, S., & Hyde, T. (1997, October). Psychiatric assessments of nursing home residents under OBRA-87: Should PASARR be reformed? *Journal of the American Geriatrics Society, 45,* 1173–1181.

Braun, J. A., & Capezuti, E. A. (2000, Fall). The legal and medical aspects of physical restraints and bed siderails and their relationship to falls and fall-related injuries in nursing homes. *DePaul Journal of Health Care Law, 4,* 1–72.

Bright-Long, L. (2006, February). Alzheimer's treatment in nursing homes: Room for improvement. *Journal of the American Medical Directors Association, 7,* 90–95.

Camp, C. J., Cohen-Mansfield, J., & Capezuti, E. A. (2002, November). Use of nonpharmacologic interventions among nursing home residents with dementia. *Psychiatric Services, 53,* 1397–1401.

Cody, M., Beck, C., & Svarstad, B. L. (2002, November). Challenges to the use of nonpharmacologic interventions in nursing homes. *Psychiatric Services, 53,* 1402–1406.

Coleman, C. H., Menikoff, J. A., Dubler, N. N., et al. (2005). *The ethics and regulation of research with human subjects.* Newark, NJ: Matthew Bender & Company.

DeRenzo, E. & Moss, J. (2006). *Writing clinical research protocols.* Burlington, MA: Elsevier Academic Press.

Dresser, R. (2001). Dementia research: Ethics and policy for the twenty-first century. *Georgia Law Review, 35,* 661–690.

Faden, R. R., & Beauchamp, T. (1986). *A history and theory of informed consent.* New York: Oxford University Press.

Gaddy, K. (2000, Spring–Summer). Special care environments: An overview of state laws for care of persons with Alzheimer's disease. *Bifocal: Newsletter of the American Bar Association Commission on Legal Problems of the Elderly, 21,* 1, 8, 12, 18–24.

Gatter, R. (2003). Walking the talk of trust in human subjects research: The challenge of regulating financial conflicts of interest. *Emory Law Journal, 52,* 327–401.

Grisso, T., & Appelbaum, P. S. (1998). *Assessing competence to consent to treatment.* New York: Oxford University Press.

Hughes, C. M., Lapane, K. L., Mor, V., et al. (2000, August). The impact of legislation on psychotropic drug use in nursing homes: A cross-national perspective. *Journal of the American Geriatrics Society, 48,* 931–937.

Institute of Medicine. (1986). *Improving the quality of care in nursing homes.* Washington, DC: National Academy Press.

Kapp, M. B. (1998, March/April). Editorial, families can help reduce the use of nursing home restraints. *American Journal of Alzheimer's Disease, 13,* 105–106.

Kapp, M. B. (1999, March). Restraint reduction and legal risk management. *Journal of the American Geriatrics Society, 47,* 375–376.

Kapp, M. B. (2002a, November). Decisional capacity in theory and practice: Legal process versus 'bumbling through'." *Aging and Mental Health, 6,* 413–417.

Kapp, M. B. (Ed.). (2002b). *Issues in conducting research with and about older persons. Ethics, law, and aging review* (Vol. 8). New York: Springer Publishing Company.

Kapp, M. B. (2003). *The law and older persons: Is geriatric jurisprudence therapeutic?* Durham, NC: Carolina Academic Press.

Kapp, M. B. (Ed.). (2004a). *Decision-making capacity and older persons. Ethics, law, and aging review* (Vol. 10). New York: Springer.

Kapp, M. B. (2004b). Protecting human participants in long-term care research: The role of state law and policy. *Journal of Aging and Social Policy, 16,* 13–33.

Kapp, M. B. (Ed.). (2005). *Deinstitutionalizing long-term care: Making legal strides, avoiding policy errors. Ethics, law, and aging review* (Vol. 11). New York: Springer.

Kapp, M. B., & Mossman, D. (1996). "Measuring decisional capacity: Cautions on the construction of a 'capacimeter'." *Psychology, Public Policy, and Law, 2,* 73–95.

Karlawish, J. H. T., Casarett, D., Propert, K. J., et al. (2002, Summer). Relationship between Alzheimer's disease severity and resident participation in decisions about their medical care. *Journal of Geriatric Psychiatry and Neurology, 15,* 68–72.

Lamberg, J. L., Person, C. J., Kiely, D. K., et al. (2005, August). Decisions to hospitalize nursing home residents dying with advanced dementia. *Journal of the American Geriatrics Society, 53,* 1396–1401.

Linkins, K., Robinson, G., Karp, J., et al. (2001). *Screening for mental illness in nursing facility applicants: Understanding federal requirements.* SAMHSA Publication No. (SMA) 01-3543. Rockville, MD: Center for Mental Health Services, Substance Abuse and Mental Health Services Administration.

Loue, S. (2004). The participation of cognitively impaired elderly in research. *Journal of Long Term Home Health Care, 5,* 245–257.

Mitchell, S. L, Teno, J., Miller, S. C., et al. (2005, February). A national study of the location of death for older persons with dementia. *Journal of the American Geriatrics Society, 53,* 299–305.

Moody, L. E., Small, B. J., & Jones, C. B. (2002, March). Advance directives preferences of functionally and cognitively impaired nursing home residents in the United States. *Journal of Applied Gerontology, 21,* 103–118.

National Bioethics Advisory Commission. (1998). *Research involving persons with mental disorders that may affect decisionmaking capacity: Report and recommendations.* Washington, DC: Author.

Nedza, S. (2005, March). Driving improvement in long-term care: Enforcement and quality initiatives. *Journal of Legal Medicine, 26,* 61–68.

Palmer, B. W., Dunn, L. B., Appelbaum, P. S., et al. (2005, July). Assessment of capacity to consent to research among older persons with schizophrenia, Alzheimer disease, or diabetes mellitus. *Archives of General Psychiatry, 62,* 726–733.

Ryan, J. M., Kidder, S. W., Daiello, L. A., et al. (2002, November). Psychopharmacologic interventions in nursing homes: What do we know and where should we go? *Psychiatric Services, 53,* 1407–1413.

Snowden, M., Piacitelli, J., & Keopsell, T. (1998, September). Compliance with PASARR recommendations for Medicaid recipients in nursing homes. *Journal of the American Geriatrics Society, 46,* 1132–1136.

Spillman, B. C., & Lubitz, J. (2002). New estimates of lifetime nursing home use: Have patterns of use changed? *Medical Care, 40,* 965–975.

State Department of Human Services v. Northern, 563 S.W.2d 197 (Tenn.Ct.App. 1978).

Streim, J. E., Beckwith, E. W., Arapakos, D., et al. (2002, November). Regulatory oversight, payment policy, and quality improvement in mental health care in nursing homes. *Psychiatric Services, 53,* 1414–1418.

Svarstad, B. L., & Mount, J. K. (2001, December). Chronic benzodiazepine use in nursing homes: Effects of federal guidelines, resident mix, and nurse staffing. *Journal of the American Geriatrics Society, 49,* 1673–1678.

Svarstad, B. L., Mount, J. K., & Bigelow, W. (2001, May). Variations in the treatment culture of nursing homes and responses to regulations to reduce drug use. *Psychiatric Services, 52,* 666–672.

Ulrich, L. P. (1999). *The resident self-determination act: Meeting the challenges in resident care.* Washington, DC: Georgetown University Press.

U.S. Department of Health and Human Services, Office of Inspector General (2001a, January). *Younger nursing home residents with mental illness: An unidentified population.* Washington, DC. OEI-05-99-00701.

U.S. Department of Health and Human Services, Office of Inspector General. (2001b, January). *Younger nursing home residents with mental illness: Preadmission screening and resident review (PASRR) implementation and oversight.* Washington, DC. OEI-05-99-00700.

U.S. Department of Health and Human Services, Office of Inspector General. (2003, March). *Psychosocial services in skilled nursing facilities*. Washington, DC. OEI-02-01-00610.

Van Haaren, A. M., Lapane, K. L., & Hughes, C. M. (2001). Effect of triplicate prescription policy on benzodiazepine administration in nursing home residents. *Pharmacotherapy, 21*, 1159–1166.

Wagner v. Fair Acres Geriatric Center, 49 F.3d 1002 (3d Cir. 1995).

Woods, B. & Rebekah, P. (2005, September) Awareness in dementia: Ethical and legal issues in relation to people with dementia. *Aging and Mental Health, 9*, 423–429.

Yaffe, K., et al. (2002). Resident and caregiver characteristics and nursing home placement in residents with dementia. *Journal of the American Medical Association, 287*, 2090–2097.

22

Mental Health in the Assisted Living Setting

Quincy M. Samus and *Adam Rosenblatt*

Assisted living (AL) has been the most rapidly expanding form of residential long-term care in the United States over the past 20 years (American Association for Retired Persons, AARP, 2002; National Center for Assisted Living, NCAL, 2001). Its expansion has been driven largely by state and private sector interest in the reduction of long-term care expenditures as well as consumer backlash toward the nursing home (NH) industry (Hawes, 2001). AL is now widely viewed as an integral, intermediary component of the long-term care continuum that fills the gap between home-delivered care and institutional-style care for many elders who cannot live independently in the community (Figure 22.1). Best estimates suggest that over 1 million elders are living in more than 35,000 AL facilities nationwide (Hawes, 2001; Mollica, 2002) and one study of residential care (RC) usage predicts that by the year 2010, more elders will be cared for in the AL setting than in nursing homes (Promatura Group, 2000). In concept, AL is meant to epitomize a "social" model of care, focusing primarily on the creation of a physical and social environment that promotes independence, health, and quality of life and allows residents to "age in place," minimizing the need to move to another setting (Assisted Living Quality Coalition, ALQC, 1998; NCAL, 2001). This is in contrast to the "medical" model of care typically found in other institutional settings like skilled nursing facilities (SNFs) that make the provision of health-care services the primary aim (Coleman, 1995;

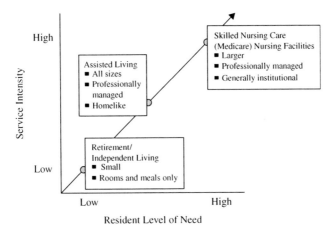

FIGURE 22.1. The continuum of residential long-term care (Source: NCAL, 2001 Assisted Living Sourcebook).

Hawes et al., 1999). As a result, AL has often been viewed as an alternative *housing option* rather than as a *health-care system*.

This perception is, however, changing. Emerging data has documented substantial psychiatric morbidity in the AL population, resulting especially from dementia and depression. In fact, dementia appears to be more common than any other chronic health condition in AL, including heart disease (Rosenblatt et al., 2004). This revelation can be understood in the context of changes in long-term care utilization patterns that have accompanied the introduction of AL to the care continuum (Bishop, 1999; Spillman et al., 2002). In the past, RC placement for people with dementia and other mental conditions often meant admission to SNFs. Yet, owing to a myriad of factors including pressure for shorter hospital stays and more restrictive SNF entry standards, SNFs now serve primarily subacute patients and those with the highest medical needs (Spillman & Black, 2006). Concomitantly, the broadening of state-directed Medicaid reimbursement policies for AL in the United States (Nolin & Mollica, 2001) and elders' desire to be cared for in a more homelike and less institutional environment (Morgan et al., 2001) have made AL an appealing alternative to SNFs. Thus, elders with fewer medical problems but who need a supervised and supportive care environment because of dementia or other mental health problems have entered AL.

As the appreciation of the prevalence and severity of mental health conditions in AL has increased, so has unease about whether AL is equipped to meet the needs of this population. Unlike nursing homes, oversight and licensure of AL is undertaken at the state rather than the federal level. This introduces a considerable amount of variability in the definitions, practices, and standards of care employed among settings that fall under the large umbrella of "assisted living" and complicates efforts to assess the totality of the burden of mental health conditions as well as the quality of care being delivered (Hawes, 2001; Hawes & Phillips, 2007; Wilson, 2007). Understanding the epidemiology of mental health conditions in this population and how well they are currently being recognized and managed is a priority among stakeholders of all types and is germane to the continued evolution of AL and in the shaping of policies that govern it.

In this chapter we will provide a comprehensive overview of the epidemiology, consequences, and management of mental health conditions in the context of AL, as it is understood today. Specifically, we will use the empirical data available to discuss the epidemiology of specific mental health disorders and the effects of these disorders on key outcomes such as quality of life, length of stay, and facility resource use. We will also identify elements of quality care relevant in AL, discuss current practices in the detection and management of mental health disorders, and review the implications of these practices and directions for the future.

EPIDEMIOLOGY OF MENTAL HEALTH DISORDERS IN ASSISTED LIVING

A number of studies have attempted to describe the demographic and health characteristics of AL residents quantitatively, including mental health conditions (Golant, 2004). Because of the definitional ambiguity of AL, these studies developed differing strategies to estimate the overall statistical population, to select study samples, and to measure resident characteristics (Golant, 2004). This may explain some of the variability in results.

Published studies reporting on the prevalence of mental health conditions in AL, commonly, estimates of "cognitive impairment," have generally provided indirect estimates, based on interviews with AL staff or on medical chart reviews. Because conditions like dementia are known to be under-recognized and undertreated in elders in the primary care setting (Solomon et al., 2000) it is reasonable to expect indirect estimates of this type in AL to be similarly low. In evidence of this, one study found that 63% of AL residents determined to have cognitive impairment by direct assessment on the Mini-Mental State Examination (MMSE) did not have a diagnosis of dementia listed in their AL facility chart (Magsi & Malloy, 2005).

Direct assessment techniques, which likely provide more realistic estimates, have been employed by far fewer studies in AL. The largest direct study of AL conducted to date, The Collaborative Studies of Long-Term Care (CS-LTC), included 2,078 AL/RC residents from 197 AL/RC facilities across four states (i.e., North Carolina, Maryland, Florida, and New Jersey) (Zimmerman et al., 2001). This broadly focused study used on-site resident interviews, observations, and staff interviews to examine a number of resident health characteristics and outcomes including cognitive impairment, behavioral problems, and depression. Follow-up data were gathered by telephone interview every 3 months for up to 1 year. Another direct study conducted by Magsi and Malloy (2005) examined 230 AL residents from seven ALs in Nebraska and was focused on the prevalence of cognitive impairment and dementia diagnosis and treatment. Finally, the Maryland Assisted Living (MD-AL) study, an ongoing longitudinal investigation of the epidemiology of psychiatric disorders in AL, is arguably the most in-depth evaluation of psychiatric conditions in AL conducted thus far. MD-AL uses physician-based examinations to determine the prevalence, incidence, detection, and treatment of these conditions in a total sample of 401 AL residents from 28 AL facilities in Maryland. Residents are evaluated in-person semiannually for 3 years after admission to AL. Together, these studies provide most of the epidemiological data to be discussed.

Cognitive Impairment, Dementia, and Related Neuropsychiatric Symptoms

Cognitive impairment and dementia

Assisted living serves a population of elders at the highest risk for having or developing cognitive impairment or dementia. In the United States, the average age of an AL resident is 85 years, with 54% being 85 and older and 5% to 10% being over 95 (Hawes et al., 2000; Zimmerman et al., 2001). A prevalence of dementia of about 30% would be expected on the basis of age alone (Small et al., 1997), but because the presence of cognitive impairment is highly predictive of need for residential long-term care like AL (Hawes et al., 2000), it is not surprising that dementia is common in the AL cohort.

Dementia is a clinical syndrome characterized by impairment in multiple cognitive domains (including memory), resulting in impairment in social or occupational functioning, which represents a significant decline from previous function (American Psychiatric Association, APA, 2000). Alzheimer's disease (AD) is the most common form of dementia in older people (65%–70% of all cases; Brookmeyer et al., 1998; Katzman & Fox, 1999). Vascular dementia is probably the second most prevalent form of dementia in older adults. Other less common forms of dementia, occasionally found in AL, include dementia with lewy bodies (DLB) and frontotemporal dementia (FTD).

In contrast to dementia, cognitive impairment is a much broader term that is used to describe a whole range of presentations of abnormal declines in one or more cognitive domains. Mild cognitive impairment (MCI) or cognitive impairment, not dementia (CIND) are two frequently used terms for conditions that do not meet clinical criteria for a dementia syndrome. The predictive validity of constructs such as MCI or CIND as a prodrome for later dementia varies substantially by the definitional criteria used (Albert & Blacker, 2006).

Prevalence.   Prevalence rates of cognitive impairment and dementia in AL have varied substantially by assessment method and criteria. Indirect estimates obtained through reporting by facility administrators and primary care physician surveys range from 20% to 50% (Hawes et al., 1995; Lair & Lefkowitz, 1990), but these data may be affected by underreporting, underrecognition, or chart inaccuracies. Studies using direct estimates of cognitive impairment by a priori scale cutoff scores have suggested generally higher estimates than indirect studies, ranging from 40% to 63% (Hawes et al., 1995; Magsi & Malloy, 2005; Morgan et al., 2001; Quinn et al., 1999).

Table 22.1 shows directly assessed prevalence estimates of cognitive impairment in AL by study, setting, and impairment criteria. The MD-AL study is currently the only study available that has incorporated a comprehensive in-person assessment (including a geriatric psychiatrist exam and a detailed cognitive battery) so that the *Diagnostic and statistical manual of mental disorders, fourth edition, text revision (DSM-IV-TR)* criteria (APA, 2000) could be applied. This study found that among the 198 participants who were selected at random, 134 (68%) met DSM-IV-TR criteria for dementia. Of the cases with dementia, probable Alzheimer's disease (AD) was the most common type of dementia (69%) followed by mixed dementia or dementia not otherwise specific (NOS) (28%), vascular dementia (13%), and Lewy Body disease (<1%) (Rosenblatt et al., 2004). Additionally, almost 7% of residents who did not meet criteria for dementia were diagnosed with another clinically significant cognitive disorder, most commonly, *cognitive disorder not otherwise specified (NOS)*. Thus, 74% of the total sample of residents met DSM-IV criteria for some type of cognitive dysfunction (Rosenblatt et al., 2004).

In all studies, the majority of residents who were cognitively impaired were in the mild to moderate range of severity (Magsi & Malloy, 2005; Morgan et al., 2001) (Table 22.2). Nevertheless, a sizable minority of AL residents (between 15% and 31%) were characterized as having severe cognitive impairment in the CS-LTC (Morgan et al., 2001). Similarly, in residents determined to have dementia in the MD-AL study, over a quarter had a MMSE score less than 10, with an average score of 3.9 (SD 3.1). Scores below 24 are typically indicative of dementia.

Despite the high prevalence rates estimated from cross-sectional studies, few studies have looked at the incidence of dementia as AL residents' age in place. The longitudinal phase of the MD-AL study currently underway will provide this estimate as well an estimate of the incidence of other psychiatric conditions, such as depression. This study will also describe the trajectory of cognitive decline in those already suffering from dementia from the outset.

TABLE 22.1. Direct Assessment Estimates of Cognitive Impairment from Studies of AL Residents

AUTHOR(S)	YEAR	STUDY	POPULATION	CRITERIA	PREVALENCE (%)
Cognitive impairment					
Hawes et al.	1995		Board and care homes	Short Blessed exam, Cognitive Performance Scale—Cut-off scores not reported.	40
Quinn et al.	1999		Personal care homes (n = 80)	Short Orientation-Memory-Concentration Test score >8	60
Morgan et al.	2001	Collaborative Studies of Long-Term Care	Residential care/AL (n = 2078)	MDS-COGS score ≥2	45–63[a]
Rosenblatt et al.	2004	Maryland Assisted Living Study	Assisted living (n = 198)	DSM-IV-TR criteria	74
Magsi & Malloy	2005		Assisted living (n = 230)	MMSE score ≥23	58
Dementia					
Rosenblatt et al.	2004	Maryland Assisted Living Study	Assisted living (n = 198)	DSM-IV-TR criteria	68

[a] Prevalence rate varied by type of facility.

TABLE 22.2. Cognitive Impairment by Severity among Direct-Assessment Studies

AUTHOR(S)	YEAR	STUDY	POPULATION	CRITERIA	PREVALENCE (%)
Mild/moderate					
Morgan et al. aziner	2001	Collaborative Studies of Long-Term Care	All residential care/AL (n = 2078)	MDS-COGS score 2–4	25–32[a]
Sloane et al.	2005	Collaborative Studies of Long-Term Care	RC/AL residents with dementia[c] (n = 773)	Independent in all: locomotion, transfer, feeding	71[b]
Magsi & Malloy	2005		All AL (n = 230)	MMSE score ≥10	95
Rosenblatt, et al.	Unpublished	Maryland Assisted Living Study	All AL (n = 198)	MMSE score ≥10	81
	Unpublished		AL residents with dementia (n = 134)	MMSE score ≥10	74
Moderate/severe					
Hawes et al.	2000	A National Survey of Assisted Living for the Frail Elderly	All AL/RC residents (sample size not reported)	Short Blessed exam, Cognitive Performance Scale (CPS)-Cut-off scores not reported.	27
Sloane et al.	2005	Collaborative Studies of Long-Term Care	RC/AL residents with dementia[c] (n = 773)	Assistance with one or more: locomotion, transfer, feeding	29

Severe

Morgan et al.	2001	Collaborative Studies of Long-Term Care	Residential care/AL (n = 2078)	MDS-COGS ≥ 5	15–31[a]
Magsi & Malloy	2005		All assisted living (n = 230)	MMSE score < 10	5
Rosenblatt et al.	Unpublished	Maryland Assisted Living Study	Assisted living (n = 198)	MMSE score < 10	19
	Unpublished		Assisted living residents with dementia (n = 134)	MMSE score < 10	26

[a] Prevalence rate varied by type of facility.

[b] Only included "Mild Cases."

[c] Dementia defined as individuals with (a) medical record diagnosis of a form of dementia and (b) scored > 2 on MDS-COGS.

Smaller facilities, sometimes known as "mom and pop homes" or "domiciliary homes for the elderly," appear to care for greater proportions of elders with dementia and cognitive impairment, compared to the larger AL facilities. For instance, in the CS-LTC, "traditional facilities" operationalized as "larger homes of the traditional board and care type" (Zimmerman et al., 2001) had the lowest overall rate of cognitive impairment (45%) among the resident population when compared with the two other facility types. "New-model facilities" (i.e., facilities meeting several criteria including having more than 15 beds and being built after January 1, 1987), had a rate of 52%, while smaller facilities (i.e., those having fewer than 16 beds) had the highest prevalence of cognitive impairment (63%) (Zimmerman et al., 2001). The MD-AL study, which used the same definition for "smaller" facilities (i.e., <16 beds), also found that 81% of residents of small facilities had dementia compared to 63% in large facilities (i.e., > 15 beds). Further, the severity of cognitive impairment among all residents, as measured by Mini-Mental State Exam scores, was markedly worse among residents of small facilities (mean 13.0) compared to that among residents of larger facilities (mean 19.9) (Leroi et al., 2006).

Dementia-related neuropsychiatric symptoms

Neuropsychiatric symptoms, sometimes known as behavioral and psychological symptoms of dementia (BPSD), behavioral symptoms related to dementia (BSRD), or the noncognitive features of dementia (Boustani et al., 2005; Karlsson, 1996; Rabins et al., 2006; Turner, 2005), are commonly associated with dementia and occur at some point in 90% of dementia cases (Steinberg et al., 2003). Neuropsychiatric symptoms can include hallucinations, delusions, aggressive behaviors, anxiety, motor disturbances, and mood-related problems like sadness, irritability, and sleep disturbances.

Prevalence.   Not surprisingly, given the high prevalence of dementia, behavioral disturbances are common in AL, with cross-sectional prevalence rates from the CS-LTC ranging from 36% to 49% among *all* AL residents, depending on type of facility (Morgan et al., 2001). AL providers in this study reported that about 34% of all AL residents had weekly episodes of BPSD (Gruber-Baldini et al., 2004) and that between 42% and 56% of residents *with dementia* had had a behavioral disturbance in the past 2 weeks (Boustani et al., 2005). In the MD-AL study, 83% of residents with dementia were reported by their primary formal caregivers to have had at least one neuropsychiatric symptom in the past month, with 70% having clinically significant symptoms (i.e., Neuropsychiatric Inventory score >4) (Leroi et al., 2006; Rosenblatt et al., 2004).

The prevalence of *specific* neuropsychiatric symptoms by study is presented in Table 22.3. The evidence suggests that agitation including resistance to care, aggressive behaviors such as hitting or kicking, aberrant motor behaviors such

TABLE 22.3. Prevalence of Selected Behaviors by Study of AL Residents

AUTHOR(S)	AGITATION/ AGGRESSION (%)	DELUSIONS/ HALLUCINATION (%)	ANXIETY (%)	IRRITABILITY (%)	VERBAL BEHAVIOR (REP. STATEMENTS, SCREAMING, STRANGE NOISES) (%)	PHYSICAL NONAGGRESSIVE (PACING, HOARDING, REPETITIOUS MANNERISMS) (%)
All residents						
Morgan et al. 2001[a]		11–18	35–38	24–31		
Dementia residents						
Gruber-Baldini et al.2004[a]	13				22	20
Unpublished MD-AL[b]	27	22	11	22		14

[a] Data are from the CSLTC. Two-week retrospective time frame for behavior reported.
[b] Unpublished data from MD-AL Phase II (n = 266) study. Based on presence of symptoms on Neuropsychiatric Inventory domains. One-month retrospective time frame for behaviors reported.

as wandering, and irritability, anxiety, and psychosis appear to be the most common neuropsychiatric symptoms in AL. One survey suggests that from the AL facility administrators' perspective, resistance to care and wandering are the most problematic (Wagenaar et al., 2003). Aggressive behaviors that result in violence are often cited as a special concern among administrators and front-line care workers in residential care settings. In a Swedish study of violent behaviors in residential care involving individuals with dementia, 11% of staff reported they had been exposed to a violent incident and nearly one-third had had a subsequent physical wound or bruise (Astrom et al., 2004).

Correlates. Several studies have examined the cross-sectional correlates of neuropsychiatric symptoms in AL residents. The presence of depression, dementia, worse overall cognitive impairment, and functional impairment were strongly associated with behavioral symptoms of all types in the CS-LTC (Gruber-Baldini et al., 2004). Similarly, in a study sample that included AL and NH residents with dementia from the CS-LTC, the prevalence of BSRD was associated with several resident-level characteristics, including worse overall cognitive impairment, impaired mobility, low mood, and treatment with psychotropic medications. Residents of facilities that had supervisory staff trained to detect and treat these behaviors had lower prevalence rates. Facility size did not appear to play a role (Boustani et al., 2005). In analyses that include only AL, residents of smaller facilities have consistently greater mean scores on measures of neuropsychiatric symptoms (Gruber-Baldini et al., 2004; Leroi et al., 2006) and psychosis in particular (Leroi et al., 2006) than those in larger facilities.

Consequences. Dementia and related neuropsychiatric disturbances can lead to a number of adverse outcomes in AL. They are highly related to the need to move individuals to higher, more intensive and expensive care levels such as SNFs. For example, AL facility discharge policies hinge almost universally on residents' need for daily assistance, usually specifying ADL domains with heavy caregiver demands such as incontinence, and on behavioral symptoms (Hawes et al., 2000), both of which may be regarded as essential features of dementia. In a national survey of facility administrators, 76% reported that they would discharge residents due to behavioral issues (Hawes et al., 2000). Similarly, an exploratory qualitative study on factors that contributed to administrators' decisions to discharge AL residents with dementia to skilled nursing facilities reported that the progression of dementia, need for more assistance with activities of daily living, incontinence, wandering, and aggressive behaviors often influenced discharge decisions (Wagenaar et al., 2003). Recent empirical data suggest that these stated policies are put into practice. Data from The National Study of Assisted Living for the Frail Elderly, a large nationally representative study of AL with 11 beds or more, reported that AL residents with severe cognitive impairment were over two times as likely to be discharged to a nursing home over a 7-month follow-up period as compared to residents who were either cognitively intact or mildly cognitively impaired (Hawes et al., 2003). In the MD-AL study, residents with dementia exited the AL facility an average of 209 days, or about 7 months, sooner than those without dementia (Lyketsos et al., 2007) over a follow-up period of 2 years.

Dementia is also a strong independent predictor of disability in AL (Burdick et al., 2005), disproportionate use of facility resources such as staff time resource use (Arling & Williams, 2003; Rosenblatt et al., 2004), and caregiver stress (Bruce et al., 2005). Beyond these effects, dementia and related neuropsychiatric disturbances are also related to quality of life (González-Salvador et al., 2000; Samus et al., 2005) among AL residents. Agitation, aggression, apathy, and irritability explained about 30% of the variance in quality of life for AL residents with dementia in the MD-AL study (Samus et al., 2005).

Depression

Depression and other mood disorders are common among residents of residential care settings. In AL, mood disorders are the most common type of noncognitive psychiatric condition, and depressive disorders are the most common type of mood disorder. Some evidence suggests that symptom expression of depression may be age dependent. For example, elders may not complain of sadness or low mood but may instead be more irritable or socially withdrawn (Salzman, 2000). Medical comorbidity, cognitive impairment, and disability further complicate detection and diagnosis (Alexopoulos, 2005).

Prevalence. When understanding prevalence estimates, it is important to consider that "depression," as used in the literature, can refer to *symptoms* or to disorders. Prevalence rates of depressive symptoms and diagnosed depressive disorders in AL have been reported by several studies. In most studies, clinically significant depressive symptoms were classified on the basis of a depression scale cutoff score, usually the Cornell Scale for Depression in Dementia (CSDD) (Alexopoulos et al., 1988), administered to the participant and/or a knowledgeable staff member. Table 22.4 shows the prevalence rates using various diagnostic criteria for depression by study for all residents. In general, prevalence rates using scale cutoff scores range from 13% to 24% and vary by criteria. In the only study to have applied DSM-IV-TR standards, the prevalence of mood disorders was 18% (Rosenblatt et al., 2004), falling approximately in the middle of the scale estimates range. The most frequently endorsed symptoms on the CSDD scale were (in residents not necessarily clinically depressed) mood-related items such as anxious expression, rumination, worrying (37%); irritability, easy annoyance (28%); sad expression, sad voice, tearfulness (25%); and lack of reactivity to pleasant events (18%).

TABLE 22.4. Prevalence of Depressive Symptoms and Depression Diagnosis by Study

AUTHOR(S)	YEAR	STUDY	POPULATION	CRITERIA	PREVALENCE (%)
All AL residents					
Hawes et al.	1995		Board and care homes	CAI	21
Watson et al.	2003	Collaborative Studies of Long-Term Care	AL residents (n = 2078)	Cornell > 7	13
Watson et al.	2006	Maryland Assisted Living Study	AL residents (n = 198)	Cornell > 7	24
Rosenblatt et al.	2004	Maryland Assisted Living Study	AL residents (n = 198)	DSM-IV-TR criteria mood disorder	19
Dobbs et al.	2006		AL/RC residents (n = 366)	Chart review of diagnosed depression	22
Residents with dementia					
Edelman et al.	2004		Day care, NH, AL	Cornell > 7	24
Unpublished		Maryland Assisted Living Study	AL residents (n = 132)	Cornell ≥ 7	26
Gruber-Baldini et al.	2005	Collaborative Studies of Long-Term Care	Assisted living (n = 347)	Cornell ≥ 7	24

[a] Prevalence rate varied by type of facility.

Psychomotor changes and somatic items (i.e., multiple medical complaints) were also endorsed by 15% to 20% of residents (Watson et al., 2003).

Depressive disorders or symptoms often co-occur in individuals with dementia (Alexopoulos, 2005). Among residents with normal cognitive functioning (using a score of 1 or less on the MDS-COGS), one study found that approximately 7% of AL residents had clinically significant symptoms of depression, but rates were elevated significantly with increasing cognitive impairment (Watson et al., 2003). The prevalence of depression in the early stages of dementia (mild or moderate), such as that typically found in the AL population, is approximately 40% (Holtzer et al., 2005). The prevalence rates for depressive symptoms among residents with dementia by study are shown in Table 22.4. In all three studies, approximately one-quarter of residents with dementia had clinically significant depressive symptoms at the time of assessment.

A special consideration for AL residents is the potential for adjustment disorders that may be precipitated by the stress of moving from one setting to another. Adjustment disorders may present with features of mood, anxiety, or conduct disturbances and occur within 3 months of the stressor. While it makes sense intuitively that this would be a common condition given the magnitude of the life change for elders who move into AL, data on newly-admitted residents from the MD-AL study show that the prevalence is actually fairly low (4/202; 2% prevalence). This has also been corroborated by findings of low incident relocation stress among newly admitted nursing home and AL residents (Walker et al., 2007).

Correlates.   The presence of clinically significant depression has been associated with several resident characteristics including actual and perceived medical comorbidity, greater dependency in activities of daily living, less social participation/contact/support, less satisfaction with living environment, and shorter duration of stay in AL (Cummings & Cockerham, 2004; Watson et al., 2003, 2006). It has been suggested that those who have more negative internalized health beliefs are more likely to have greater depression than individuals with similar medical morbidity and dependency (Jang et al., 2007). Some new evidence suggests that greater resident influence over facility policies and involvement in facility administration is significantly associated with lower levels of depressive symptoms (Chen et al., 2007). In residents with dementia, depression appears to be related to severe cognitive impairment, behavioral symptoms, pain, and living in a for-profit facility (Gruber-Baldini et al., 2005).

Outcomes in AL Setting.   Several studies have shown that depression is related to discharge from AL to higher levels of care. For instance, AL residents with a psychiatric disorder (largely, mood disorders) were 1.78 times more likely to be discharged to a nursing home compared to residents without a psychiatric disorder (Dobbs et al., 2006). In another study, residents with depression were

1.5 times as likely to be discharged to a nursing home compared to nondepressed AL residents (Watson et al., 2003). Depression is also related to both subjective and proxy-rated quality of life (Samus et al., 2006; unpublished MD-AL data).

Anxiety Disorders, Psychotic Disorder, and Other Psychiatric Disorders

Anxiety disorders and primary psychotic disorders such as schizophrenia are less common than dementia or mood disorders in AL but are still an important consideration. In older adults in the community, the prevalence of diagnosable anxiety disorders is about 10%, with generalized anxiety disorders and specific phobias being the most prevalent (Ayers et al., 2007); however, 20% of older adults may experience clinically relevant symptoms of anxiety but do not meet criteria for a disorder (Himmelfarb & Murrell, 1984). Anxiety is often comorbid with depression and dementia, conditions very common in AL. Schizophrenia of all types is fairly uncommon in older adults in the community setting with estimates from the Epidemiologic Catchment Area of 0.1% (Regier et al., 1988). However, the disorder may be more common in residential care settings like AL where individuals receive more support.

Prevalence, Correlates, and Outcomes. Very few studies have examined the prevalence of these disorders in AL. One study based on chart review suggested that approximately 9% of AL residents had a diagnosed anxiety disorder. The MD-AL study, which used physician-directed clinical assessment, found that 13% of residents met DSM-IV criteria for an anxiety disorder (Rosenblatt et al., 2004) and 22% of all AL residents sampled suffered from at least one symptom of anxiety (Smith et al., unpublished). Similarly, this study found a prevalence rate of 12% for psychotic disorders (Rosenblatt et al., 2004). Sixteen percent of those with an active psychotic disorder, or 2% of the total sample, had schizophrenia (unpublished MD-AL data) and the prevalence of a psychotic disorder was much more common in smaller homes compared to large homes (Leroi et al., 2006). Individuals with schizophrenia in AL facilities tend to be younger, never married, males with less than high school education, who have suffered from a psychiatric illness for more than 21 years (Cadena, 2006). There are no published data available that assess outcomes related to anxiety disorders or psychotic disorders in the AL setting.

CARE OF MENTAL HEALTH CONDITIONS IN ASSISTED LIVING

The provision of person-centered care and individualized services that accommodate changing needs is a core principle of AL (ALQC, 1998; NCAL, 2001).

However, the adequacy and quality of care provided by AL in meeting this goal has been increasingly scrutinized, in part due to growing appreciation of the magnitude and consequences of mental health morbidity in this setting. Specifically, some policy makers worry that in the absence of uniform care standards, such as those implemented in NHs, ALs are poorly equipped to detect and manage residents who suffer from mental disorders. Others contend that regulation is best performed at the state-level and cite the problems created when SNFs were over-regulated. In making these decisions, several questions must be weighed. What are the elements that comprise "quality" care in the context of AL? What are the current practices for the provision of mental health care in AL? How do various elements of care affect AL resident outcomes and to what extent are they modifiable? In the following section, we address these questions by drawing on data from several empirical studies as well as evidence-based guidelines on the care of older adults with mental disorders.

Elements and Measures of Quality Mental Health Care in AL

Defining and measuring quality care in AL presents a formidable challenge because resident needs are so multifaceted and diverse (Sloane, Zimmerman, & Ory, 2001). For example, mental health conditions among assisted living residents are not only highly prevalent but are also of diverse types and severity. This diversity exists not only between individuals (such as the differences in characteristics and needs between a resident with mild AD and one with severe AD), but also within individuals over time as conditions change and progress. Psychiatric conditions also interact with residents' medical and functional comorbidities, further compounding variability. As a result, AL residents' care needs, treatment options, and goals are heterogeneous as a group and can be divergent with the passage of time. This presents AL with a significant challenge in providing appropriate and quality individualized care.

The first step is to identify basic elements that comprise appropriate mental health care in AL. We will focus on the example of dementia since it is the most common disorder in AL and highly prevalent in all types of facilities, but these principles can apply generally to many other mental health disorders prevalent in AL. The elements presented here are based on basic principles of dementia care and are not exhaustive, but they include what we consider the essential components of care *for the AL setting*. For example, we will not discuss the safety issue of living alone, because residents of AL no longer have this need.

These elements are based on several sources including Practical Dementia Care (Rabins et al., 2006), the position statement for the American Association for Geriatric Psychiatry (Lyketsos et al., 2006), and the Alzheimer's Association (Alzheimer's Association, 2007). The elements and measures specific to AL are given in Table 22.5. From a clinical standpoint, these elements are targeted at

TABLE 22.5. Mental Health-Related Components and Measures of Care Used in the Study

KEY CARE COMPONENT	EXAMPLES OF MEASURES OF CARE
Structure	
Care setting philosophy that addresses mental health needs	Tolerant admission and discharge policies for residents exhibiting cognitive, psychological, and behavioral symptoms of mental health disorders; the degree of freedom choice and privacy
Therapeutic physical environment	Features that provide safety and security, orientation, sensory stimulation, comfort, social and assistive resources
External mental health-related support	Linkages with home health agencies, mental health providers, family support networks such as the Alzheimer's association; Proximity of health care facilities, senior centers, day care
Administrative environment	Direct care staff levels/ratios, turnover, salary
Revenues	Fee scale structure, rates, payer mix
Caregiver training and support in mental health disorders	AL staff certification, frequency and type of training, knowledge, levels/ratios, schedules, and turnover
Process	
Providing for general non-health-related needs	Provision of services such as meal preparation, housekeeping, laundry
Providing therapeutic and stimulating activities	Access to various leisure and therapeutic activities such as exercise class, current event discussions; active encouragement of family involvement; Access to physical therapy, speech therapy, occupational therapy
Providing for general health-related needs	Routine medical assessment; Medication assistance/administration, wellness checks, access to on-site medical care
Providing therapy for mental health-specific needs	Routine assessment of cognitive and behavioral symptoms; care planning for mental health evaluations; Use of specific non-pharmacological interventions and pharmacological therapies for specific disorders and symptoms

Source: Zimmerman, Sheryl, PhD, Philip D. Sloane, MD, MPH, and J. Kevin Eckert, PhD, eds. Foreword by M. Powell Lawton. *Assisted Living: Needs, Practices, and Policies in Residential Care for the Elderly.* p. 256. Table 11.4. © 2001 The Johns Hopkins University Press. Reprinted with permission of The Johns Hopkins University Press.

several crucial activities of care including recognition and assessment, management and treatment, and prevention. In addressing each of these elements, it is prudent (as well as challenging) to consider the influence of social, environmental, medical, and psychological factors since these often affect the course, treatment options, and outcomes (Rabins et al., 2006).

Sloane and colleagues (2001) have applied a popular theoretical approach to organize elements of quality care in the AL setting on the basis of three dimensions: structure, process, and outcome (Donabedian, 1966). Using their framework and conceptualizations (Sloane et al., 2001), structure (input) represents characteristics of the setting in which care is provided. Process relates to the actions and procedures that comprise the actual delivery of care. Finally, outcomes refer to resident characteristics that are hypothesized to be impacted by care. In the context of mental health care, examples of outcomes may be the presence and severity of psychiatric or cognitive symptoms, degree of functional impairment, retention in AL, suicidalty, quality of life, and satisfaction with care. This organizational scheme is employed in Table 22.5.

We will also use this framework to augment the presentation of data on current AL practices in relation to mental health care, beginning with those currently being practiced by AL that are theorized to represent good general mental health care for the broad gamut of psychiatric conditions, followed by a discussion of care elements regarded as important for the treatment of dementia and depression. We focus on these conditions since these are the two most common in AL. As Sloane and colleagues (2001) caution, these care elements are based on theory and practice guidelines, but their effects on actual resident outcomes have not yet been empirically validated in many cases.

Elements of General Mental Health Care in Current Practice

Structure of care elements

Several structure elements are germane to general mental health. These include formal AL policies that address mental health needs, the therapeutic attributes of the physical environment, and characteristics of the care providers. AL admission and discharge policies are variable at the state and provider level that usually take into account a broad range of factors related to resident health-care needs (Mollica et al., 2005). Survey data suggest that issues related to mental health are a major focus of admission and discharge policies that are in place based on responses from AL providers. For example, in a survey of 94 AL administrators in Michigan, slightly less than half (47%) reported they would be willing to admit or retain an individual who had recently had a psychiatric hospitalization (Wagenaar et al., 2003). On the other hand, specific behavioral disturbances such as physical aggressiveness, social or sexual inappropriateness, and verbally abusive behaviors have been identified by approximately three quarters of the facilities in surveys as problems that would hamper the admittance and subsequent retention of residents (Hawes et al., 2000; Wagenaar et al., 2003). Other behaviors linked to denial of admission and premature discharge included wandering, screaming, and resistance to help with ADLs (Hawes et al., 2000; Wagenaar et al., 2003).

Impairment in activities of daily living is also routinely considered in admittance and discharge policies. This impairment must be understood as a frequent complication of dementia, and not only as a result of orthopedic or general health problems. Greater than one-third of large facilities from a national survey reported that they were not willing to admit residents who were incontinent or needed help with locomotion and over half of these facilities reported that they were unwilling to admit an individual who needed assistance in transferring (Hawes et al., 2000). In an earlier national study, Kane and Wilson (1993) reported that only 50% of assisted living facilities would retain residents who needed help eating. National survey results suggest that slightly over one half of facilities had policies in place that would impede the admission and retention of individuals with moderate to severe cognitive impairment (Hawes et al., 2000).

Physical plant characteristics that provide comfort, safety, and sensory stimulation are also highly variable in AL. The most common type of living arrangements are a one bedroom studio or efficiency unit with a full private bathroom (Hawes et al., 2000; Sloane, Zimmerman, & Walsh, 2001; NCAL, 2006), and a significant minority (41%) of resident accommodations are apartment type units (Hawes et al., 2001). Sharing with an unrelated individual is uncommon but not unheard of; 21% of apartments were found to be shared by unrelated individuals (Hawes et al., 2000). Not surprisingly, the majority (80%) of smaller homes tended to have "very homelike" public areas compared to 30% in traditional and 58% in new model facilities, respectively (Sloane, Zimmerman, & Walsh, 2001).

Use of safety devices that may benefit those with mental health conditions is common in AL environments. In a national survey of facilities with more than 10 beds, 82% of residents had access to a call button in their bedrooms and 78% had handrails in their bathrooms. Data from the CS-LTC suggests that use of safety devices may vary by setting type. For instance, only 23% of AL rooms in small facilities (<16 beds) had call buttons, whereas 64% and 73% were equipped with that feature in traditional and new-model homes, respectively (Sloane, Zimmerman, & Walsh, 2001). This trend also applies to the moderate or extensive use of handrails in hallways where 32%, 71%, and 83% of small, traditional, and new-model facilities respectively had this safety feature in place (Sloane, Zimmerman, & Walsh, 2001).

The minimization of adverse sensory stimulation is another important environmental feature for individuals with mental disorders. Data from the CS-LTC show that in the majority of facilities (>75%), residents screaming or calling, staff talking loudly, loudspeaker/intercom, or alarm bells were not heard in most public areas. However, loud noise from a TV or radio was quite common (60%–79%) (Sloane, Zimmerman, & Walsh, 2001). On the whole, about half of the facilities from this study provided pleasant or engaging tactile stimuli (public areas rated as having "extensive" or "quite a bit" of) and about two-thirds had visual stimuli that met this criterion (Sloane, Zimmerman, & Walsh, 2001).

Staff characteristics relevant to the care of residents with mental health problems can be divided into several categories: certification, specific training/ knowledge, and staff levels/ratios. Certification requirements for direct care staff in AL are determined by state regulations and, in fact, as of 2000 most states did not require this certification (Hodlewsky, 2001). Available data suggests that approximately 71% of AL facilities have an RN or LPN on staff either full-time or part-time (Hawes et al., 1999) and that between 40% and 47% have at least one full-time staff member of this type (Hawes et al., 1999; Zimmerman, Sloane, Eckert et al., 2005). The majority of staff in AL are those that provide hands-on care (Hawes et al., 2000). These staff have various designations including nursing or resident care assistants, medication technicians, or resident care coordinators (Hawes et al., 2000). Some states require either a certified nursing assistant certificate or the completion of some other comparable training program for an individual to be involved in direct care (Hodlewsky, 2001).

The content and extent of training required for AL staff is regulated by the states, but varies to a large degree (Hodlewsky, 2001). For the most part, very little training is required. One survey reported that the most common extent ranged from 1 to 16 training hours and the majority of the training was provided on the job (Hawes et al., 2000). The most common training topics included resident rights (96%), how to provide personal care (92%), information about dealing with behavior problems (83%), information about Alzheimer's disease (80%), and first aid (79%). Skill training related to medication management was less common (67%) (Hawes et al., 2000). There are little data available on requirements for follow-up or ongoing training.

As part of the same survey, staff training and knowledge about mental health issues was assessed (Hawes et al., 2000). Surprisingly, 88% of staff reported that symptoms of confusion were a normal part of aging. Further, 78% and 63% of staff reported that depression and anger, respectively, were normal for older persons. Staff were even less informed about psychotropic medications. Less than half of staff (48%) involved in medication administration were able to identify psychotropic medication side effects that should be reported to supervisory staff and 21% reported that they had no idea what adverse symptoms should be reported when administrating these types of medications (Hawes et al., 2000). This is particularly troubling because prevalence estimates show that 47% of residents are on at least one psychotropic agent (Lakey et al., 2006).

In terms of staff ratios, nearly all facilities have 24-h staff on duty (NCAL, 2001) and the median staff ratios for direct care staff in facilities with 11 beds or more is about 1:14 (Hawes et al., 2000). Staff ratios are generally highest during the first shift (early morning to late afternoon) and lowest at night (Hawes et al., 2000). In the CS-LTC, the number of care hours per resident per day was calculated for various staff types. Levels for RN and LPNs ranged from 0.11 to 0.17 care h/resident/day. The average aide care hours per resident per day were approximately 1.52 (Zimmerman et al., 2005). Interestingly, data from the MD-AL study suggests that for residents without dementia, a little over 2 h per day of care was required but, if dementia was present, this care time more than doubled (4.3 h) (Rosenblatt et al., 2004). This suggests that the current staff ratios may be overburdening workers. In fact, some residents with greater needs are contracting with nonfacility staff for care.

Consistency of staff may also be related to the quality of mental health care. Turnover of direct staff is considered a major issue in the AL industry. In a national survey of administrators, about 50% of the entire staff had been employed by the facility for 2 years or more, but turnover for the aides (direct care staff) was estimated at 25% and one in five aides had only been on the job less than 6 months (Hawes et al., 2000). Data from the CS-LTC suggests an even higher turnover rate among care aides, up to 68% (Zimmerman et al., 2005).

Process of care elements for dementia

Elements associated with the process of care in AL include services targeted at both non–health- and health-related needs and the provision of therapeutic and stimulating activities. Non–health-related services frequently provided by ALs include the provision of meals and snacks, housekeeping and laundry services, as well as transportation to locations off site (Hawes et al., 1995, 1999; NCAL, 2001). The vast majority of ALs report providing health care–related services including assistance with ADLs, medication administration and storage, nursing services, resident health assessments, health monitoring/wellness checks, and transportation to medical care (Hawes, et al., 1999; NCAL, 2001). Skilled nursing care and hospice services are available in the majority of facilities, 60% and 75% respectively, but these services are contracted out with home health agencies. Provisions for these services also vary on the basis of individual state policy (NCAL, 2001). Various forms of therapeutic services such as speech, occupational, physical therapy are seldom provided by facility staff but are often available through arrangement with contract staff (Hawes et al., 1999; NCAL, 2001). Virtually all facilities taking part in the NCAL survey in 2000 reported offering organized social and recreational activities (100%), exercise classes (93%), and group outings (92%); however, this is likely variable by definition since other estimates suggest that social and recreational activities are available in about 51% of facilities (Zimmerman et al., 2005).

There are little available data on mental health specific services. One small survey from a single state suggests that 66% of facilities perform some type of mental health assessment at admission and 54% of these reassess either quarterly or yearly. Sixty percent of providers in this study identified the residents' primary care physician as the most common provider of mental health service followed by 48% by a psychiatrist and 43% by community mental health agencies (Wagenaar et al., 2003). Only a little over a quarter (28%) of AL facilities in the CS-LTC study involved a mental health professional in formal care planning (Gruber-Baldini et al., 2005).

Care Specific to Residents with Dementia and Related Neuropsychiatric symptoms

Overview of principles of dementia management

The guiding principles for the management of dementia and related neuropsychiatric symptoms, including the use of medications have been discussed in detail in other works (Lyketsos et al., 2006; Rabins et al., 2006; Waldemar et al., 2007) and will not be discussed here in depth.

In a residential setting, such as an AL, nonpharmacological interventions are a crucial component of the overall management of dementia. These techniques include the creation of a routine daily schedule, environmental modifications, attention to safety for the prevention of accidents and falls, adequate nutrition and hydration, support in ADLs, good sleeping habits, access to primary care with follow-up as needed, and the employment of specific interpersonal approaches by caregivers (Buhr & White, 2006; Rabins et al., 2006). According to a recent systematic review, cognitive stimulation, improved socialization, and behavior management techniques centered on the patient's behaviors were some of the most effective interventions for neuropsychiatric symptoms in randomized controlled trials (Livingston et al., 2005). These therapies are especially effective when applied as part of a multicomponent disease management regimen. Selection of pharmacologic and nonpharmacologic therapies should be based on the unique characteristics of the patient, the facility-specific setting, the severity of the symptoms, and the likelihood of a therapeutic response (Lyketsos et al., 2006). When applied appropriately and systematically, the cumulative effects of these interventions can be quite significant.

Structure of care elements for dementia

Staff training and knowledge regarding the detection of dementia is highly pertinent. States are increasingly mandating dementia training requirements for both new and existing AL care staff (Mollica et al., 2005). Studies show that the majority of direct care staff in AL report that they have received some type of training or information on dementia and behavior management (Hawes et al., 2000; Sloane, Zimmerman, & Ory, 2001), and one study reported that the vast majority (97%) felt they were able to assess these problems adequately (Boustani et al., 2005). However, the content of the training varies greatly and it remains unclear how effectively the training translates into practice. There is evidence that despite training staff are still not well equipped to differentiate dementia from other conditions including normal aging (Hawes et al., 2000). Data from the MD-AL study show that direct care staff failed to detect dementia in nearly one-quarter (22%) of residents who met DSM-IV criteria for dementia, residents who had an average MMSE score of 18.6. Dementia detection rates were slightly better in smaller facilities compared to larger facilities (87% vs. 74%, respectively), a finding that may be related to the increased amount of daily resident-caregiver contact in smaller homes (Leroi et al., 2006). Caregiver unawareness of dementia was predicted by several resident characteristics including being male, better cognition, fewer neuropsychiatric symptoms, and less functional impairment (Maust et al., 2006). Staff education on recognition, in tandem with routine use of cognitive screening measures such as the MMSE or the MDS-COGS, may improve detection in AL, especially since these measures have been shown to have reasonable sensitivity and specificity in this population (Zimmerman et al., 2007).

Environmental modifications are another structural element of dementia care in AL. These may include use of controlled exits to reduce chances of elopement (34%–56% prevalence; Sloane, Zimmerman, & Ory, 2001) , use of strategic lay-out of the living space (e.g., open doors, bathrooms in line of sight), objects for visual cueing to improve orientation, specialized lighting, and provision of objects that promote continuity with the past for the individual with dementia (Day et al., 2000; Sloane, Zimmerman, & Ory, 2001).

Process of care elements for dementia

Elements associated with the process of care for AL residents include the evaluation of dementia and related neuropsychiatric symptoms and the subsequent provision of therapy. In the only study to have estimated the completeness of dementia evaluation, Rosenblatt and colleagues (2004) reported that 73% of residents with dementia had a complete evaluation as determined by the study's interdisciplinary consensus panel, 13% had only a partial evaluation, and 14% had no discernible evaluation. Overall treatment of dementia was also rated in this study and included the consideration of both pharmacological and nonpharmacological treatments. A little over half (52%) of residents with dementia were rated as being completely treated, 33% were partially treated, and 15% were receiving no treatment at all (Rosenblatt et al., 2004). Predictors of nontreatment of dementia in this study included family and caregiver unawareness of dementia (Maust et al., 2006). This study also demonstrated that among individuals with dementia who were followed for approximately 18 months, those who had received dementia treatment remained in AL an average of 7 months longer than those who received no treatment (Lyketsos et al., 2007). Together these findings suggest that appropriate dementia treatment has beneficial effects on resident-level outcomes such as the ability to age in place but is contingent on staff and family recognition of the disorder.

Nonpharmacological interventions *specific to dementia care* such as bedrails, physical restraints, and wandering protection are used fairly infrequently in ALs that are not designated as dementia-specific care areas (DSCAs) (DSCAs will be discussed subsequently). The use of bedrails among residents with dementia in the MD-AL study was about 12%, with smaller facilities being more likely to employ them (17%) compared to larger facilities (6%) (Leroi et al., 2006). Observational data show that rates of use of restraints for persons with moderate to severe dementia is also low, ranging from 2% to 11% depending on facility type (i.e., traditional, new model, small) (Leroi et al., 2006; Sloane et al., 2001). This may be a desirable finding since it suggests that ALs are managing symptoms without compromising individual freedom of movement.

Safety measures related to elopement and wandering are also important elements of care for individuals with dementia. Such measures may include items of clothing or jewelry that make high-risk residents identifiable by AL staff (such as a brightly colored bracelet), video surveillance systems, electronic bracelets that alert staff if a resident enters certain areas, or bed alarms. However, we could find no data on the prevalence of use of such device in AL.

Several studies have documented the use of pharmacological therapies among AL residents with dementia. In studies of AL residents with a documented chart diagnosis of dementia, the prevalence of ACI (acetylcholinesterase) prescriptions ranged from 35% to 59% (Boustani et al., 2005; Carlson et al., 2005; Magsi & Malloy, 2006). However, these figures may be overestimates of ACI treatment since evidence suggests that up to 63% of residents with cognitive impairment do not have a chart diagnosis (Magsi & Malloy, 2006). In the MD-AL study, which used DSM-IV criteria to determine the dementia diagnosis and sub-type, 33% of residents with a dementia of any type were taking an ACI, and the specificity of ACI use (32% use prevalence) did not improve among residents regarded by the study as having AD. Rates of ACI treatment did rise to 50%, however among those with AD who had a MMSE of greater than 16 (Rosenblatt et al., 2007). ACI use among residents with AD, the type of dementia for which these agents are currently indicated, was significantly associated with better retention in AL at 6 months compared to residents with AD who were not taking those agents. Further, it has been found that when these agents are prescribed, the dose is not fully titrated in a significant number of patients (Rosenblatt et al., 2004; Magsi & Malloy, 2006), bringing into question whether the potentially beneficial effects of these medications in this setting could be optimized with more vigilance on the part of the prescriber. There are no data yet on the patterns of memantine use (another, more recently introduced therapeutic agent for AD) in the AL setting.

In regard the to the nonpharmacological treatment of neuropsychiatric symptoms, one long-term care study found that comprehensive behavioral management techniques carried out principally by direct care workers (CNAs) during ADL care resulted in impressive improvements in disruptive vocalizations, restlessness, and physical aggression among nursing home residents (Burgio et al., 2002). However, a randomized trial testing an approach such as this has not yet been undertaken in AL. This should be viewed as a priority, since for reasons of safety, effective nonpharmacological interventions are usually the initial focus of treatment care plans.

Pharmacological treatment of dementia-related neuropsychiatric symptoms with psychotropic medication is fairly common in AL. Among residents with neuropsychiatric disturbances who had a mental health diagnosis (i.e., dementia, depression, psychosis, other psychiatric disorder by chart review), the CS-LTC study found that 68% of residents were receiving a psychotropic medication (Gruber-Baldini et al., 2004). Among those in this sample with an active neuropsychiatric disturbance who had dementia specifically, 43% were taking a neuroleptic, 37% an antidepressant, and 26% a hypnotic (Boustani et al., 2005). Of note, this study also reported that 9% of those who did not have a mental diagnosis or evidence of a behavioral disturbance were taking a psychotropic medication (Gruber-Baldini et al., 2004). At this point it is difficult to draw conclusions regarding the quality of psychotropic use, but longitudinal studies are underway that may shed more light on this question.

Structure and process of dementia care in dementia-specific special care units

Dementia-specific special care units (SCUs) in AL have proliferated and are being increasingly marketed (Davis et al., 2000). Generally, dementia SCUs are segregated areas that accommodate only cognitively impaired persons and that offer one or more special features specific to dementia care, such as specialized activity programming, staff selection and training, and special design features such as controlled or camouflaged exits (Day et al., 2000). Despite the recent increase in popularity of SCUs for the care of individuals with dementia, there is a dearth of information on the structure and process of care for persons with dementia within these settings. What few data exist come from the CS-LTC. Policies for admission and retention of individuals in relation to behavioral disturbances were observed to be more flexible in SCUs as compared to non-SCUs, yet the prevalence of therapeutic modifications of the physical environment did not appear to differ much between settings, with the exception of a higher use of controlled exits in SCUs (Sloane et al., 2001). Resident-level process of care elements such as physical restraints, ACI use, antipsychotic use (i.e., neuroleptics), or use of other psychotropic medications did not appear to differ between settings either (Sloane et al., 2001; Zimmerman et al., 2005) nor were any differences found in 1-year health or functional outcomes between residents in SCUs and in non-SCUs. However, as the authors imply, further and more extensive examinations of SCUs are needed to better understand the potential benefits of these environments on other types of outcomes.

Care Specific to Residents with Depression

Overview of management of depression among older adults

In general, the principles guiding the care of older adults with depression are similar to those in younger adults and are described in detail elsewhere (Salzman, 2000; Alexopoulos, 2005). Treatments for depression include behavioral rehabilitation, psychotherapy, and pharmacotherapy and are aimed at alleviation of symptoms of depression and prevention of relapse, prevention of suicidal ideation, improvement of cognition and function, and development of appropriate coping skills for affected individuals who are dealing with psychosocial adversity or disability (Bartels et al., 2003).

Structure and process of care elements for depression

Although depression is the second most prevalent psychiatric disorder in AL, data are scant on the elements of structure and process for care of depression in this setting. As in other mental health disorders, staff training for the detection of depression is crucial for treatment. In the CS-LTC, less than half (48%) of AL facilities had >75% of all supervisory staff or direct care staff participate in formalized training (Gruber-Baldini et al., 2005). Despite this, the majority of staff felt that they were able to detect depression. However, in a sample of AL residents with dementia found to be currently depressed using a CSDD cutoff of >7, only 42% were recognized by staff. Of this group, 44% had a professional mental health workup and fewer (40%) had a written or standardized assessment in the past year (Gruber-Baldini et al., 2005).

Rates for the provision of treatment for depression are similar to those for dementia. Among AL residents with dementia who were currently depressed, only 28% had any formal mental health treatment by a professional (could include psychiatrist, psychologist, mental health social workers, physician or anyone defined as a professional mental health worker by facility supervisor). However, 37% had a mental health professional involved in care planning (Gruber-Baldini et al., 2005).

Treatment rates for nonpharmacological interventions (defined as any other reported nonpharmaceutical treatment including medical care, emotional or social support, and recreational activities) among those with dementia who were currently depressed was 58%. By comparison, 54% of this depressed group was receiving antidepressant pharmacotherapy (Gruber-Baldini et al., 2005). In contrast, among all AL residents with current depression (regardless of dementia status) in the CS-LTC, where the cutoff for depression was 1-point higher, only 18% were taking antidepressants. This treatment rate rose to just 38% in severe cases (CSDD >12) (Watson et al., 2003). Treatment rates for depression in the MD-AL study were somewhat higher even when applying the same CSDD criteria. Forty-three percent of those currently depressed were receiving antidepressants (Watson et al., 2006). Residents with depression had poorer outcomes than those not depressed and were 1.5 times more likely to be discharged to nursing homes. Rates of mortality were also higher for depressed residents, but only those with severe depression (CSDD >12) had a statistically significant increased rate of death (Watson et al., 2006).

CONCLUSIONS AND IMPLICATIONS

Mental health conditions, particularly dementia and depression, are extremely common in the AL setting and have serious adverse consequences, most notably risk of discharge to nursing homes and decreased quality of life. Available evidence suggests that these conditions are being under-recognized, and that many ALs lack adequate structure of care elements such as staff programming and training protocols, which are effective in the detection of these conditions. The treatment of these disorders, including process of care elements such as symptom evaluation, mental health services, and the provision of specific pharmacological and nonpharamacological interventions, is often problematic.

Given this situation, what are the implications for the future of AL? First, AL continues to grapple with its de facto role as a *setting of health care* and is in a state of continual evolution. At this point, state policies are beginning to reflect and respond to new data as they become available from public health researchers, and thus far the AL industry has avoided federal regulations in the United States—but for how long is unknown. Regulatory decisions are best made in the presence of sound empirical data; thus, interested stakeholders would benefit from more research on how well specific elements of care predict important resident outcomes. These data will come in the form of further longitudinal studies, which relate resident outcomes to elements of structure and process of care and from randomized controlled trials testing interventions that could be implemented in this setting. In the meantime, discussions should continue between the AL industry, professional health care providers, consumer advocacy groups, policy makers, and public health researchers about how quality mental health care can be delivered in a cost-effective and efficient manner. Finally, concerted efforts must be made to link ALs with the other health systems such as primary and community mental health care. These natural and sustainable collaborations would promote a higher level of coordinated care for the AL resident.

Acknowledgments   We wish to thank Megan Schultz and Kelly Sloane for their assistance.

REFERENCES

Albert, M. S., & Blacker, D. (2006). Mild cognitive impairment and dementia. *Annual Review of Clinical Psychology, 2*(1), 379–388.

Alexopoulos, G. (2005). Depression in the elderly. *The Lancet, 365*, 1961–1970.

Alexopoulos, G. S., Abrams, R. C., Young, R. C., & Shamoian, C. A. (1988). Cornell scale for depression in dementia. *Biological Psychiatry, 23*(3), 271.

Alzheimer's Association. (2007). Dementia Care Practice Recommendations for Assisted Living Residences and Nursing Homes: Phase 3 End of Life Care [Electronic Version]. *Alzheimer's Association Campaign for Quality Residential Care.* Retrieved January 10, 2008 from http://www.alz.org/documents/DCPRPhase3_.pdf.

American Association for Retired Persons. (2002). *In brief: Before the boom: Trends in long-term supportive services for older Americans with disabilities.* Washington, DC: Author.

American Psychiatric Association. (2000). *(DSM-IV-TR) Diagnostic and statistical manual of mental disorders,* (4th ed.). text revision. Washington, DC: American Psychiatric Press.

Assisted Living Quality Coalition. (1998). *Assisted living quality initiative: Building a structure that promotes quality.* Washington, DC .

Arling, G., & Williams, A. (2003). Cognitive impairment and resource use of nursing home residents: A structural equation model. *Medical Care, 41*(7), 802–812.

Assisted Living Quality Coalition. (1998). *Assisted living quality initiative: Building a structure that promotes quality.* Washington, DC.

Astrom, S., Karlsson, S., Sandvide, A., Bucht, G., Eisemann, M., Norberg, A., et al. (2004). Staff's experience of and the management of violent incidents in elderly care. *Scandinavian Journal of Caring Sciences, 18*(4), 410–416.

Ayers, C. R., Sorrell, J. T., Thorp, S. R., & Wetherell, J. L. (2007). Evidence-based psychological treatments for late-life anxiety. *Psychology and Aging, 22*(1), 8–17.

Bartels, S., Dums, A., Oxman, T., Schneider, L., Areán, P., Alexopoulos, G., et al. (2003). Evidence-based practices in geriatric mental health care: An overview of systematic reviews and meta-analyses. *Psychiatry Clinics of North America, 26*(4), 971–990.

Bishop, C. E. (1999). Where are the missing elders? The decline in nursing home use, 1985 and 1995. *Health Affairs, 18*(4), 146–155.

Boustani, M., Zimmerman, S., Williams, C. S., Gruber-Baldini, A. L., Watson, L., Reed, P. S., et al. (2005). Characteristics associated with behavioral symptoms related to dementia in long-term care residents. *Gerontologist, 45*(suppl_1), 56–61.

Brookmeyer, R., Gray, S., & Kawas, C. (1998). Projections of Alzheimer's disease in the United States and the public health impact of delaying onset. *American Journal of Public Health, 88* (9), 1337–1342.

Bruce, D. G., Paley, G. A., Nichols, P., Roberts, D., Underwood, P. J., & Schaper, F. (2005). Physical disability contributes to caregiver stress in dementia caregivers. *Journals of Gerontology series A: Biological Sciences and Medical Sciences, 60*(3), 345–349.

Burdick, D. J., Rosenblatt, A., Samus, Q. M., Steele, C., Baker, A., Harper, M., et al. (2005). Predictors of functional impairment in residents of assisted-living facilities: The Maryland Assisted Living Study. *Journals of Gerontology series A: Biological Sciences and Medical Sciences, 60*(2), 258–264.

Burgio, L. D., Fisher, S. E., Fairchild, J. K., Scilley, K., & Hardin, J. M. (2004). Quality of care in the nursing home: Effects of staff assignment and work shift. *Gerontologist, 44*(3), 368–377.

Buhr, G. T., & White, H. K. (2006). Difficult behaviors in long-term care patients with dementia. *Journal of the American Medical Directors Association, 7*(3), 180–192.

Burgio, L. D., Stevens, A., Burgio, K. L., Roth, D. L., Paul, P., & Gerstle, J. (2002). Teaching and maintaining behavior management skills in the nursing home. *Gerontologist, 42*(4), 487–496.

Cadena, S. V. (2006). Living among strangers: The needs and functioning of persons with schizophrenia residing in an assisted living facility. *Issues in Mental Health Nursing, 27*(1), 25–41.

Carlson, J. M., Gerding, G., Estoup, M. W. (2005). Evaluation of demographics and medication use in patients with dementia in assisted living and skilled nursing facilities. *The Consultant Pharmacist, 20*(7), 584–594.

Chen, C. K., Zimmerman, S., Sloane, P. D., & Barrick, A. L. (2007). Assisted living policies promoting autonomy and their relationship to resident depressive symptoms. *American Journal of Geriatric Psychiatry, 15*(2), 122–129.

Coleman, B.J. (1995). European models of long-term care in the home and community. *International Journal of Health Services, 25*(3), 255–74.

Cummings, S., & Cockerham, C. (2004). Depression and life satisfaction in assisted living residents: Impact of health and social support. *Clinical Gerontologist, 27,* 25–42.

Davis, K. J., Sloane, P. D., Mitchell, C. M., Preisser, J., Grant, L., Hawes, M. C., et al. (2000). Specialized dementia programs in residential care settings. *Gerontologist, 40*(1), 32–42.

Day, K., Carreon, D., & Stump, C. (2000). The therapeutic design of environments for people with dementia: A review of the empirical research. *Gerontologist, 40*(4), 397–416.

Dobbs, D., Hayes, J., Chapin, R., & Oslund, P. (2006). The relationship between psychiatric disorders and the ability to age in place in assisted living. *American Journal of Geriatric Psychiatry , 14*(7), 613–620.

Donabedian, A. (1966). Evaluating the quality of medical care. *Milbank Memorial Fund Quarterly, 44,* 166–206.

Edelman, P., Kuhn, D., & Fulton, B. (2004). Influence of cognitive impairment, functional impairment and care setting on dementia care mapping results. *Aging Mental Health, 8*(6), 514–523.

Golant, S. M. (2004). Do impaired older persons with health care needs occupy U.S. Assisted living facilities? An analysis of six national studies. *Journal of Gerontology Series B Psychological Sciences and Social Sciences, 59*(2), S68–79.

González-Salvador, T., Lyketsos, C. G., Baker, A., Hovanec, L., Roques, C., Brandt, J., et al. (2000). Quality of life in dementia patients in long-term care. *International Journal of Geriatric Psychiatry, 15*(2), 181–189.

Gruber-Baldini, A. L., Boustani, M., Sloane, P. D., & Zimmerman, S. (2004). Behavioral symptoms in residential care/assisted living facilities: prevalence, risk factors, and medication management. *Journal of the American Geriatrics Society, 52*(10), 1610–1617.

Gruber-Baldini, A. L., Zimmerman, S., Boustani, M., Watson, L. C., Williams, C. S., & Reed, P. S. (2005). characteristics associated with depression in long-term care residents with dementia. *Gerontologist, 45*(suppl_1), 50–55.

Hawes, C. (2001). Introduction. In S. Zimmerman, P. D. Sloane & J. K. Eckert (Eds.), *Assisted living: Needs, practices, and policies in residential care for the elderly.* Baltimore, MD: The Johns Hopkins University Press.

Hawes, C., Lux, L., Wildfire, J., Green, R., Mor, V., Greene, A., et al. (1995). *A description of board and care facilities, operators, and residents.* Research Triangle Park, N.C.: U.S. Department of Health and Human Services, Research Triangle Institute, Brown University.

Hawes, C., & Phillips, C. (2007). Defining quality in assisted living: Comparing apples, oranges, and broccoli. *The Gerontologist, 47*(Special Issue III), 40–50.

Hawes, C., Phillips, C. D., & Rose, M. (2000). *High service or high privacy assisted living facilities, their residents and staff: Results from a national survey*: Washington, DC: Myers Research Institute.

Hawes, C., Phillips, C. D., Rose, M., Holan, S., & Sherman, M. (2003). A national survey of assisted living facilities. *Gerontologist, 43*(6), 875–882.

Hawes, C., Rose, M., & Phillips, C. (1999). *A national study of assisted living for the frail elderly: Results from a national survey of facilities.* Washington, DC: Myers Research Institute.

Himmelfarb, S., & Murrell, S. (1984). The prevalence and correlates of anxiety symptoms in older adults. *The Journal of psychology., 116*((2d Half)), 159–167.

Hodlewsky, R. (2001). Staffing problems and strategies in assisted living. In S. Zimmerman, P. D. Sloane & J. K. Eckert (Eds.), *Assisted living: Needs, practices, and policies in residential care for the elderly* (pp. 78–91). Baltimore: The Johns Hopkins University Press.

Holtzer, R., Scarmeas, N., Wegesin, D. J., Albert, M., Brandt, J., Dubois, B., et al. (2005). Depressive symptoms in Alzheimer's disease: Natural course and temporal relation to function and cognitive status. *Journal of the American Geriatrics Society, 53*(12), 2083–2089.

Jang, Y., Bergman, E., Schonfeld, L., & Molinari, V. (2007). The mediating role of health perceptions in the relation between physical and mental health: A study of older residents in assisted living facilities. *Journal of Aging and Health, 19*(3), 439–452.

Kane, R., & Wilson, K. (1993). *Assisted living in the United States: A new paradigm for residential care for frail older people?* American Association for Retired Persons.

Karlsson. (1996). Treatment of noncognitive symptoms in dementia. *Acta Neurologica Scandinavica, 168*, 93–95.

Katzman, R. & Fox, P. (1999). The worldwide impact of dementia in the next fifty years. In R. Mayeux, Y. Christen (Eds), *Epidemiology of Alzheimer's disease: From gene to prevention.* New York: Springer-Verlag.

Lair, T., & Lefkowitz, D. (1990). *Mental Health and Functional Status of Residents of Nursing and Personal Care Homes (DHHS): National Medical Expenditure Survey Research Findings,* (No. PHS-90-3470). Rockville, MD: Department of Health and Human Services.

Lakey, S. L., Gray, S. L., Sales, A. E. B., Sullivan, J., & Hedrick, S. C. (2006). Psychotropic use in community residential care facilities: A prospective cohort study. *The American Journal of Geriatric Pharmacotherapy, 4*(3), 227–235.

Leroi, I., Samus, Q. M., Rosenblatt, A., Onyike, C. U., Brandt, J., Baker, A. S., et al. (2006). A comparison of small and large assisted living facilities for the diagnosis and care of dementia: The Maryland Assisted Living Study. *International Journal of Geriatric Psychiatry, 22*(3), n/a.

Livingston, G., Johnston, K., Katona, C., Paton, J., Lyketsos, C. G., & Old Age Task Force of the World Federation of Biological, P. (2005). Systematic review of psychological approaches to the management of neuropsychiatric symptoms of dementia. *American Journal of Psychiatry, 162*(11), 1996–2021.

Lyketsos, C., Colenda, C., Beck, C., Blank, K., Doraiswamy, M., Kalunian, D., et al. (2006). Task Force of American Association for Geriatric Psychiatry position statement of the American Association for Geriatric Psychiatry regarding principles of care for patients with dementia resulting from Alzheimer disease. *American Journal of Geriatric Psychiatry, 14*(7), 561–572.

Lyketsos, C. G., Samus, Q. M., Baker, A., McNabney, M., Onyike, C. U., Mayer, L. S., et al. (2007). Effect of dementia and treatment of dementia on time to discharge from assisted living facilities: The Maryland Assisted Living Study. *Journal of the American Geriatrics Society, 55*(7), 1031–1037.

Magsi, H., & Malloy, T. (2005). Underrecognition of cognitive impairment in assisted living facilities. *Journal of the American Geriatrics Society, 53*(2), 295–298.

Maust, D. T., Onyike, C. U., Sheppard, J.-M. E., Mayer, L. S., Samus, Q. M., Brandt, J., et al. (2006). Predictors of caregiver unawareness and nontreatment of dementia among residents of assisted living facilities: The Maryland Assisted Living Study. *American Journal of Geriatric Psychiatry, 14*(8), 668–675.

Mollica, R. (2002). State assisted living policy: 2002. Retrieved January 19, 2007, from http://www.nashp.org/Files/ltc_15_AL_2002.pdf

Mollica, R., Johnson-Lamarche, H., & O'Keeffe, J. (2005). *State residential care and assisted living policy: 2004.* Washington, D.C.: U.S. Department of Health and Human Services.

Morgan, L. A., Gruber-Baldini, A., & Magaziner, J. (2001). Resident characteristics. In S. Zimmerman, P. D. Sloane & J. K. Eckert (Eds.), *Assisted living: Needs, practices, and policies in residential care for the elderly* (pp. 117–143). Baltimore, MD: The Johns Hopkins University Press.

National Center For Assisted Living. (2001). Facts and trends: The assisted living sourcebook. Retrieved December 18, 2006, from http://www.ncal.org/about/resident.htm

National Center for Assisted Living. (2006). Assisted Living Resident Profile. Retrieved December 18, 2006, from http://www.ncal.org/about/resident.htm

Nolin, M., & Mollica, R. (2001). Residential care/assisted living in the changing health care environment. In S. Zimmerman, P. D. Sloane & J. K. Eckert (Eds.), *Assisted living: Needs, practices, and policies in residential care for the elderly.* Baltimore: The Johns Hopkins University Press.

Promatura Group, LLC. 2000. *NIC national supply estimate of seniors housing & care properties.* Annapolis, MD: National Investment Center for the Seniors Housing and Care Industries

Quinn, M. E., Johnson, M. A., Andress, E. L., McGinnis, P., & Ramesh, M. (1999). Health characteristics of elderly personal care home residents. *Journal of Advanced Nursing, 30*(2), 410–417.

Rabins, P., Lyketsos, C., & Steele, C. (2006). *Practical dementia care*, (2nd ed.). New York: Oxford University Press.

Regier, D., Boyd, J., Burke, J., Rae, D., Myers, J., Kramer, M., et al. (1988). One-month prevalence of mental disorders in the United States. Based on five Epidemiologic Catchment Area sites. *45*(11), 977–986.

Rosenblatt, A., Samus, Q. M., Onyike, C. U., Baker, A. S., McNabney, M., Mayer, L. S., et al. (2007). Acetylcholinesterase inhibitors in assisted living: patterns of use and association with retention. *International Journal of Geriatric Psychiatry, 23*(2), 178–184.

Rosenblatt, A., Samus, Q. M., Steele, C. D., Baker, A. S., Harper, M. G., Brandt, J., et al. (2004). The Maryland Assisted Living Study: Prevalence, recognition, and treatment of dementia and other psychiatric disorders in the assisted living population of central Maryland. *Journal of the American Geriatrics Society, 52*(10), 1618–1625.

Samus, Q. M., Rosenblatt, A., Steele, C., Baker, A., Harper, M., Brandt, J., et al. (2005). The Association of Neuropsychiatric symptoms and environment with quality of life in assisted living residents with dementia. *Gerontologist, 45*(suppl_1), 19–26.

Samus, Q. M., Rosenblatt, A., Onyike, C., Steele, C., Baker, A., Harper, M., et al. (2006). Correlates of caregiver-rated quality of life in assisted living: The Maryland Assisted Living Study. *Journal of Gerontology Series B Psychological Sciences and Social sciences, 61*(5), P311–314.

Salzman, C. (2000). Mood disorders. In C. Coffey & J. L. Cummings (Eds.), *Textbook of Geriatric Neuropsychiatry* (2nd ed., pp. 313–328). New York: The American Psychiatric Publishers, Inc.

Sloane, P. D., Zimmerman, S., Gruber-Baldini, A. L., Hebel, J. R., Magaziner, J., & Konrad, T. R. (2005). Health and functional outcomes and health care utilization of persons with dementia in residential care and assisted living facilities: Comparison with nursing homes. *Gerontologist, 45*(suppl_1), 124–134.

Sloane, P. D., Zimmerman, S., & Ory, M. G. (2001). Care for persons with dementia. In S. Zimmerman, P. D. Sloane & F. K. Eckert (Eds.), *Assisted Living: Needs, practices, and policies in residential care for the elderly* (pp. 242–270). Baltimore, MD: Johns Hopkins University Press.

Sloane, P. D., Zimmerman, S., & Walsh, J. F. (2001). The physical environment. In S. Zimmerman, P. D. Sloane & J. K. Eckert (Eds.), *Assisted Living: Needs, practices, and policies in residential care for the elderly* (pp. 173–197). Baltimore: The Johns Hopkins University Press.

Small, G., Rabins, P., Barry, P., Buckholtz, N., DeKosky, S., Ferris, S., et al. (1997). Diagnosis and treatment of Alzheimer disease and related disorders. Consensus statement of the American Association for Geriatric Psychiatry, the Alzheimer's Association, and the American Geriatrics Society. *Journal of the American Geriatric Society, 278*(16), 1363–1371.

Smith, M., Samus, Q.M., Steele, C., Baker, A., Brandt, J., Rabins, P.V., Lyketsos, C.G., & Rosenblatt, A. Anxiety symptoms among assisted living residents: Implications of the "no difference" finding for subjects with and without dementia. (Unpublished manuscript).

Solomon, P. R., Brush, M., Calvo, V., Adams, F., DeVeaux, R. D., Pendlebury, W. W., et al. (2000). Identifying dementia in primary care practice. *International Psychogeriatrics, 12*, 483–493.

Spillman, B. C., & Black, K. J. (2006). *The size and characteristics of the residential care population: Evidence from three national surveys.* Washington, DC: U.S. Department of Health and Human Services.

Spillman, B., Liu, K., & McGilliard, C. (2002). Trends in residential long-term care: Use of nursing homes and assisted living and characteristics of facilities and residents. Washington, DC: Assistant Secretary for Planning and Evaluation, U.S. Department of Health & Human Services.

Steinberg, M., Sheppard, J.-M., Tschanz, J. T., Norton, M. C., Steffens, D. C., Breitner, J. C. S., et al. (2003). The incidence of mental and behavioral disturbances in dementia: The cache county study. *Journal of Neuropsychiatry and Clinical Neuroscience, 15*(3), 340–345.

Turner, S. (2005). Behavioural symptoms of dementia in residential settings: A selective review of nonpharmacological interventions. *Aging and Mental Health, 9,* 93–104.

Wagenaar, D. B., Mickus, M., Luz, C., Kreft, M., & Sawade, J. (2003). An administrator's perspective on mental health in assisted living. *Psychiatric Services, 54*(12), 1644–1646.

Waldemar, G., Dubois, B., Emre, M., Georges, J., McKeith, I. G., Rossor, M., et al. (2007).

Recommendations for the diagnosis and management of Alzheimer's disease and other disorders associated with dementia: EFNS guideline. *European Journal of Neurology, 14*(1), e1–e26.

Walker, C., Curry, L., & Hogstel, M. (2007). Relocation stress syndrome in older adults transitioning from home to a long-term care facility. *Journal of Psychosocial Nursing and Mental Health Services.*

Watson, L. C., Garrett, J. M., Sloane, P. D., Gruber-Baldini, A. L., & Zimmerman, S. (2003). Depression in assisted living: Results from a four-state study. *American Journal of Geriatric Psychiatry, 11*(5), 534–542.

Watson, L. C., Lehmann, S., Mayer, L., Samus, Q., Baker, A., Brandt, J., et al. (2006). Depression in assisted living is common and related to physical burden. *American Journal of Geriatric Psychiatry, 14*(10), 876–883.

Wilson, K. (2007). Historical Evolution of Assisted Living in the United States, 1979 to the present. *The Gerontologist, 47*(Special Issue III), 8–22.

Zimmerman, S., Sloane, P. D., Eckert, J. K., Buie, V. C., Walsh, J. F., Koch, G. G., et al. (2001). An overview of the collaborative studies of long-term care. In S. Zimmerman, P. D. Sloane & J. K. Eckert (Eds.), *Assisted living: Needs, practices, and policies in residential care for the elderly* (pp. 117–143). Baltimore, MD: The Johns Hopkins University Press.

Zimmerman, S., Sloane, P. D., Eckert, J. K., Gruber-Baldini, A. L., Morgan, L. A., Hebel, J. R., et al. (2005). How good is assisted living? Findings and implications from an outcomes study. *Journal of Gerontology Series B Psychological Sciences and Social Sciences, 60*(4), 195–204.

Zimmerman, S., Sloane, P. D., Williams, C. S., Dobbs, D., Ellajosyula, R., Braaten, A., et al. (2007). Residential care/assisted living staff may detect undiagnosed dementia using the minimum data set cognition scale. *Journal of the American Geriatrics Society, 55*(9), 1349–1355.

Zimmerman, S., Sloane, P. D., Williams, C. S., Reed, P. S., Preisser, J. S., Eckert, J. K., et al. (2005). Dementia care and quality of life in assisted living and nursing homes. *Gerontologist, 45*(Suppl 1), 133–146.

Zimmerman, S., Williams, C. S., Reed, P. S., Boustani, M., Preisser, J. S., Heck, E., et al. (2005). Attitudes, stress, and satisfaction of staff who care for residents with dementia. *Gerontologist, 45*(Suppl 1), 96–105.

Index

CPSIA information can be obtained at www.ICGtesting.com
Printed in the USA
BVOW051240171211

278602BV00005B/66/P